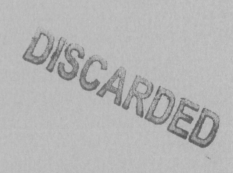

International Encyclopedia

of PSYCHIATRY, PSYCHOLOGY, PSYCHOANALYSIS, & NEUROLOGY

International Encyclopedia

of

PSYCHIATRY,
PSYCHOLOGY,
PSYCHOANALYSIS,
& NEUROLOGY

BENJAMIN B. WOLMAN

Editor

Volume 7

Produced for
Aesculapius Publishers, Inc.

by
Van Nostrand Reinhold Company

Library of Congress Catalog Card Number: 76-54527
ISBN: 0–918228–01–8

Manufactured in the United States of America

Produced by Van Nostrand Reinhold Company
450 West 33rd Street, New York, N.Y. 10001

For Aesculapius Publishers, Inc.
10 West 66th Street, New York, N.Y. 10023

10 9 8 7 6 5 4 3 2 1

Library of Congress Cataloging in Publication Data

Main entry under title:

International Encyclopedia of Psychiatry, Psychology, Psychoanalysis, & Neurology
    Bibliography:
    Includes index.
    1. Psychiatry—Dictionaries. 2. Psychology—Dictionaries.
3. Psychoanalysis—Dictionaries. 4. Neurology—Dictionaries.
I. Wolman, Benjamin B.
RC334.I57   1977   616.8′9′003   76-54527

International Encyclopedia

of PSYCHIATRY, PSYCHOLOGY, PSYCHOANALYSIS, & NEUROLOGY

M

MARATHON GROUP MEETINGS

A marathon group meeting is one that lasts for a significantly longer period of time than a usual group meeting. The sacrosanct 90-minute group therapy hour has been extended to include such time intervals as 6 hours, 12 hours, or more commonly 24 or more consecutive hours or several days in a row with breaks for sleep.

The distinction between the encounter group and a therapy group is perhaps somewhat spurious, and a marathon group may be said to be both a growth-enhancing experience for healthy people or a therapeutic experience for people with emotional difficulties. *Therapy groups* are viewed as following the medical model, in that the members are patients who are seeking relief from an illness, and treatment is directed at alleviating an abnormality. *Encounter groups,* on the other hand, are composed of "normal people" who seek to enhance their personal growth and improve their social skills. Perhaps the main reason for the vast popularity of this movement is that it helps to supply an answer to a societal need for more intimacy in spite of the fear of it, and helps in achieving a more satisfactory balance between the individual's dependency and assertiveness and an increased ability to relate more directly to others. These generally are problems of alienation that are not necessarily socially aberrant, but do contribute significantly to emotional disorders.

There have been several paths or precursors which have been determinants in the evolution of the marathon group movement. From psychoanalytic group psychotherapy have come ideas of "group-as-a-whole." The humanistic psychology movement has introduced greater involvement of the leader as a person. The encounter group movement, drawing on these, is particularly an outgrowth of the small group movement which started in 1946 at the National Training Laboratories where the laboratory method of learning and research has been emphasized. These innovations and special attentions have included a here-and-now orientation, marked emphasis on feelings and emotions, feedback procedures, interpersonal learning, and even formation of leaderless groups. The work of Fritz Perls and the Gestalt orientation has placed particular emphasis on the "here and now," and the idea of personal responsibility of feelings and actions. In addition, starting in the late 1950s, the increasing importance of the therapeutic community and the milieu, where a full 24-hour therapeutic approach to hospitalized patients was encouraged, highlighted the value of a prolonged therapeutic contact. Also a form of "multiple impact therapy" had been described by Mac-Gregor (1962) whereby a family received the full attention of a psychiatric team for two or three full days. These factors have all been instrumental in determining the rationale, approach, and philosophy of marathon groups.

Early investigators have included Bach, Casriel, and Stoller, who have helped to define the accelerated interaction said to be characteristic of this format. With the phenomenal growth in the late 1960s of the small-group movement, marathon meetings became increasingly popular. These have been conducted in the usual meeting-rooms of organizations and therapists, in more faraway and idyllic meeting areas (such as homes, motels, or special conference grounds), and especially in the burgeoning "growth centers," both in remote tranquil settings and also in urban areas.

From various backgrounds and answering individual and cultural needs, marathon group meetings have become an established phenomenon of current society.

Rationale and Characteristics of Marathon Groups

Many of the general considerations concerning group therapy and encounter groups apply with equal validity to marathon groups. Confidentiality, physical restraints, no drugs or alcohol, and an attempt to present oneself honestly apply to most groups, though there are some definite exceptions. What then are the specific variables which, because of the extended time feature, make for the unique contribution of the marathon group experience? A marathon, unlike many open-ended groups, has two unique features: (1) a limited number of hours, usually more than 6, or perhaps 12 or 24 hours, a weekend, five 12-hour days, or some other precisely defined time limit; and (2) these hours are fairly consecutive and whatever momentum is built up is not allowed to dissipate during long periods when the group is apart.

The marathon group therefore quickly becomes a world unto itself with a specific life-span. The participant is encouraged to accept the responsibility for himself and for his fate in the group. It is emphasized that there are correlations between the paths he chooses in the group and those he traverses in the world. He is made keenly aware that he has alternatives, and he is encouraged to risk and experiment to find newer and perhaps better methods of relating with others. Change in the undesirable aspects of his initial presentation is acknowledged and approved by the group, thereby encouraging further attempts at change.

Some people come for a marathon group experience by self-referral, having heard about it from others or read about it. They come out of a desire to be given an opportunity to relate more closely and directly to others and to "grow." Others come on referral by therapists. The patient may be someone who is "stuck" in individual or group therapy, and who also shares a desire to "grow" and to interact more directly and intimately with others. In addition, there are organizational groups (churches, businesses, schools, civic groups, etc.) where participation is strongly encouraged or even demanded.

There are many factors that enter into selection and admission into a group. Perhaps the most important are the motivation and informed consent of the person, and his awareness of the option to leave should he consider the experience undesirable. (Though this is rarely exercised, the explicit awareness of this opportunity may "permit" a person to work through his anxieties.) Finally, the awareness of an opportunity to discuss the group further after the meeting with a nonparticipant also helps to maintain perspective on the experience and to lessen the likelihood of an undesirable result.

It is common practice to have a pregroup screening meeting, where expectations of the leader and the participants may be explored and the "rules" briefly reviewed. Though the rules vary widely, the generally accepted philosophy includes such ideas as no drinking or drugs, no physical violence, and the direct and honest open expression of feelings and ideas. Confidentiality of information and events is agreed upon and the participants are encouraged to avoid any subgrouping. The primary affiliation is to the entire group. These or similar rules are stressed either before the main meeting or very early at the start of the meeting.

Many of the following features have become associated with this experience. A more relaxed informal setting, frequently a home, and the availability of creature comforts (such as food and bathroom facilities) make for a less artificial or clinical environment. Within this universe, a group life emerges which is available to the scrutiny of all. Subgrouping, whispering, or experiencing meaningfully outside of the group is strongly discouraged. Within the microcosm that emerges, less and less attention tends to be paid to the genetic antecedents. Generally, the "here-and-now" is of greatest concern. Frequently an attempt is made to draw up a contract as to what changes are desired during the life of the group. A participant then has the benefit of experiencing directly his own changes and the effect of these on others. He is able to discover immediately the consequences of his action, and to consider the desire of any further change.

A sense of belonging and cohesiveness develops during the course of the group. Attempts at "instant intimacy" do not succeed as well as allowing the group to experience for itself and to deal with its frustrations, stresses, and strains, and for members to accept each other and to feel related. Intensive interpersonal confrontation and most particularly expressions of intense emotions accompanied by anger and tears appear to be part of the necessary steps toward achieving the desired and necessary cohesiveness.

The group experience may be seen as dividing itself roughly into four phases. Initially, there is apprehension and anxiety, even in members who have previously experienced marathon meetings, at the prospect of the new and unknown. With this anxiety and the attendant insecurity, the participants are defensive and "closed." After the initial transactions when many of the expectations and fantasies are not met, a sense of disappointment characterized by increasing aggression and hostility is arrived at. This second phase is important in demonstrating the open and honest tone that had previously been described but is now happening. When the participants have reacted intensely and genuinely over a period of time, an increasing emotional and physical closeness develops with a shift in the defensive structure of the individuals, and the potent force of the group becomes evident. The group usually actively seeks out and expresses concern about those members who have not actively participated, and every attempt is made to include them and to have them join in. The sense of intimacy, trust, cohesiveness, and belonging is paramount. The final phase of the marathon meeting concerns its impending dissolution and the separation anxieties this provokes. As the final hours of the marathon approach, the sense of urgency increases, the fatigue factor becomes more important, and the cohesiveness within the group is such that there is an even more meaningful and accelerated rate of interaction. There are various "go arounds" with one person either telling the others his reactions or receiving from them their impressions. Almost always the participants, though physically fatigued, feel exhilarated and significantly related with one another as the group ends at its predetermined time. There is frequently a reluctance to separate, and any evaluations done at this time usually reflect the positive feelings and exhilarations of the majority of the people. At this time the participant is under strong pressure, both personal and from the group, to report a positive experience. After his investment of time, money, and energy it would be difficult to be critical and feel that it was all a bad expenditure. Furthermore, there are strong group pressures for all to share in the positive cohesive feelings. These pressures lessen in time, and a follow-up meeting, perhaps several weeks later, can give a more accurate appraisal of the longer-term effects of the marathon meeting. At the follow-up meeting, many of the participants are likely to report a sense of letdown and depression for several days after the main meetings. This is probably related somewhat to physiological factors, as from sleep deprivation, unusual diet, and atypical emotional and perhaps physical experiences, but also due to the reentering into the world and having the many expectations and fantasies of change disappointed. The result is that the report at the follow-up meeting is less glowing and having a quality of a religious experience, but more realistic, though generally still of a positive nature.

The overall marathon experience may then be said to consist of three related events. Initially, a participant prepares for the event. This may be done by hearing of a brief description of the meeting and applying for it, by being referred to it and being seen by a leader, or even by experiencing a brief preliminary group meeting. Then there is the marathon meeting itself, with its various phases. Finally there is the post-marathon situation. The participant may go off and only retain memories of the meeting for himself, he may share it with important others, including other groups he may be in or individual therapists, or he may subsequently attend a follow-up meeting with the original marathon members where, with the additional perspective of time, the relevance and meaning of the marathon event can be reviewed. It is desirable at the close of the marathon meeting to have some resource available for the participant, be it an ongoing therapist, the group leader himself, or some other experienced person who would be available, if necessary, to help the participant integrate the marathon experience into his everyday world.

Techniques, Methods, and Approaches

Specific techniques, methods, or approaches vary with the nature of the individual leaders. No single correct methodology can emerge.

Instead of the standard question of "Why are you here?" a more precise definition and contract is required. Specifically, something of the nature of, "What is it you want to get out of this experience?" or "How do you hope to be different at the end of the group?" may be demanded of the participants early in the meeting. An answer may be satisfactory only if it is acceptable to the rest of the group. Toward the end of the session, these "contracts" are reviewed, and a final opportunity to fulfill them is afforded, or they may be modified.

Developments in electronic audio-visual media have been used, and these include lighting effects and music. Particularly for psychodrama situations or for structured fantasy experiences, these devices help in setting a mood. Sound and video recorders and their immediate playback capabilities provide objective feedback to enhance the interpersonal feedback of the group members.

Various encounter techniques are widely used. There is a marked tendency for nonverbal behavior to be observed, emphasized, and interpreted, and for varieties of this behavior to be encouraged. The "language of the body" is not only observed and interpreted, but the use of the body is encouraged by asking someone to reach out to someone else or by a variety of physical exercises, particularly when the verbal mode of communication has become less effective.

Schutz and Mintz have compiled many of these structured exercises or situations. The use of many physical interactions become part of the group, and may be used effectively if comfortably applied by the leader at the appropriate time. The rationale for these activities is that they provide an additional means to help set a more open and intimate tone and also to circumvent the usual verbal barriers. Additionally, they may help in the clarification and resolution of issues that had been unsuccessfully attempted by the more usual verbal means. Finally, information obtained can be conceptualized and verbalized and make a valuable contribution to the overall marathon experience. If these structured exercises, be they verbal or physical interactions, or use of some art media, are applied arbitrarily and insensitively, they may serve as a disruption to the ongoing group process and be experienced by the members as being either valueless and inappropriate or threatening and damaging, either psychically or physically.

Leader Considerations

It has generally been recommended that at least two leaders participate in the group because of the extra demands being made on the leader by the extended time format. Ideally, these leaders represent both sexes. This then gives the participant a richer authority stimulus to which he can react and after which he can model himself.

The duty of the leaders is to create an atmosphere in which the participants can relate as meaningfully as possible with each other. They therefore introduce techniques to enhance this and to intensify the immediate experience. In addition, they also attempt to clarify the meaning of the happenings.

Relative to ongoing weekly groups, the role of the marathon leader as an involved participant and a model of expected behavior is a more vital one, and generally more directly revealing of himself. The meeting may even take place at his home. He shares his feelings and reactions with the group, and when appropriately stimulated, may feel free to express a problem area or dilemma of his own. These all have a tendency to make him all the more human and less a blank or aloof authority. It is this ability of the therapist to be involved and authentic, rather than autocratic and intolerant, which serves as a model for the other participants and encourages the honest and nondefensive behavior which helps to achieve the direct group goals. Each leader must develop an approach and a style of interaction that is unique to him. He should be a person with clinical experience, but without a "clinical approach," a person acceptable to himself and with a desire to help others, and a willingness to be responsible, not only for his own behavior, but for the group and its results. The extent of leader involvement is likely to vary at different times during the meeting. This may range from withdrawing and letting the members deal with their feelings, to commenting on the group process, to participating actively and intensely with a single or several participants.

Responsibility and Results

Are encounter groups to be considered group therapy, and is a leader in an encounter group a "therapist?" A task-force of the American Psychiatric Association concluded:

In our opinion a physician, even though he involves himself in a group nominally non-therapy in nature, still may not divorce himself from his traditional continuing responsibility to the participants whether or not they are specifically labeled his patients. (Members may join a human awareness group led by a psychiatrist because of covert expectations of the psychotherapy experience.) Encounter group trainers . . . are not legally responsible for possible detrimental effects of the group on a member unless the leaders are specifically advertised as mental health experts. . . . It would seem probable that the psychiatrist retains his "mental health expert" designation even when leading a group which is not specifically labeled as therapy, but which may be a potent influence both positively and negatively upon the mental health of the participants.

This implied burden of responsibility may partially help to account for the relatively lesser participation by psychiatrists in marathon group experiences.

Many of the group leaders who have emerged are individuals without any formal educational background in a behavioral science. Instead, they claim that their life experiences and their prior group experiences are sufficient to allow them to lead groups. Some disclaim any idea of responsibility for the participants, stating that each person is basically in charge of himself and responsible for his own fate.

The majority of the leaders do seem to have an educational qualification for the role. Of the traditional psychotherapists, social workers and psychologists are more involved in encounter and marathon groups. The lesser involvement by psychiatrists is complex, but some of the considerations include the specific medical model and training of the physician which appears antithetical to some of the desired traits of a group leader, for example, clinical experience but not a clinical approach. The psychiatrist's traditional role is a distant, frequently enigmatic, self-reserving one and more in line with the classically powerful authoritarian and sagacious physician. The trainer or leader is more self-disclosing and personally involved with a willingness to be less of an authority. However, there are significant variations and overlapping in various leaders' and therapists' styles, and the specific professional background may be of less importance than the leader's clinical experience and his ethics and philosophy. Similarly, the outcome and results seem less related to the individual leader's formal background and more to his personal orientation and style.

The leadership functions basically include emotional stimulation (revealing feeling, challenging, exhorting), caring (offering protection, affection, and concern), meaning-attribution (intellectual appreciation and understanding), and an executive function (setting rules and limits, managing and commanding time and action). Leaders from the same schools and theoretical background do not necessarily behave similarly in terms of their basic leadership function. Generally, leaders who emphasize meaning-attribution and caring seem to have better results with their groups in terms of more desirable short- and long-term effects and fewer undesirable results and casualties. Those leaders emphasizing an impersonal executive function with much emotional stimulation are most likely to have the participants who may become casualties, or at least remember the experience as threatening and undesirable.

Not every intense and emotional experience, even if it is labeled as a part of therapy, is necessarily corrective and desirable. Undoubtedly the structure of a marathon group does encourage and beget many intense emotional expressions, which hopefully is of benefit to the participants, but this may not always be so. Attempts have been made to define what aspects of an encounter group experience are potentially most harmful, what individuals are most likely to be hurt by such an experience, and how to eliminate and "screen out" these potentially undesirable events. Here again, the ability of the leader is of paramount importance in initially screening out the potential casualties, and also in evaluating and supporting such people once they are in the group. However, it has also been shown that leaders are at times not as aware of the detrimental effects on a participant as are some of the other members.

What then may be expected after participation in a marathon group meeting? There is certainly no basis for the claim of an enduring and permanent change in one's personality pattern from this single event. Some have suggested that people periodically attend, perhaps at regular intervals, a number of such meetings as a method of maximizing the benefits of the experience. Others have used the marathon meeting as a valuable adjunct to ongoing individual or group psychotherapy, as a diagnostic situation before therapy, or as an intensive means of getting involved in either individual or group therapy. Perhaps a realistic expectation of one marathon experience is that the participant would become more aware of his own feelings, experience a sense of well-being and relatedness to others, and acquire some insight which would make for more satisfactory functioning. For those in ongoing psychotherapy, the experience could provide valuable material to be further explored. Frequently, important decisions are arrived at during the intensive meeting, and a proper balance between premature and impulsive action and a well-thought-out and advised plan of action are achieved.

A marathon group meeting may offer a unique and powerful experience, the benefits and values of which are partially inherent in the structure of the group. These benefits also depend on the ability of the individual to help assimilate the experiences both within the group and later, and on the skill of the therapist.

BIBLIOGRAPHY

BACH, G. R. The marathon group: Intensive practice in intimate interaction. *Psychological Reports*, 1967, *20*, 995–999.

GENDZEL, I. B. Marathon group therapy: Rationale and techniques. In J. H. Masserman (Ed.), *Current psychiatric therapies* (Vol. 12). New York: Grune & Stratton, 1972. Pp. 151–160.

LIEBERMAN, M. A.; YALOM, I. D.; and MILES, M. B. *Encounter groups: First facts.* New York: Basic Books, 1972.

MINTZ, E. E. *Marathon groups—reality and symbol.* New York: Avon Books, 1971.

SCHUTZ, W. *Joy: Expanding human awareness.* New York: Grove Press, 1967.

IVAN B. GENDZEL

MARGINAL MAN

See ROLE CONFLICT, MOBILITY, AND MARGINAL MAN

MARITAL CHOICE: DETERMINANTS

The determinants of marital choice may be conveniently separated into two classifications: (1) factors determining a "field of eligibles," and (2) factors determining the choice of partner within a field of eligibles.

The Field of Eligibles

The evidence influencing the field of eligibles has been rather apparent throughout history ("birds of a feather flock together"), but quantitative evidence supporting homogamy has been gathered mainly since the end of World War II. It has been found that individuals tend to marry those of the same race, age, education, socioeconomic status, locale, intelligence, attitudes and values, and religion at a greater than chance rate.

Of the foregoing variables, the tendency to marry someone who lives very close to oneself (most often within one mile) operates in a different manner from the other variables in which similarity may serve to attract the individuals to each other. The degree of propinquity of itself does not attract. Rather, it serves as a possible suppressor of other variables. If two individuals live very far apart, the cost in fatigue, time, and expense will serve to inhibit courtship unless there is an unusually strong attraction. Hence, all things being equal, those possessing the proper homogamous characteristics *and* living close together will be preferred to potential partners living further away.

That individuals tend to marry others of similar characteristics does not necessarily imply that they actively seek these characteristics in others. Often, homogamy occurs inevitably by the nature of their associations. Parents may send their daughter to a small liberal arts college for which one may suggest the name "Selecto." Colleges are generally regarded as the top marriage markets in the United States. Here, daughter finds those of her own age. Her parents have heard that their friends and offspring liked Selecto; consequently, it should come as no surprise that most students of Selecto are of the same race and religion, because the parents' friends tend to be of the same race and religion. Since tuition of Selecto is rather high, most students from Selecto are of the same or similar socioeconomic class.

To a lesser but still greater than chance probability, boy-girl pairs from the college will have the same intelligence level and the same values. The reason for this is that the aptitude scores required to get into Selecto are high, and Selecto has the reputation of being liberal. Last, there are no problems of propinquity in courtship on a college campus. Thus, without any conscious effort toward homogamy, courtship in a college will generally follow a homogamous trend.

However, even where environments are not strongly screened to produce homogeneity of background, the individuals often seek it themselves. Although the facts of *homogamy* have been with us for many years, little attention has been given to why, to the individuals concerned, homogamy is preferable to heterogeneity. Although there are little or no data on this question, it is probable that homogamy serves several important functions. First, it is easier to relate to someone similar, because similarity provides a sociopsychological environment which is comfortable and readily mastered. Where another is of the same race, religion, age, class, education, and values, tension regarding guiding philosophies of life, choice of everyday activities, career goals, and the like are less apt to cause conflict between members of a couple. Second, if another holds similar values and, for example, has made a similar commitment to education, association with such an individual is rewarding because he (she) provides confirming evidence that the individual is attuned to the important commitments in life and is living "correctly."

Homogamy of background, nevertheless, does not signify that the individuals are alike as peas in a pod, because there is generally room for variability in physique, temperament, and personality.

Selecting From the Field of Eligibles

Although in a general sense individuals marry homogamously, there are two problems with depending on homogamy as the sole determinant of marital choice. First, there may be several marital possibilities with very similar backgrounds. Second, there are always a number of examples of individuals who depart from homogamous norms in one or more important respects. An old "geezer" may marry a "pretty young thing." A white marries a black, a Jew a Gentile, a prince a pauper, and, rather more rarely, an heiress a gasoline attendant. These exceptions are often treated as no more than "errata" in sociological textbooks, but a number of researchers have constructed theories to account for individual selection from among the field of eligibles. These theories have focused on *values* (individuals are drawn together by similar value systems), the *completion principle* (it does not matter whether the man or woman is adequate to deal with a given problem or task as long as one or both members of the couple can handle any given task the two are apt to face as a couple). There are also *filter* theories (individuals are at first selected for similar values, but later in courtship, values are no longer selective—those of disparate values tend to eventually break up—and psychological compatibility takes over). Finally, there are *process* theories in which the nature of the interaction between the members of a couple and between them and their environment are considered more important than any given personality traits or features they may possess as individuals.

These theories have drawn relatively little attention, because they were either so loosely formulated as to fail to appeal to many workers in the field, or because they have inspired little or no research by either the authors themselves, or other researchers. Two theories, however, have been more extensively developed by their authors, and have been tested empirically; consequently, they will be briefly covered. The two theories are *complementary needs* by the sociologist Robert F. Winch, and the *stimulus-value-role* theory by Bernard I. Murstein, a psychologist. Both are psychological theories, but they differ radically in that complementary needs is a single principle theory, whereas stimulus-value-role is a relatively complex process-exchange theory.

Complementary Needs

The theory of complementary needs states that "each individual seeks within his or her field of eligibles for that person who gives the greatest promise of providing him or her with maximum need gratification" (Winch, 1958, p. 89). However, individuals are drawn together by complementary needs, which are defined as "*A*'s behavior in acting out *A*'s need *X* is gratifying to *B*'s need *Y,* and *B*'s behavior in acting out *B*'s need *Y* is gratifying to *A*'s need *X*" (Winch, 1958, p. 93). In practice, Winch expects that a couple should be negatively correlated for a given need (e.g., dominance) and positively correlated for complementary needs (if the man is high on dominance, the woman should be high on submissiveness).

Winch tested his theory with 25 young married couples at Northwestern University in the early 1950s. He reported statistical support for the theory, but his methodology has been strongly criticized (Murstein, 1976). Moreover, the majority of other researchers have failed to verify his findings.

Winch believes that his theory failed to consider attraction based on the partner's adherence to role norms; hence, he has revised his theory and now believes that complementarity should lead to stability if it accords with role norms, but not if it contradicts them. Thus, a dominant husband and a submissive wife would constitute a stable pair in a patriarchal society, but a dominant wife and a submissive husband would not. Although the original theory has lost favor in recent years, Winch's position as the first person to put forth an empirically testable theory has earned him a secure place among marital researchers.

Stimulus-Value-Role

Two basic principles underly the stimulus-value-role theory, first formulated in 1970: (1) marital courtship involves a series of sequential stages which are labeled *stimulus, value,* and *role,* and (2) at any given point in the courtship, its viability is dependent on the equity of exchange experienced by the participants. Exchange relates to the assets and liabilities each member of the potential couple sees in the other. The assets minus liabilities determine an individual's profitability, and the more profitable the interaction with an individual, the more his company is desired. Nevertheless, it does little good to pine after a desirable person if one's own profitability to the other is far below the other's profitability to oneself; hence, equity of profitability is generally most conducive to long-lasting relationships.

Concerning the sequential aspects of the theory, the stimulus stage is determined by the perception of the other's physical, social, mental, or reputational attributes. It is what determines whether extensive interaction will be desired. If there is equity in stimulus attributes, the second, value comparison stage follows, in which the values of each are tested for compatibility. The role stage involves the ability of each to function in roles compatible with desirable spousal images.

The theory has led to the formulation of 39 hypotheses which have been tested with several hundred subjects in three populations. The majority of these have been supported (Murstein, 1976). One of the most important findings was that with respect to personality characteristics, neither complementarity nor homogamy of itself could predict marital choice. Instead, individuals high in self-acceptance were drawn to partners who were perceived as similar to themselves, whereas those dissatisfied with themselves were drawn to opposite-appearing partners.

Neither Winch nor Murstein dwell heavily

on love in the formal properties of their theories. However, love is incorporated into the fabric of Winch's theory. To Winch, love is experienced by an individual when the other meets his needs or appears to embody highly desired personal attributes. Murstein is more apt to view love as a label popularly used to describe a vast number of different reasons for marriage including equity of exchange, passion, rationalization, and fantasy projection. Since it is used widely to describe a vast array of different and often contradictory behaviors, its heuristic utility in understanding marital choice is limited.

BIBLIOGRAPHY

MURSTEIN, B. I. *Who will marry whom? Theories and research in marital choice.* New York: Springer, 1976.
WINCH, R. F. *Mate-selection: A study of complementary needs.* New York: Harper, 1958.

BERNARD I. MURSTEIN

MARITAL CONFLICT

The term *marital conflict* denotes a state of marital dissatisfaction—which dissatisfaction, however, may or may not be shared by the spouses, may or may not be openly expressed, and may or may not be focused on specific issues. In some instances, *marital conflict* refers to a diagnosis made by an outside observer and not to any initial perception of marital difficulty on the part of the couple.

While there are no theories of marital conflict resolution in any strict sense of the word, three distinctive orientations to intervention have emerged. They may be identified, after their characteristic foci, as the *insight, communication,* and *behavioral* approaches. The descriptions which follow aim to capture the major thrust and flavor of each approach. Much is common to all three, and within each approach there are distinctive differences in emphasis and technique.

Insight Approaches

The insight approach is the oldest and most widespread orientation to marital conflict resolution. It began in the late 1940s around efforts to understand and treat childhood schizophrenia, but has since been extended to a wide range of marital and family problems.

Characteristically, marital conflict is viewed in terms of a *manifest* and a *latent* dimension. The manifest dimension involves the issues about which the couple is explicitly concerned. These may include fights over specific matters like sex or money management, symptom formation in one spouse or in a child, or vague complaints such as "inability to communicate."

The latent conflict concerns more profound issues in the marital relationship. It is grounded in each spouse's unsuccessful experiences in his own family of origin which produce unrealistic marital expectations and the projection onto the other of malevolent parental introjections.

The latent conflict remains unresolved because it lies beneath the level of conscious awareness and because it is maintained by unrecognized, maladaptive patterns of marital interaction. In addition, low self-esteem in both partners favors avoidance of highly charged issues because of anxiety that open confrontation will lead to loss of the other.

The role of the therapist is to assist in the constructive resolution of the latent conflicts. This being done, the manifest issues will be found to have either disappeared or lost their significance. In some instances the marriage may end in a constructive, unembittered divorce in which each spouse has been strengthened by new self-understanding.

Since marriage is viewed as an interactive system in which the behavior of one spouse affects and is affected by the behavior of the other, the preferred therapeutic modality is the conjoint session. By encouraging interaction in his presence, the therapist obtains information on the nature of the latent conflict and the ways in which it inhibits the marital relationship. He may attempt to convey his understanding directly via interpretations of the family-of-origin sources of the conflict, or more obliquely by pointing out the maladaptive patterns of interaction to which he has been witness and by encouraging new patterns of interaction. Ancillary techniques such as videotape feedback or group sessions with the couple's parents or other married couples may be used to focus on the unrecognized sources of difficulty and to produce more veridical awareness of self and spouse.

Of the three approaches to reducing marital conflict, the insight approach is most likely to aim for a reassent and restructuring of the entire basis of the marriage. It is most often the treatment of choice for verbal couples where the motivation and potential for self-observation and change are high.

Communication Approaches

The communication approach reflects most clearly the influence of Carl Rogers and non-directive psychotherapy, but has also drawn upon the encounter and personal growth movements, social and organizational psychology, and those insight therapists who have emphasized patterns of marital communication.

Marital conflict is seen as the consequence of impaired communication skills and/or problem-solving ability rather than of conflicts rooted in past experiences. The aim of intervention is not to correct serious pathology, but to enhance relatively stable marriages in terms of such factors as increased mutual empathy, heightened ability to express feelings, enhanced sense of marital intimacy, and autonomous growth within the context of the marriage.

Certain characteristic assumptions about marriage are made:

1. Marital conflict is inevitable. The goal is not to eliminate differences but to channel their expression along constructive lines.

2. Communication occurs on both verbal and nonverbal levels. A source of marital friction is an incongruity in the messages being transmitted at these two levels. Incongruities are most likely to result when open expression of differences is inhibited.

3. Spouses frequently differ in their styles of relating. Such differences are to be expected, but can be a source of difficulty if the differences are not recognized and each style not accepted as equally valid. The most common stylistic differences represent some variant of the task-versus-socioemotional orientation. One spouse, often the husband, is seen as paying more attention to "getting things done" and the "facts," while the other, usually the wife, is thought to be more attuned to the relationship-oriented aspects of marital interchanges.

Intervention strategies emphasize the development of rules and skills that will better equip the couple to master the complex task of successful marital communication. The methods are presented didactically rather than emerging gradually in the course of treatment, the latter approach being more common in the insight approach. Since the aim is to assist normal couples, interventions may take the form of self-help manuals in which specific exercises and recommendations are set forth. Two typical methods will serve to illustrate the general orientation.

In *conjugal therapy,* marital dialogues over actual or simulated differences are used to train husband and wife to listen to one another in a more empathic, nonjudgmental manner. Thus, after listening to his wife present her viewpoint, the husband is asked to demonstrate that he has understood her by reflecting back what she has said as accurately as possible. The trainer may intervene by suggesting that the husband make the nonverbal or feeling quality of his remarks congruent with his presumed desire to indicate to his wife that she has been understood. Sessions may be supplemented by assigned readings or at-home exercises.

In Bach's *fight therapy,* couples are encouraged to actively seek out and argue over their differences, but within a framework of rules designed to make such fights productive of increased marital intimacy. These rules include such concepts as not hitting "below the other's belt"; fighting to communicate rather than to win; and sticking to current sources of dissatisfaction rather than calling forth old grievances. Here, too, the emphasis is on quasi-formal teaching, supervised dialogue, and home practice.

Behavioral Approaches

The use of behavioral techniques to reduce marital conflict is in its infancy. Only a relative handful of reports of its use have appeared. The approach promises to become increasingly popular, both on its own merits and as a source of adjunctive techniques for therapists of differing theoretical persuasions. Its widest application is to marriages in which some clear impairment of function exists.

Marital conflict is seen in terms of inadequate levels of positive mutual reinforcement. (Therapists with a more purely behavioral orientation talk of "unfavorable contingencies of reinforcement," while others speak simply of a breakdown in the marital quid pro quo.) The goal of intervention is to alter the reward characteristics of marital interaction. Insight into unconscious dynamics is considered irrelevant.

Although commonly employing the language of behavior modification, behavioral approaches to marital conflict are characterized more by common procedures than by common adherence to any systematic theory of learning. Among the more typical procedures may be included:

1. *Identification of the target behaviors to be changed.* Target goals are explicitly identified in consultation with the couple. In some cases, the initiative for identifying problematic behaviors is placed directly with husband and wife. A therapeutic "contract" in the form of an agreement between the spouses and therapist to produce the desired change(s) may be spelled out.

2. *Observation and analysis of target behaviors.* When and where do the symptomatic behaviors occur? With what frequency? What are the behaviors which maintain them? These questions are answered objectively by observers or by self-report on the part of the couple.

3. *Devising a treatment plan.* The treatment plan is stated in terms of new behaviors which are to be introduced into the marital interaction and specific techniques for increasing the frequency of these behaviors. Techniques may include well-known behavior modification methods such as assertiveness training or symptom desensitization; the introduction of token economies by which the spouses earn points from one another by producing behaviors desired by the other; or the use of technical adjuncts such as videotape feedback or electromechanical signaling devices to help couples gain control of undesirable behaviors.

4. *Measuring the effects of treatment.* Objective comparisons of the post- with the pretreatment situation are made in terms of the initial target goals.

Summary

Approaches to reducing marital conflict have been characterized by a high degree of clinical inventiveness. Theory and research have not shown a corresponding level of development. Several conceptual and empirical issues are especially in need of clarification:

1. *Effects of intervention.* There is little reliable evidence that the methods reviewed are effective. Much of the evaluative research which has been done suffers from inadequate methodology, including lack of relevant control groups and vague, subjective outcome measures.

2. *Treatment-conflict-specificity.* Marital conflict is an umbrella term covering a wide variety of marital difficulties. Whether these difficulties can be fruitfully conceptualized in identical terms and be treated with equal success by the same approach is an important question which has been little discussed. It is plausible to suggest that different types of marital conflict may require different types of intervention.

3. *Integration of research on conflict resolution and clinical practice.* Little is presently known about the nature of unassisted conflict resolution in marriage. Controlled studies of marital conflict are necessary as a check on notions derived exclusively from clinical practice. Thus, the assumption that avoidance of conflict produces unstable marriages has not been supported by the research of Raush, Barry, Hertel, and Swain (1974) on styles of marital communication. Their study also found that an issue-oriented rather than a relationship-oriented focus was more productive of mutually satisfying outcomes. More such studies are needed.

4. *"Pathological" versus "normal" conflicts.* It is a widely held assumption that the specific contents of marital conflicts are rarely, if ever, crucial in themselves, but are the secondary manifestations of "something deeper"—that is, a latent, unperceived conflict of a pathological nature. That marital conflicts can be addressed effectively at the level of the manifest conflict is still a minority viewpoint, but one that merits further consideration. (A notable example is the work of Masters and Johnson in treating sexual dysfunction.)

Another consequence of the "something deeper" orientation has been neglect of the highly predictable stresses of normal married life. The birth of a child; the decision of the wife to seek employment; the departure of grown children from the home; planning for retirement—even a decision to divorce: all require renegotiation of sometimes complex substantive issues as well as previous styles of marital relating. It would seem desirable to begin to explore the parameters of major marital life events and methods by which the likelihood of a constructive, problem-solving orientation to them might be fostered.

BIBLIOGRAPHY

BACH, G. R., and WYDEN, P. *The intimate enemy: How to fight fair in love and marriage.* New York: Avon, 1968.

BOSZORMENYI-NAGY, I., and FRAMO, J. L. (Eds.). *Intensive family therapy.* New York: Harper & Row, 1965.

ELY, A. L.; GUERNEY, B. C.; and STOVER, L. Efficacy of the training phase of conjugal therapy. *Psychotherapy: Theory, Research, and Practice,* 1973, *10,* 201–207.

GURMAN, A. S. The effects and effectiveness of marital therapy: A review of outcome research. *Family Process,* 1973, *12,* 145–170.

HALEY, J., and GLICK, I. *Psychiatry and the family: An annotated bibliography of articles published, 1960–1964.* Palo Alto, Calif.: Family Process, 1965.

MOUTON, J. S., and BLAKE, R. R. *The marriage grid.* New York: McGraw-Hill, 1971.

OLSON, D. H., and DAHL, N. S. *Inventory of marriage and family literature, 1973 and 1974* (Vol. 3). St. Paul: University of Minnesota, 1975.

O'NEIL, N., and O'NEIL, G. *Open marriage.* New York: Avon, 1972.

RAUSH, H. L.; BARRY, W. A.; HERTEL, R. K.; and SWAIN, M. A. *Communication, conflict, and marriage.* San Francisco: Jossey-Bass, 1974.

SATIR, V. *Conjoint family therapy* (Rev. ed.). Palo Alto, Calif.: Science and Behavior Books, 1967.

KENNETH KRESSEL

MARITAL AND FAMILY THERAPY

The Family System

The family has at least two major functions. One is organized around the *nurturing* and *rearing* of children, and the second concerns the provision of an ongoing network from which they can venture into the wider world, and yet return for renewal and continuity of relationship. Children become parents and then grandparents, and the caring, customs, and traditions are passed through generations.

In addition to nurturing the child through an extremely long latency period, the family has to prepare him for self-sufficiency, and to teach the child how to fill the multifaceted roles he will have to take as a mature person. He may have to be taught forcibly the difference between me and not-me and he may also have to be restrained from doing what may seem like fun (leaping onto the glass top table, for example). Some renunciations may come hard, to be rewarded only by the subtle but heady thrill of mastery and the freedom it gives.

The child needs to feel that he has an effect on his environment; this comes from being responded to in an appropriate way with relevance to both manifest content of his communication and its intent. Communication which is severely skewed often results in the tragic human being who cannot trust any input from without or any action which he himself makes.

The learning of *role-oriented* behavior is the second major child-rearing task of the family. In an increasingly complex society, the individual is asked to take on more and more roles, more and more varied ways of interacting in a situation and with other people. The paradigm for his later assumption of those roles is the roleplaying in the family of origin. The child is taught, either subtly or explicitly, that certain behaviors are expected of him as his parents' child. His father may expect him to be "a chip off the old block" and his mother may expect him to be well behaved and a good student.

Much of the learning comes in observing the parents' marriage as his example of how two adults live together. A child can learn respect and love from the parents' marital style or he can learn contempt and exploitation. He may learn intimacy from the way parents interact or he can learn that sexuality has hostile connotations.

The second major family function is in providing an ongoing network and base from which members of the family can venture into the world, and return for sustenance. The most common family organization, based on monogamous marriage, provides the possibility of a continuity of relationship, but also creates the danger of a narrow and constricted family unit, parochial and isolated from other people in the larger society. Loyalty to membership in such a closed system may lead to extreme constriction and limitation of growth for the individual family members. The monogamous structure has favored men, and the implications of this domination have become increasingly clear as women's liberation has grown more articulate. Larger social forces including the revolution in electronic communication and the shrinking of the world community because of modern transportation (resulting in massive shifting of population) have posed great threats to the orderly family structure. The result is that crisis in the family is now commonplace, and breakdown in marriage relationships is nearing the point where over half of all marriages in some regions of the United States end in divorce.

Evaluating the Family

How well does the family do the tasks that are set out for it and at what cost to the total organism and its constituent individual parts?

To understand the family it is necessary to see that it is the product of its context and does not exist in isolation from that context. The way people act as wife, husband, and parent is partly determined by class, for example. If the therapy is to be useful to the family, the therapist who may come from an entirely different social situation from that of his client family, must bring his own experience but must also recall that the client will return to a different setting. The aim of the therapy may sometimes be to help the family be more adaptive to that setting.

The two individuals who get married bring with them all their past experience and all the needs anyone has for intimacy-distance, affirmation, nurture and caring. The marriage is more than just the personalities that two individuals bring with them, however. There is a kind of new being that comes out of their relating and a process of confirmation-disconfirmation in the marriage relationship. The two partners court and decourt each other, reinforcing elements in each other which are concordant with their ideas of what a marriage is and is not. If the people have complementary concepts of marriage, then the process may be accomplished without major violence to the other's selfhood. If the two individuals are not complementary, the result may be a pitched battle wherein each serves as adversary, trying to force the other into fulfilling his own needs.

The exact nature of the problems in a family will be related to many factors. These include the evolutionary phase in which the family finds itself. Marital problems may be the focus of concern at any phase. Early in a marriage problems may focus on new adaptations, and the necessity of creating an entire new home structure. Issues of intimacy and sexuality have to be resolved, and sharing of the mutual work load has to be negotiated. With children, the marital system changes radically, and reaction to the new stresses may be the development of symptomatic behavior in family members. As the marriage continues, problems of chronicity may appear, related to the erosion of the romantic mantle which may have obscured some of the realities that the friction of life eventually exposes. Increase of financial burdens, the complexity of life with children, and the complications of three generational family networks (parents, children and grandparents), lead to a multiplicity of situations which can create intense dysfunctions. These, of course, can be signalled by a member of the family, who indeed may pay a severe personal penalty as he sees his role as obscuring the realities from the consciousness of the rest of the family group.

As children grow and have increased interaction with others outside the nuclear family, further stresses may occur. The school period brings its own stresses, and then adolescence carries a threat not only for the individual children, but also for the parents who now may feel competitive with their own children and lost in some despair themselves as they compare their own development, and possibly their own lost chances, with the new life opening up for the younger generation. After the children are grown, a new dilemma faces the marital system, since they now must face their own relationship, and in that confrontation at middle age, many marriages no longer hold together. Men also grapple with the realization that career goals are never going to be fulfilled, and their middle-age depression may linger into the future. On the other hand, women who have been tied to a mother role now feel a deep loss of their own utility, and go through a crisis which often finds little relief in reality, since so many are ill-equipped for a new kind of fulfilling life, and may also have to face abandonment as husbands try for rejuvenation with a younger mate. Of special interest in the changing social atmosphere is the fact that many women now are actually taking initiative in leaving their marriages, and finding a new basis of existence for themselves free from the bonds of unsatisfying marriages in which they have remained until the children are no longer in need of their support.

Eventually the crises connected with physical illness come to each family, and these may put unbearable stresses on a system. A further phase which must follow if the union holds is the aging of the main family members, with the associated problems of retirement, financing, and the illnesses and loneliness which may very well become a continuing part of the total context.

Indications for Therapy

There are several ways a family may come to the attention of the family therapist. The *index,* or "identified" patient may be a young child with behavior problems, or a child with somatic complaints; the patient may be an older child with a school phobia, or a delinquent adolescent. Again, the patient may be the mother, referred for dyspareunia, or the husband referred by the urologist with a problem of impotence. The dysfunction may be seen as the consequence of the scapegoating of the particular member, and his "problem behavior" may actually serve to keep an equilibrium going which hides more crucial conflicts within the system, conflicts which threaten the very basis of the family functioning, and which all conspire, albeit frequently unconsciously, to keep hidden. The family therapist is consulted, and the family agrees to come "to help Sam."

In other cases, the family may recognize that there is something in their interactions which is uncomfortable, wearing, and in need of change. In such an instance, the family comes with a *system problem,* already identified, and the therapist acts as a consultant to the system, thereby beginning his intervention. Often the two marriage partners will seek counsel because they recognize a relationship or system problem. In the same way, a family may recog-

nize a *generational* problem in sieges of conflict between parents and adolescent children, or between parents and grandparents. On the other hand, dysfunctional marriages may be signalled by phobias or psychosomatic symptoms in one partner, and dysfunctional families may be identified by the psychosis in one member. In these latter cases the marriage partners, or the members of the entire family need assistance in developing awareness that the problem lies not in the one "sick" member, but rather in the total family system.

Interventions

As noted earlier, any therapeutic move made results in some effect on the total system, so that even individual therapy can be classed as an intervention which produces change in the whole family. Although this is true, most family therapists prefer to see all the members of a family, or may selectively see groupings of family members, such as parents, older children, one parent and the children, or any other grouping.

In marital therapy, many therapists have preferred to see only one spouse, advising that the other be sent to a different therapist. These therapists cite reasons such as difficulty in maintaining objectivity, and problems in encouraging differentiation of the individual partners as reasons for such a separate treatment program. Others, however, find that the involvement of the therapist in joint sessions facilitates a more rapid comprehension of the relationship difficulties, and permits more effective intervention. Some use cotherapists to meet the concern that loss of objectivity on the part of the therapist may result, and this method is also favored by many as providing a better empathetic and modelling system when cotherapists of opposite sex work together.

The use of *couples group* therapy has also found wide acceptance, and provides the double benefit of treating the couple as a system, while at the same time providing an opportunity for experimentation by both partners in forming other relationships, which can be observed and discussed by both of them.

Multiple family groups are also being more widely initiated, and provide many of the advantages of couples groups. In multiple family groups each family member can make alliances with members of other families, and find new ways to resolve old conflicts, and also to discover new connections with members of other families in positions similar to their own.

An additional contribution to family systems method has been made by the introduction of network therapy, in which not only members of a nuclear family, but also members of the extended family and members of the various networks associated with the family (such as work, school, neighbors) are all convened, in groups numbering as large as forty or fifty. In such a marathon meeting the focus is started on the problem of the index patient, and from the input of the network, forces come to light which may have been most relevant in regard to the appearance of the symptomatic behavior, but which are also of tremendous potential therapeutic value in mobilizing the family and the total system toward a resolution of major problems in the total network.

When the therapist enters into the life of an ill-functioning family, he becomes part of that family's interaction system. He is not the detached observer nor even necessarily the facilitator of the group. He interjects his own personal relationship style into an ongoing system which, while it welcomes him as helping person, may in fact resent and resist him bitterly.

This may be why some of the best change in family therapy comes about during a period of crisis. The already disturbed family homeostatic patterns and mechanisms may be just ready to let in someone who is willing to help. The therapist may be able to convince the index patient and the family that the problem and the solution is best shared among them. An individual in distress may be better able to hear what is going on than a family, wherein the mechanisms which perpetuated the pathology have a sort of redundance and self-perpetuating feedback.

The therapist may share himself openly and thereby challenge members to an openness that they have not had before. He may model other roles and thereby change the way the family related to each other. He may get people to switch places and see what it is like on the other side. He may turn the consulting room into the studio for a real-life soap opera, or to clarify what has probably gone on the whole life of the system without ever having been looked at from a third-person point of view.

This may allow the family to take over the work of being its own therapist. Above all, he allows the family to see that there are possibilities of moving outward from a compressed situation to a more open experimentation with pleasanter relationships.

Special Techniques

Family therapists are much more active in their therapeutic style than therapists who traditionally see individuals in an analytically oriented model. In addition to this more personally involving style, the family therapist may use any number of special techniques including paradoxical behavioral methods, *role-play* and *psychodrama, sculpting, home visits,* and *videotape* playback.

In the *sculpting* technique, one member of the family is asked to create a living sculpture using actual members of the family to depict in a human three-dimensional way the emotional relationships existing in the family. The instructions are that the family members are to be placed in relationship to one another so that their body postures and facial expressions portray the emotional climate, such as personal and emotional distance, bonding, exclusions, triangular alliances, dominance-submission patterns, and so on. The method can be used in an ongoing way to express nonverbally the evolution of a sequence in the life behavior of the family, and is often extremely powerful in evoking new awareness in a way which is connected with the affect of all the family members.

Home visits have become another valuable mode of intervening in the family system, but must be kept on a professional basis to enable the therapist to maintain a perspective, and to help him avoid being too quickly and too thoroughly caught up in the family system. This latter eventuality renders the therapist powerless as an important influence in intervening in an ongoing family situation, and the old and dysfunctional family equilibrium is thereby maintained.

The technique of *videotape playback* in marital therapy has been described (Alger, 1969). In brief, segments of a family session are recorded on videotape, and then played back to the family in a selected way, so that nonverbal and contextual cues are made apparent to family members with a relevance that has a unique possibility. For example, discrepancies between verbal and nonverbal messages can be easily demonstrated, and one can become aware of unrecognized affect when behavior and facial expression are reviewed on an instant replay. A further advantage of the method is that all members of the family can become involved in the mutually cooperative activity of reviewing the playback, and the often pejorative quality present in hierarchical interpretations can be avoided since each person has equal access to the data, and any attempt by one member to exert authoritarian control can be countered by reviewing the data once more.

Conclusions

Family therapy is both a technique and a theory of understanding human behavior. As a technique it may include the husband and wife or three generations, and relatives as distant as second cousins. The technique may be expanded to other important members with whom the identified patient is involved, as in network therapy. The therapist is involved personally, providing an effective method of gaining a wider awareness of the contexts and dynamics in a family, and of providing an effective intervention. Consequently the operation of that system is altered, and so are the lives of each member of the system, including the therapist himself.

The theoretical position of family therapy is that no one person's behavior can be understood without an understanding of the context in which that person is living, and of the human interactions in which he is involved. By this understanding, then, all therapy can be seen as family therapy, or systems therapy, in that any change in any member person of a system must of necessity result in an alteration in the total system, with effects on all other members.

This new way of comprehending human behavior makes one more aware of one's dependence, and also more aware that the sense of individuality and self-will may be more illusory than one had ever imagined. On the other hand, although family therapists deal with systems, and say that the system is the patient, the final human concern is also for each member of the system. Only when the system provides

for the development of the greatest possible potential of each of its members can it be considered on any human scale to be operating in an optimal way. It is to this end that family therapists devote their efforts, and in that attempt they too are brought to the possibility of achieving the fulfillment of their own potential.

BIBLIOGRAPHY

ACKERMAN, N. W. *Family therapy in transition.* Boston: Little, Brown, 1970.

ALGER, I. Joint psychotherapy of marital problems. *Current Psychiatric Therapies,* 1967, *7,* 112–117.

ALGER, I. Therapeutic use of videotape playback. *The Journal of Nervous and Mental Disease,* 1969, *148,* 430–436.

BLOCH, D. *Techniques of family therapy.* New York: Grune & Stratton, 1973.

BOSZORMENYI-NAGY, I., and FRAMO, J. (Eds.). *Intensive family therapy.* New York: Harper and Row, 1973.

HALEY, J. *Changing families: A family therapy reader.* New York: Grune & Stratton, 1971.

MINUCHIN, S.; MONTALVO, B.; GURNEY, B.; ROSSMAN, B.; and SCHUMER, F. *Families of the slums.* New York: Basic Books, 1967.

SPECK, R., and ALTNEAVE, C. Network therapy. In D. Bloch (Ed.), *Techniques of family therapy.* New York: Grune & Stratton, 1973.

IAN ALGER

MARRIAGE

MARRIAGE: CURRENT ASPECTS

Despite the appearance in recent years of books bearing such titles as *The Death of the Family* and *Is Marriage Necessary?,* the data on marriage indicate little cause for concern for the viability of marriage. A Roper poll conducted in 1974 indicated that more than nine out of ten American women prefer marriage to any other life-style. Given a choice, only 2% of the women surveyed would prefer a career to marriage and children. This in no way suggests a preference for marriage rather than a career, for the majority of women preferred combining marriage, children, and a career. Women thus want a departure from the traditional stereotyped roles of women as housekeepers and men as breadwinners. Housework is now viewed as androgynous, with either husband or wife, sons or daughters, doing such chores as laundry, cooking, and lawnmowing.

The divorce rate has continued to rise at a steady rate to the highest point in the nation's history. Back in 1860, when divorce statistics were first kept in the United States, some 7,380 divorces were recorded, representing a rate of 0.2 per 1,000 population. In 1974, the United States crossed the million mark for the first time (1,026,000 divorces) representing a rate of 4.8 per 1,000 population. The increase in divorce is not just an American phenomenon. A rise has been apparent around the world, with the greatest acceleration among the industrialized nations. The Soviet Union, for example, showed a modest rate of 0.4 per 1,000 in 1950. By 1967, when the Soviets had eased the difficulties in obtaining a divorce, the official rate (acknowledged to be an underestimate by the leading Soviet expert) was 2.7 per 1,000 population, the rate in Moscow being 6.0 (Murstein, 1974).

A common mistake made by laymen is concluding that this still-burgeoning divorce rate presages the breakdown of the institution of marriage. In fact, however, the available evidence does not suggest this conclusion. In any given year (in recent decades) about 98% of married Americans do not seek divorce. The number of individuals who never marry has gone down steadily since 1890. Today it is estimated that well over 95% of the population will eventually marry. Making allowances for severe physical and mental incapacity and for homosexuality, it would seem that most everyone who wishes to marry can and does so.

Despite the high divorce rate, divorced persons appear to express dissatisfaction with the partner more than with the institution by virtue of their high remarriage rate. At any age, the divorced are more likely to remarry than are single persons.

The birth rate in the United States has been steadily falling in recent years, and in 1973 reached its lowest point ever, 15 births per 1,000 population. In practical terms, the fertility rate has dropped to 1.9 children per family, a figure substantially below the "replacement level" of 2.1 children. Should this trend continue, the United States would in the early twenty-first century reach zero population growth followed by a slow decline. The major reasons for the decline in fertility are the decline in interest in large families, perfection of contraception, increase in sterilization, and the later marrying age of the population. Americans were marrying at steadily younger ages until 1950; since then, the median age at marriage has slowly increased.

Sex and Marriage

The 1960s and 1970s have seen an increase in sexual emphasis in the American culture. A normal probability survey undertaken in the early 1970s indicated that "married people today have intercourse more often, take longer to do so, use more variations and get greater satisfaction from it than did the married people surveyed by Dr. Alfred Kinsey from 1938 through 1949" (Hunt, 1973).

Surprisingly, the rate of extramarital sex has not risen appreciably. Between 80% and 90% of husbands and wives say that they and their spouses would object to such activity. A majority of disapproval is found among the young as among the old. It is difficult to know precisely the percentage of individuals who engage in extramarital sex. In the 1950's Kinsey estimated that about half the men and a quarter of the women engage in extramarital sex at least once in their lives. The best available indices suggest that the figure for men today has risen only slightly, but that for women it is somewhat greater, though still below that for men.

The biggest change in the attitude toward sexual behavior seems to have occurred in the incidence of premarital sex. Here the change is so rapid that even the most recent figures become outdated by the time they reach print. In 1937 and again in 1959, the Roper agency asked the question, "Do you think it is all right for either or both parties to a marriage to have had previous sexual intercourse?" In both samples, 22% said yes for both men and women, with another 8% agreeing that it was all right for men only. In 1969, 68% of the normal probability sample in a Gallup poll thought premarital sex wrong. When Gallup repeated his poll four years later, only 48% disapproved—an unprecedented change of 20% in only four years.

Regarding premarital sexual behavior, Kinsey reported that about 9 out of 10 men and half of the women in his sample engaged in sex before marriage. About 20% of his women respondents had engaged in premarital sex while in college. The *Playboy* survey (Hunt, 1973) shows a relentless upsurge in premarital sex for both sexes as one compares the premarital behavior of older and successively younger married persons. Of those men over 55 years of age, 84% have engaged in premarital sex. The current figure for married men under 25 is 95%. The modest increase is due to the fact that the figure for males was already close to the ceiling. Women over 55 had a 31% incidence, but those under 25 had an 81% incidence. As to college behavior, several probability surveys indicate that currently 70–85% of both sexes have already engaged in premarital sex. By the time the typical college student graduates, therefore, possibly 90% will have engaged in premarital sex.

There is absolutely no evidence, however, that this permissiveness has been accompanied by promiscuity. The average number of premarital partners has not gone up compared to the generation of the 1950s. More of the young have intercourse today only with their future marriage partner than was true in Kinsey's time, according to the *Playboy* survey. At least one survey indicates that the youth of today are more faithful to their premarital partners than are married persons. They may go with several partners before marriage, but while they are doing so, they are generally faithful.

Innovative Marriage Styles

Within the last decade, a number of marital and quasi-marital variations have gained attention: cohabitation, group marriage, "swinging," and "open marriage." The simplest definition of *cohabitation* is two people spending most of their nights together in the same bedroom and having a sexual relationship. Cohabitation is fast becoming a replacement for "going steady" in American colleges. About a quarter to a third of a representative college population report having cohabited. By the time they graduate, more than 50% have cohabited at least once. Cohabiting both in and out of college does not at present constitute a threat to marriage. Most cohabitors marry their partners or break up and move on to other relationships which eventually lead to marriage.

Group marriage is a rare phenomenon which (as far as is known) has involved no more than a few thousand persons. Most group marriages break up quickly—within weeks or months. It is difficult enough for two people to live together for a long period of time; for 4 to 6 persons, it apparently is practically impossible.

Swinging, the exchange of sexual partners (spouse or friend) for recreational sex, has probably involved 1–2% of the population. However, many of these individuals have had only one such experience. Although the number of devoted hard-core swingers is well publicized, their numbers are infinitesimal.

The term *open marriage* has been bandied about by many, but its definition remains fuzzy. Presumably, it refers to a departure from conventional norms for spousal behavior, with the exact amount of freedom to be determined by agreement between the spouses. Thus, open marriage blends easily into *contract marriage* in which the parties agree in advance on certain duties and rights for each member of the marriage.

BIBLIOGRAPHY

HUNT, M. Sexual behavior in the 1970s, part III: Sex and marriage. *Playboy,* December 1973, pp. 90–91, 256.
MURSTEIN, B. I. *Love, sex, and marriage through the ages.* New York: Springer, 1974.

BERNARD I. MURSTEIN

MARRIAGE AND FAMILY ROLES OF THE AGED

Aged conjugal families can best be understood by utilizing the concept of the family life cycle of eight stages. This cycle begins with marriage and proceeds with the expansion of the family through the bearing and socialization of children with subsequent contraction when children reach adulthood and marry. The eighth stage begins with retirement and terminates with the death of the spouses. As the person moves through this life cycle, he or she experiences role entrances and exits. In order to accomplish successful role transits, the earlier demands and expectations are redefined, relinquished, or restructured.

Preretirement Roles

During the first seven stages of the family life cycle, male social roles are usually sharply differentiated from those of the female. Although the situation may be modified as more married women enter the work force, for the majority of couples the instrumental (occupational) role is a major focus for the male, followed by his marital and familial roles as husband and father. The primary female role throughout the cycle is a more expressive one, centered in the internal affairs of the growing family.

Because of the centrality of the work role for the male (it is considered the single best indicator of social class) many males come to equate self-worth with occupational mobility and prestige. The occupational status not only functions to maintain self-respect, but it also represents the principal source of income and prestige for the male, and indirectly for his wife and offspring. This occupational role also affects the male's influence in decision making in marriage—the higher the husband's occupational status and income, the greater is his marital authority as a decision maker. Thus, the male's two major roles are interdependent, since his "success" in his marital and familial roles is partially defined in terms of his achievement in his occupational role.

In the stage of the family life cycle prior to retirement, following the launching of the last child, situational imperatives require distinct role reorientations. The marital partners must now shift their focus of attention from children to one another. This functions to ease the trauma of the female role exit from the socializing mother role, and also represents a transitional stage for the male from his pre- to postretirement familial role.

Postretirement Roles

If the occupational role was a satisfactory one and the husband was compelled to relinquish it rather than left it voluntarily, then role exit of the male from the occupational sphere can involve feelings of deprivation, sadness, depression, and uncertainty—much the same feelings that are involved in bereavement, but on a less intense level. In general, wives tend to be less deeply involved in the process of retirement, both in expectations and reactions, than do their husbands. The male's major problem is finding a replacement for the purposeful activity, satisfaction, and maintenance of self-respect accorded him by his former occupational role. Concurrently, the female is faced with the tension-producing adjustment of incorporating the male's extended presence in the home and coordinating his activities there with her own. One of the consequences of this adjustment is a modification in the location of power in decision making. There is an increase in the wife's influence in decision making, a concomitant decrease in husband-centeredness, and equalitarianism.

After retirement, the formerly rigidly differentiated and dichotomized roles of the husband and wife become blurred. Role conventionality diminishes, and in place of the traditional stereotyped sex roles there is a division of tasks based on the interpersonal relationships of the couple; there is a fluidity of role allocation where each contributes what he or she can to the family functioning, and the wife's power in decision making is intensified. Role differentiation by gender is thus reduced with retirement and increasing age.

Role Redefinition

A major adaptive mechanism for the retired male is the creation of a new meaningful role to replace the occupational one. There is a deliberate acceptance of a substitute task-sharing role by the husband that is also inadvertently expressive in relation to the wife. Studies indicate that after retirement this new task-sharing role for the retired husband involves the performance of many household chores, which for the male usually requires little specialized skill and knowledge and which at times can be participated in jointly. This behavioral acquisition and sharing of household duties, although more normatively acceptable by upper-occupational than lower-occupational strata, does not differ behaviorally between these two groups. The task-sharing role adds a new dimension of common interests for the husband and wife, solidifies emotional bonds, and is viewed as functionally related both to the aged male's increasing emphasis on expressive roles and his marital adjustment. Some writers have described the reciprocity of the aged marital pair in this eighth stage as a *state of symbiosis*.

Since any change in behavior of one spouse also alters the reciprocal behavior of the other, the wife must adjust to a readjusting husband. Given his involvement in household activities, her traditional role orientation of "good housewife and homemaker" can no longer be the major distinction between her role and that of her retired spouse. She must coordinate her role with his and, like her husband, emphasize the expressive qualities of love, affection, and companionship. The departure of children, by denying outlets for these role sets, intensifies her dependence on the husband as an object of expressive satisfactions. Most wives of retired husbands are generally satisfied with the extent of their spouses' participation in household tasks, and studies indicate that no major disharmony arises or is created between husband and wife as a result of these household role adjustments.

Research Findings

Limited empirical studies of "marital satisfaction" show variations in different stages of the family life cycle. After an initially happy beginning, these studies find, there is a consistent decline in marital satisfaction and a progressive disenchantment with marriage, peaking in the middle years. For those marriages which survive, however, there is a qualitative improvement in the eighth stage for both husband and wife.

As age assaults the individual, society withdraws many of its primary-group supports. Peers die off, occupational associations cease with retirement, children move away, and the old neighborhood (where most individuals continue to reside) changes. The aged couple comes closer together to create their own affectively supportive relations. Studies show that aging retired couples demonstrate a general feeling of peacefulness and marital satisfaction which approaches the level of the newly married couple.

Although there has been a redefinition of roles within the household, older conjugal couples still maintain ties with their kinship network. Most elderly couples do not suffer from an extreme sense of isolation and loneliness. While the parents prefer to (and generally do) live in their own homes, there is a two-directional flow of support between aged parents and their offspring. Because of greater residential propinquity, as well as lower income, working-class couples, who see their children more frequently, tend to exchange services, while middle-class couples, whose married children more often live apart from them and at a greater distance, exchange money and gifts. There is a tendency for this extended family linkage to be stronger on the female line of the family. Aged parents are much more prone to call on their daughters than on their sons or daughters-in-law when they need assistance. Not only is mutual aid more frequent along the female line, but evidence indicates that interaction is greater with the wife's relatives, and residences are usually closer to the wife's parents. In that ultimate and most severe role crisis of widowhood and bereavement, wives seem better able to adjust because of these closer kinship ties and their skills in forming intimate and expressive relationships.

BIBLIOGRAPHY

Bott, E. J. *Family and social network.* London: Tavistock, 1957.

Lipman, A. Role conceptions and morale of couples in retirement. *Journal of Gerontology,* 1961, *16,* 267–271.

Shanas, E., and Streib, G. F. (Eds.). *Social structure and the family: Generational relations.* Englewood Cliffs, N.J.: Prentice-Hall, 1965.

Shanas, E. et al. *Old people in three industrial societies.* New York: Atherton, 1968.

Troll, L. E. The family of later life: A decade review. *Journal of Marriage and the Family,* 1971, *33,* 263–290.

Aaron Lipman

MARRIAGE THERAPY: ADLERIAN

Adlerians rely on four processes in their therapeutic approach to marriage: marriage therapy, marriage counseling, marriage education, and marriage study groups. Working with a marriage is called *marriage therapy* when it is done in private by a psychotherapist; it is called *marriage counseling* when done in private by a counselor. *Marriage education* takes place in a public setting, and can be conducted by those trained as psychotherapists or as counselors. *Marriage study groups* can be conducted either by professionals or by a lay person.

Adler delineated three life tasks: work, friendship, and love. He saw marriage as the natural solution to the life task, love, and viewed marriage as the ultimate test of two people's social interest and courage. Sexual intercourse, to Adler, represents the ultimate test of two people's ability to demonstrate interest in self, and one another, to cooperate, and to contribute to the welfare of one another.

Choice of a Mate

"We fell in love" is often given as the reason for a man and a woman to decide on marriage. Acknowledgment that one chooses the direction of his love, in accordance with his fundamental purposes, makes it possible to say that he even decides upon whether or not to fall in love (Dreikurs, 1946). "We are not in love" is often given as a reason for separation or divorce. Married people can discover that love is a by-product of a cooperative relationship.

Mates are chosen on the basis of much more knowledge than a person is aware of on a conscious level. One tends to chose someone who will treat him as he expects to be treated. When one accepts a person as an intimate other, it is not on the basis of common sense, but more on the basis of that person who offers

an opportunity to realize our personal pattern, who responds to our outlook and conception of life, who permits us to continue or to revive plans which we have carried since childhood. We even play a very important part in evoking and stimulating in the other person precisely the behavior which we expect and need (Dreikurs, 1946, pp. 68–69).

After living together for a while, when couples discuss the problems in their relationship, they state that the very attributes that attracted them might be the same that presently create dissonance. A quiet man may be attracted to a gregarious woman. Later, he may complain, "She never wants to leave the party." She may complain, "He is too quiet to be fun at the party." A passive woman may be attracted to an aggressive man and later complain that he wants to control their lives.

Conflict Resolution

Adlerian therapists see problems that develop in a marriage as in the relationship, and which ultimately have to do with the difficulty encountered by two people who may have a goal of an equalitarian relationship, but who have little background for living with other people as equals. Most human relationships are characterized by some degree of superiority-inferiority, but Adler held that whenever one partner elevates himself, or herself, above the other partner, that relationship is always temporary, and the partner in the inferior position will always attempt to reverse the balance. This is most clearly etched in the marriage relationship.

Intramarital fighting does not lead to a solution of the problem, but only lays the groundwork for the next conflict. Only with courage and self-confidence can people face the difficulties of cooperation. Dreikurs (1946) cited two misconceptions regarding human cooperation.

One is the belief that resentment can lead to improvement or that it is even a prerequisite for actions directed toward improvement . . . the husband will gladly adjust himself to his wife's desires if he feels fully accepted by her, but he may drive in the opposite direction if he senses her resentment and rejection. [And the second belief that] when interests clash, nothing can be done except to fight or yield. (Pp. 103–105)

Whatever complaints a couple presents in therapy, counseling, or the marriage education center, will be dealt with by utilizing Dreikurs's four principles of democratic resolution: mutual respect; pinpointing the issue; reaching a new agreement; and participation in decision making.

Every marriage conflict will include violation of one, or more, of these principles. Mutual respect means neither fighting nor giving in; it is neither overpowering one's partner, nor capitulating. For example, a couple may complain about sex, in-laws, work, money, or child-rearing. Behind the complaint there will be some threat to personal status, prestige, superiority, some concern with who is winning, or who is going to decide, or who is right. Reaching a new agreement is based on the understanding that, when there is conflict in the marriage, and the couple is fighting, they have reached an agreement to fight. If conflict is to be resolved, a new agreement must be reached, ultimately, each party stating, "This I am willing to do, with no strings attached." Both parties in a marriage must participate in mutual decisions, not only in the decision making process, but in the responsibility for the decision. This principle is regularly violated, reflecting lack of respect for one's partner.

One of the key questions in marriage is, "How much allowance for individual differences will be acceptable in the relationship?" When couples are getting along, they are accepting one another as they are. When couples are not getting along, they are not tolerant and both people feel misunderstood. Solutions to marriage problems come about through mutual understanding.

Marriage Therapy

As often as possible marriage therapy is conducted with both parties present. Reluctant partners are asked to attend.

The phases of therapy include establishing a working relationship, which often includes a contract for a definite number of sessions, followed by an evaluation of progress, and the possibility of negotiation of a further contract; an evaluation of both the individuals, through the formulation of the personal life style, as well as of the marital relationship itself; the results of the interpretations and evaluations are presented to the couple and further work is continued through the process of reorientation and reeducation.

Rudolph Dreikurs introduced *multiple therapy* in 1946; subsequently, a number of Adlerian therapists have found that two therapists, preferably a man and a woman, can work most efficiently with a couple.

The Process of the Life Style. When doing personal life styles, data collection and interpretation is often done in the presence of both spouses. This process is a learning experience in itself. Even those couples who have been married for many years, may learn unexpected nuances about the personalities of their mates. Data is collected in an organized fashion. The partner's childhood family constellation is diagrammed. The relationships between the members of the childhood family are clarified

as each family member is described. In this part of the data collection, the family atmosphere, that is, the shared family values, become clear. After asking about childhood talents, ambitions, illnesses, fears, and habits, the partner whose life style is being formulated is asked to rate himself or herself in comparison to the siblings close in age. A list of thirty attributes is used to indicate how this particular person sought to find a position in the childhood family. Next, a brief inquiry is directed toward physical, sexual, and social development, and school and work experience. Early childhood dreams are recorded verbatim. These give the subjective themes and melodies, in the person's view of himself and how he finds his place in life. Each person is asked to recall, from childhood, a song, a fairy tale, a nursery rhyme, a poem, a Bible personality, a Bible story, a television show, a radio show, and a movie, and to describe what impressed him.

The therapist summarizes the collected data and interprets the early childhood recollections and dreams. After listing the primary themes and melodies which emerge (the individual's convictions and guidelines about who he or she is, what life is, what one's expectations are, and what ethical considerations one operates with), both partners and the therapist cooperate in listing the strengths of the person who has had his or her life style done.

After personal life style formulations are completed, the therapist considers the recurrent questions presented by both partners. These questions are considered in light of the personal life styles of the partners. Sometimes, one, or both partners may choose to work on changing basic aspects of the personal life style.

Recommendations are commonly given which the couple can put into practice on their own. Marriage therapy usually is a relatively brief therapy—under 12 to 18 hours.

Recommendations/Home Work Assignments. Adler recommended *prescribing the symptom.* Dreikurs called this *antisuggestion,* and Frankl (1971) used the term, *paradoxical intention.* On the surface, a paradoxical recommendation appears simple enough, since people are asked to do what they are already doing, especially those things they may be complaining about. If a couple states that they disagree about money, the recommendation is given to disagree, in exactly the way they described their money fights, at a certain time each day. When this recommendation is followed, the problem often begins to appear ridiculous, and even humorous which may encourage them to try new behaviors. In a conflict, there often is some issue of who is in control. With a paradoxical recommendation, the therapists are taking control from both partners by recommending their behavior.

Recommendations are used regularly in marriage therapy, marriage counseling and marriage education centers. In marriage study groups couples often decide on some homework assignment to carry out as a couple or the whole group may decide on an assignment.

Couples are asked if they are willing to take turns at being in charge. For example, if leisure and recreation, or sex, or money, are listed as problems, the therapists may ask that one spouse be in charge of sex or money for one week, and the next week, the other partner will take the leadership role.

Marriage conferences, as outlined by Corsini, are a favorite self-help assignment. A couple is asked to make an hour appointment with one another. One person speaks first, for exactly one-half hour, with no interruptions from the spouse. The conference is often improved if the partners sit so that they cannot see one another. This eliminates nonverbal disapproval. After 30 minutes, the second person speaks, until the time is up. The 30 minutes are kept, whether filled with speech, or not. No controversial subjects brought up in the conference are to be discussed between conferences. Conferences can be held from one, to three times, per week.

Couple councils are also recommended. Councils are conducted like a business meeting, with minutes recorded, a chairperson, meeting at a regular time each week, and with an agenda.

Couples are asked to write, in private, their expectations for: the self; the other; and their relationship. These expectations are to be brought to the next session, where they are shared, and discussed. Partners are often asked if they would be willing to carry out a spouse's expectation for one week.

Communication, with paraphrasing, is rec-

ommended when couples have difficulty listening. After one person speaks, the partner must paraphrase to the other partner's satisfaction, before being able to answer back.

Another technique is to ask couples to communicate by writing, to explain a point of view, to bring up a delicate subject, or to express encouragement to the other.

Couples are invited to read articles or books and underline, with different colors, ideas important to them and to discuss these with the counselors or therapists.

It is common for the therapist to ask couples what they have learned and, if they are in a group or marriage center, to share their new knowledge. This is often helpful to others. They may be asked to reverse roles during the session, sitting like the spouse sits, and imitating, as carefully as possible, his/her actions and behaviors (Moreno, 1953). This enables one to think and feel the way the partner does. Couples can also use role reversal at home.

Life Task Ratings. A simple rating procedure allows marriage partners to rate themselves and one another; to predict how they will be rated; and to hear, in fact, how the partner does rate each in the life task areas. The life tasks, expanded from Adler, are work, friendship, love, spouse, relating to the other sex, getting along with spouse, the search for meaning, leisure and recreation, and parenting. The partner is asked to rate himself or herself on a scale of 1 to 5 (1 the highest) as to functioning in each of these areas. After the prediction of one partner's rating is recorded, the other responds, and the process is reversed. This process, referred to as "taking the temperature of the marriage," (Pew, 1974) often pinpoints trouble areas in the marriage or reveals areas that need to be more fully explored. The therapist gets some idea of how well the partners know themselves, and each other, and is provided a base reading which can be referred to, later on in therapy, to give some indication of the success of the therapy.

If the couple want to remain married, the goals in therapy are clear: to enhance the relationship and to work out trouble areas. If one, or both, partners are in doubt about remaining married, and a clear decision has not been made to dissolve the marriage, life style formulations can be done, and discussion of the decision is part of therapy. Goals in marriage therapy must constantly be renegotiated and shared; or resistance may develop a difference in goals between the therapists and the married pair, who have come for therapy.

It is common to ask a married pair to suspend any major life decision until the personal life style formulations have been completed. If dissolution is the choice of the married pair, therapy can be conducted toward a goal of friendly and cooperative dissolution which is least hurtful to either party or to the children.

Although marriage therapy is usually focused on the current problems presented by the couple, sometimes a detailed history of the marriage is necessary to understand what is going on in the present. Most sexual complaints are seen as relationship problems. At times, a detailed sexual history is indicated. Sexual, and other, fantasies are discussed, and current dreams are interpreted. Cotherapists rely heavily on establishing their own warm and trusting relationship, and attempt to model for the couple such a relationship. At the same time, the therapists model a couple who can disagree and also communicate clearly and constructively.

The Number One Priority. A relatively new addition to Adlerian theory, and practice, is the *number one priority.* The number one priority concept is particularly useful in marriage therapy, marriage counseling, and marriage education centers. Four parts of number one priority have been identified: (1) comfort, (2) pleasing, (3) control, and (4) superiority. Each person has all four, but in transactions and interactions with other people each moves toward his number one priority first. It would appear that among many other factors people choose marriage partners on the basis of number one priority. That is, a person chooses someone with whom he or she can be oneself, which means to move toward the number one priority.

A person with a number one priority of comfort most wants to avoid pain and stress; a person with a number one priority of pleasing most wants to avoid rejection; a person with a number one priority of control most wants to avoid humiliation; and the person with a number one priority of superiority most wants to avoid meaninglessness. The four priorities are neither good nor bad. Problems develop when

an individual moves toward the "only if" absurdity. For example, "Only if I am comfortable do I really belong." The more an individual moves toward the "only if" absurdity, the higher the price paid.

In general, people with a number one priority of comfort pay a price of reduced productivity; those with a number one priority of pleasing pay a price of self-abnegation, and some reduction in personal growth; those with a number one priority of control pay a price of social distance or reduced spontaneity; and those with a number one priority of superiority pay a price of being overloaded.

As marriage partners learn about their own and their partner's number one priority, certain vulnerabilities of the partner become clear. The therapists teach each partner to be an effective agent of encouragement, rather than attacking vulnerabilities. Married couples seldom have the same number one priority. The most common pairings are control and superiority; and comfort and pleasing. If the therapists are skilled at pinpointing the number one priority very early in an initial interview, they are getting at one facet of the life style, and can help their clients to feel understood.

Frequently, the goal of private marriage therapy is to help the couple get to the point where they can deal with their problems in the public setting of a marriage education center. Often couples are urged to attend a marriage education center as an adjunct to private therapy. Private marriage therapy is more often used in situations of complex, personal problems.

Marriage Counseling

In marriage counseling, the concentration is on current conflict resolution, that is, teaching couples to live together more cooperatively using the four principles of conflict resolution. Often counseling does not emphasize life style work but counselors may utilize the life style.

In marriage counseling, as well as in a marriage education center and marriage therapy, the counselors make use of various recommendations. In all approaches to marriage, the therapists rely heavily on humor. No matter how tragic a relationship may seem, if partners can learn to laugh at their foibles, to increase their "courage to be imperfect," the groundwork is laid for a better relationship.

Marriage Education

The purpose of marriage education centers is to disseminate basic mental health principles which lead to more harmonious living, to a large audience; to provide a resource for troubled couples; and to train other counselors to work more effectively with couples. Marriage education centers may be housed in hospitals, churches, schools, or other public sites. Funding sources are varied, but in many centers, much of the work is done by volunteers. The staff of a marriage education center includes the director or codirectors, who are professionals in the mental health field, and who have had extensive additional training and experience with the Adlerian model. In some communities, however, lay people have been trained to direct marriage education centers with professional supervision. Other staff usually include the coordinator, an intake worker, a recorder, and staff members for an activity center for children and adolescents.

Admission is free in most marriage education centers. Participants can simply observe; they may ask questions; or they may be the volunteer (demonstration) couple who is counseled in front of the group just as Adler counseled families in child guidance clinics. The volunteer couple actually helps the cocounselors teach Adlerian principles to the larger group through the interview process. The volunteer couples will have been in the audience for several weeks before becoming a demonstration couple. They usually will have learned some basic Adlerian principles of democratic living. They often learn more after returning to the audience, which gives them an opportunity to see themselves reflected in further interviews. Couples learn that they are not alone with their concerns, and also that some couples in the group have discovered satisfactory solutions.

An interview in a marriage education center is often relatively brief, and ends with specific recommendations given to the couple. Some of the recommendations are generated through discussion with the audience. The couple agree to carry out the recommendations, for a specified time, usually one week.

Although audience participation is encouraged, cocounselors are vigorous in ensuring that the couple is in no way put on the spot. A counseling session with a couple often ends with the audience participating in an encouragement session. The audience is invited to give their honest reactions to the couple regarding the strengths and assets in the marriage relationship. The couple are (usually) asked to return, for follow-up sessions, to describe their successes and failures in applying the new techniques and principles.

A marriage education center is an example of primary preventive mental health. The counselors are able to reach many more people than they could by talking with individual couples. This preventive aspect, and the aspect of community outreach, and community education, have particularly interested a number of hospitals.

The marriage education center becomes a referral agent to other community agencies, as well as a community resource.

Marriage Study Groups

An outgrowth of marriage education centers, and an emphasis in general on the benefits of study groups, is the marriage study group. A group of couples meets weekly for eight to ten weeks to study a book like Dreikurs's *The Challenge of Marriage*. The study groups are lay led; and they depend upon the ability of couples to learn principles, and put them into practice on their own. When couples find this difficult, marriage therapy or marriage counseling, may be indicated.

Couple Group Therapy

Adlerians have adapted marriage therapy to the group process. A group of five or six married couples are seen for two hours a week, usually for a time limited period, for example, ten weeks. Couples benefit from the group by identifying with, and getting ideas from, peers. They discover that they are not alone, and they may broaden their sense of belonging to a wider sphere. Ideally, such couples will have had some private sessions, including formulation of their life styles. Couple group therapy may take place in conjunction with attendance at a marriage education center.

BIBLIOGRAPHY

ANSBACHER, H. and ANSBACHER, R. *The individual psychology of Alfred Adler.* New York: Harper & Row, 1956.
ANSBACHER, H., and ANSBACHER, R. *Superiority and social interest.* Evanston, Ill.: Northwestern University Press, 1964.
DEUTSCH, D. Group therapy with the married couple. *The Individual Psychologist,* 1967, *4,* 56–62.
DREIKURS, R. *The challenge of marriage.* New York: Sloan and Pearce, 1946.
DREIKURS, R. The choice of a mate. *International Journal of Individual Psychology,* 1935, *1* (4).
DREIKURS, R., and SONSTEGARD, M. A. The Adlerian or teleoanalysis group counseling approach. In G. M. Gazda (Ed.), *Basic approaches to group psychotherapy and group counseling.* Springfield, Ill.: Thomas, 1968. Pp. 197–232.
PEW, W. L., and PEW, M. L. Adlerian marriage counseling. *Journal of Individual Psychology,* 1972, *28,* 192–202.
PEW, W. L. Taking your own psychological temperature. *Single Parent,* April 1974, pp. 5–7.
PEW, W. L., and PEW, M. L. Marital therapy. In A. G. Nikelly (Ed.), *Techniques for behavior change.* Springfield, Ill.: Thomas, 1971. Pp. 125–128.

MIRIAM L. PEW

MASKING PROCEDURE IN CONDITIONING

One problem associated with the classical conditioning of human subjects is that the procedures are so simple and obvious that the human participant may bring a variety of voluntary processes to bear on the procedure. For example, when the individual notices the change from conditioning to extinction procedures he purposefully inhibits responses. If one views classical conditioning as an involuntary and automatic process, such voluntary interventions are a cause for concern because they may distort the natural conditioning processes.

In the case of eyelid conditioning, masking procedures were developed as a way of overcoming this difficulty by distracting the subject of the experiment. The method involved embedding the conditioning experiment in some other task that might even seem more important to the subject. One typical masking task was that of predicting which of two lights would come on after a given signal. In such a

procedure the conditioning trial could be administered while the individual was making his choice.

The results of experiments carried out to compare conditioning with and without a masking task have been quite consistent. Acquisition is very slightly retarded and extinction is much slower.

GREGORY A. KIMBLE

MASLOW, ABRAHAM H. (1908–1970)

Maslow, known as the founder of humanistic psychology, is noted for his hierarchical theory of motivation and his description of the characteristics of self-actualizing people. Probably more than anyone else, he is responsible for turning the attention of psychologists and social scientists toward the often-neglected potentialities of human beings.

Maslow was born in Brooklyn on April 1, 1908. He attended the University of Wisconsin for both undergraduate and graduate work, receiving his doctorate of psychology in 1934 for a study of the social characteristics of monkeys. After a fellowship at Columbia, he taught at Brooklyn College for almost 15 years, then was called to the new Brandeis University where he became chairman of the Psychology Department and taught from 1951 to 1969. Maslow was elected president of the American Psychological Association for 1967–68. He later became a Resident Fellow of the W. P. Laughlin Charitable Foundation in Menlo Park, California, where he died of a heart attack on June 8, 1970. He had married Bertha Goodman in 1928 and they had two daughters, Ann and Ellen.

Hierarchy of Motives

Already known by the early 1950s as a thought-provoking teacher of psychology and coauthor of a popular textbook in abnormal psychology, Maslow began to impress his colleagues with a new classification of motives. He had been dissatisfied with the piecemeal and unsystematic treatment of motivation by psychologists, and with their overemphasis on physiological drives. In 1943, he proposed a "holistic-dynamic" theory of motivation, which he elaborated ten years later and included in his *Motivation and Personality*. He set up a hierarchy of motives, starting with physiological needs (food, air, water, fairly constant temperature, etc.); their satisfaction permits other needs to emerge, such as safety and the avoidance of danger. If physiological and safety drives are gratified, higher needs come into play, for example, belonging and love, followed by the need for self-esteem, whose satisfaction leads to feelings of adequacy and self-confidence, and whose thwarting to feelings of inferiority and helplessness. But even if all these needs are satisfied, continued Maslow, discontent and restlessness may develop (he later called these "grumbles") "unless the individual is doing what he is fitted for. A musician must make music, an artist must paint, a poet must write, if he is to be ultimately at peace with himself. What a man *can* be, he *must* be. This need we may call self-actualization" (Maslow, 1954, p. 91). The term self-actualization had been coined by Kurt Goldstein in his book, *The Organism;* Maslow used it in the more specific sense of man's desire for self-fulfillment, "the tendency for him to become actualized in what he is potentially. This tendency might be phrased as the desire to become more and more what one is, to become everything that one is capable of becoming" (Maslow, 1954, pp. 91–2).

Maslow criticized the psychologists for "their pessimistic, negative and limited conception of the full height to which the human being can attain" and their "setting of his psychological limits at too low a level." Too often, he stated, they pursue trivial goals with limited methods. Thus

the science of psychology has been far more successful on the negative than on the positive side; it has revealed to us much about man's shortcomings, his illnesses, his sins, but little about his potentialities, his virtues, his achievable aspirations, or his full psychological height. It is as if psychology had voluntarily restricted itself to only half its rightful jurisdiction, and that the darker, meaner half (Maslow, 1954, pp. 353–54).

Self-Actualization

To support his views, Maslow presented studies of "self-actualizing people." Some were famous, like Lincoln, Thomas Jefferson, Einstein, Eleanor Roosevelt, or Beethoven, Thoreau, Walt Whitman, and Albert Schweitzer. Others were chosen from Maslow's friends and acquaintances. The main criterion was "full use and exploitation of talents, capacities, potentialities, etc. Such people seem to be fulfilling themselves and to be doing the best that they are capable of doing" (Maslow, 1954, pp. 200–201). Analysis of the characteristics of self-actualizing people, as compared with ordinary persons showed:

1. More efficient perception of reality and more comfortable relations with it;
2. Greater acceptance of self, others and nature;
3. More spontaneity, simplicity and naturalness;
4. Stronger focus on problems outside themselves;
5. A quality of detachment and need for privacy;
6. Greater autonomy, and independence of culture and environment;
7. Continued freshness of appreciation and richness of feeling;
8. More frequent mystic or transcendent experience;
9. A deep feeling of identification with mankind (Adler's "Gemeinschaftsgefühl");
10. Deeper and more profound interpersonal relations;
11. A more democratic character structure;
12. Greater ability to discriminate between means and ends;
13. A philosophical, whimsical, unhostile sense of humor;
14. Without exception: creativeness, originality or inventiveness;
15. Resistance to cultural conformity.

Maslow noted that self-actualizing people are not free from imperfections; they are strong people and can be vain, irritating, or cold, or uncritical and overgenerous. They are not free from guilt, anxiety, and conflict; but their values are different from those of conventional and deprived people. They are more completely individual, yet also more completely socialized. In them major polarities have been resolved, for example, between heart and head, acceptance and rebellion, introversion and extraversion. Such people are different in kind from the immature and unhealthy specimens usually studied; Maslow insisted that the study of self-actualizing people should be the basis for a more universal science of psychology.

Humanistic Psychology

Maslow had used the term *holistic-dynamic* to describe his organismic approach to psychology, but it soon came to be called *humanistic.* In 1961, in collaboration with Anthony J. Sutich, he founded the *Journal of Humanistic Psychology,* and the following year, along with Carl Rogers, Rollo May, Charlotte Bühler, and other psychologists and social scientists, the American Association for Humanistic Psychology (later shortened to the Association for Humanistic Psychology). Humanistic psychology was defined as the

third main branch of the general field of Psychology (the two already in existence being the psychoanalytical and the behavioristic) and as such, is primarily concerned with those human capacities and potentialities that have no systematic place, either in positivistic or behavioristic theory or in classical psychoanalytic theory, e.g., creativity, love, self, growth, . . . self-actualization, higher values, being, becoming, spontaneity, play, humor, affection, ego-transcendence, . . . responsibility, psychological health, and related concepts.

The new organization grew rapidly and Maslow was active in it, contributing to most issues of its journal, and speaking at its meetings and conferences. Here and in his books, notably *Toward a Psychology of Being* (1962, 1968), he developed his ideas and theories, contrasting the usual "deficiency motivation" with the Being or Growth type of motivation, which is best shown in self-actualizing people. He also described what he called the "cognition of Being in the peak-experiences"—those happiest and most ecstatic moments that have an almost mystical quality and are so rich and intense that each one seems an end in itself.

Neurosis is a failure of personal growth, as Maslow saw it—a blocking of self-actualization. He disliked the words *therapy, psychotherapy,* and *patient,* because they represent the medical model and pathology. "What the good clinical therapist does," he wrote, "is to help his particular client to unfold, to break through the defenses against his own self-knowledge, to recover himself, and to get to know himself" (Maslow, 1967, p. 285). Health is not mere adjustment to environment but involves transcendence or independence of the environment. Not extrapsychic success but intropsychic strength is the secret of mental health. However, in the preface to his revised *Motivation and Personality* (1970), Maslow warned that personal growth is a painful process and will be shunned by some persons. Knowledge of psychodynamics is still necessary to combat regressive, fearful, and self-diminishing tendencies.

Maslow strove to extend his ideas beyond the confines of classroom and clinic. He visited industry, for example, and wrote a book called *Eupsychian Management* (1965), exploring ways in which conditions of work can satisfy the individual's personal fulfillment and also the health and prosperity of the organization. In *Religions, Values and Peak-Experiences* (1964, 1970) he discussed man's transcendent nature and proposed that religious experience can be studied scientifically.

There are many indications that the humanistic psychology of Abraham Maslow has made a real difference in American psychology and through it, in other aspects of our life as well.

BIBLIOGRAPHY

GOBLE, F. G., *The third force; the psychology of Abraham Maslow.* New York: Pocket Books, 1971.

LOWRY, A. *A. H. Maslow: An intellectual portrait.* Monterey, Calif.: Brooks/Cole, 1973.

MASLOW, A. H. *Motivation and personality.* New York: Harper, 1954; Rev. ed., 1970.

MASLOW, A. H. *Toward a psychology of being* (2nd ed.). Princeton, N.J.: Van Nostrand, 1968.

MASLOW, A. H. *The psychology of science: A reconnaissance.* New York: Harper & Row, 1965.

MASLOW, A. H. Self-actualization and beyond. In J. F. T. Bugental (Ed.), *Challenges of humanistic psychology.* New York: McGraw-Hill, 1967. Chap. 29.

S. STANSFELD SARGENT

MASOCHISM: HORNEY'S VIEW

According to Horney, *masochism* is neither a love of suffering for its own sake nor a biologically predetermined self-negating process. It is a form of relating, and its essence is the weakening or extinction of the individual self and merging with a person or power believed to be greater than oneself. Masochism is a way of coping with life through dependency and self-minimizing. Though it is most obvious in the sexual area, it encompasses the total range of human relations.

As part of a neurotic character development, masochism has its own special purposes and value system. The neurotic suffering may serve the defensive purposes of avoiding recriminations, competition, and responsibility. It is a way of expressing accusations and vindictiveness in disguised form. By exaggerating and inviting suffering, it justifies demands for affection, control, and reparations. In the distorted value system of the masochist, suffering is raised to a virtue and serves as the basis for claims to love, acceptance, and rewards.

Since the masochist takes pride in and identifies with the self-effacing, suffering, subdued self, an awareness of conflicting drives toward expansiveness and self-glorification as well as a healthy striving for growth would be destructive to his self-image. By abandoning himself to uncompromising hatred for the intolerable side of himself, the masochist attempts to eliminate the conflict of contradictory impulses. Thus, a masochist has engulfed himself in self-hate and suffering.

As Horney's (1950) ideas on neurosis evolved, the concept of masochism was incorporated into the more inclusive *self-effacing* character structure and its extreme end stage, *morbid dependency*. Masochism is best understood, in this context, as part of a particular attempted solution to the conflicts engendered by the neurotic process.

BIBLIOGRAPHY

HORNEY, K. *Neurosis and human growth.* New York: Norton, 1950.

ARNOLD MITCHELL
HAROLD KELMAN

MASS MEDIA

MASS MEDIA: THEIR IMPACT
MASS MEDIA AND THEIR INFLUENCE
MASS MEDIA AND VIOLENCE

MOTION PICTURES AND PSYCHIATRY
TELEVISION AND PSYCHIATRY

MASS MEDIA: THEIR IMPACT

An important way we come to know the external world is through the mass media. It has been reported, (Baker and Ball, 1969), that the average American spends one-quarter to one-half of each waking day attending to some form of the mass media. It seems that one uses radio and television both for comfort during lonelier hours and as an important source of information. The media present a constant nexus among people living in an increasingly complex world. The pervasiveness of the encounter with the mass media justifies reflections on its possible influence on human lives.

An element which is not generally considered a major factor in media impact is the news event. However, research indicates that remote social events, reported by the media as "news," have significant effects on our judgments and behavior toward absolute strangers.

American preoccupations are reflected in the organization of media newscasts. The "big news" story seems to be crime, sex, novelty and conflict (Baker and Ball). The frequency, time, location and pictorial content in presenting the news have been found by Booth (1970–1971) to be critical factors in the extent to which news items will be recalled. Thus, news items dealing with violent episodes in close proximity to the viewing audience seem to interest many and have a greater probability of being remembered.

According to some investigators, American news, as compared with that of other countries, contains more violence. This is significant when considered in the light of research findings which suggest that riots, aggressive crimes, mass murders and the like show an increase after these events are publicized (Berkowitz, 1970).

Violence has been linked to television drama. *U.S. News and World Report* reported that two nights after the movie *Fuzz* was viewed on television, a crime similar to that shown in the movie was committed in Boston. However, Feshbach demonstrated that realistic aggression shown on television had an even stronger impact on the audience than fictional programs which portray the fantasy of aggressive acts. A case can thus be made that television and radio news broadcasts impact behavior even more significantly than television drama or serial presentations.

Considering the concern about the possible influence of dramatic television violence on aggression, it is surprising that the resulting research has not addressed the impact of media news presentations on the attending public. As stories concerning crimes of assault, murder, and arson are tossed at the public in quick succession, their possible influence on behavior and attitudes deserves attention.

The Impact of "The News"

The assassination of John F. Kennedy stunned the nation. Schramm (1971) found that less than one-half of the people in his national sample could continue their usual activities after hearing reports of the event. According to a "National Survey of Public Reactions and Behavior" conducted by Sheatsley and Feldman, many reported physical symptoms following the tragic event. Sears found that some people identified themselves as being less politically partisan, but Wrightsman and Noble (1965) demonstrated the less obvious. The news of Kennedy's assassination altered people's conceptions of prevailing moral and ethical dispositions.

Hornstein (1976) ascribed the findings he obtained immediately following reports of the assassination of Robert F. Kennedy to a similar effect. His research involved "losing" wallets on the streets of New York City to be found by unsuspecting strangers. On the average, 45% of the people who found these wallets would return them. The day the Kennedy assassination was reported, not a single wallet was returned. Hornstein suggested that the news caused subconscious alterations in people's conceptions of the moral-ethical dispositions of the community at large, resulting in less helping behavior than ordinary. This idea was more systematically explored by Hornstein, LaKind, Frankel, and Manne (1975) who reported that subjects who were exposed to reports of prosocial events behaved more cooperatively toward strangers (measured by one round of a nonzero sum game) than did subjects exposed to news broadcasts reporting antisocial events.

Singer (Hornstein, 1976) reported a similar effect in the case of jury decisions in a mock courtroom trial situation. Exposure to "bad" news or reports of antisocial events increased the likelihood that guilty verdicts would be delivered by the mock jury. In a similar study, LaKind (Hornstein, 1976) found that subjects who heard "good" news were far more disposed to judge alleged murderers innocent than those who heard "bad" news. Further laboratory confirmation of the impact of newscasts' reporting of remote social events was offered by Kaplan (Hornstein, 1976) who noted that after hearing bad news, boys discriminated sharply between similar and dissimilar others, showing favoritism for the similar others. This did not occur with exposure to "good" news or no news.

Explanations for these findings indicate that news reports have more psychological meaning than simply serving notice of one or another event. There is compelling evidence that people draw from such reports of remote social events, at least temporarily, generalizations *about people in general,* and apply these generalizations in their behavior toward particular strangers. Such information becomes a significant input in determining whether the next stranger we encounter will be considered "we" or "they." Knowledge of remote social events is a source of influence on our understanding of the surrounding social environment. Specifically, this knowledge has critical impact because it alters beliefs, if only temporarily, about the extent to which the surrounding community is composed of people who hold pro- or antisocial dispositions, and one's assessment of the community determines inferences about particular strangers and whether they will cooperate or compete, help or harm, thereby affecting one's behavior toward particular others. The news, then, effects our assessment of others in general which in turn influences our behavior toward particular strangers whom we encounter.

Support for the first point in the above rationale is provided in an experiment by Hornstein and his colleagues (1975) in which subjects exposed to the prosocial newscast estimated that greater percentages of the population subscribe to prosocial values and beliefs than did subjects exposed to antisocial newscasts. Subjects viewed the public as more honest, cleaner and more altruistic after hearing the "good" news. Findings from several naturalistic studies supported the second point in the rationale by demonstrating that specific information about the community at large affected whether a subject behaved altruistically toward a particular stranger. This finding, together with data gathered by other investigators indicates that an individual's general social outlook affects behavior toward complete strangers.

To verify the assumption that it is the *social* component of the remote event which causes the observed alterations in behavior and judgment, a study was conducted which exposed subjects to newscasts which reported "good" and "bad" news involving acts of man (social) and "good" and "bad" news involving natural events. The consequences of these events—the "good" and "bad" news stories—were identical. Only the causes—natural or social—were varied. In the case of the social events, findings replicated those of Hornstein and his colleagues (1975) and those of Kaplan, both of which had reflected increased cooperative behavior toward strangers after "good" news. This effect did not emerge in the natural events newscast, lending further support to the idea that it is the social component of the reported event which is the critical factor influencing behavior.

The idea that behavior is affected by the inferences one draws concerning the social universe is supported by work in related areas. Sales (1973) has accumulated extensive archival data from contrasting historical periods which document a rise in authoritarianism during periods which were characterized by threatening events. The impact of the Soviet launching of the *Sputnik I* in the fall of 1957 has been well documented by educational as well as cold war historians. The consequences of that event for American school children of the period were a marked institutional emphasis on discipline, academic rigor, and a new era of institutionally induced competition. Escalona (1963) linked the threat of thermonuclear war communicated by mass media with alterations in adolescent development during the 1950s.

The data received from the media, in the absence of specific information about particular strangers, dispose one to classify strangers as "we" or "they." Apparently after "bad" news the boundaries of "they"—those perceived to be dissimilar—grow larger. After "good" news the boundaries of "we" grow larger. Our attitudes and behavior toward strangers about whom we know nothing are influenced by this irrelevant information concerning unrelated remote social events.

Newscasts are typically saturated with "bad" news, such as stories of murder, armed robbery, rape, and the like. The reporting of these events captures the attention of many. Some investigators have suggested that tragic events should be juxtaposed with life-saving ones, and they criticize newscasting for the indifferent reporting of violent events.

BIBLIOGRAPHY

BAKER, R. K., and BALL, S. *Violence and the mass media.* Washington, D.C.: U.S. Government Printing Office, 1969.

BERKOWITZ, L. The contagion of violence: An S-R mediational analysis of some effects of observed aggression. *Symposium on Motivation,* 1970, *18,* 95–135.

BOOTH, A. The recall of news items. *Public Opinion Quarterly,* 1970–71, *34,* 604–616.

ESCALONA, S. Children's responses to the nuclear war threat. *Children,* 1963, *10,* 137–142.

HORNSTEIN, H. A. *Cruelty and kindness: A new look at aggression and altruism.* Englewood Cliffs, N.J.: Prentice-Hall, 1976.

HORNSTEIN, H. A.; LAKIND, E.; FRANKEL, G.; and MANNE, S. The effects of knowledge about remote social events on prosocial behavior, social conception and mood. *Journal of Personality and Social Psychology,* 1975, *32,* 1038–1046.

SALES, S. M. Threat as a factor in authoritarianism: An analysis of archival data. *Journal of Personality and Social Psychology,* 1973, *38,* 344–355.

SCHRAMM, W. *The process and effects of mass communications* (2nd ed.). Urbana: University of Illinois Press, 1971.

WRIGHTSMAN, L., and NOBLE, F. C. Reactions to the president's assassination. *Psychological Reports,* 1965, *16,* 159–162.

LYLE TUCKER
STEPHEN M. HOLLOWAY

MASS MEDIA AND THEIR INFLUENCE

Instructional Effects of Media Entertainment

Perhaps the most obvious way that media entertainment may contribute to socialization is by providing instruction to young viewers.

Recognizing this possibility, investigators and public authorities have expressed active interest in educational television since the medium rose to popularity in the mid-1950s; the very palpable success of *Sesame Street* stands as clear testimony that the entertainment media can be powerful teachers of cognitive skills. They can teach social lessons as well.

Most children certainly understand that television and movie plays are fictional in the sense that the particular events shown did not actually happen to the individuals appearing on the screen; nonetheless, they believe that television is real in other ways and are instructed by it regardless of what writers or broadcasters may intend. Fully 40% of a sample of white elementary school-age children in one study said they had learned more about how blacks look, talk, and act from entertainment television than from any other source (Greenberg, 1972), and an even larger percentage of adolescents in a second investigation stated that television crime shows "tell about life the way it really is" (McLeod, Atkin, and Chaffee, 1972). In a third study (Defleur and Defleur, 1967), children between the ages of 6 and 13 were interviewed and tested about their knowledge and impressions of various jobs and professions; the results led the investigators to conclude that "within the present samples of children and occupations, television is a more potent source of occupational status knowledge than either personal contact or the general community culture" (p. 787).

The Impact of Television

In contrast to other media, television is a serious contender as the most important socializing force during the formative years; by age 16 most children in the United States will have spent more time watching television than going to school, so the question of what they see assumes considerable importance. Content analyses reveal that portrayals of minority groups and women on television are limited and stereotyped and that violence and aggression tend to be the medium's dominant entertainment themes. It has been realistically estimated that the average child will watch the violent destruction of more than 13,400 persons on television entertainment between the ages of 5 and 15, a concern heightened by the fact that most often aggressive acts are portrayed on entertainment television as potent and successful tactics for achieving the protagonist's goals (Stein, 1972).

Under the auspices of an intensive inquiry by the United States National Institute of Mental Health, a series of correlational field studies involving thousands of children and adolescents was completed in 1971. The thrust of these findings was clear and uniform: for youngsters of both sexes and a variety of backgrounds, the amount of aggressive material an individual views on television is positively related to the person's acceptance of aggression as a mode of behavior (Chaffee, 1972). A major longitudinal study in the series also provided more direct confirmation that, at least for males, exposure to large doses of televised aggression in middle childhood is causally linked to aggressive behavior in late adolescence (Huesmann, Eron, Lefkowitz and Walder, 1973). Experimental studies further confirm the causal link by showing that exposure to examples of aggressive behavior in entertainment taken directly from broadcast television increases aggressiveness in viewers throughout the entire age span from early childhood to late adolescence (Ellis and Sekyra, 1972; Leifer and Roberts, 1972; Stein and Friedrich, 1972; Steuer, Applefield, and Smith, 1971).

Correlational and experimental evidence further converge on the effects of televised aggression by showing that its impact is not limited to stimulating overt aggressive behavior; greater willingness to approve or tolerate the aggressive acts of others, a lowered sensitivity to real-life aggression, expectations of personal victimization, and decrements in cooperative behavior all have been shown to be indirect manifestations of the original input (Drabman and Thomas, 1974; Gerbner and Gross, 1974; Hapkiewicz and Roden, 1971).

Though less fully researched, exposure to televised sex, race, and role stereotypes seems to lead to direct acceptance of them in a manner generally paralleling the more extensive violence findings. However, socially desired changes in values and behavior can also be cultivated by television entertainment, including the acquisition of useful social skills and the development of cooperation and self-control (Liebert and Poulos, 1975).

BIBLIOGRAPHY

CHAFFEE, S. H. Television and adolescent aggressiveness (overview). In G. A. Comstock and E. A. Rubinstein (Eds.), *Television and social behavior,* vol. 3: *Television and adolescent aggressiveness.* Washington, D.C.: U.S. Government Printing Office, 1972. Pp. 1–34.

DeFLEUR, M. L., and DeFLEUR, L. The relative contribution of television as a learning source for children's occupational knowledge. *American Sociological Review,* 1967, *32,* 777–789.

DRABMAN, R. S., and THOMAS, M. H. Does media violence increase children's toleration of real life aggression? *Developmental Psychology,* 1974, *10,* 418–421.

ELLIS, G. T., and SEKYRA, F. The effect of aggressive cartoons on the behavior of first grade children. *Journal of Psychology,* 1972, *81,* 37–43.

HAPKIEWICZ, W. G., and RODEN, A. H. The effects of aggressive cartoons on children's interpersonal play. *Child Development,* 1971, *42,* 1583–1585.

HUESMANN, L. R.; ERON, L. D.; LEFKOWITZ, M. M.; and WALDER, L. O. Television violence and aggression: The causal effect remains. *American Psychologist,* 1973, *28,* 617–620.

LEIFER, A., and ROBERTS, D. Children's responses to television violence. In J. P. Murray, E. A. Rubinstein, and G. A. Comstock (Eds.), *Television and social behavior,* vol. 2: *Television and social learning.* Washington, D.C.: U.S. Government Printing Office, 1972. Pp. 43–180.

LIEBERT, R. M.; NEALE, J. M.; and DAVIDSON, E. S. *The early window: Effects of television on children and youth.* New York: Pergamon Press, 1973.

LIEBERT, R. M., and POULOS, R. W. Television and personality development: Socializing effects of an entertainment medium. In A. Davids (Ed.), *Child personality and psychopathology: Current topics.* New York: Wiley, 1975.

McLEOD, J. M.; ATKIN, C. K.; and CHAFFEE, S. H. Adolescents, parents, and television use: Adolescent self-report measures from Maryland and Wisconsin samples. In G. A. Comstock and E. A. Rubinstein (Eds.), *Television and social behavior,* vol. 3: *Television and adolescent aggressiveness.* Washington, D.C.: U.S. Government Printing Office, 1972. Pp. 173–238.

STEIN, A. H., and FRIEDRICH, L. K. Television content and young children's behavior. In J. P. Murray, E. A. Rubinstein, and G. A. Comstock (Eds.), *Television and social behavior,* vol. 2: *Television and social learning.* Washington, D.C.: U.S. Government Printing Office, 1972. Pp. 202–317.

STEUER, F. B.; APPLEFIELD, J. M.; and SMITH, R. Televised aggression and the interpersonal aggression of preschool children. *Journal of Experimental Child Psychology,* 1971, *11,* 442–447.

ROBERT M. LIEBERT

MASS MEDIA AND VIOLENCE

The coupling of a salient social concern with a pervasive set of theoretical interests can be expected to generate a substantial amount of speculation and research—and even policy recommendations. It is accordingly not surprising that few topics have received the degree of attention that has been accorded the portrayal of violence in the mass media. The issue derives from the public's heavy reliance on the media, especially television, for entertainment and information, and the relatively rich diet of mayhem and hostility embedded in standard TV fare. Children are of special concern, both because they use TV to an inordinately high degree and because they are presumed to be particularly vulnerable to realistic interpretations of fantasy materials. Public concern with the issue is amply attested to by the variety of governmental committees and commissions that have considered the issue over the past two decades or so, often lamenting the lack of definitive evidence on which to base possible policy decisions. Under the prodding of the United States Senate Subcommittee on Communications, this led to a more concerted research effort—a well-funded program encompassing over 20 new studies, along with a report of a specially-appointed scientific advisory committee.

Cathartic Model

This effort was preceded by a considerable volume of social science research dealing with various aspects of the issue—probably more than on most social issues in the recent past. After the dismissal of earlier claims of adverse effects due to inadequate data, the results of several survey studies in the early 1960s generally contended that televised violence had neither harmful nor beneficial effects except possibly on a small minority of particularly susceptible children. Additional research, mostly experimental in nature, led to more partisan positions. The possibility of favorable consequences of mediated violence stemmed from a catharsis theory of media exposure, particularly to fantasy material, as advanced by Feshbach. It was argued with some supportive evidence that pent-up hostility in the viewer could be reduced or eliminated through vicarious participation in violent actions presented on television drama and the like.

Most of the subsequent research, however, has tended to reject such a cathartic model, suggesting the opposite interpretation of an increased predisposition toward aggressiveness following exposure to violence. Such an instigational effect is most apparent in the work of Bandura and others on social learning and the imitation of observed behavior. This approach suggests that children (and adults, to a lesser degree) repeatedly exposed to a steady diet of apparently instrumental and rewarding aggression will tend to adopt such behavior patterns and adapt them to their own environmental circumstances.

Berkowitz

Another major impetus came from the numerous studies by Berkowitz and his followers demonstrating a tendency toward more aggressive responses after exposure to a violent film (e.g., a boxing sequence) as compared to a more neutral (e.g., a track race) one. Berkowitz accordingly argues for a generalized cue model of aggression in which incidences of depicted violent behavior, by serving as cues, raise the probability of an aggressive response in the individual's hierarchy of possible responses. While the greater the similarity between the depicted behavior and the individual's particular environment, the greater the likelihood of the observed behavior being emulated, both theoretical positions allow for rather liberal generalizations from the observed behavior to that which the viewer enacts.

The Advisory Committee

Such research findings constitute a reasonable basis for genuine concern about antisocial consequences of media violence, and have spurred demands that at least the gratuitous violence so prevalent in standard TV program offerings be substantially reduced. The results of many of the studies sponsored by the Surgeon General's Advisory Committee lent further emphasis to such a recommendation. Although convincing proof was still lacking, there was an extensive array of different studies by different investigators, working in different research settings, and using different research methodologies and measurement techniques—all pointing toward heightened antisocial tendencies related to selective viewing of violent TV and film materials. Especially when it is difficult to reproduce findings in a

replication of the same experiment, such cumulative evidence was rather impressive, to the advisory committee as well as others. Despite a somewhat ambiguous formal report, individual committee members publicly testified, under questioning by Senator Pastore at a hearing of his subcommittee following the issuance of the report in 1972, that the time had arrived for some definitive action.

An obvious focus for remedial activity was to reduce the incidence and intensity of violent episodes. But this would involve tampering with content, something the TV networks tend to avoid for fear of reducing program appeal and popularity, and government bodies are reluctant to do lest they violate the free speech and free press provision of the first amendment. Thus, while still more research added to the mounting evidence (still circumstantial, as was apt to be the case from the outset), change was slow in coming. Finally, in early 1975, the Federal Commission offered a compromise of sorts, readily endorsed by Senator Pastore and accepted by the networks. So-called family programming was extended until 9 p.m. on the assumption that few children will be watching beyond that hour. This is obviously not designed to reduce the amount of violent content as such, but to relegate most of it (and probably more explicit sexual content as well) beyond the conventional reach of the more vulnerable children's audience.

Current Research

At that, there is some question whether reducing the incidence of violent episodes will lead to any lessening of aggression, individually, let alone socially. A different theoretical position advanced by Tannenbaum and Zillman focuses on the emotional arousal produced by different TV content, including violence, that is largely responsible for any heightening in subsequent antisocial behavior. It is assumed that individuals in a state of arousal, whatever its source, will be more responsive in any behavior situation they find themselves. In this case, they would more readily attribute the excitation to the anger felt against some legitimatized target—for example, another person who angered the individual earlier and toward whom they can now retaliate, as in most experiments to date—

and thus be inclined to respond more aggressively toward that target. Given the nature of the TV industry, especially the need to produce a substantial volume of programming to fill the screen hours on end, it is likely that some other form of formula programming featuring conflict and action would be substituted for any explicit violence deleted. According to the theory at least, to the degree that the substitute material would be arousing, it would be just as instigational.

In this connection, it is important to recognize that few research studies report significant increases in spontaneous aggression in the absence of some sanctioned target. In the typical experiment, there are usually three phases: the first, in which the subject is either angered or not by another person; a second step, during which the subject is exposed to one of several TV or film stimuli, usually some violent versus nonviolent episode, and a third during which the subject can react against his original tormentor, for example, by ostensibly sending mild electric shocks. The critical conditions for producing significant increments in aggressive responses is the presence of both the angering and violent communication content, neither being adequate in itself. Only rarely has there been such an effect in the absence of the angering condition, or even when the angering agent is not the object of the later shocks. Similarly, there is no research evidence of a person deliberately seeking just anybody to beat after an exciting violent program.

No consideration of media violence and its consequences is complete without recognizing that such portrayals tend to occur in fairly consistent program contexts and are accompanied by consistent presentational characteristics. In a sense, each such regular pattern of presentation can be viewed as an instance of an implicit policy, even of censorship, in the sense that some systematic selection is being consistently exercised.

A case in point concerns the issue of justification, as when the violence is commonly presented as a means toward a socially legitimate end, often as the administration of justice itself. In a number of investigations in which the degree of justification has been systematically varied—for example, in terms of a simple good-guy versus bad-guy dichotomy, or as vengeance or self-defense—more, rather than less, subsequent aggressive behavior was found where the justification was more explicit.

A related issue concerns the "sanitization" of violence. Often, as a result of the industry production code, it is portrayed without its more brutal negative consequences—the blood and gore, mutilated bodies, faces of dead people, and so forth. While one expectation is that the presence of such explicit visual content would evoke more aggression, the results of several studies suggest an opposite effect.

In a similar vein, it has been found that under certain conditions partial censorship in the form of deletion of explicit violent (or sexual) scenes can actually be more stimulating, both in the sense of being more physiologically arousing and in the subsequent aggressive behavior. The critical conditions appear to concern the cues provided in the antecedent and/or subsequent content as to the nature of the missing material. Under such circumstances, the individual has to do the filling in for himself, engaging his own imagination and fantasy. What he fills in may be more vivid than what was omitted. More to the point, theoretically, the viewer can become a more actively involved participant rather than a relatively passive receiver.

Current TV industry practice tends to encourage the increased instigation of aggressive dispositions. This is not to imply that such practices are deliberate; quite the opposite is probably true. But some selection has to be made, and the tendency in any organization is for such patterns of selective treatment to become regularized over time. An important policy issue is thus who makes the selection and by what criteria, and to what degree those criteria can be informed by appropriate social psychological research.

BIBLIOGRAPHY

BANDURA, A. *Aggression: A social learning analysis.* Englewood Cliffs, N.J.: Prentice-Hall, 1973.

BERKOWITZ, L. The frustration-aggression hypothesis revised. In L. Berkowitz (Ed.), *Roots of aggression: A reexamination of the frustration-aggression hypothesis.* New York: Atherton Press, 1969.

CATER, D., and STRICKLAND, S. *TV violence and the child: The evolution and fate of the surgeon general's report.* New York: Russell Sage Foundation, 1975.

FESHBACH, S., and SINGER, R. *Television and aggression.* San Francisco: Jossey-Bass, 1971.

HOWITT, D., and CUMBERBATCH, G. *Mass media violence and society.* London: Paul Elek, 1975.

TANNENBAUM, P. H., and ZILLMAN, D. Emotional arousal in the facilitation of aggression through communication. In L. Berkowitz (Ed.), *Advances in experimental social psychology* (Vol. 9). New York: Academic Press, 1975.

Television and growing up: The impact of televised violence. Report to the Surgeon General of the United States Public Health Service from the Surgeon General's Scientific Advisory Committee on Television and Social Behavior. Washington: Government Printing Office, 1971.

PERCY H. TANNENBAUM

MASTERY MOTIVE

Mastery motive is a generic term used to cover a variety of different possible motives, postulated by different theorists, concerning the attempts of organisms, particularly man, to exercise control over their environments. The first explicit statement of this specific motive was made in 1942 by the psychoanalyst Ives Hendrick. He posited the existence in man of an "instinct to master," through the operation of which infants obtain pleasure from such behaviors as learning to suck, to manipulate, to walk, and to speak. Adults, too, receive pleasure from successful task performances. Although this formulation was rejected by many orthodox Freudians, a more positive reception was given to the conception of Heinz Hartmann and others that the ego has an autonomous sphere of development, that is, that certain adaptive skills have an inherent basis.

Abraham Kardiner, in a somewhat different sense, emphasized the gratification of children in carrying out successful actions. Bela Mittleman maintained that motility, as manifested in such skilled acts as walking and manipulating objects, constitutes a basic motivation. Somewhat similar is Erik Erikson's position that children express a "sense of industry" in seeking mastery over objects. Also pertinent here is Henry Murray's concept of "modal needs"—the tendency of persons to carry out activities, e.g., the playing of a game, with a degree of excellence. Finally, somewhat similar concepts, such as the idea of "function pleasure," was suggested by Karl Bühler, and "activity drive" was proposed by Gardner Murphy.

It is to be emphasized that the concept of a mastery motive, as represented by the theorists noted above, is different from the more restricted idea that persons are, or may be, motivated to seek power, as exemplified in different ways, e.g., in the writings of Machiavelli, Hobbes, Nietzsche, and others, or to seek superiority, as posited by Adler. There is, nevertheless, some familial relation among the several sets of concepts, since all concern the successful exercise of one's capacities. Closer to the notion of a mastery motive is Robert White's concept of competence motivation, or "effectance"; indeed, White considered the views of Hendrick, Hartmann, Mittleman and Erikson as support for his competence concept. Also very close is R. S. Woodworth's much earlier (1918) behavior-primacy theory of motivation, which posits a basic tendency of higher animals to deal successfully with their environments. It is interesting to note that Woodworth originally put forth this conception in 1918.

In evaluation of the concept of a mastery motive, along with other, similar notions, it seems clear that they all point up an important aspect of behavior. At the present time, however, none of these concepts has attained a rigorous stature in a methodological sense.

BIBLIOGRAPHY

HENDRICK, I. Instinct and the ego during infancy. *Psychoanalytical Quarterly,* 1942, *11,* 33–50.

WHITE, R. W. Motivation reconsidered: The concept of competence. *Psychological Review,* 1959, *66,* 297–333.

See also COMPETENCE MOTIVATION

PAUL MCREYNOLDS

MATCHING-TO-SAMPLE

Matching-to-sample and oddity learning are instances of relational learning paradigms in which the correct response is based upon some relationship among the stimuli present in a display rather than upon their absolute properties. In order to demonstrate successful solution of such problems, the subject *(S)* must respond correctly when specific elements of the display are replaced or their reward value reversed. In a typical matching-to-sample experiment, on a given trial a single standard (sample) stimulus is first presented. After one or more responses to the sample, two or more comparison stimuli are presented, one of which, the correct choice, is physically identical to the standard. In simultaneous matching, the sample and comparison stimuli are simultaneously present; in successive matching the comparison stimuli may be introduced as the sample is terminated (zero delay) or after some interval (delayed matching).

Like oddity learning, matching-to-sample may be performed as a group of specific conditional discrimination problems (e.g., if sample is green, respond to green comparison stimulus), or on the basis of a more general rule. To demonstrate the acquisition of a rule, it is necessary to use a transfer test with different stimuli from those used in original acquisition. Typically the training stimuli are taken from a single stimulus dimension (e.g., color). Successful transfer to the matching of stimuli according to their form would signify broader application of the matching rule than if transfer were shown to other colors.

Because matching-to-sample performance presumably reflects "higher mental processes," it has been widely used as a comparative-developmental tool. It has been determined, for example, that monkeys perform better than pigeons but not as well as young children. Within the human species, the ability to solve matching-to-sample problems seems to develop gradually with most children successful by the age of six years. Whereas children who perform well in a matching-to-sample task typically show substantial transfer, animals do not, suggesting rule learning in the former case but not in the latter.

In animal research, the matching-to-sample problem has sometimes been used to distinguish between differing functions of stimuli. The comparison stimuli are simple discriminative stimuli, signalling the availability of reward, whereas the sample stimuli are instructional stimuli which give the comparison stimuli their significance. These differing functions of stimuli may be differentiated on the basis of the way they are influenced by drugs, reinforcement schedules and other experimental manipulations.

In the more recent literature, delayed matching-to-sample has proved to be a fruitful paradigm in the investigation of short-term memory in animals. Performance is based upon

recognition memory, since one of the available comparison stimuli is identical to the standard. A variation of the matching-to-sample procedure called symbolic matching (or conditional matching) provides an analogy to a recall test. With this procedure the match is based upon an arbitrary association between the sample and the comparison stimuli, rather than upon physical identity, thus the correct choice requires recall of the value of the standard.

BIBLIOGRAPHY

CUMMING, W. W., and BERRYMAN, R. The complex discriminated operant: Studies of matching-to-sample and related problems. In D. I. Mostofsky (Ed.), *Stimulus generalization.* Stanford, Calif.: Stanford University Press, 1965.

D'AMATO, M. R. Delayed matching and short-term memory in monkeys. In G. H. Bower, *The psychology of learning and motivation* (Vol. 7). New York: Academic Press, 1973.

HOUSE, B. J.; BROWN, A. L.; and SCOTT, M. S. Children's discrimination learning based on identity or difference. In H. W. Reese (Ed.), *Advances in child development and behavior* (Vol. 9). New York: Academic Press, 1974.

DAVID R. THOMAS

MATERNAL BEHAVIOR

While it is true that mothers in most cultures and in most historical periods have been the primary caretakers of children, until only three generations ago in the Western hemisphere the worlds of family and work were closely integrated so that fathers played more of a role in the rearing of children, especially of sons. This involvement notwithstanding, much more discussion has been centered on mother-infant interactions, perhaps reflecting the still pervasive belief that the role of the father is relatively unimportant as a source of influence on the young child's development. However, until a decade ago even research on mothers' behavior had been rather scarce. Empirical studies on father-infant interactions have been almost nonexistent until even more recently.

As a result of the primacy of interest given the mother's activities, the term *maternal behavior* has been overextended with regard to the person performing it, and has taken on the connotation of any nurturant behavior toward the infant, even if sometimes performed by the father or other caretaker. The usage of the term has also often been constricted with regard to the age of the child receiving nurturance, which is usually confined to two years or younger. For the present purpose, maternal behavior is defined as nurturant, caregiving behavior toward a child by its female caretaker.

While females may have a lower threshold of response to infants than do males in the view of Maccoby and Jacklin (1974), there may also be a critical postnatal period for mother-infant contact during which conditions conducive to high levels of maternal behavior are established. The results of research showing cross-sex effects in attempts by children to dominate adults, and a tendency for adults to yield to these attempts more readily when initiated by their opposite sex children, have led these authors to suggest that the conditions for rearing of children of both sexes is optimized when both parents are actively involved. There are some data to suggest that fathers, if given the opportunity, are capable of showing high levels of nurturant behavior toward their newborn infants. Much of what has been found to be characteristic of maternal behavior is not particular to female caretakers, and in such instances the term *parenting* is more appropriate. Of course, even this term can refer to behavior not necessarily performed by the child's own parents.

Biological Factors

Some aspects of maternal behavior have been related to the hormonal changes of childbirth in biological mothers. Among these is postpartum lability. It has been estimated that about 30% of normal mothers experience such emotional upset. So many other factors are confounded with the hormonal changes that accompany giving birth that it is difficult to establish threads of causality between variables. While the most prevalent opinion is that such postpartum emotional changes are organically determined, Thomas and Gordon (1959) found a number of exogenous factors to be significantly related to it. These included home background of the mother, a history of previous emotional disorder or physical illness, and changes in social or economic status. These researchers gave advice and guidance to one

group of new mothers and found the incidence of emotional upset six months later to be only 2% as compared to 28% in a control group. In addition, the babies of the experimental group mothers were significantly less irritable and had significantly fewer feeding and sleeping problems than the infants of the control mothers at age six months, and again at four to six years.

The effect of breastfeeding on the female caretaker's nurturant behavior has generated more research among subhuman species than among humans. Increased levels of prolactin produced in subhuman mothers during breastfeeding have been shown to influence some maternal behaviors. In studies with humans, it has been found that mothers who breastfeed show an increased need for body contact with their infants above that shown by mothers who bottlefeed. In these studies, however, it has been impossible to show whether the differences are due to hormones produced during lactation or to the more intimate pleasurable associations learned during breastfeeding as opposed to bottlefeeding. The quality of the feeding experience, not the type of feeding, is significantly related to positive psychological effects on the infant. Sherman (1971), who has reviewed the literature on the effects of hormonal changes involved in childbirth and lactation, concluded that these effects are almost certainly not crucial to the display of maternal behavior, but that the kind and extent of their importance is not known.

Initial Responses

Klaus and his co-workers (1970) have described the characteristic pattern of responses which mothers make when they are first presented with their infants. This pattern is especially conducive to infant-mother eye contact, and thus interaction sequences are highly likely. As Richards (1974) has pointed out, however, psychologists know very little about the effects of different methods of caretaking within the normal range. Nevertheless, the infant's behavior is patterned even during the last months of prenatal life, and these patterns are assigned meaning by the caregiver. Likewise, the infant selectively attends to stimulation that is conducive to communication as demonstrated by the infant's tendency to attend to faces. The problem for the understanding of maternal behavior is thus to observe what aspects of the caretaker's behaviors contribute to this communication.

Dunn and Richards (1975) reported results from a longitudinal study of 68 home-delivered mother-child pairs in Cambridge, England. They found evidence to suggest that the frequency of affectionate talking by the mother to her baby during the first 10 days of feeding sessions was the most important variable associated with the infant's rate of sucking. Type of feeding (breast versus bottle) controlled a negligible amount of the variance in rate of sucking. They concluded that "warm" maternal behavior could not be defined by a unitary measure, and that differences in maternal styles during the first ten days are affected by labor and delivery factors which affect the arousal level of the baby, and in turn, affect the behavior of the mother toward her child. While no significant relationship has been found between the tendency of the mother to respond to crying by the infant and her tendency to exhibit affectionate mothering during the first ten days, a positive relationship between these variables is found by the time the infants are three weeks old. The work at Cambridge suggests that during the first ten days, the probability that a mother will pick up her baby to feed it is not primarily dependent on crying, but on the time of the last feeding. The context in which the cry is heard is thus more important than what the infant is doing.

Ainsworth and her co-workers (1974) have emphasized the mother's contribution to the quality of the mother-infant relationship in the first year of life. They have found four characteristics of maternal behavior which are significantly related to the quality of these interactions: sensitivity, acceptance, cooperation, and accessibility. Mothers rated high on sensitivity (perceiving and responding promptly and appropriately to infants' signals) also rated high on the other three variables. With regard to crying, Ainsworth and her co-workers found that the more quickly the mother responds to her child's crying during one quarter of the first year, the less crying the infant shows during the subsequent quarter of observation. Speaking more generally, she concluded that maternal responsiveness fosters infant development in the direction of being less demanding and

impatient. Maternal sensitivity was also positively related to infant's compliance to commands in the first year and to the frequency of exhibiting behaviors indicative of internalized control during the fourth quarter of the first year. Ainsworth concludes that infant socialization results from reciprocal mother-infant responsiveness, which is clearly facilitated by the mother's sensitivity and responsiveness to her infant. In her view, differences in infant behavior are more influenced by maternal responsiveness than maternal behavior is influenced by infant characteristics. Infants of mothers who respond reciprocally then become increasingly able to respond to the communication aspects of the mother's behavior.

Infant's Effect on Parent

A number of authors have pointed out that research on parenting has emphasized the effects of parent behaviors on the infant and has neglected the effects of infant behavior on the parent. Moss's (1967) study clearly shows the effects of babies on their mothers. In this study it was shown that the boy babies were more irritable and received more response from their mothers than did the girls during the third week, but that by the twelfth week the mothers of the boys had tired of trying to pacify them and were spending less time responding to them than were the mothers of girls.

Sander and his co-workers (1970) reported a study in which two nurses cared for one or the other of two babies. While one nurse's baby showed much less crying than the other, she responded less quickly and less frequently to the cry of her baby than did the other nurse to her baby. The one factor which distinguished the care of the nurse whose baby cried less was that her caretaking responses to crying were longer in duration. Thus, as Bernal (1974) has suggested, differences in crying between infants seem to be related more to what goes on during the caretaking than to how quickly the caretaker comes when the infant signals. The quality of the parent-child interaction is obviously affected by feedback emanating from both sources. In the case of the nurse whose baby cried more, it also slept much longer than the other baby, thus illustrating a further point concerning the importance of observing a variety of maternal and child behaviors rather than isolating only one or two of each.

The importance of physical contact between child and caregiver, over such other factors as reduction in hunger, has formed the basis of Bowlby's (1958) theory of attachment. The results of Harlow's research with rhesus monkeys, in which dramatic decrements in later social behavior were shown as a result of having been reared in isolation with a wire mother surrogate as opposed to a cloth mother surrogate, have been used to illustrate the importance of intimate physical contact. Nevertheless, nurturant parenting behaviors which facilitate reduction in infant pain and distress have also been shown to play an important role in the development of caretaker-infant attachment. Rheingold and co-workers' (1959) controlled study of institutionalized infants dramatically illustrates the effect of amount of nurturance shown by a caretaker on the infant's social responsiveness to the caretaker and to a stranger. However, while Schaffer (1971) views mother-infant relations in the first year as of great importance to later social relationships, Kohlberg (1969) deemphasizes its importance to later social behavior.

Social Class

Kagen and co-workers (1962) have studied social class differences in maternal behavior toward 10-month-old girls. While no differences were found between middle class and working class mothers with regard to the frequency of nonverbal behaviors directed toward their infants, every category of verbal behavior was more frequent among the former group. Since there was no difference in the infant's tendency to spontaneously vocalize, the differences are not attributable to infant differences to which the mothers could have responded. In addition, middle class mothers gave their infants things to play with more often than the working class mothers. However, the latter group of children interacted with adults other than the mother to a greater extent than the middle class children did, so the working class children could not be said to be deprived of verbal interactions. Obviously, focusing on maternal behavior to the exclusion of interactions with other individuals is inadequate for giving a view of the interactions in which the child is a participant.

A number of studies have shown that the affective elements of mother-child interactions are not much different between social classes, and that the working class mothers actually provide more physical stimulation than middle class mothers. Thus the extensiveness of the care given by mothers, and certainly the mothers and others taken together, does not differ by social class.

Adequacy of maternal care must always confront the question of adequacy with regard to what? Studies using a number of measures of infant exploratory behavior and social responsiveness have demonstrated, as Schaffer (1971) has pointed out, that an essential aspect of parenting may be the stimulation the parent provides. Whether defined as "attentiveness," "sensitivity," or "patterned reciprocity," a number of researchers have emphasized its importance. Unfortunately, the upper and lower boundaries of these terms, beyond which such stimulation is less than optimal, are not well understood. Furthermore, it is acknowledged by many that while the mother's role involves modulating the amount of stimulation her infant receives, an even more important skill may be her ability to vary or pattern her interactive stimulation to the needs of her individual infant in all of his many states of arousal, thus providing familiarity of stimulation source but variation in its level and type. Both the familiarity and variability thus provided may be reinforcing to the infant.

The work of Richards and Dunn suggests that timing of stimulation in relation to the infant's responses by the caregiver also contributes to the reciprocality of the interaction and thus to the acquisition by the infant of an awareness that his actions successfully affect his environment. In this sense, the infant is socializing the caregiver and is an active participant in his own socialization. This sense of power to effect change in one's environment has recently been emphasized by investigators of development at every level from infancy through aging. It is becoming increasingly apparent that such a sense of control is beneficial to humans at every developmental stage, and that fostering it is a goal which might appropriately concern mental health practitioners. Yet the numerous reports generated by the classic studies (e.g., Jones and Bayley, 1941; Kagen and Moss, 1962; and Sears, Maccoby, and Levin,

1957) of the effects of maternal behavior on child development have deemphasized mental growth as defined by increasing control over one's environment in favor of adaptation to one's existing niche. Perhaps this is because an infant's or child's bids for control often conflict with those of the parents, who believe they have the right and duty to maintain power over their children.

Various groups have emerged that have taken on the task of defining and supporting legislation to protect the rights of children. Inevitably, some of these rights come into direct conflict with those of the persons who have control over them. Resolving these conflicts is one of the tasks of extrafamilial institutions. These political institutions are the same ones which determine what the mother will require of her children in her role as socializer, and they stand ready to deprive her of her authority over her child if she deviates from her expected role sometimes in ways which have nothing to do with what is in the best interest of the child, but rather what is in the best interests of the segment of society that is in a position to impose its views on the rest. The question needs to be raised as to whether the definition of socialization prevalent in one segment of a particular society is the only one possible or allowable to the members of that society as a whole. Maternal behavior can only be successful in assisting the growing child acquire a sense of control over his environment if the child (and the mother) are allowed to share increasingly in the making of that world.

BIBLIOGRAPHY

AINSWORTH, M. D. S.; BELL, S. M.; and STAYTON, D. J. Infant-mother attachment and social development: 'Socialisation' as a product of reciprocal responsiveness to signals. In M. P. M. Richards (Ed.), *The integration of a child into a social world.* New York: Cambridge University Press, 1974.

BERNAL, J. Attachment: Some problems and possibilities. In M. P. M. Richards (Ed.), *The integration of a child into a social world.* New York: Cambridge University Press, 1974.

JONES, H. E., and BAYLEY, N. The Berkeley growth study. *Child Development,* 1941, *12,* 167–173.

KAGEN, J., and MOSS, H. *Birth to maturity.* New York: Wiley, 1962.

KLAUS, M. H.; KENNEL, J. H.; PLUMB, N.; and ZUEHLKE, S. Human maternal behavior at the first contact with her young. *Pediatrics,* 1970, *46,* 187–192.

KOHLBERG, L. Stage and sequence: The cognitive-developmental approach to socialization. In D. A. Goslin (Ed.), *Handbook of socialization: Theory and research.* Chicago: Rand-McNally, 1969.

MACCOBY, E. E., and JACKLIN, C. N. *The psychology of sex differences.* Stanford: Stanford University Press, 1974.

RHEINGOLD, H. L.; GEWIRTZ, J. L.; and ROSS, H. W. Social conditioning of vocalizations in infants. *Journal of Comparative and Physiological Psychology,* 1959, *52,* 68–73.

RICHARDS, M. P. M. First steps in becoming social. In M. P. M. Richards (Ed.), *The integration of a child into a social world.* New York: Cambridge University Press, 1974.

SANDER, L. W.; STECHLER, G.; BURNS, P.; and JULIA, H. Early mother-infant interaction and 24-hour patterns of activity and sleep. *Journal of the American Academy of Child Psychiatry,* 1970, *9,* 103–123.

SCHAFFER, H. R. *The growth of sociability.* Baltimore: Penguin, 1971.

SEARS, R. R.; MACCOBY, E. E.; and LEVIN, H. *Patterns of child rearing.* New York: Harper & Row, 1957.

SHERMAN, J. *On the psychology of women.* Springfield, Ill.: Thomas, 1971.

THOMAS, C. L., and GORDON, J. E. Psychosis after childbirth: Ecological aspects of a single impact stress. *American Journal of Medical Science,* 1959, *238,* 363–388.

See also FATHERS AND CHILDREN; EARLY EXPERIENCE: MATERNAL DEPRIVATION

MICHELE ANDRISIN WITTIG

MATERNAL EMPLOYMENT: EFFECTS

Over half of the mothers in the United States with children of school age but none younger are gainfully employed. While the percentage of employed women with preschool children is less, even for this group an estimated 47% work for pay at least part of the year. Furthermore, the percentage of mothers employed continues to increase and the rate of increase is higher for those with preschoolers.

As maternal employment becomes a more common pattern than fulltime housewife, the effects of employment may also be expected to change. As a deviant pattern, maternal employment was often greeted with censure by others and guilt on the part of the mother. Working mothers, particularly in the middle class, tried to compensate for their employment—for example, by setting aside special times for interaction with the child. In some cases the mother's concern about the possible adverse effects of her employment on the child led to constructive action on her part that may have helped avoid such effects. In other cases, the mothers appear to have overcompensated out of guilt with less beneficial results. Both compensatory patterns, as well as other aspects of the previous maternal employment situation, may change. Thus it is difficult to generalize the research findings already obtained to the future situation.

Most of the research to date, however, is reassuring to the working mother. There is little evidence that the children of working mothers are either emotionally neglected or unsupervised. Although there is some evidence that the mother who is dissatisfied with her role—whether working or not—is apt to be a less adequate mother, there is very little support for the notion that maternal employment itself has a negative effect. The research suggests, in fact, that employment may have a positive effect on girls.

Working mothers, their husbands, and their children tend to have less traditional sex-role concepts and are more likely to approve of maternal employment. The husbands are more likely than husbands of nonworking women to help with household chores and child-care activities. In general, the research indicates that maternal employment has a more clear-cut effect on the female role in the family than on the male role and a greater effect on daughters than sons. The daughters of working mothers, in comparison to the daughters of full-time housewives, are more likely to name their mother as the person they most admire, to think of women in general as competent, and to have higher academic and professional aspirations for themselves. There is some evidence that the daughters of working mothers are also more independent and that they perform better academically than daughters of nonworking women.

The data for sons, however, are more ambiguous. Research suggests that, in the lower class, the sons of working mothers are less likely than the sons of nonworking mothers to choose their father as the person they most admire. On the other hand, they also show higher school performance than the sons of nonworking mothers. In the middle class, neither of these relationships are found, and there is some evidence that the sons of middle class working mothers do not do so well academically as the sons of the nonworking mothers.

The effects of maternal employment are usually not direct but mediated by other factors. Thus, in addition to the sex of the child, other important aspects of the situation are the mother's attitude about employment, the nature of her child-care arrangements, the amount of strain involved in handling the dual roles of worker and mother, whether employment is full-time or part-time, and a host of other conditions. Positive effects of employment are enhanced when the employment is accompanied by a minimum of conflict and strain for the mother. Part-time employment, perhaps because it involves role satisfaction with minimum strain, often compares favorably to both nonemployment and full-time employment.

A very important factor is the age of the child. Most of the existing data were obtained from studies of school-age children and almost no research has been carried out on the effects of maternal employment on the infant and preschool child. Recent child development research has indicated the importance of the early mother-child interaction. No data are available, however, on whether maternal employment affects the amount of stimulation and person-to-person interaction available to the infant, whether the mother's absence interferes with her serving as the stable adult figure needed by the infant, or whether the attachment of the infant to the mother or the mother to the infant is jeopardized.

BIBLIOGRAPHY

HOFFMAN, L. W. and NYE, F. I. *Working mothers*. San Francisco: Jossey-Bass, 1974.

LOIS WLADIS HOFFMAN

MATESHIP SYSTEMS

The sexual relationships within individual species have been studied for their intrinsic interest and because these relationships are a fundamental aspect of the entire social organization of any species. Although there is not good agreement in the way these relationships are defined, there are three basic types of relationships: (1) *monogamy* in which one male and one female restrict their copulatory behavior to one another. (2) *Polygamy* in which one individual mates with two or more members of the opposite sex. Two forms of polygamy are found: *polygyny,* the more common form, in which one male copulates with two or more females, and *polyandry,* the much rarer form, in which a single female copulates with two or more males. Implicit in all polygamous relationships is the notion that copulation is restricted to the members of the polygamous group. (3) In *promiscuous* mateship systems the sexes come together, copulate, and separate again. It is implied that one or both of these individuals will copulate with additional individuals.

There are several problems in attempting to apply these terms to a variety of animals. Monogamous relationships vary in duration from less than an hour to a life-time. Polygamous relationships may vary from less than an hour to the duration of the breeding season, and therefore in some tropical species may extend year-round.

Pair Bond

Many authors include the duration of the pair bond as part of their criteria for classification and clearly the pair bond is an important aspect of the relationship between the male and the female. However, pair bonding is a little understood phenomenon. Clearly more is involved in a pair bond than simply restricting copulation to the mate. A great many social interactions occur only between the mates and other social interactions, such as aggression, may be inhibited between them. The bond may be very longlasting and copulation restricted to only a short period. Selander (1972) has classified mating systems on the basis of pair bond duration. He reserves the terms defined above (except for promiscuity) for mating relationships which include pair bonds of at least a few days duration, and proposes new terms (*monobrachygamy, polybrachygamy, polybrachygyny,* and *polybrachyandry*) for relationships in which the pair bond is missing or lasts less than an hour. In his scheme the polygamous systems with short pair bonds are synonymous with promiscuity.

The relative participation of the two sexes in rearing the young is also considered in some definitions. It is true that mating systems and parental behavior are often related especially in those cases where the sexes remain together for long periods of time. For example, a polygynous male or polyandrous female has less time available to devote to each group of young than does a monogamous parent. In polygamous systems an individual with many mates, regardless of its sex, participates minimally or not at all in parental behavior. Such considerations are of significance in understanding the reproductive behavior and social organization of the species but are not helpful in understanding the mating system itself. Parental care is an important factor in the evolution of mating systems (Orians 1969; Jenni, 1974), and it is generally assumed that in birds at least the primitive system was monogamy with shared parental responsibility. To the extent that deviation from monogamy reduces the parental contribution of one of the parents, changes in parental behavior must coevolve with or evolve before changes in the mating system.

Part of the confusion arises from the use of the term *pair bond.* Although the notion of pair bond is very widely used it is practically never defined. Pair bonding remains at best a poorly known phenomenon. Another problem is the use of euphemisms such as mating, breeding, and pairing when the authors really mean copulation or insemination.

Intraspecific Systems

Researchers in this field have generally considered the mateship system a characteristic of the entire species rather than as a characteristic of the individual members of the species. Wiley (1973) has extended this notion and classified mating systems on the basis of the ratios between the sexes actually contributing genes to the next generation. Thus he takes an extreme population viewpoint. Wiley classified as polyandrous, for example, any species in which more males than females contribute genetic material to the next generation regardless of pair bond duration. Any mating system can also be characterized by durable pair bonds or promiscuity. Although he placed emphasis on differential genic contribution to the next generation, Wiley's classification scheme is essentially identical to that of Selander who placed primary emphasis on duration of the pair bond.

Except for man, polyandrous relationships

are not found in mammals. Most mammalian mating relationships are relatively brief, and polygyny or promiscuity are common. Eisenberg (1966) classified mammalian mating systems as *brief pairing,* typical of solitary species; *consortship,* temporary pairing within a social group; *harem* formation, male defense of a group of females; and *pair bonding* in which the male and the female remain together after copulation. In addition some mammals, such as the chimpanzee *(Pan troglodytes)* (Lawick-Goodall, 1968) are promiscuous. Each female in estrus, copulates with several or all of the sexually mature males in the group. There is little or no aggression or interference among the males as different ones copulate with the receptive females.

When classifying mating systems it is important to distinguish between simultaneous and sequential relationships. Sequentially polygamous relationships are, for example, little different from sequentially monogamous ones, especially if the relationship covers the entire period of potential fertilization. In sage grouse *(Centrocercus urophasianus)* each female copulates only once unless she renests. A very few of the males perform essentially all the copulations and most of the males do not copulate. This is clearly a polygynous mateship system. The fact that this system is the one usually described by ornithologists as a classic example of promiscuity is based on the emphasis placed on the pair bond which in the case of sage grouse does not form, at least reciprocally. In this system we find copulation without pair bonding.

Although each species is considered to have one or another kind of mateship system, it is self-evident that the sexual relations which are the basis of the mateship systems are relationships between individual members of the species. Within polygamous and promiscuous species there is often great variation in the number of individuals copulating with one another. Even in species which form pair bonds there may be great variation in number of mates. For example in the best known polyandrous system (Jenni and Collier 1972; Jenni 1974), 21% of the females are monogamous 46% have two mates, 25% have three mates, and 7% have four mates. In monogamous species there appears to be little deviation from monogamy although individuals may occa-

sionally form sequentially polygynous or polyandrous relationships (Jenni, 1974). The animals appear to be more flexible in their sexual relations than the classification system biologists use. It is clear that all individuals within a species do not necessarily behave exactly alike.

BIBLIOGRAPHY

Eisenberg, J. F. The social organizations of mammals. *Handbuch der Zoologie,* 1966, *8*(39), 1–92.
Jenni, D. A. Evolution of polyandry in birds. *American Zoologist,* 1974, *14,* 129–144.
Jenni, D. A., and Collier, G. Polyandry in the American jacana. *Auk,* 1972, *89,* 743–765.
Lawick-Goodall, J. van. The behaviour of free-living chimpanzees in the Gambe Stream Reserve. *Animal Behaviour Monographs,* 1968, *1,* 161–311.
Orians, G. H. On the evolution of mating systems in birds and mammals. *American Naturalist,* 1969, *103,* 589–603.
Selander, R. K. Sexual selection and dimorphism in birds. In B. Campbell (Ed.), *Sexual selection and the descent of man 1871–1971.* Chicago: Aldine, 1972. Pp. 180–230.
Wiley, R. H. Territoriality and non-random mating in sage grouse, *Centrocercus urophasianus. Animal Behaviour Monographs,* 1973, *6,* 85–169.

Donald A. Jenni

MATHEMATICAL BASIS OF STATISTICS

The existence of errors of measurement and inherent differences over the objects of study creates obvious difficulties in inductive inference. It is clear that the course of knowledge acquisition and theory development is rocky indeed when one can be sure that a given set of observations will vary considerably when made on another group of similar objects or subjects, or even on reevaluation of the same objects or subjects. That is indeed the case in such disciplines of human behavior as psychology and psychiatry.

To take a simple illustration of the problem, consider the early work of psychologists in the area of juvenile delinquency. Armed with their newly developed measuring instruments, intelligence tests, these psychologists determined the intelligence quotients of juvenile delinquents who were apprehended and, in many cases, placed in detention facilities. They found that these IQs were, in general, considerably below average. This led to the inference that juvenile offenders were of defective intelligence, and, even further, that because of the defective intelligence the delinquents could not command the finer moral and legal distinctions.

We now know that the particular observations of these early psychologists stemmed from a lack of motivation of the delinquents to perform well on the tests (error of measurement) and the high selection in terms of those delinquents apprehended and subjected to court action (subject differences). Lack of motivation leads to lower observed IQ and the duller offenders are those less likely to beat the justice system.

Statistics is that branch of mathematics widely used in the empirical sciences to reach plausible inferences when the data are subject to the above types of distortions. The core of statistics is the theory of probability which is the formal counterpart of the intuitive notion of likelihood. It is not that probability and statistics prevent inferential errors like that of the early psychologists on juvenile delinquency and defective intelligence, but they do provide one important tool in the battle.

Probability

Modern probability theory is based upon the concepts sample space, event, and probability function. The space is the abstract representation of all possible outcomes to a given set of manipulations in the empirical world; elements in the space correspond to possible real world outcomes. An event represents all outcomes that are similar in some designated way; it consists of all elements in the space corresponding to those similar outcomes. And a probability function is a rule that assigns numbers equal or greater than zero to all events under the restrictions: (1) the probability assigned to the event representing all possible outcomes (that is, the entire space) is equal to one, and (2) if two events have no elements or outcomes in common, the probability of either event is equal to the sum of the separate probabilities.

The foregoing summarizes the axioms originally formulated in 1933 by Kolmogorov (translated into English, 1950). He introduced an axiomatic foundation for probability theory as a special case of more general notions of mathematics. The more general notions of particular relevance were measure of a set (analogous to probability of an event) and integral of a function (analogous to expected value of a random variable).

The theory of probability (and, in subsequent development, of statistics) could then be developed from a basic set of axioms in exactly the same way as such clearly mathematical disciplines as geometry and algebra. That is, the basic elements of interest were defined, their interrelationships specified in axioms, and the axioms used to deduce consequences (theorems) that were independent of concrete meanings assigned to the elements. Like every axiomatic theory, moreover, an unlimited number of concrete meanings could be assigned to the elements, and, as a consequence, the theorems can be interpreted in the resulting concrete terms. Thus, the same abstract expressions of probability and statistics have applications in such diverse fields as psychology, psychiatry, engineering, sociology, physics and chemistry.

As a first step in expanding the basic axiom set, we define the conditional probability of an event, *A*, given that another event, *B*, has occurred as the probability of both events occurring simultaneously over the probability of *B* alone. The concept of independence of events flows directly from the definition of conditional probability. Two events are independent if the conditional probability of one event, say *A*, given the occurrence of another event, say *B*, is equal to its probability before *B* occurred. That is to say, *A* and *B* are independent if the probability of *A* remains the same whether or not *B* has occurred.

Using the basic axioms plus the definition of conditional probability, it is easy to deduce a theorem that expresses the conditional probability of *B* given *A* when the conditional probability of *A* given *B* is known. This is the well-known Bayes' theorem; if the events represented by *B* are called "hypotheses" and *A* is a type of empirical outcome, Bayes' theorem may be interpreted as a formula for the probability that hypothesis *B* "caused" the outcome. The assignment of certain concrete meanings to Bayes's theorem produces Bayesian statistical theory. More will be said about that development later.

Distributions

The concept of distributions provides the critical bridge between probability theory and more general statistical theory. A distribution specifies a range of possible numerical outcomes and associated probabilities of occurrence; this specification is accomplished by the assignment of numerical values to outcomes in the probability space and thereby producing what is called a random variable. The assignment is usually by equation but may be by a simple listing, a graph, or a table.

A simple example is the Bernoulli distribution. The relevant sample space contains two elements for the outcomes *success* and *failure*. This space might represent the experimental trial tossing a coin once, where a head is considered a success and a tail a failure. The probability of a success (or a head) is given by $P[s]$ and a failure (or a tail) is given by $P[f]$. A distribution is specified when it is stated that a success takes on the value 1 and a failure the value 0, and that $P[s]$ is equal to a particular value like ½ and $P[f]$ is equal to a particular value like ½. The 1 and 0 are values of the random variable. The specified distribution could of course be put in the form of a table.

If a Bernoulli trial is repeated more than once (that is, for example, a coin is tossed two or more times) and the values of interest are the numbers of successes (or heads) in set of trials (tosses), the resulting distribution is of the binomial type. It specifies the probabilities for the various values of the random variable number of successes in n trials, where n is an integer larger than 1.

If instead of using number of successes in n trials as the values of the random variable, we use average successes (that is, number of successes divided by n), an interesting distribution results as n becomes infinitely large. It is called the normal distribution. Its widespread interest results from the fact that the likelihoods of occurrence of many natural phenomena are well-approximated by its specified probabilities.

Other important distributions may be derived on the basis of the normal distribution. If $a, b, c, d,$ and so forth up to a total of m letters are each normally distributed (and independent of each other), then $y = a^2 + b^2 + c^2 + d^2 + \ldots$ has what is referred to as chi-square (χ^2)

distribution with m degrees of freedom (it is actually a special case of the gamma distribution).

If x is distributed as χ^2 with l degrees of freedom, and y is distributed as χ^2 with m degrees of freedom, and x and y are independent, then the ratio $F = mx/ly$ follows an F-distribution. This is perhaps the critical distribution for experimental work in psychology and psychiatry since it is the basis of the analysis of variance.

Finally, if z is normally distributed, and if y has a χ^2 distribution with m degrees of freedom, and z and y are independent, then the ratio $t = z/\sqrt{y/m}$ has Student's t-distribution. It is not difficult to note that t^2 has an F-distribution, since t^2 is the ratio of two independent χ^2 variables (with one degree of freedom in the numerator and m degrees in the denominator).

Population and Sample

In constructing specific theories, no matter how rudimentary, one specifies generalized groups to which certain theoretical statements apply. A given group may consist of schizophrenics, or American children, or mentally retarded children, or people above the age of 70. Each such group is called a population. A central problem in advancing knowledge consists in drawing inferences about an entire population when only a selected few of its elements are available for observation. The available elements compose what is called a sample.

If the sample is selected in a random fashion, the methods of statistics, using distribution theory, permit one to infer characteristics of the population. To illustrate, suppose the variable of interest is the number of hostile adjectives used by paranoid schizophrenics in a fixed period of open-ended discussion. A random sample of the population of paranoid schizophrenics is drawn and their hostile word counts are determined. Assuming that an infinite repetition of the sampling process is conceivable, one uses the distribution of possible sampling values as a basis for determining the likelihoods that a given sample value came from populations with various alternative possible characteristics.

Although that may seem reasonable enough, one might immediately question how it is possible to know the distribution of sampling values. It turns out that God is on the side of the statistician in many instances. For example, if the variable of interest is normally distributed in the population, which is indeed the case for many of the populations in nature, then the average of each sample in a series of infinitely repeated samples will be normally distributed. And that is independent of sample size. But even if the population distribution is not normal, the central limit theorem tells us that the average of a random sample is approximately normal with a large enough sample size. Note that the normal approximation to the binomial distribution, as discussed previously, is an example of this limiting process.

Classical Statistical Inference

The central issue in statistical inference is the effort to determine characteristics of a population by observing only a random sample from that population. The process in classical theory is divided into three categories: point estimation, confidence intervals, and hypothesis testing—in accord with the type of conclusion the investigator aims at. Important landmarks in the development of the theory may be found in Fisher (1922) on point estimation, in Neyman (1937) on confidence intervals, and in Neyman and Pearson (1928) on testing statistical hypotheses.

In the case of point estimation the aim is to infer a central determining characteristic of the population distribution; this type of central characteristic is called a parameter. In the case of the Bernoulli distribution, for example, there is one parameter—the probability of success (the probability of failure is simply one minus that probability).

Statistical theory specifies both desirable properties of an estimation process and algebraic methods for achieving optimum results. Thus, the method called maximum likelihood estimation produces a point estimate that, when used as a parameter, leads to the highest probability for the obtained sample results.

Clearly, a point estimate differs from the parameter value in all but the rarest of cases, and we have no way of knowing the extent of that discrepancy. The method of confidence intervals provides an estimate of the extent of that error by providing a range of values within which the parameter lies with a specified probability. To understand the method, imagine the possibility of an infinite repetition of the sampling process, exactly as discussed for sampling distributions. For each sample, a boundary is set around the specific value used as an estimator of the parameter. The boundary is of the form $\bar{X} \pm 1.96c$, where $\bar{X}$ is the mean of the sample and c is an attribute expressing the concentration or spread of values. A certain proportion of these boundaries—or confidence limits—will encompass the parameter, and the remaining proportion will not. The probability associated with a given confidence set is simply the expected proportion that will encompass the parameter, over infinite repetitions of the sampling process.

The most widely used aspect of statistical inference in psychiatry and psychology is hypothesis testing. A hypothesis, in this context, is a statement about one or more population distributions, and a test is simply a rule for deciding to accept or reject the hypothesis. As an illustration of the method, suppose an empirical question is whether or not two treatment methods, say A and B, differ in effectiveness, where effectiveness is measured by a certain variable. One must imagine a population treated by method A, and a population treated by method B. We will agree that there is no difference between populations A and B if the distributions of the variable of interest do not differ in mean value between A and B. Clearly, the investigation must be restricted to samples from these populations. The statistical hypothesis is, then: population A mean is equal to population mean B, and acceptance or rejection of the hypothesis is made on the basis of the sample values.

If the variable of interest is normally distributed, the testing will be accomplished by the t-distribution. The test or rule will be of the form: if t is too large in a positive or negative direction the statistical hypothesis (frequently called the null hypothesis) should be rejected. The variable t will be too large if the mean of sample A differs from the mean of sample B more than the chance fluctuation predicted by the probability distribution.

If there are three or more treatment populations having normal distributions with the empirical question of differential effectiveness as above, the method of procedure is the analysis of variance and the *F*-distribution. If one is dealing with data in the form of frequencies, the distribution used would be χ^2.

There are two types of errors that might be committed in hypothesis testing. We might reject the statistical or null hypothesis when it is true, which is called a *type I* error, or we might accept the hypothesis when it is false, which is called a *type II* error. Tests (rules of procedure) are selected to minimize the magnitudes of these errors. The principally used such procedures are based upon the Neyman-Pearson lemma (theorem) which specifies the method for finding the best test among all those with the same probability of a type I error (which can be set suitably low).

Decision Theory

This approach focuses upon possible states of nature and possible action decisions of the investigator, and is applicable in the classical contexts of point estimation and hypothesis testing. The method was partly motivated by the theory of games and initiated by the pioneering work of Wald (1947).

Suppose appropriate action depends upon an unknown parameter that completely specifies a distribution. Three spaces are assumed: one containing an element representing each possible value of the parameter (these are the states of nature), one containing an element representing each possible sampling outcome, and a third containing an element for each possible action decision. A decision rule links sampling outcomes with action decisions, with decision theory oriented toward developing good rules and the methods of evaluating them. A central tool toward that end is the "loss function" which specifies a relationship between possible states of nature and alternative action decisions. The function is in loss form because its value is zero when the decision is correct or optimum, and gets larger as the discrepancy between nature and decision becomes more gross (and uncomfortable for the investigator).

The elements of the decision space depend upon the type of problem under consideration. In point estimation, the decision space is exactly equal to the parameter (states of nature) space; in hypothesis testing, the decision space

has only two elements, representing accept or reject the statistical hypothesis.

Bayesian Inference

Bayesian inference is based upon decision theory, but extends it by using subjective probability to measure the degree of belief that particular elements of the parameter space represent the true states of nature. The approach had its origins in a book published by Savage in 1954. Savage defined subjective probability as a measure of the confidence that a person has in the truth of a particular statement, and used Bayes' theorem as the basis for revising subjective probability as observational data become available.

Classical theory, in contrast, is based on a relative frequency interpretation of probability —that is, the concrete meanings assigned to expressions of probability in the basic axioms are in terms of the relative frequencies of events. Thus, one speaks, as above, of the probability (or proportion of times) that a set of confidence limits will encompass a parameter in infinitely repeated samplings. The frequency interpretation is indeed consistent with the popular notion of probability since when a gambler, for example, considers a probability associated with a roll of the dice he immediately thinks of the relative frequency of occurrence.

The Bayesian approach provides a means of associating a probability distribution with the parameter space. The task is at best cumbersome with a frequency interpretation of probability since parameters represent fixed, not random properties of nature. But if probability is degree of belief, one can easily imagine different degrees of belief in the array of parameters, and thereby probabilities (subjective) become assigned to parameter values.

Correlation and Prediction

The mathematical basis for most problems of correlation and prediction in the behavioral sciences is the regression equation. Its most widely used form is the linear model, expressing the variable of central interest as a weighted sum of concomitant variables. For example, if the variable of interest is scholastic performance *(S)*, related variables which could be used to predict scholastic performance include intelligence *(I)*, motivation *(M)*, persistence *(P)* and aspiration *(A)*. In linear equation form, the relationship would be expressed $S = W_1 I + W_2 M + W_3 P + W_4 A + e$, where W_1, and so on are weights and e is an error component.

The correlation coefficient is a measure of the degree to which the variability of the central variable is represented in the set of concomitant variables. In the special case where there is only one concomitant variable, this gives the product-moment correlation coefficient; more generally it gives the multiple correlation coefficient.

In the case of using the linear model for prediction, it is possible to allow for error by obtaining a prediction interval that is analogous to a confidence interval. A special use of the prediction equation is for discrimination or classification. Thus, for example, a psychiatrist could use the linear model to classify a patient on a certain aspect of biochemistry on the basis of observed behavior.

BIBLIOGRAPHY

FISHER, R. A.   On the mathematical foundations of theoretical statistics. *Philosophical Transactions of the Royal Society, London, Series A,* 1922, *222,* 309–368.

KOLMOGOROV, A. N.   *Foundations of the theory of probability.* New York: Chelsea, 1950.

NEYMAN, J.   Outline of a theory of statistical estimation based on the classical theory of probability. *Philosophical Transactions of the Royal Society, London, Series A,* 1937, *236,* 333–380.

NEYMAN, J., and PEARSON, E. S.   On the use and interpretation of certain test criteria for purposes of statistical inference. *Biometrika,* 1928, *20* A, Part I, 175–240; and Part II, 263–294.

SAVAGE, L. J.   *The foundations of statistics.* New York: Wiley, 1954.

WALD, A.   Foundations of a general theory of statistical decision functions. *Econometrica,* 1947, *15,* 279–313.

ARNOLD BINDER

MATHEMATICAL MODELS IN EXPERIMENTAL PSYCHOLOGY

Almost all substantive areas of experimental psychology by now have seen efforts to construct formal, substantively based, mathematical models. Mathematically based theories have been in psychology since the time of Fechner and Helmholtz in the nineteenth cen-

tury and were occasionally advocated by Thurstone and his co-workers in the first half of the twentieth century. However, the area of psychology known as mathematical models (or mathematical psychology) was really begun in 1950 with the paper by W. K. Estes entitled "Toward a Statistical Theory of Learning," which appeared in *Psychological Review.* Estes's paper was followed shortly by two other papers by Bush and Mosteller which appeared in the same journal in 1951, entitled "A Mathematical Model for Simple Learning" and "A Model for Stimulus Generalization and Discrimination."

Estes's and Bush and Mosteller's ideas were closely tied to the then relatively new set-theoretic approach to the areas of probability, statistics, and stochastic processes. Their basic idea was this: Any paradigm in experimental psychology gives rise in a natural way to a sample space consisting of all possible observable data complexes for a subject. The aim of a model is to predict a probability distribution for the sample space that is in general accord with the properties (events) of data generated in an actual experiment. The assumptions of a mathematical model are grounded in substantive psychological considerations. Thus rationally motivated postulates lead to the derivation of probabilities of various experimentally determined events usually as functions of theoretically meaningful parameters such as learning rate, reinforcement effectiveness, temporal spacing, memory capabilities. Finally parameter estimation and goodness of fit are obtained using principles of mathematical statistics now commonplace in psychology.

It is useful to contrast the mathematical models approach with the functionalist tradition of employing analysis of variance models for the interpretation of psychological data. The analysis of variance employs the general linear model, regardless of content considerations, in order to infer the existence of *differences between groups* of subjects run under variations of a common paradigm. In contrast, a mathematical model attempts to predict the pattern of data in a *single group* as arising naturally from psychologically motivated processes. Differences between groups are traceable to variations in meaningful parameter values for the underlying process. Variability of data is an intrinsic attribute of the underlying psychological process rather than the random or uncontrollable error variance envisioned in analysis of variance.

Learning Theory

By far the greatest influx of mathematical models into psychology has been in the learning area. In fact, as we have seen, the origins of mathematical models can be traced to the pioneering articles of Estes (1950), which introduced stimulus sampling theory, and the two papers by Bush and Mosteller (1951), which introduced linear-operator theory. Estes and his co-workers continued to develop stimulus sampling theory into a comprehensive framework for generating specific models for a variety of learning paradigms, and Bush and Mosteller (1955) similarly developed their linear-operator framework. Finally in the 1960s, the small state Markov model framework came to replace its two natural parents as the dominant variety of statistical learning theory. Markov models have had a considerable impact on the areas of concept identification and memory as well as learning.

To gain an insight into these three approaches to learning theory, this study will analyze the simple situation of learning to connect a single correct response to a stimulus. Suppose an organism is in a discrete trial learning situation, S (e.g., T-maze learning, paired associate learning) where one response, R, is the correct one. The core assumption of statistical learning theory for this setting is that for any trial number n the organism's response strength can be measured by

$$p_n = p(R_n \mid S)$$

the probability of the correct response on the nth trial, $n \geq 1$.

Stimulus sampling theory represents an effort to formalize and objectify the framework of Edwin Guthrie, a major learning theorist for the first half of the twentieth century. Basically a learning situation is represented by a population of stimulus elements to each of which a response is connected. On any trial the organism samples a subset of the population and p_n is determined by the proportion of stimulus elements in the sample connected to response R. Feedback (or reinforcement) of a particular response on that trial has the effect of connecting

all stimulus elements in the sample to that response, thus increasing the representation of that response in the population itself.

In order to utilize the framework one must specify several things:

1. the response alternatives and associated reinforcement operations
2. the theoretical size of the population, and the proportions of elements connected to the various response alternatives on the first trial
3. a mechanism of trial to trial sampling from the population.

In practice, feedback of responses is tied to experimental operations such as indicator lights or money. The population size and initial trial settings are generally left as estimable parameters in the model. Usually one of two sampling schemes is employed—the *fixed sample size* and the *variable sample size*. The fixed sample size assumption is that a constant proportion of the population is sampled independently and with replacement from trial to trial. The variable sample size assumption is that each population element has a constant probability of getting into the sample on any trial.

To illustrate a computation with the model, suppose that there are N elements in the population, half of which are initially connected to response R, and the rest to various alternatives. Suppose the fixed sample size assumption with r the sample size. Suppose on the first two trials response R is reinforced. Then it is an easy computation to show that the expected values of p_1, p_2, and p_3 are given by

$$p_1 = \frac{1}{2}$$

$$p_2 = \frac{1}{2}\left(1 + \frac{r}{N}\right)$$

$$p_3 = \frac{1}{2}\left(1 + \frac{2r}{N} - \frac{r^2}{N^2}\right)$$

Clearly by equating these and other theoretical expressions to corresponding data values, the predictive adequacy of the scheme is assessable (Atkinson, Bower, and Crothers, 1965, Chap. 8; Atkinson and Estes, 1963; and Levine and Burke, 1972).

The linear-operator framework of Bush and Mosteller postulates that each set of external contingencies x on a trial (such as the subject's response combined with feedback selection) gives rise to an operator Q_x which (deterministically computes p_{n+1} from p_n according to an equation of the form

$$Q_x(p_n) = (1 - \theta_x)p_n + \theta_x\lambda_x$$

where $0 \le \theta_x, \lambda_x \le 1$. In the simple case where each trial presents positive reinforcement for response R, the same operator with $\theta_x = \theta$ applies (with $\lambda_x = 1$) to yield the expression

$$p_n = 1 - (1 - \theta)^{n-1}(1 - p_1)$$

for $n \ge 1$. This simple model predicts that an individual organism's trial-ordered, error-success protocol is generated by a nonstationary Bernoulli process with success probability given by the preceding equation. It is easy to estimate the parameters θ and p_1 from data statistics and provide a strong statistical test for the model. While the linear-operator framework has attracted extensive and deep mathematical analysis, as in Norman (1972), few psychologists have continued to employ the framework for substantive problems. An exception is Lovejoy (1968).

The small state Markov model framework popularized by the success of the all-or-none or one element model (Bower, 1961) supposes that a learner can be thought of as occupying, on any trial, exactly one of a small number of *states of learning.* Each state has its own probability distribution over the set of response alternatives, and learning is reflected in trial-to-trial transitions among the states of learning. On any trial, a subject's response is represented as a random draw from the response distribution associated with his current learning state. After feedback, the subject may make a transition to a new learning state. The probabilities of these transitions among learning states are governed by a first order Markov chain (Atkinson, Bower, and Crothers, 1965, Chap. 2).

A theorist wishing to apply the approach has merely to specify several rational stages in a learning process (e.g., stimulus familiarity, response differentiation, short-term memory, stimulus confusion, etc.) and postulate the form of the response probability distributions for each state as well as the state-to-state transition matrix. By now extremely powerful and general statistical techniques exist for estimating parameters and evaluating goodness of fit of such models. The considerable successes of this approach to theorizing are documented in

Greeno (1974) and Restle and Greeno (1970).

The Markov model approach has proven more tractable mathematically, more flexible psychologically, and a more successful predictor of data than either of its predecessor frameworks. While the framework is likely to give way to the more general but compatible framework of finite state (probabilistic) automata (Suppes, 1969; Kieras, 1976), it has definitely had a great impact on experimental work in learning, memory, and concept identification since the beginnings of statistical learning theory.

Choice Theory

A considerable number of substantitively different experimental paradigms involve at some stage the task of an individual subject choosing one member from a set of discrete, well-defined choice alternatives, U. In 1959, Luce's book, *Individual Choice Behavior: A Theoretical Analysis,* attempted to mathematically capture this common theme at a sufficiently general level to be applicable to such disparate fields as paired comparison, psychophysical scaling, utility theory, signal detection, and learning.

At the basis of Luce's approach is the notion that choice behavior is probabilistic in character (an assumption traceable to Thurstone in the early 1920s). Thus if A is a finite subset of choice alternatives in U, one can denote by $p(x|A)$ the probability that x is picked from A. In addition to the elementary axioms of discrete probability theory for each $A \subseteq U$, Luce postulates an additional consistency axiom which serves to tie the probability measures from different subsets of U together. The essence of the axiom is that for all nested sequences of choice sets $R \subseteq S \subseteq T \subseteq U$, $p(R|T) = p(R|S)p(S|T)$, where, for example,

$$p(R|T) = \sum_{x \in R} p(x|T).$$

This axiom, which is designed to tie choice tendencies from different situations together, has an innocent enough appearance; however, if it holds for a subject, a number of surprisingly strong predictions are possible. Most of these can be seen as consequences of the fact that Luce's axiom system permits choice objects to be measured on a ratio scale, $v{:}U{\to}$Reals, such that

$$p(x|A) = \frac{v(x)}{\sum\limits_{y \epsilon A} v(y)}$$

The literature on mathematical choice theory has been very considerable since Luce's book. Suffice it to say that highly mathematical, probabilistic as well as algebraic, choice models exist for a variety of paradigms. Further, a great deal is known about the mathematical interrelationships between such models. The reader wishing an up-to-date coverage of the choice area is urged to read relevant articles which appear occasionally in *Psychological Review* and, more frequently, in the *Journal of Mathematical Psychology*. Notable is the work by Tversky (1972) who has developed a choice theory in which subjects select an alternative by paying attention to unshared features of the choice alternatives. This approach represents a formal development of an idea presented in Restle's book *Psychology of Judgment and Choice* (1961).

Reaction Time

Most experimental tasks that involve response selection yield measurable response latencies or reaction times. A considerable modeling effort has taken place in the reaction time area ranging from simple reaction time and choice reaction time to reaction time predictions in complex cognitive tasks involving memory and reasoning.

In a simple reaction time experiment, a subject responds as quickly as possible to the onset of a stimulus. Restle (1961) proposed that the observed reaction time T is composed of r unobservable and hypothetical components T_i such that

$$T = \sum_{i=1}^{r} T_i$$

where each T_i is the time to traverse the ith "neural stage." Restle assumes that the T_i random variables are independent and identically distributed exponentials, that is the distribution function for each T_i is given by

$$F_i(t) = p(T_i \le t) = 1 - e^{-\lambda_i t}$$

From this "neural series" assumption and constant λ_i, Restle derives that T is gamma distributed with mean r/λ and variance r/λ^2.

While Restle's simple stage model was successful in accounting for several sets of data, it gave way to a more general framework which allowed λ_i to vary from stage to stage (McGill, 1963).

A more interesting problem is choice reaction time. In this paradigm one of several stimuli, S_j, is presented to the subject and he must accurately and rapidly make the correct response, R_j, to S_j, $1 \le j \le J$ (often $J=2$). An adequate model of choice reaction time must account for the effects of variables like the presentation probabilities and sequential effects of past stimuli and responses on the reaction time as well as the error frequencies.

Since 1960 there have been a wide variety of detailed models for choice reaction time ranging in underpinnings from information theory to the theory of random walks in stochastic processes. The information-theoretic approach attempts to relate the *uncertainty* in which a stimulus will appear on the nth trial to the reaction time. The random walk models generally postulate *sensory counters* for each stimulus. Following presentation of a stimulus, all counters begin stochastically incrementing with different rates (naturally the rate for the presented stimulus is assumed to be highest). The subject responds when some function of the counter readings reaches a critical value, for example in the case of $J=2$, the difference in counts. The functional values constitute a random walk. Laming (1973, Chap. 8–11) presents a comprehensive review of many of these models. More recently, Luce and Green (1974) developed a neural response time model that, unlike Restle's primitive neural stage model of 1961, takes into account detailed neural and sensory information.

An increasing and very popular recent trend in experimental psychology is the development of paradigms for studying the reaction time to complete nontrivial cognitive tasks, for example recognition of set membership (Sternberg, 1969), the determination of truth or falsity of a sentence (Collins and Quillian, 1969), the solution of elementary problems in reasoning

(Clark, 1969), and many more. The usual approach to model construction is to decompose the cognitive task into a number of hypothetical stages each of which is theoretically grounded in information processing notions. The object of the analysis is to predict reaction time differences between related tasks as a function of the unshared stages in the two tasks. Such models generally postulate that a subject completes the stages serially; however, parallel processing models are also in evidence.

While information processing models for reaction times have been generally elementary from a mathematical standpoint, their analysis is complicated from a statistical viewpoint. Basically errors due to fast guesses or imperfect processing prove difficult to analyze and contaminate the interpretation of the reaction times on success trials. In an effort to cope with the problem of errors, theorists have developed the notion of a speed-accuracy tradeoff for a cognitive task (Pachella, 1974). The basic idea of a speed-accuracy tradeoff function is that in order for a subject to speed up his reaction time he must tolerate more errors and vice versa. Thus the subtraction of mean reaction times between two tasks must take into account where on the speed-accuracy function both tasks are. The analysis of such data is aided by a direct application of models from the choice reaction time area. In this case, detailed modeling efforts in simple paradigms have definitely aided in the formulation of theory for more cognitively rich phenomena.

Visual Search

In a visual search experiment, subjects are presented with a visual display (letters, objects, pictures, etc.) for a brief period of time (usually tachistoscopically) and asked to comply with some task such as to indicate the presence or absence of a critical item. Sperling (1960) popularized the paradigm in order to study brief visual memory (of approximately a second in duration). Estes and his students (Estes and Taylor, 1966) have developed a number of serial processing models that permit the recovery of the (hypothetical) time to process a single letter into short-term memory from data involving detection accuracy for different display sizes.

A substantively interesting parallel processing model for the same task was developed by Rumelhart (1970) which attempts to decompose the process into sensory information storage, feature extraction, construction of perceptual vectors, and letter naming through accessing a sensory-memory dictionary stored in long-term memory. Rumelhart's model is the "front-end" of a detailed information processing theory for the integration of a number of different memory systems. The theory is capable of generating mathematical models for a great variety of experimental paradigms in the memory area (Norman and Rumelhart, 1971). This theory, along with the buffer model of Atkinson and Shiffrin (1968), represents major efforts to tie a number of situational models to a common theoretical framework deriving in part from notions in computer simulation. Primary source material is necessary to gain the flavor of the considerable literature in this area of mathematical models.

Other Topics

This brief survey of mathematical models would be incomplete in important ways without briefly mentioning two other major areas of modeling. The first is the area of *signal detection,* introduced into psychology by Tanner and Swets (1954). The area concerns modeling the behavior of subjects attempting to detect sensory signals embedded in noisy backgrounds. The aim of a model is to recover psychologically meaningful parameters from the subject's "hit" (correct detection) and "false alarm" (false detection) probabilities. These two probabilities vary systematically with both sensory and decision-theoretic variables.

The dominant theory in the area has been the theory of signal detection (Green and Swets, 1966). However, a number of discrete state detection models (Atkinson, Bower, and Crothers, 1965, Chap. 5) have also been developed. These models have been employed successfully in recognition memory paradigms to separate recognition accuracy from guessing processes.

A second area that can receive only passing mention is the considerable effort to model *psychophysical scaling* (Laming, 1973, Chap. 3–7).

Experimental Paradigms

An appreciation of the vast extent to which viable, substantive, mathematical models exist for various paradigms in experimental psychology, is facilitated by presenting a taxonomy of experimental paradigms. Each entry is an area or paradigm in experimental psychology where a considerable effort to construct substantive models has been made.

I. Animal Learning Paradigms
  A. Avoidance learning
  B. Escape learning
  C. Classical conditioning
  D. Operant learning (schedules of reinforcement)
  E. Discrimination and generalization
  F. Reversal shifts
  G. Extinction and spontaneous recovery
  H. Maze learning
II. Human Learning Paradigms
  A. Verbal learning
    1. Paired associate learning
    2. Verbal discrimination learning
    3. Serial list learning
    4. List transfer paradigms
    5. Massed and spaced practice
    6. Probability learning
  B. Concept identification and reasoning
    1. Affirmative concepts
    2. Conjunctive concepts
    3. Reversal and nonreversal shifts
    4. Disjunctive concepts
    5. Two- and three-term series
    6. Syllogistic reasoning
    7. Bayesian inference
    8. Group problem solving
    9. Deductive logic
  C. Memory
    1. Free recall
    2. Recognition memory
    3. Iconic memory
    4. High speed scanning
    5. Free and constrained association
    6. Long term memory
    7. Naming
    8. Probe digit technique
III. Choice
  A. Paired comparison
  B. Ranking
  C. Choice among gambles
  D. Portfolio selection
  E. Two person gaming
IV. Psychophysics
  A. Magnitude estimation
  B. Sensory threshold determination
  C. Auditory signal detection
  D. Psychophysical scaling
V. Reaction time
  A. Simple reaction time
  B. Choice reaction time
  C. Visual search
  D. Comprehension of sentences
  E. Question answering
  F. Triad judgments for semantic systems
VI. Miscellany
  A. Impression formation
  B. Clinical assessment
  C. Medical diagnosis
  D. Asch paradigm
  E. Binary choice in children
  F. Attitude change

Summary

The field of mathematical models in experimental psychology was initiated in the early 1950s by the pioneering work of Estes and Bush and Mosteller on statistical learning theory. The aim was and has continued to be the development of substantive models for various psychological phenomena. The area is characterized by eclectic utilization of mathematical notions tailored to specific psychological assumptions. Since its inception in 1950, a literature of several thousand items has grown and invaded almost all psychological paradigms under investigation. Today the all pervasive, general linear model of the analysis of variance is no longer the theoretical catchall that it was for the early functional psychologists. Strong psychological inference demands serious psychological models, and the mathematical models area has provided them.

In the 1970s psychology turned to cognitively richer paradigms such as reasoning, psycholinguistics, question answering, chess playing, complex motor skills, neural processing. To keep abreast of these developments modelers employ a richer variety of mathematical formalisms in model construction such as graph theory, automata theory, predicate and modal logic, generative grammar, computer languages, information theory, systems theory, topology, and algebra. Many of these frameworks lack direct statistical underpinnings and these will have to be developed to permit prediction.

BIBLIOGRAPHY

ATKINSON, R. C.; BOWER, G. H.; and CROTHERS, E. J. *An introduction to mathematical learning theory.* New York: Wiley, 1965.

ATKINSON, R. C., and ESTES, W. K. Stimulus sampling theory. In R. D. Luce, R. R. Bush, and E. Galanter (Eds.), *Handbook of mathematical psychology.* Vol. 2. New York: Wiley, 1963. Pp. 121–268.

BOWER, G. H. Application of a model to paired-associate learning. *Psychometrika,* 1961, *26,* 255–280.

BUSH, R. R., and MOSTELLER, F. *Stochastic models for learning.* New York: Wiley, 1955.

COOMBS, C. H., DAWES, R. M., and TVERSKY, A. *Mathematical psychology: An elementary introduction.* Englewood Cliffs, N.J.: Prentice-Hall, 1970.

GREEN, D. M., and SWETS, J. A. *Signal detection theory in psychophysics.* New York: Wiley, 1966.

GREENO, J. G. Representation of learning as discrete transition in a finite state space. In D. H. Krantz, R. C. Atkinson, R. D. Luce, and P. Suppes (Eds.), *Contemporary developments in mathematical psychology.* Vol. 1. San Francisco: W. H. Freeman, 1974. Pp. 1–43.

LAMING, D. *Mathematical psychology.* New York: Academic Press, 1973.

LEVINE, G., and BURKE, C. J. *Mathematical model techniques for learning theories.* New York: Academic Press, 1972.

LOVEJOY, E. *Attention in discrimination learning.* San Francisco: Holden Day, 1968.

McGILL, W. J. Stochastic latency mechanisms. In R. D. Luce, R. R. Bush, and E. Galanter (Eds.), *Handbook of mathematical psychology,* Vol. 1. New York: Wiley, 1963. Pp. 309–360.

NORMAN, D. A., and RUMELHART, D. E. A system for perception and memory. In D. A. Norman (Ed.), *Models of human memory.* New York: Academic Press, 1971. Pp. 21–63.

NORMAN, M. F. *Markov processes and learning models.* New York: Academic Press, 1972.

RESTLE, F. *Psychology of judgment and choice.* New York: Wiley, 1961.

RESTLE, F., and GREENO, J. G. *Introduction to mathematical psychology.* Reading, Mass.: Addison-Wesley, 1970.

WILLIAM H. BATCHELDER

MATHEMATICAL MODELS IN LEARNING

See MATHEMATICAL MODELS IN EXPERIMENTAL PSYCHOLOGY

MATHEMATICS LEARNING AND INSTRUCTION

Research in the area of early mathematics learning during the first half of this century was mostly concerned with the mathematical abilities of entering school-age children. Such skills included the ability to identify numbers, count various object arrays, and add and compare small quantities. This orientation for learning early number concepts was the product of certain prerequisite skills defined by the mathematics curriculum. From this perspective, mathematics learning is a hierarchical network of capabilities; a set of terminal behaviors or abilities to perform certain specific functions under specified conditions (Gelman, 1972).

Gagné (1970) developed a model for analysis of the different levels of mathematical learning in terms of an instructional hierarchy. The model suggests that if the final skill desired is a problem-solving capability, then the scope and sequence of the mathematics curriculum is determined by a task analysis of the subordinate capabilities that are prerequisite to the attainment of the given objective. The hierarchical structure of mathematics greatly aids the formulation of the sequence, although the resultant structure of prerequisites is not necessarily universal. Readiness is essentially a function of the presence or absence of prerequisite learning. Thus, mathematics instruction is viewed as the product of effective problem-solving behaviors.

Piaget's developmental research has had a pronounced effect on mathematical learning and instruction. Piaget's (1952) theory of number conservation has directed attention to the stages through which young children pass in arriving at the knowledge of number. Research in the cognitive area of number conservation has changed and broadened the emphasis of mathematics education for young children from the attainment of narrowly defined mathematics skills to the development of broad intellectual powers. From this perspective, mathematics learning becomes a discipline reflecting the nature of the knowledge-acquisition processes that makes possible the understanding of knowledge.

Bruner (1966) also views mathematics from

the perspective of the inherent processes of learning. The learner begins with the manipulation of materials or tasks in order to present a problem. This problem may take the form of (1) goals to be achieved in the absence of readily discernible means for reaching these goals; (2) contradictions between sources of information of apparent equal creditability; or (3) the quest for structure or symmetry in situations where such order is not readily apparent. The process then becomes more systematic as the learner is led to move back through the needed associations and concepts to finally derive the appropriate rules for solving the problem.

The current focus of early mathematics learning seems to be combining the best of the product and process approaches to instruction. For example, Lazarus (1974) reported on the goals of a federally funded elementary mathematics program called Project One, which views math as a living subject whose context is real life situations. Mathematical concepts are taught within the framework of science, technology, and the arts. The aim of the Project One mathematics program is effective quantitative thinking. This includes two kinds of abilities: (1) familiarity and competence with specific mathematical concepts: numbers and arithmetic, measurement, estimation, mapping and scaling, and graphing; (2) a set of cognitive skills: strategies for organizing experiences in such a way as to facilitate reasoning, problem solving, and analytic thinking.

BIBLIOGRAPHY

Bruner, J. S. *Toward a theory of instruction.* New York: Norton, 1966.

Gagné, R. M. *The conditions of learning.* New York: Holt, Rinehart and Winston, 1970.

Gelman, R. The nature and development of early number concepts. In H. W. Reese (Ed.), *Advances in child development and behavior* (Vol. 7). New York: Academic Press, 1972. Pp. 115–167.

Lazarus, M. Toward a new program in mathematics. *The National Elementary Principal,* 1974, *53,* 72–81.

Piaget, J. *The child's conception of number.* London: Routledge and Kegan Paul, 1952.

Jerome Bernstein

MATING AND COURTSHIP
See Courtship and Mating

MATSUMOTO, MATATARO (1865–1943)

A Japanese psychologist, Matsumoto received a Ph.D. from Yale University and studied with W. Wundt at Leipzig. He became professor of psychology at Tokyo Higher Normal College (presently Tokyo University of Education), Kyoto Imperial University, and Tokyo Imperial University. He was originally interested in auditory perception and perceptual-motor learning and skills, but later became interested in mental development, intelligence and psychology of arts. Matsumoto has founded the first psychological laboratories in Tokyo and Kyoto.

Shinkuro Iwahara

MAUDSLEY, HENRY (1835–1918)

An English psychiatrist, Maudsley believed, as did Thomas Huxley, in consciousness as epiphenomenon (mind as by-product of nervous processes, although belonging to different basic reality). Maudsley supported the somatic view of mental illness, conceiving of insanity as "failure in organic adaptation to external nature." He is the author of *The Physiology and Pathology of the Mind* (1867). The Maudsley psychiatric hospital in London was named for him and is considered today as one of the best-conducted institutions of its kind in the United Kingdom.

Patrick J. Capretta

MAZE LEARNING

In 1902, W. S. Small at Clark University constructed a replica in miniature of the Hampton Court maze and studied the progress of rats learning to find their way through it. This rat-in-maze methodology became the hallmark of the scientific study of learning for half a century. Unfortunately, the method turned out to be a scientific cul de sac. The method is rarely used these days.

In general terms, a maze consists of four components: a starting box, a true path to a goal, blind alleys, and a goal compartment. The simplest maze of all has just the true path, a straight alley leading from a starting box to the goal. Other simple mazes are in the form of a T or a Y, where there is just one correct turn and one incorrect turn at a choice point. More complex mazes were constructed by linking several Ts or Ys together to make a multiunit maze. Such mazes were used widely until it became clear that the complex maze is not a very useful piece of scientific apparatus.

The problem is that maze behavior is incredibly complex. In just two papers, those on the goal gradient and the habit-family hierarchy, Hull dealt with almost three dozen phenomena of such learning. Such complexity led many psychologists to use the simpler mazes mentioned above. Even these have now nearly disappeared from the literature, which is dominated by work with the Skinner box and other possibly simpler methods.

GREGORY A. KIMBLE

MEASUREMENT; MENTAL TESTS

MECHANICAL APTITUDE: MEASUREMENT METHODS

Mechanical ability is popularly thought of as concerning the making and fixing of things, as distinct from clerical, sales, administrative and professional abilities. In general, we speak of mechanical ability in relation to *trades* and various levels of skilled work. There is no fine dividing line between mechanical occupations and those which are not mechanical. Some occupations that most of us would classify as mechanical are those of a plumber, carpenter, automobile mechanic, and boatbuilder.

There is no one type of test function which underlies mechanical work to the same extent that the general intelligence tests relate to schoolwork. In order satisfactorily to predict a particular mechanical job, a range of different kinds of tests must be used in a battery. Different combinations of tests are usually needed for different jobs. Some of the kinds of tests that have proved useful in the prediction of success at mechanical work and in vocational guidance are described in the following sections.

Intelligence Tests

The fact that an individual is involved in making and fixing things does not mean that intelligence is an unimportant attribute. When it is possible to do so, either a battery of the major intellectual factors or at least a general intelligence test should be tried as a predictor. The spatial and perceptual factors are very useful in predicting success in many mechanical jobs. Some tests embodying these functions will be considered in the subsequent discussion. However, it is important to consider the verbal, numerical, and reasoning factors as well in the prediction of success in mechanical work. Because general intelligence tests are composed mainly of these factors, a good general intelligence test is often one of the best predictors of job success.

General intelligence tests tend to be more predictive of how well the individual will do in job training than of how well he will perform subsequently on the job. This is probably due to the fact that the training phase requires more abstract ability. In many cases, the training program involves classroom-like procedures, the reading of materials, and the learning of machine operations. Success at activities of this sort is what intelligence tests predict best.

A second major reason why intelligence tests (and all other types of tests as well) tend to correlate more highly with performance in training than with later job performance is because, as a rule, performance is more reliably measured in training than on the job. Progress in training is usually graded more carefully. There is a greater opportunity to observe the worker, and in many cases achievement tests are used to assess progress in training.

The general intelligence tests tend to be more predictive of success in high-skill than in low-skill jobs. That is, validities are usually higher for jobs such as that of electrical technician or complex machine operator than for jobs such as that of truck driver or furniture mover. The difference in validity is probably due to the increased importance of abstract ability in more highly skilled work. In selecting people for unskilled work, the problem is to set up minimum standards of intelligence rather than to seek persons of high intelligence.

Spatial and Perceptual Tests

A wide variety of mechanical work requires spatial and perceptual abilities. For example, the automobile mechanic needs *spatial orientation* in his work. In a typical job situation, he is lying under the automobile and must remove a nut from the engine above him. The nut is slanted at a 45–degree angle, and he must remove it with a wrench that has two joints. He must orient himself spatially to the complex of angles and movements in order to do such work. In draftsmanship, it is necessary to portray three-dimensional objects on two-dimensional pieces of paper. In some drawings, the objects must be shown in tilted positions or partially disassembled. Spatial ability, both *spatial orientation* and *visualization,* is required to work as a draftsman and at many other jobs.

One of the best-known spatial tests for mechanical aptitude is the Minnesota Paper Form Board Test. This is a printed test in which each item consists of cut-out pieces from a geometrical form, and the subject is required to choose from a number of composite forms what the pieces would look like when put together. It is a useful predictor of grades in shop courses, supervisors' ratings of workmanship, objective production records, and many other measures of mechanical performance.

In addition to the spatial abilities mentioned above, perceptual abilities also are required in a variety of jobs. The *perceptual speed* factor has been used as a predictor for many jobs. This requires the rapid recognition of details, as in quickly judging whether pairs of telephone numbers are the same or different. Such measures of perceptual speed are useful in the selection of office clerks and for numerous other jobs. The individual who sits by a fast-moving conveyor belt and looks for flaws in manufactured products must use perceptual speed. It is possible that other types of spatial and perceptual abilities will prove useful in the measurement of mechanical aptitude.

Mechanical Comprehension. Among the most successful tests of mechanical aptitude are those designed to measure the mastery of mechanical principles, or the ability to reason with mechanical problems. In a typical problem, a truck driver is rushing medical supplies to a fire-damaged town. He discovers that his truck is about an inch too tall to clear a bridge leading to the town. What should he do? The answer is to let some air out of the tires. In another example, a motorist must remove a boulder that blocks the road. He finds a long, stout pole to do the job. He must then decide whether to use the pole as a pry or a lever. He can construct a lever by balancing the pole on a rock placed between the boulder and himself (the lever exerts more force than a pry). After deciding to use the lever action with the rock as a balancer (a *fulcrum*), he must then decide where to place the balancer (rock) and how to exert his strength best against the pole. As a third example, a hoist is being built to lift three trunks into the bed of a truck. A system of gears and chains is set up to transfer the power from an electric motor to the hoist. It must be decided how large the different gears should be to give the desired power to the hoist.

The three examples above are typical of the items found in tests of mechanical comprehension. Essentially these are reasoning tests concerning the ability to solve mechanical problems. Such tests tend to be more predictive of job success when the problem situations relate directly to the job in question, for example, questions concerning dysfunctions of automobiles as a test for trainees as automobile mechanics.

Mechanical Information. One of the most useful measures for the selection of skilled and semiskilled workers is a test of information, or knowledge, about tools and machinery. For example, a set of questions, such as the following, would be useful in the selection of automobile mechanics:

1. What is a torque converter?
2. What is a ratchet?
3. Where is the "needle valve" in an automobile?
4. What source of power is used to run the alternator in most automobiles?
5. How do you recognize "preignition"?

Each of these questions would have a number of alternative answers, and the subject would be required to mark the correct answer in each case.

Information tests can be constructed to measure either general knowledge of mechanical work or knowledge of one particular job. It is usually the case that a test constructed specifically for one job, such as television repairman, will be more predictive than a test of knowledge in general about mechanical work. However, the test which is constructed specifically for one job is likely to be useful only for selecting personnel for that job or for closely related jobs. Also, because of the specific knowledge which the instrument measures, it is of little use in vocational guidance, where it is usually necessary to measure broad functions rather than highly specialized information. A more general measure of mechanical knowledge is often useful in vocational guidance.

Analysis of Mechanical Aptitude Tests. A sufficient personnel-selection program usually requires a careful study of the particular industrial setting. The diversity of psychological functions required by different jobs makes it necessary to try out a range of tests to find the one that will work well in practice. Also, it is often necessary to invent and construct tests for particular jobs.

Few of the mechanical aptitude tests have been studied as extensively as the tests of intellectual ability. Consequently, it is usually necessary to perform considerable research in the job setting to determine the utility of particular tests. In few cases have norms for the tests been obtained on a sufficiently representative sample to allow their use as dependable guides. It is generally more meaningful to obtain local norms for particular personnel selection or school programs.

Mechanical aptitude tests have modest validity for many different jobs, the amount varying considerably with the job. The seemingly small validities for some jobs should be regarded from a number of standpoints. Primarily there is the possibility that formal abilities, such as those measured in psychological tests, have little to do with job success. Another possibility is that the criterion of job success is unreliable and consequently cannot be predicted. If the criterion is determined only from the sketchy impressions of foremen and managers, it is seldom very reliable. Because of the unreliability inherent in most criteria, mechanical aptitude tests are often more valid than is apparent from the correlation coefficients. The third point to consider is that the modest to low individual validities should not obscure the fact that a combination of several tests in a battery will often produce reasonably good predictive efficiency.

BIBLIOGRAPHY

ANASTASI, A. *Psychological testing* (3rd ed.). New York: Macmillan, 1968.
CRONBACH, L. J. *Essentials of psychological testing* (3rd ed.). New York: Harper & Row, 1970.
THORNDIKE, R. L., and HAGEN, E. *Measurement and evaluation in psychology and education* (3rd ed.). New York: Wiley, 1969.

JUM C. NUNNALLY

MEDIATION IN LEARNING

The concept of mediation plays a very significant role in stimulus-response theories where it is important in the explanation of such "mentalistic" phenomena as thinking, concept formation, and problem solving. For the S-R theorist, the problem with such behavior is that there appears always to be a large ideational gap between the objective stimulus situation and the objective behavior which reveals that the individual has been thinking, formed a concept, or solved a problem. The theoretical contribution of mechanisms of mediation is to bridge this gap.

The simplest and most important mediational concept is that of the *fractional anticipatory goal response,* developed by Hull to account for certain phenomena of maze learning in the rat. When the rat is reinforced for completing a run through the maze, its final responses are those of seizing, chewing, and swallowing food, collectively referred to as a goal response and symbolized R_G. Since R_G is a response, it can be conditioned to the stimuli that are present when it occurs by the process of classical conditioning. The CS would be the stimuli in the goal box and the US would be food.

By the mechanism of *stimulus generalization,* the conditioned R_G would transfer to any stimuli resembling those in the goal box. In a maze, the segments all resemble the goal box, being made of wood, painted black, covered with wire screen, and the like. Hence R_G could occur anywhere in the maze except for the fact that the critical stimulus for its full elicitation, food, is missing. Fractional components of R_G (symbolized r_g), such as salivation and chewing movements could occur, however. Mediational theory assumes these components occur before the animal reaches a goal and are thus fractional *anticipatory* goal responses.

Beyond this, the theory assumes that r_gs have characteristic proprioceptive stimulus consequences, s_gs, which become a part of the general stimulus situation controlling behavior. Thus the simplest possible mediated bit of behavior could be diagrammed.

$$S-r_g-s_g-R$$

Other applications of this r_g-s_g mechanism have been widely used to account for cognitive activity in lower organisms and in man. Such applications in general involve the conception that not just goal responses, but also other elements of a complex set of reactions can function as mediators.

More recent theorizing has tended to reject such conceptions in favor of admittedly mentalistic interpretations. These newer theories treat complex behavior in terms of overall "plans" or "programs" that guide complex acts.

BIBLIOGRAPHY

HULSE, S. H.; DEESE, J.; and EGETH, H. *The psychology of learning.* New York: McGraw-Hill, 1975. Pp. 90–92.

See also FRACTIONAL ANTICIPATORY GOAL RESPONSE; PROBLEM SOLVING

GREGORY A. KIMBLE

MEDITATION, TRANSCENDENTAL
See TRANSCENDENTAL MEDITATION

MEDITATION AS A THERAPEUTIC AGENT

Recent years have seen a growing popular interest in self-administered techniques aimed at personal growth such as hatha yoga, meditation, and certain relaxation exercises. Paralleling this popular movement has been an increased use of these and other self-administered relaxation techniques with psychiatric patients. Alpha biofeedback training aims at equipping the patient with a technique which he can eventually use by himself to produce a relaxing state said to accompany the production of alpha waves on the EEG, and training in progressive relaxation is designed to help patients achieve deep relaxation through their own efforts by alternately tensing and relaxing various muscle groups. Similarly, *autogenic training* (more recently a type of autogenic training combined with biofeedback) is being used for a home program of therapy. Following this trend, the discipline of meditation has begun to be studied by clinicians interested in its potential as a self-administered therapeutic technique.

Research

Several factors have lent momentum to this consideration of meditative techniques. Laboratory studies have indicated that meditation often produces profound physiological changes and at least one standardized meditative technique has become readily available for use in scientific research. These factors, together with the widespread concern within the medical and mental health fields about the prevalence of stress-related diseases, has led to an upsurge of interest in studies investigating the properties and potential therapeutic uses of meditation. The present article will review these studies, with emphasis on research relating to the value of meditation for the mental health field.

The first scientific investigations of meditation used Japanese Zen masters and Indian yogis as subjects. Difficult as these investigations often were to conduct, they yielded some interesting results. Physiological measurements on yogis typically showed a decrease (often dramatic) of respiration and heart rates during meditation and an increase in the electrical resistance of the skin, while electroencephalographic investigations suggested some differences between the traditional schools of meditation. When repeated trials of a click stimulus were administered during deep meditation, for example, Zen masters were found to show no habituation of their response to the clicks (as measured by alpha blocking on the EEG), while yogis in meditation failed to show any indication that they were registering stimuli much more intense than clicks (e.g., loud banging noises, being touched with a hot glass tube)—that is, they habituated completely. Such differences in response have been linked to differences in philosophical approach between the two meditative disciplines, Zen masters being trained to be fully "open" to nature, ever reviewing the world with "the eye of a beginner," and the yogi being trained to withdraw his senses from contact with the outer world. A direct relationship between the philosophy and physiology of meditative techniques is thus suggested.

Transcendental Meditation

Full-scale scientific investigation of meditation awaited the development of a simple standardized technique suitable for widespread experimental use, since investigators could not rely for their subject population on a few practitioners who might take as much as 20 years to master the art of meditation. A simple westernized form of *mantra* meditation, known as transcendental meditation (TM), developed in 1958 by an Indian monk, Maharishi Mahesh Yogi, fulfilled the above criteria and has been used in over 300 experimental investigations on the effects of meditation. Studies of this form of meditation are still proliferating thanks to the zeal of an organization of teachers of transcendental meditation (The Students International Meditation Society or SIMS) and to the current interest of the scientific community in the study of relaxation techniques in general.

Since TM's standardization and wide availability make it the first meditative technique to be scientifically feasible to study on a wide scale, it will be the subject of the bulk of the present discussion. Our focus on this technique, however, should not be construed as indicating that other equally effective meditative techniques may not be standardized in the future, becoming also available for research purposes.

Persons who have learned TM are expected to practice the technique 20 minutes twice daily by sitting upright in a chair, eyes closed, and mentally repeating a "mantra" (a Sanskrit sound considered soothing) while effort or striving of any sort during this experience is discouraged. Although it bears some resemblance to the process of free association, the mental state achieved through meditation is far more global and diffuse, being primarily nonverbal and nonconceptual in nature. Unlike free association, TM has no "goal" or "purpose" (even a therapeutic one) for which the practitioner strives, and it is entirely an intrapersonal experience, not involving communication with any other person.

Physiologically, meditation seems to represent a unique state during which the body appears to be in a profound state of rest and where decreased autonomic activity, decreased emotional and sensory reactivity, and decreased muscle tension coincide with a generally wakeful and alert brain. Changes in the electrical activity of the brain, in the autonomic nervous system, and in somatosensory functions during TM show a more or less characteristic pattern. Respiration and heart rate show slight but consistent decreases during TM while cardiac output as measured by catheters may be slowed by as much as 25%. Oxygen consumption during TM tends to decrease as much as or more than it does during deep NREM (quiescent) sleep. In general it might be said that decreases in total oxygen consumption and cardiac output during both TM and sleep appear to be of the same order of magnitude, with the difference that during TM the decreases take place within a few minutes, while in sleep the drop usually requires considerable time (often several hours). Unlike sleep, the brain waves during TM tend to show a semialert pattern.

A decrease in tension during meditation has been suggested by studies of skin resistance. Wallace (1970) and Wallace et al. (1971) have reported that within minutes after starting meditation, their subjects' skin resistance increased on the average by 160%. This is reminiscent of the 130% rise in skin resistance above waking level which may occur after several hours of sleep, although the increase, when it occurs, is much more rapid during meditation than during sleep, suggesting that an unusually rapidly induced general relaxation is characteristic of the former state. Although two recent studies have failed to replicate the dramatic rise in skin resistance reported by the Wallace group, all researchers have noted *some* rise in skin resistance during TM, and Glueck (1974) reports that an increase in skin resistance was seen in all of the meditating psychiatric patients in his study *at every session where this was monitored,* a surprisingly consistent finding.

Lactate concentration in the blood has been found to decrease markedly during TM, possibly indicative of lowered anxiety at this time, and several studies have found blood flow to be augmented in forearms and forehead. No consistent changes in blood pressure have been identified during the TM state, although longitudinal studies have shown that hypertensive patients meditating over a period of time may show an average reduction in systolic and diastolic blood pressures of 9mm and 6mm respectively.

Brain Waves

Brain waves recorded from well-practiced meditators during TM appear to be characterized by a "marked" increase in the intensity of alpha wave trains in the central and frontal regions of the brain (although *total* alpha may not necessarily increase). These may be followed later by bursts of theta waves. Like Zen meditators, TM meditators have been reported to show no habituation to sound and light stimuli administered during meditation. Drowsiness and light sleep also frequently appear in the EEG records of subjects during TM, although in general the meditative state appears to differ from both that of sleep and of ordinary rest with eyes closed. For example, whereas most subjects show spindles in alpha waves (10 cycles per second) during rest, during TM the EEG also shows periods of beta spindles (22 cycles per second) which are said to be synchronized and in phase from all points on the scalp, suggesting a unique condition of orderliness in the brain physiology. At the same time the relatively high frequency of this very ordered pattern indicates a state of wakefulness. Occurring simultaneously with deep metabolic rest, this strikingly ordered yet alert brain wave pattern may conceivably perform a function distinct from that of either sleep or ordinary wakefulness.

Longitudinal EEG studies have also shown that longer term meditators tend to produce more spontaneous alpha (when they are not meditating) than they did several months previously (before learning to meditate) and other studies have shown that meditators, as compared to nonmeditators, can learn to control their alpha waves more quickly during biofeedback training.

Psychological Factors

Psychological correlates have also been studied although relatively few published articles are as yet available in this area. One study reports meditators performing significantly better on a perceptual-motor task than nonmeditators. Another study has shown significant improvement on a simple perceptual-motor task following a session of meditation, as compared to test scores after a session of simple rest, in two groups of experienced meditators. Also of interest are preliminary studies which suggest that experienced meditators show keener auditory discrimination following a 20-minute session of meditating than they do following 20 minutes of reading a book.

A consistent and reliable change found over time in persons who meditate is marked reduction in anxiety levels. This finding has been investigated in a number of laboratories with no failure to replicate. TM seems to reduce anxiety in a majority of those who practice it, although when groups practicing other relaxation techniques were used as controls, several recent studies have indicated that similar reductions in anxiety may result from the continued practice of such techniques as progressive relaxation or alpha biofeedback. An apparent difference between meditation and the latter techniques, however, is the relatively low attrition rate for TM practitioners ranging from 30% to 50% as compared to the generally high attrition rates (ranging from 70% to 100%) for the control groups practicing either progressive relaxation or alpha biofeedback. The latter techniques appear to be only minimally attractive to subjects who are asked to continue them outside the laboratory setting, while TM appears to be self-reinforcing when practiced alone.

A number of questionnaire surveys have suggested that the regular practice of TM has an antiaddictive effect, tending to reduce abuse of such drugs as marijuana, LSD, barbiturates, amphetamines, alcohol and cigarettes. Many of these drug studies have been flawed, however, by the self-selection involved in the populations studied, only those persons who stick with meditation over a long period of time being chosen as respondents. A lack of control groups has also been a conspicuous feature in most of the surveys. A more recent study (Shafii et al.,

1974), designed to overcome these difficulties, used a matched control group. These researchers found that while only 15% of the non-meditating control group had decreased or stopped their use of marijuana during the preceding three months, between one-half to three-quarters of the meditators (depending on the length of time since their initiation, the longer the time the greater the decrease) had decreased or stopped their use of marijuana during the first three months after initiation into mediation. The authors found that the longer a person had practiced meditation, the more likely it was that he had decreased or stopped his use of marijuana. The same authors, studying the relationship between cigarette smoking and meditation, found that 71% of persons who had practiced meditation more than two years had significantly decreased their use of cigarettes and 57% had stopped smoking altogether (while cigarette usage figures for a control group of nonmeditators remained the same over a two-year period).

These findings suggest obvious clinical applications of meditation and studies investigating these possibilities are now underway in a number of hospital settings. Some pioneering studies are also being undertaken in prisons and in connection with drug rehabilitation programs. Meditation is currently being investigated as an adjunct in the treatment of such diseases as bronchial asthma, hypertension, aphasia following stroke, cancer, and certain speech disorders. Its potential use in hospital psychiatry and outpatient psychotherapy is also being studied.

Psychotherapy

The Institute of Living in Hartford, Connecticut, has been conducting a long-term study on the use of self-achieved relaxation techniques in the treatment of psychiatric illness (Glueck, 1974). Initially comparing three matched groups of psychiatric inpatients—patients who learned alpha biofeedback, patients who learned progressive relaxation, and patients who learned TM, the research team found the attrition rate so high among the first two groups that the study had to be redesigned, retaining only the meditating patient group who remained faithful to their technique and comparing them with matched twin controls selected

from the hospital population at large. Among the findings to date, the Hartford research team reports a significantly greater level of improvement on discharge among meditating patients as compared to the rate of improvement of hospital discharges in general or of the matched twin comparison group. Preliminary data for this study, as yet incomplete, also suggests a reduction among meditating patients in the total amounts of psychotropic and sedative drugs they require, as well as a reduction in levels of pathology as measured by the MMPI. Final results await termination of the three-year study and accumulated data from a much larger number of subjects. At the present time the research team considers the meditation program a promising one and well suited for use with psychiatric inpatients suffering from character disorders, schizophrenia, psychotic depression and organic brain syndrome, among others. It appears that most seriously ill psychiatric patients can learn to meditate, providing that adequate attention is given to the various problems that may arise during the first several weeks of meditation.

Addressing themselves to the adjunctive use of meditation with patients in outpatient psychotherapy, a psychologist-psychiatrist team has classified clinical responses to meditation on the basis of anecdotal evidence accumulated from their own and colleagues' case material (Carrington and Ephron, 1976). These authors list the following personality changes as noted in meditating patients:

1. *Tension reduction:* a general lessening of anxiety, disappearance of inappropriate startle responses, improvement in psychosomatic conditions (e.g., tension headaches, hypertension, insomnias and hypersomnias), reduced need for psychotropic medication.

2. *Energy release:* increased physical stamina, increased creative productivity, increased productiveness of free associations during the therapeutic session.

3. *Superego amelioration:* lessened tendencies towards self-recrimination, lessened paranoid tendencies.

4. *Mood stabilization:* elevation and stabilization of mood in patients with neurotically determined depressions (although not, in their experience, in patients with acute depressive reactions. The latter tended to stop meditating

even though they might be showing beneficial results from the meditation.).

5. *Availability of affect:* increased affective relatedness to others, increased availability of affect during psychotherapeutic sessions.

6. *Individuation:* increased sense of separate identity, increased self-assertiveness (the self rather than the expectations of others becoming the point of reference).

7. *Antiaddictive properties:* lessening of tendencies toward the abuse of marijuana, alcohol or cigarettes.

The authors warn against overmeditation (i.e., meditating for several hours a day rather than the prescribed two 20-minute sessions) which may cause decompensation in borderline patients. They also identify a number of forms of resistance to meditation which may require working through in psychotherapy. If meditation alters a pathological lifestyle in a manner for which the patient is emotionally unprepared, the patient may stop meditating unless he is helped therapeutically to adjust to the change in self-image. Several advantages for the meditating psychotherapist are noted: increased sensitivity to unconscious processes, increased empathy, reduced fatigue after long hours of work, and greater tolerance of patients' negative transference reactions. These observations are consistent with studies of Zazen meditation (a more demanding form of meditation than TM), concerning the development of empathy in psychological counselor trainees. In one study, significant improvement in empathic ability was seen in those counselors who regularly practiced meditation during the course of the study, as compared to two control groups of counselor trainees who did *not* practice meditation.

BIBLIOGRAPHY

BANQUET, J. P. Spectral analysis of the EEG in meditation. *Electroencephalography and Clinical Neurophysiology*, 1973, *33*, 454.

CARRINGTON, P., and EPHRON, H. S. Meditation as an adjunct to psychotherapy. In S. Arieti and G. Chrzanowski (Eds.), *New demensions in psychiatry: A world view.* New York: Wiley, 1976.

SHAFII, M.; LAVELY, R.; and JAFFE, R. Meditation and marijuana. *American Journal of Psychiatry*, 1974, *131*, 60–63.

WALLACE, R. K. Physiological effects of transcendental meditation. *Science*, 1970, *167*, 1751–1754.

WALLACE, R. K.; BENSON, H.; and WILSON, A. F. A wakeful hypometabolic state. *American Journal of Physiology*, 1971, *221*, 795–799.

PATRICIA CARRINGTON
HARMON S. EPHRON

MEDUNA, LADISLAUS JOSEPH VON (1896–1964)

Ladislaus Joseph von Meduna was born March 27, 1896, in Budapest, Hungary. His family had originated in Papal nobility. He attended the medical school in Budapest, graduating from there in 1921 and then served in the Research Institute for Neuropathology under Karl Schaeffer. In 1927 he received an appointment as assistant professor in the University Clinic for Nervous and Mental Diseases, and director of its outpatient department, but also he continued his studies in neuropathology.

While at the National Hospital for Nervous and Mental Diseases (famous also for the work of Pandy on CSF protein and Hollos for his psychoanalytic work with psychotics) von Meduna was said to have noted the difference in the amount of glial tissue in the brain of a patient with epilepsy and those with schizophrenia. He had other reasons to believe that these two conditions were incompatible and he began to produce convulsions in schizophrenics. At first he used injections of camphor and in 1933 began using pentamethylene tetrazol (Metrazol) as a convulsive agent. He published papers on this in 1934 and 1935 and an extended monograph in 1937.

In 1939 he emigrated to the United States and became affiliated with Loyola University in Chicago. In 1943 he joined the Department of Psychiatry of the University of Illinois and the Illinois Neuropsychiatric Institute. Here he studied and promoted the use of CO_2 for psychoneurosis. He published numerous papers and several books, organized a research association for CO_2 therapy, was president of the American Society of Medical Psychiatry and founded the *Journal of Neuropsychiatry*.

Meduna's highly significant paper is "General Discussion of Cardiazol Treatment," in the *Journal of the American Psychiatric Association* (supplement), 1938, *94*, 40.

LEO H. BERMAN

MELANIN IN NEURAL TISSUES

The term, melanin, is applied to a group of brown or black pigments associated with protein and not often derived from tyrosine (monohydroxyphenylalanine) or from dihydroxyphenylalanine (DOPA) by the action of tyrosinase (DOPA oxidase), a copper-containing oxidative enzyme. The chemical mechanisms are complex, with many intermediate products formed and with other substances and processes also playing a role, and other synthetic mechanisms may exist. It is nonetheless of interest to incubate sections in a solution containing DOPA to determine the activity of tyrosinase (dopa oxidase), as manifested by the production of brown or black pigments, presumably melanin. It should be kept in mind that atmospheric oxygen oxidizes DOPA, particularly when it is in alkaline solution; also that DOPA can be oxidized by other enzyme systems.

Melanin is not soluble in organic solvents or in most aqueous solutions; tends to be darkened by many silver staining techniques; may be stained by basic dyes including the Nissl dyes; and is bleached by hydrogen peroxide, permanganate, and other oxidizing agents. A useful identifying technique is that described by Lillie which utilizes the capacity of melanin to absorb ferrous ions; the latter are then demonstrated by acidified ferricyanide solutions.

Melanin is normally found in some of the mesenchymal cells of the leptomeninges, especially at the base of the brain, but it is not limited to this area. It is also present in the cytoplasm of many neurons particularly those in the substantia nigra; the locus ceruleus and rostrocaudal column of nerve cells caudal to the locus coeruleus in the pons and medulla oblongata; scattered nerve cells in the roof of the IVth ventricle; in dorsal and sympathetic ganglia; and in dorsal autonomic ganglia.

In such intraneuronal sites, the melanin tends to be unstained by Nissl dyes in acid solutions, at a pH at which melanin at other sites are stained. This difference, and some others, have led to its designation as "neuromelanin," though the melanins at other sites are heterogenous and also vary in their properties. In disease states in which these neurons are destroyed, such as Parkinson's disease, the melanin is liberated into the tissues, partially engulfed by phagocytes, carried toward the blood vessels and then into the reticuloendothelial system for disposal. In this circumstance, some of the melanin becomes more basophilic with Nissl dyes in acid solution. Melanin may also be found in tumors, such as metastatic melanomas, melanosarcomas (tumors presumably arising from the melanin-containing mesenchymal cells of the leptomeninges), and rarely in meningiomas.

BIBLIOGRAPHY

BARDEN, H. The histochemical relationship of neuromelanin and lipofuscin. *Journal of Neuropathology and Experimental Neurology,* 1969, *28,* 419–441.

LILLIE, R. D. Ferrous ion uptake; a specific reaction of the melanins. *Archives of Pathology,* 1957, *64,* 100–104.

LILLIE, R. D. The basophilia of melanins. *Journal of Histochemistry and Cytochemistry,* 1955, *3,* 453–545.

IRWIN FEIGIN
ABNER WOLF

MEMORY

MEMORY: ANIMAL STUDIES

Collecting "all of the experiments in which retention data could be found after a diligent search of the literature," Schneck and Warden (1929), in the first comprehensive survey of the experimental literature on animal memory, uncovered 30 studies published in the period 1898 to 1926, based on subjects ranging from worms to primates. Interestingly, not a single study employing the delayed-response task was included in their review, although Hunter's classic paper appeared in 1913 and variations of the delayed-response paradigm had been explicitly used to assess animal memory. Possibly an implicit distinction between short-term and long-term memory—a distinction which later came to command such attention in studies of human memory—was partially responsible for this oversight, inasmuch as all of the studies cited by Schneck and Warden used retention intervals of at least 24 hours, whereas far shorter intervals were used with the delayed-response task, often only a matter of seconds. In any case, the early interest shown in animal memory, particularly by the comparative psychologists of the first quarter of the twentieth century, though not extinguished, had to smolder for more than three decades before igniting into a substantial research effort.

Methods of Studying Retention in Animals

For convenience we may classify the great variety of available methods into *acquisition* and *performance* techniques. In the former, the animal is trained on one or more tasks to some acquisition criterion, and after a period of time has elapsed retention of the previously learned material is assessed by one means or another, often by relearning. Because they do not lend themselves to repeated retesting, and because they often are obliged to employ substantial retention intervals, acquisition techniques find their greatest use in studies of long-term memory (LTM).

Performance techniques capitalize on an already-existing, well-learned relationship, established either experimentally or by the animal's ordinary experience. The degree to which an animal can maintain a given instance of this relationship over a time interval devoid of supporting cues constitutes the test of retention. In delayed matching-to-sample (DMTS), for example, the animal is first taught to choose from among a group of alternatives the stimulus that is identical to the sample, usually with the sample and alternative stimuli simultaneously available. After this relationship is well established, the effect of interposing retention intervals between removal of the sample stimulus and presentation of the alternatives is evaluated. In one version of the direct delayed-response technique, one of two food wells is simply baited with food in full view of the animal, who requires little if any training to choose the baited food well if allowed to do so immediately. Retention of this information is assessed by delaying the opportunity for choice over an interval during which the food wells are blocked from view. Obviously the performance techniques lend themselves to repeated tests of retention in the same animal without the necessity of acquisition training before each test and are therefore very useful for studying short-term memory (STM) functions in animals. A similar distinction, it might be noted, can be applied to the methods used to study STM and LTM in humans.

Animal Short-Term Memory

It was only natural that the enormous interest, empirical and theoretical, captured by human STM would soon invade the domain of animal behavior. A substantial number of studies, largely based on the DMTS paradigm, have provided us with data regarding the STM capacity of animals and some amount of theory. We know that the STM of monkeys as revealed by DMTS is not a fixed quantity but rather can be increased tenfold and more by accumulated practice (D'Amato, 1973). It has been established that under favorable conditions monkeys will show substantial retention after delay intervals of 3 minutes or more (D'Amato, 1973), while pigeons are far less gifted in this regard, often displaying little retention after only 5–15 seconds. In one study a dolphin produced almost perfect DMTS performance with a 2-minute retention interval, the longest at which it was tested.

A number of parallels in the operation of animal and human STM have recently been identified. Retention, as reflected by DMTS performance, can be impeded by presenting interfering materials either before or after the sample stimulus (proactive and retroactive interference, respectively). On the other hand, increasing the number of sample presentations or increasing the duration of the intertrial interval serves to enhance short-term retention. And there is even a hint of modality-specific interference, not unlike that which occurs in humans (D'Amato, 1973).

With all these points of contact it is somewhat surprising that the animal and human STM data depart so when it comes to the matter of the temporal capacity of STM, which a number of theorists have placed at a mere 30 seconds or less for human STM. That DMTS is a recognition task whereas most of human STM studies are based on recall seems not to be an important consideration, for there exists evidence that monkeys do equally well on STM tasks that are more analogous to recall than to recognition (D'Amato, 1973). Moreover, when assessed by methods other than DMTS, animal STM often appears even more impressive. More than half a century ago Köhler, in what was essentially a variation of the delayed-response task, found that chimpanzees were capable of remembering the spot where fruit had been buried 16½ hours earlier, although they had been ushered away from that location immediately after the food was buried. Under somewhat more controlled conditions, Yerkes and Yerkes (1928) extended this result to 48 hours. Because only a single "trial" was involved in these retention tests, they appear (at least according to some models) to qualify as assessments of STM; if so, they testify to an extraordinary STM capacity in higher infrahuman primates.

Apparently, even rats are capable of retaining for long periods of time information presented on a single trial. These results were obtained in reward-alternation studies (another performance technique) in which reward and nonreward alternated regularly, either at the end of a straight-alley apparatus or in the two arms of a T-maze. The rats' behavior clearly showed that, to some degree at least, they were able to remember the outcome of the previous trial for hours, perhaps even for 24 hours,

though the latter claim has been contested. In contrast, goldfish require special training procedures to produce evidence of retention after an interval of only 20 seconds.

One way of resolving the apparent disparity between human and animal STM with regard to temporal capacity is by granting animals the ability to engage in rehearsal or some such equivalent process. There is, however, very little evidence to support this assumption. The "rehearsal" studied by Wagner, Rudy, and Whitlow (1973) in rabbits subjected to Pavlovian conditioning of the nictitating membrane is better thought of as consolidation, a topic on which there is, of course, a considerable literature. *Rehearsal* differs from consolidation in that it implies an active—in humans, often verbally mediated—process by means of which received information can be maintained for an indefinite period of time. *Consolidation,* on the other hand, has generally referred to the passive continuation of a self-limiting process that is subject to premature termination by outside intervention. Unlike consolidation, rehearsal may be based on quite different neurological processes than those initiated by the received information. Indeed, rehearsal can and often does take place in a different modality from that in which the original information was encoded.

Be that as it may, if the formidable STM displayed by animals in DMTS and other tasks is the result of rehearsal (or more neutrally, "recycling"), it should be possible to steepen sharply the short-term retention gradient by interposing tasks that block the recycling process. Unfortunately, the scraps of relevant evidence currently available do not permit any conclusions on this score. If it turns out, as recently suggested, that animal STM is based on temporal discrimination processes rather than on limited-capacity storage mechanisms, the apparent disparity between the temporal capacity of animal and human STM can be reconciled without the postulation of recycling processes (D'Amato, 1973).

Long-Term Memory

A reader of the animal retention literature should be aware that what is left in the animal's head at the end of a retention interval is, like the partially filled cup, subject to different interpretations. An animal that has half-forgotten something has half-remembered it, too. But judging from the quite disparate conclusions sometimes drawn by different writers from the very same data, this reciprocity is not beyond being completely forgotten. Consequently, quantitative estimates of retention should be consulted wherever possible.

Long-term memory (LTM) has been studied experimentally in a wide variety of organisms, employing behaviors ranging from simple Pavlovian conditioned responses to the far more complex discrimination learning sets. In general, the results of this research parallel those obtained with humans: under favorable circumstances the LTM of animals is impressively durable, but after sufficiently long intervals some retention loss, even of well-learned behaviors, is inevitable.

To cite just a few illustrations, pigeons trained on a conditioned emotional response showed no retention loss whatever when tested 2½ years later, nor was a subsequent 1½-year interval effective in inducing forgetting. Pigeons have also displayed good—but by no means perfect—retention of a food-motivated response after a four-year retention interval. There is a hint here and there that retention of aversive events might generally be more lasting than retention of positive events, but it is difficult to investigate this important issue properly, and as yet no convincing data exist one way or the other.

The monkey's retention of object discriminations is also quite impressive, frequently remaining at very high levels for many months (Medin and Davis, 1974). Discrimination learning sets, which constitute a form of rule learning, have been shown to be retained with little or no loss for as long as seven months in monkeys and for five months in blue jays. However, with a long enough retention interval (up to six years), they too succumb to substantial forgetting (Bessemer and Stollnitz, 1971; Kamil, Lougee, and Shulman, 1973). Interestingly, monkeys and blue jays that enjoy the benefit of strongly established learning *sets* for object discriminations show quite significant forgetting of recent discriminations after intervals of as short as two or three minutes, as if the price exacted by well-developed learning sets for rapid learning of the new was accelerated forgetting of the old.

Forgetting in animals can be greatly encouraged in a variety of LTM tasks—perhaps including learning sets—by the simple expedient of introducing competing tasks either before or during the retention interval, the familiar processes of proactive and retroactive interference (Gleitman, 1971). Ontogenetic status is another significant variable in animal LTM. Despite the fact that early experiences often have profound effects on adult behavior organization, retention of specific experiences is relatively poor in very young rats and monkeys, improving with maturity.

Referred to Tulving's (1972) distinction between "episodic" and "semantic" memory, virtually all animal memory research falls into the first category, inasmuch as the to-be-remembered material is almost always an "autobiographical" event with specific temporal and spatial designations. Retention of learning sets, however, seems to be another matter. Here we are dealing with the retention of a rule that has no delimited spatiotemporal references, a rule that may be perfectly retained while the specific experiences upon which it was formulated fade rapidly from memory. Inappropriateness of nomenclature notwithstanding, we may have here an instance of semantic memory in animals.

Mechanisms of Animal Memory

Given the many congruences among the laboratory findings of human and animal memory research, it is not surprising that the conceptual accounting of animal memory has borrowed heavily from the human literature (e.g., Spear, 1973). As pointed out by Medin and Davis (1974), however, apart from hypotheses regarding the physical basis of memory, there has been little theorizing about the structure of animal memory. This may prove a fortunate omission. The kinds of questions that are interesting and relevant for animal memory are not necessarily those which are appropriate for human memory. For one thing, memory, like any other behavioral function in animals, has a survival value. This immediately raises the question of what memory is good for. An animal that forgets the meaning of the cues that signal a stalking predator is not likely to get the opportunity to relearn their significance. Consequently, we might expect that aversive events will generally prove unusually resistant to forgetting, a possibility that was mentioned earlier. The spatial location of the vital necessities of life also ought not to be easily forgotten, which is in keeping not only with the chimpanzee's remarkable STM for buried food, but also with the fact that animals perform far better on spatial delayed-response tasks than on the nonspatial variety.

On the other hand, remembering that it was chased by the farmer's dog the day before yesterday just as the sun was setting may not be of any particular advantage to the rabbit. Memory for the precise ordering of temporal events is a peculiarly human concern, possibly developed because of man's ability to contemplate and manipulate future events. Such capacities exist in animals at a very rudimentary level, if at all. Consequently, it is not surprising that evolution has not provided us with the faculty for performing exquisite discriminations with regard to the temporal ordering of past events, an oversight for which we have learned to compensate by means of clocks, calendars, and related devices. For their part, animals must rely on whatever temporal discriminative skills they might possess, plus assistance from such natural time-markers as the day-night cycle, the seasons of the year, and the cyclic changes in the habitat which they occasion. Viewed in this light, studies of animal retention may prove useful more for the information they yield about the temporal discrimination capacities of animals than for any insights into the limited-capacity storage-rehearsal devices thought to play so crucial a role in human memory.

Investigators of animal memory must also be alert to the various ways in which this function expresses itself in different species of animals. Because of the logical and physiological intimacy of learning and memory, species-specific learning implies species-specific memory. The preferences established by imprinting, for example, are often unusually resistant to forgetting. Certain facts of migration behavior imply an almost immutable LTM for events experienced in early life, prompting Thorpe (1963) to conclude that some strains of salmon and trout must be able to remember characteristics of their home stream for four years or more. At a less instinctive level, bees are reputed to remember the location of a food source for more than 30 days. Clearly these facts, and many others like them in the ethological literature, cannot safely be ignored by the student of animal memory. Only through the integration of evolutionary, ethological, and laboratory contributions will a coherent and comprehensive portrait of animal memory become discernible.

BIBLIOGRAPHY

Bessemer, D. W., and Stollnitz, F. Retention of discriminations and an analysis of learning set. In A. M. Schrier and F. Stollnitz (Eds.), *Behavior of nonhuman primates* (Vol. 4). New York: Academic Press, 1971. Pp. 1–58.

D'Amato, M. R. Delayed matching and short-term memory in monkeys. In G. H. Bower (Ed.), *The psychology of learning and motivation: Advances in research and theory* (Vol. 7). New York: Academic Press, 1973. Pp. 227–269.

Gleitman, H. Forgetting of long-term memories in animals. In W. K. Honig and P. H. R. James (Eds.), *Animal memory.* New York: Academic Press, 1971. Pp. 1–44.

Kamil, A. C.; Lougee, M.; and Shulman, R. I. Learning-set behavior in the learning-set experienced blue jay (*Cyanocitta cristata*). *Journal of Comparative and Physiological Psychology,* 1973, *82* (3), 394–405.

Medin, D. L., and Davis, R. T. Memory. In A. M. Schrier and F. Stollnitz (Eds.), *Behavior of nonhuman primates* (Vol. 5). New York: Academic Press, 1974. Pp. 1–47.

Schneck, M. R., and Warden, C. J. A comprehensive survey of the experimental literature on animal retention. *Pedagogical Seminary and Journal of Genetic Psychology,* 1929, *36,* 1–20.

Spear, N. E. Retrieval of memory in animals. *Psychological Review,* 1973, *80,* 163–194.

Thorpe, W. H. *Learning and instinct in animals* (2nd ed.). Cambridge: Harvard University Press, 1963.

Wagner, A. R.; Rudy, J. W.; and Whitlow, J. W. Rehearsal in animal conditioning. *Journal of Experimental Psychology,* 1973, *97,* 407–426.

Yerkes, R. M., and Yerkes, D. N. Concerning memory in the chimpanzee. *Journal of Comparative Psychology,* 1928, *8,* 237–271.

See also MEMORY: PHYSIOLOGICAL BASIS

MICHAEL R. D'AMATO

MEMORY: COMPUTER SIMULATION

Background

When digital computers arrived on the scene in the 1950s, psychologists were quick to use them. Early applications were concerned primarily with data reduction and analysis—the kinds of numerical calculations for which the machines had been originally intended. It was not long, however, until other, and perhaps more interesting applications came into being. Using computers to generate stimulus materials for experimental work, and later the direct, on-line, interactive control of experiments are two such applications. While the use of computers for data analysis, stimulus production and experimental control has been extremely important in psychology, one of the most interesting application areas has been their use for constructing simulation models or theories of human cognitive processes. This application is based upon the view that the computer is much more than a numeric manipulator.

Although the computer was originally developed primarily for numerical calculations, many were quick to recognize it as a more general purpose symbol-manipulating device. Computers are basically devices for performing a variety of operations upon internally coded information. The internal codes may represent numbers, and arithmetic is one class of operations. But the codes may represent any type of symbol, and the computer may perform operations such as storing, retrieving, comparing and associating symbols. With this realization came an important insight. Psychologists had long viewed cognitive behavior or thought as the covert manipulation of symbols. It should, therefore, be possible to use the general purpose, symbol-manipulating computer to construct representations (models) of cognitive behavior.

An important point to be noted here concerns the level of analysis or representation. The simulation work to be discussed is at an *information processing* level. That is, the human is viewed as a processor of information, capable of taking in information from the environment, performing operations upon it internally, and outputting it to the environment. This level of analysis may be contrasted to the neural network simulations that have also received much attention.

A primary goal of simulation models is their potential aid in clarifying or explaining the mechanisms underlying human cognition. To the extent they are successful, they should help understand the cause-effect relationships involved. A second goal, perhaps less elegant than the first, is that a model or theory synthe-

sizes: that is, it helps pull together a variety of ideas and data. The difficult task of explaining and synthesizing phenomena as complex as human cognition calls for powerful tools of representation and analysis. The computer program provides a highly flexible language for representing theoretical concepts and at the same time demands the formality and rigor of mathematics.

Computers actually speak many languages. These are the programming languages that have been developed in order for humans to communicate with the machines. Special languages have been developed for simulation work. The programming language is the counterpart of the mathematical equation; it embodies the concepts that make up the theory. The value of the computer itself is largely the result of the complexity of the programs that are generated to model cognitive phenomena. The actual machine serves as a device that generates consequences. By executing the programmed model on the computer it is possible to determine the theory's predictions. Thus, while the computer is not central to the theory itself, it is indispensable in exploring the consequences of complex theories.

It is difficult to separate efforts to construct simulation models of memory from other simulation work. Indeed, such a partition is necessarily arbitrary, because most simulations of cognitive processes involve some sort of representation of memory. Some of the simulation efforts in which memory has been involved have been referred to as question-answering programs, theorem-proving programs, problem-solving programs, natural-language programs, and concept-formation programs. Other simulation work oriented more towards traditional social or clinical psychology has also involved the development of memory representations. Examples are Abelson's (1963) work on opinion change and Colby's (1965) efforts in the area of neurotic belief-distortion.

While virtually all of these simulations have included a representation of some aspect of memory, the primary goal was not to discover and simulate memory. Another way of thinking about this point is to note that while the above simulation programs require a memory and processes for operating on memory, their primary focus was to represent some other aspect of behavior. Here again, however, it should be noted that such a distinction is quite arbitrary, and speaks more to how the psychologist defines or views his problem than to the nature of the system being simulated.

Two additional points have been made that also contribute to a decision about what should or should not be regarded as an example of a memory simulation program. As already noted, the simulation approach of interest here views the human as an information processing system and the approach is at that level of analysis. An information processing theory, however, need not be stated in the programming language of a computer. Many mathematical models or models stated in plain old-fashioned English prose are quite properly viewed as information-processing theories. But simulation in this context means a computer program that embodies the theoretical concepts; and if it is not programmed, it is not computer simulation. The second point is closely related. Although the computer itself is not necessary to the statement of the theory, it is important in exploring and testing the theory. Many process models have been described in flow chart language but never reached the stage of a debugged, running program. If a program has not been debugged and run, it is not a simulation. So, to be accepted as a computer simulation effort, a model must be developed to the point of a running program.

There is a reason for taking this position, which is essentially the reason for turning to simulation in the first place. Human memory obviously consists of a set of very complex structures and processes. The computer program provides a powerful procedure for expressing theories of complex phenomena and for exploring the implications of such expressions. To settle for anything less than a running program is to sacrifice the basic power of the technique.

Simulation Models

The number of simulation programs directed primarily to the analysis and study of human memory is relatively small. There are about seven models to be noted:

1. Feigenbaum's (1963) work on a learning program known as *EPAM* (Elementary Perceiver and Memorizer)

2. Hintzman's (1968) learning program known as *SAL* (Stimulus and Association Learner)

3. Quillian's (1969) model of *long-term* memory structure

4. Laughery's (1969) simulation of short-term memory

5. Reitman's (1970) simulation of short-term memory

6. Rumelhart, Lindsay, and Norman's (1972) major effort to represent long-term memory structures and processes

7. Anderson and Bower's (1973) simulation called *HAM* (Human Associative Memory).

All of these theoretical efforts have resulted in subsequent activity to develop them further. Two in particular have had a notable impact on our thinking about memory; they are the simulations developed by Feigenbaum and Quillian. The models of Rumelhart, Lindsay, and Norman, and of Anderson and Bower are more recent, but they also seem destined to have a major influence on the psychology of memory.

Feigenbaum's EPAM Model. This simulation was basically an attempt to explore the addition of information to long-term memory—learning. The task environment in which the memory processes were explored was the traditional serial and paired-associate learning of nonsense syllables. The model included several fundamental concepts that are characteristic of much subsequent work. These concepts include

1. a limited size short-term memory in which new information resides while being processed for storage in long-term memory

2. a tree structure or sorting net to represent long-term memory

3. an "executive routine" or processor that controlled the sequencing of information processing

4. a time base or "clock" which enabled the model to represent the real-time aspects of the learning task.

The sorting net as a representation of long-term memory was an important contribution. Learning was viewed as a process of acquiring discriminations and associations. The nodes of the net represented decision tests to discriminate between features of the stimulus elements (syllables) being learned. The terminal cells of the net contained the letters and syllables being stored or retrieved as well as information about their associates. During learning or acquisition, new discrimination tests were developed and added as nodes in the net, and the new letters, syllables and associates were added as new terminal cells. During retrieval the available cues or stimuli were sorted through the net to find the appropriate information regarding associations and responses. There were limitations to the concepts embodied in this earlier model. For example, the discrimination net had to be entered at a given node and could be searched in only one direction. The short-term memory was defined strictly on the basis of size and was independent of the specific nature of the contents or time in residence. Yet, the model represented a significant breakthrough in theorizing about memory and set the stage for more sophisticated simulations.

Quillian's Model. This simulation focused upon the structure of long-term memory. More specifically, Quillian developed a model to explore the relational network as an appropriate representation of semantic memory. The relational structure is a network of nodes, representing concepts or entities, connected by labeled links. The links describe relationships between the nodes. It is also important to note that links are directional. An example of two elements linked by a relation would be *rose, color, red.* Any number of relations may be attached to a single node.

This type of network can be described as a directed graph. Such a structure may contain as many kinds of links as there are relations to be distinguished by the system. Property or value relationships, such as color, are typical. The classical "association by contiguity" can be represented as a relation of simultaneity or "followed by." An important relation is the subset or superset because it is this link that permits the network to represent hierarchical structure. An example would be *bird, subset, robin.* While hierarchical structure can be represented in this fashion, it is also important to note that the network itself is not a hierarchical structure. Nodes may link to other nodes in the network that in some sense are "above" them. Putting it another way, the network is a general graph, not a tree.

The relational network as a representation of long-term memory was an important development for cognitive theory in general and for simulation in particular. While Quillian's work was directly addressing the structure and functioning of human memory, and was most influential in psychology, it was primarily concerned with the representation of semantics or meaning. The relata of a particular node represents the meaning of the concept or entity. Quillian defined a node's immediate surroundings as its immediate definition and the complete field accessible from a node as its full concept.

An important dimension of Quillian's work was a series of experiments that he and Collins carried out regarding the efficacy of the relational network as a memory model. The basic paradigm of their studies involved measuring latencies in responding *yes* or *no* about the truth of statements. The assumption was that the more tracing through the network that had to be done to determine the truth of a statement, the longer the latency. For example, the statement "canaries are yellow" would produce a faster *yes* response than "canaries have wings," because the former would require only tracing the structure "canaries, color, yellow" while the latter would require tracing "canaries, superset, birds, ability, fly." The results of these and similar studies lend support for the relational network as a means of representing the complex structure of long-term memory.

Rumelhart, Lindsay, and Norman's Model. In the introduction to a paper representing their long-term memory simulation, Rumelhart, Lindsay, and Norman (1972) correctly note that psychological theories of human memory have been closely related to one type of memory function: how people remember lists of words. Yet, as they further point out, memory is required to support a large number of highly complex tasks such as answering complicated questions based upon information stored in memory, solving problems, making logical deductions and understanding ideas. Indeed, rote memorization is seldom required during the life of the average adult. In response to this observation, Rumelhart, Lindsay, and Norman take on a king-sized task: to construct a simulation model of memory whose "structure is capable of encoding and representing a reasonable range of the information it is likely to encounter, that has direct and explicit rules for translating external information into an internal representation, and that is flexible enough to support a variety of cognitive and information-processing tasks."

The basic structure of the model is the relational network, with nodes and relational connections between nodes. The nodes, of course, represent information in the memory and the relations are various types of associations. Relations have two properties, they are labeled and directed. Actually relations are bidirectional but not symmetrical. A distinction is made between primary and secondary nodes: primary nodes refer directly to words of the language while secondary nodes represent concepts as they are used in specific contexts.

This model distinguishes among three types of information: *concepts, events* and *episodes.* A concept is a particular idea, an event is an action with actors and objects, and an episode is a series of events or actions. These different types of information can be better understood by noting the kinds of relations that are used to represent them. Three types of relations are used to define concepts: *isa, is* and *has.* The *isa* relation defines set membership, such as *cat isa animal.* Keep in mind that the relations are directional which means the same connection defines the subset relationship. The *is* and *has* relations define property relations, *is* for qualities and *has* for objects. Examples are *ball is round* and *bird has wings.* An event is essentially a scenario with actors, actions and objects. The scheme for representing events is similar to Fillmore's case grammar in which the representation centers around the verb. The conceptualization of the event permits the encoding of stored information in the memory structure. An episode is a cluster of events or actions and provides temporal relations. Special relations between events called *propositional conjunctions* are used. Examples of these conjunctions are the *then* and *while* relations which define specified temporal order and unspecified temporal order respectively.

In addition to the relational network, the model contains an executive routine or interpretive system and a relatively small set of *primitive* routines. It also includes a limited-capacity short-term memory, which is essentially a working storage for holding temporary

results and information needed to keep track of where a process is in its execution. If the short-term memory is exceeded, information will be lost, and errors will occur.

The simulation work of Rumelhart, Lindsay, and Norman is a significant step in the development of memory theory. The model represents a more comprehensive theory of memory than previous efforts. The structure and processes provide both a flexibility and explicitness that enables a variety of complex memory tasks to be simulated. The power of computer simulation techniques for representing complexity is evident in this work. A second aspect of this model that provides a step forward is the conceptualization of event clusters. This technique permits procedures for retrieving, manipulating and evaluating stored information—the processes of the model—to be encoded in the memory structure in the same way as conceptual information is stored. In a sense, an *action* relation is equivalent to carrying out that action subroutine.

Although other contributions could be noted, there is one limitation that should be realized; namely, relatively little formal testing of the model has been carried out to date. This is not, of course, a criticism of the model itself. It is instead a caution that speaks to the current stage of development. However, while there is much left to be done on their model, Rumelhart, Lindsay, and Norman have clearly provided an important contribution to memory theory.

Anderson and Bower's HAM model. This simulation is an effort to develop a comprehensive theory of human associative memory. The model is in many respects similar to the Rumelhart, Lindsay, and Norman model. The memory structure is basically a relational network and there is a short-term memory with a limited capacity. There is, however, a major difference between these two modeling efforts. Rumelhart, Lindsay, and Norman have moved boldly to construct a memory model that would be much more comprehensive than any previously developed. They have not hesitated to postulate ideas, structures and processes where experimental evidence has not been available to lead the way. This comment is not to imply that they are insensitive to the need for experimental verification. They are prepared, however, to move theoretically with the understanding that experimental verification may have to await the development of new experimental paradigms and technology.

Anderson and Bower, while certainly at the forefront of theoretical developments, have attempted to maintain a closer integration of theory development and experimentation. Their successes to date are impressive. For example, a variety of experiments on learning and remembering sentences, using reaction time and recall probability measures, indicate good qualitative and quantitative fits between the model's output and the experimental results. It will be interesting to observe these two theoretical programs in the future to note where they converge or diverge.

General Comments

In the years since Feigenbaum published the EPAM model, computer simulation models of memory have evidenced considerable progress. Models now being developed enable the simulated subject to emerge from the laboratory world of nonsense syllables and sequences of digits into the real world of language comprehension, problem solving and logical reasoning with the same underlying memory structure. Obviously, the computerized human in many ways does not yet match the object of the simulation. But progress is evident. The power of the relational network is revealed by noting that virtually any concept, idea, or thought can be represented with this notation. The comprehensive nature of recent models permits the theoretical analysis of behavior in more complex, real-world tasks. This analysis in turn permits the exploration of interactions between parts of the system that previous approaches had attempted to study independently through experimental isolation.

In the future it will be more difficult to consider simulation of memory in isolation. It is more likely to be considered within the context of tasks such as comprehending language and other human functions that memory must service.

BIBLIOGRAPHY

ABELSON, R. P. Computer simulation of "hot" cognition. In S. Tomkins and S. Messick (Eds.), *Computer simulation of personality.* New York: Wiley, 1963. Pp. 277–298.
ANDERSON, J. R., and BOWER, G. H. *Human associative memory.* Washington: Winston, 1973.
COLBY, K. M. Computer simulation of neurotic processes. In R. Staay, and B. Waxman (Eds.), *Computers in biomedical research* (Vol. 1). New York: Academic Press, 1965.
FEIGENBAUM, E. A. The simulation of verbal learning behavior. In E. A. Feigenbaum, and J. Feldman (Eds.), *Computers and thought.* New York: McGraw-Hill, 1963. Pp. 297–309.
HINTZMAN, D. L. Explorations with a discrimination net model for paired-associate learning. *Journal of Mathematical Psychology,* 1968, *5,* 123–162.
LAUGHERY, K. R. Computer simulation of short-term memory: A component-decay model. In G. H. Bower, and J. T. Spence (Eds.), *The psychology of learning and motivation* (Vol. 3). New York: Academic Press, 1969. Pp. 135–200.
QUILLIAN, M. R. The teachable language comprehender: A program to understand English. *Communications of the Association for Computing Machinery,* 1969, *12,* 459–476.
REITMAN, J. Computer simulation of an information processing model of short-term memory. In D. A. Norman (Ed.), *Models of human memory.* New York: Academic Press, 1970. Pp. 117–148.
RUMELHART, D. E.; LINDSAY, P. H.; and NORMAN, D. A. A process model for long-term memory. In E. Tulving, and W. Donaldson (Eds.), *Organization and memory.* New York: Academic Press, 1972. Pp. 197–246.

KENNETH R. LAUGHERY

MEMORY: CONSOLIDATION THEORY

Consolidation theory represents a general conception that relatively permanent memories are formed by processes which require considerable time, often extending beyond active practice or experience.

This concept has been known for over the 75 years since its first clear statement in 1900, but none of the many particular hypotheses which have been put forward concerning the processes involved in the consolidation of memory is widely accepted. Knowledge of the behavioral phenomena to which consolidation theory is addressed continues to advance so rapidly as to make particular hypotheses outmoded soon after their formulation. The neurology of learning and memory, on the other hand, is still in too speculative a state to provide a firm base for theory.

History

Müller and Pilzecker are credited with the first elaboration of consolidation theory in 1900. They suggested that there was a neural process which must perseverate for some time after learning in order to consolidate memory. The perseveration was subject to disruption by new input, which would have the effect of preventing memory consolidation. Specifically they suggested that retroactive inhibition was produced by new activity interfering with the consolidation of recently learned material.

Retroactive inhibition eventually proved more amenable to other types of explanations. However, the relevance of consolidation theory to retrograde amnesia from accidental head injuries was almost immediately noted. *Retrograde amnesia,* the lack of memory for events which precede trauma or massive stimulation of the nervous system, became the primary behavioral evidence supporting consolidation theory. This amnesia frequently occurs in gradient form, with poorest memory for events immediately before the accident and progressively better memory for events more distant in time from the accident. Such evidence suggests that consolidation progresses steadily. The longer it continues before disruption, the more memory is formed. Retrograde amnesia evidence also suggests that there may be little overt sign that consolidation is proceeding, since the amnesia gradient sometimes extends over many minutes or even hours during which there is no sign of practice, rehearsal, or awareness of the memories. There are variations in degree of amnesia which are not due to the amount of time before trauma, both between individuals and between memories within an individual, so that the rate of consolidation or the amount of consolidation necessary for memory is assumed to vary.

More controlled and precise observations of retrograde amnesia began with the extensive use of electroconvulsive shock (ECS) therapy in the 1930s. ECS reliably produces retrograde amnesia. In 1949, C. P. Duncan extended the use of ECS to laboratory animals, and soon other amnesic agents (e.g., anoxia, anesthesia) were being studied in the laboratory.

A proliferation of laboratory studies of amnesia, and eventually also of memory facilitation, has continued to the present time. Added to the clinical observation of amnesias in humans, this has produced considerable data, reviewed below, on the relation of temporal, situational, behavioral, neuroanatomical, and pharmacological variables to memory phenomena.

In the same year, 1949, that laboratory research into amnesia began, D. O. Hebb, in his *Organization of Behavior,* stimulated theoretical development with specific hypotheses about neurological processes involved in consolidation. Electrical activity continuing after cessation of stimulation had been noted in spinal reflexes since Sherrington. It was hypothesized that there were neural circuits which fed back into themselves, reexciting activity in the circuit, thus producing the afterdischarges. Hebb postulated that such self-reexciting reverberating circuits kept a "memory" active although permanent neural change did not occur immediately. Further, this reverberatory activity, by producing repeated activity of synapses, was said to be responsible for the slow buildup of permanent changes in synaptic resistance, the postulated neural substrate of long-term memory. Thus, two memory processes—a transitory one for immediate memory and a permanent, structural one for long-term memory—were postulated.

Dual-process theories of memory continue to be popular, extending to cognitive theories. Consolidation theory has been one base for the hypothesis of two different memory stores: one more immediately sensory, of limited capacity and brief duration; the other more semantic, requiring processing, of great capacity and long duration. In many of these theories the short-term store is only temporary, material being lost as it is replaced by new material in the limited capacity store, while the long-term store is permanent, with lack of overt expression of memory due to retrieval failure. The cognitive analogues of consolidation theory attend to semantic and organizational processing, which within these theories is equivalent to consolidation. By contrast, most expressions of consolidation theory conceive of neural fixation of rather simple memories, the emphasis being on anatomical locations and physiological mechanisms of fixation. Interestingly, some of the earliest discussion of human amnesia spoke of consolidation as the association and organization of new learning with established learning, as opposed to simple fixation. Cognitive processing received increasing emphasis during the revival of interest in clinical evidence, to the point that some accounts of amnesia entirely ignore fixation difficulties in favor of problems of meaningful integration of new experiences into existing cognitive structures.

Several features of Hebb's general formulation remain controversial. There is as yet no direct evidence of reverberatory activity in the nervous system, and single chemical processes which grow and decline with time have been offered as alternatives to the dual process conception. In addition, dual processes which are independent, that is, with long-term storage unaffected by short-term storage, have been suggested. There is, moreover, no direct evidence yet that learning produces structural changes at the synapse. While much speculation still centers on the synapse, long-term memory has been attributed to other neural mechanisms, specifically encoding in neuronal RNA or protein synthesis, which may or may not have their effects on synaptic resistance.

Finally, there is continuing disagreement about whether the behavioral evidence should be interpreted in terms of storage at all. Disputes about whether amnesias, in particular, represent retrieval or storage failures have abounded in the behavioral literature since the 1950s. Consolidation theory attributes amnesia to a failure to store memories. Four classes of evidence have been used to bring the basic assumption of storage failure into question:

1. evidence that apparent amnesias may reflect suppression of behavior by competing demands on the animal

2. that the absent memories may recover

3. that nonperformance may reflect inappropriate cueing rather than absence of memories

4. that amnesia may reflect interference with motor mechanisms.

Clinical Amnesias

The introduction of careful control comparisons, refined techniques in the measurement of memory, and care in implicating memory as opposed to motivational or sensory variables in performance, all represent important recent methodological advances in this area.

Clinical amnesias from head and other bodily injuries, electroconvulsive therapy, epileptic seizures, and brain surgery usually have a retrograde component. There is almost always some recovery, frequently reported as working from distant memories to memories more closely preceding the trauma. However, a residual retrograde amnesia for shortly preceding events often remains. Problems with a simple consolidation interpretation come from the observation that there are often marked irregularities in the retrograde scaling of memory loss, most noticeably when distant memories may be lost although many more recent memories are not. Perhaps factors other than consolidation, such as emotional factors, are involved in these exceptions. Alternatively, perhaps a simple temporal scale of memory loss is not to be expected if consolidation is not simply a function of time, and if cerebral assaults interfere in some manner with weakly consolidated memories, regardless of their age.

Clinical retrograde amnesia is frequently accompanied by anterograde amnesia, in which the patient has difficulty in new learning. There is little problem in holding new memories temporarily, but they do not last over any period of distraction which exceeds a few minutes. It is as if the consolidation processes were inoperative, with a resulting inability to transfer short-term memory into long-term memory. Briefly, several types of patients reveal marked anterograde amnesias which are taken as strong evidence for an impaired consolidation process. A now classic case is Milner's report of H. M. Following bilateral temporal lobe lesions to correct epilepsy, H. M. had a normal IQ and good short-term memory as long as he maintained attention to the material. If he was distracted, or if too much information was presented so as to exceed a limited capacity, his forgetting was prodigious. This evidence, together with stimulation studies on lower animals (reviewed below) is responsible for the view that the temporal lobes, particularly the hippocampus, is implicated in consolidation. Also, in nonoperated epileptics, temporal lobe seizures produce both retrograde and anterograde amnesia. A related, but not easily interpreted, finding is that these patients frequently experience strong *déjà vu* phenomena associated with their seizures.

Korsakoff patients, suffering limbic system (medial dorsal neuclei, mammillary bodies) brain damage from years of alcoholism, also show impressive anterograde amnesia. Discussions of these cases emphasize retrieval problems and impairment of organizational and semantic processing. The impairment seems more general than just memory. These patients conspicuously lack initiative in planning and organizing anything in their lives, including their daily activities. Senile brain deterioration is associated with a wide spectrum of memory disorders frequently difficult to disentangle from other effects, but anterograde amnesia is often present in some degree.

Experimental Amnesia and Memory Facilitation

Retrograde amnesia in the laboratory has been most frequently and most reliably produced by ECS, but a variety of other amnestic agents have been found, including many anesthetics, radical changes in body temperature, carbon dioxide, anoxia, spreading cortical depression, protein synthesis inhibitors, RNA synthesis inhibitors, stimulation of the hippocampus, stimulation of the caudate nucleus, and anticholinesterases. Certain CNS stimulants (e.g., strychnine) at appropriate doses, and protein synthesis or RNA synthesis stimulators have also been reported to facilitate memory. Some of these agents have obvious implications for anatomical involvements in consolidation, for example, the cerebral cortex, the hippocampus, the caudate; others for possible neural mechanisms, for example, protein synthesis, RNA synthesis, synaptic transmitters. However, there is little consensus on the interpretation of the pattern of these implications, particularly when the complexity of ECS effects are included.

The complexity of findings and the diversity of hypotheses offered is exemplified by the effects of administration of anticholinesterases which enhance synaptic accumulation of acetylcholine. It has been reported that besides producing brief retrograde amnesia, they facilitate recent memory, decrease more mature memory, and again facilitate very old memory. Scopolamine, which blocks acetylcholine receptors, has opposite effects. This sort of evidence has been used to suggest a single consolidation process involving neurotransmitters such as acetylcholine, which develops and wanes over rather long periods. Within this approach there is an optimum level of neural transmitter for appropriate behavioral per-

formance, either too little or too much producing poorer performance.

Several findings have implications for the mode of action of ECS. Convulsions are not necessary; animals anesthetized before ECS (preventing convulsions) show retrograde amnesia. The degree of amnesia produced has been found to correlate with the amount of current used for ECS, and with the amount of disruption in cortical theta activity. Further, the disruption in cortical EEG patterns has been noted to last a considerable time.

Amnestic agents often do not have all-or-none effects. Two ECS treatments one hour apart produce more amnesia than either one alone, and a long period of spreading depression produces more amnesia than a short period.

Many of the procedures for investigating ECS-produced retrograde amnesia have evolved from efforts to eliminate alternative interpretations to consolidation. Almost all recent studies employ one-trial passive avoidance tasks. The animal receives one very painful experience, usually a foot shock, in a previously neutral or positive situation. A discriminated avoidance can be clearly demonstrated to follow the one foot shock. The methodological advantages are many. Only one ECS is administered; repeated ECS treatments raise questions of permanent neural damage, and demonstrably produce fear and avoidance. Since ECS can be administered in the same location as the foot shock, no behavioral competition between fear of foot shock and any possible fear of ECS could occur. In fact, whether or not the ECS occurs in the training situation appears to be inconsequential. The demonstration of discriminated avoidance is crucial in eliminating the possibility that only a general conditioned emotional response, such as freezing in the rat, is disinhibited by the ECS or countered by conditioned relaxation introduced by the ECS.

If ECS quickly follows the foot shock, amnesia in the form of approach to the foot shock situation can be reliably demonstrated the following day. The presence of a retrogradient is very reliably found, but the temporal duration of the foot shock-ECS interval gradient itself varies greatly, from 10 sec to 6 hours, and the variables involved have yet to be empirically identified.

Retrograde amnesia has only rarely been reported in an appetitive, rather than avoidance, task. Again, the variables responsible for the difference in susceptibility to retrograde amnesia have yet to be identified.

Several types of evidence are currently used to support retrieval explanations of retrograde amnesia. There have been some reports that amnesia results when ECS follows only the second of two widely spaced foot shocks. Since ample time for consolidation follows the first foot shock, this has been interpreted as evidence that ECS, through association with the reactivated foot shock memory, somehow interferes with its retrieval. This evidence has not always been replicated.

It has been suggested that in retrograde amnesia the foot shock memory is state-dependent, that is, associated with the ECS-altered state of the animal during consolidation. Failure to avoid is due to the lack of the crucial ECS-state cues at the time of the retention test. Tests soon after the ECS do, in fact, yield considerable avoidance. Other applications and tests of this notion are awaited.

Reminders, delivered before retention tests, have been highly successful in recovering avoidance from ECS-produced amnesia. The reminder may be another foot shock so small as to be almost insignificant to a control animal, or it may be another mildly fear-producing event. It may be administered in either the original foot shock situation or elsewhere. The recovery is relatively permanent.

The interpretation that memories in retrograde amnesia only require highly determined retrieval cues is also supported by the finding that amnesic memories sometimes recover with repeated exposure to the training situation.

The question of memory storage is further complicated by the fact that autonomic indicators of emotional arousal, for example, heart rate, urination and defecation, have frequently been reported in animals whose lack of avoidance defines them as amnesic in respect to a fear memory.

Finally, an amnestic agent has recently come to light which hardly shares the major characteristic of other agents; it does not involve intervention of some outside chemical or electrical event, or sudden trauma. Detention of the animal in the training situation produces retrograde amnesia, and it enhances the amnesia produced by ECS.

In conclusion, although there are serious difficulties in encompassing the data within a consolidation framework, no other general approach has been developed in sufficient detail to represent an alternative. Perhaps refinement and extension of consolidation theory will prove successful.

BIBLIOGRAPHY

GLICKMAN, S. E. Perseverative neural processes and consolidation of the memory trace. *Psychological Bulletin,* 1961, *58,* 218–233.

McGAUGH, J. L., and HERZ, M. M. (Eds.). *Memory consolidation.* San Francisco: Albion, 1972.

MILLER, R. R., and SPRINGER, A. D. Amnesia, consolidation, and retrieval. *Psychological Review,* 1973, *80,* 69–79.

SQUIRE, L. R. Short-term memory as a biological entity. In D. Deutsch and J. Deutsch (Eds.), *Short-term memory.* New York: Academic Press, 1975.

TALLAND, G. *The pathology of memory.* New York: Academic Press, 1969.

See also MEMORY: EFFECTS OF BRAIN DAMAGE; MEMORY: PHYSIOLOGICAL BASIS

RICHARD J. KOPPENAAL

MEMORY: DEVELOPMENTAL CHANGES

The number of items in a series that can be remembered and correctly recalled increases from approximately four items by a child five years of age to seven items by a child of twelve. For this reason, questions assessing memory abilities have often been included within comprehensive tests of intellectual development; memory abilities have been found to parallel many other general cognitive abilities. The importance of memory in clinical evaluations of developmental and individual differences in intelligence, and the potential significance of memory as a factor in various theories of cognition, has instigated a considerable volume of research on memory abilities in children. Most early investigators, working from an associationistic or Gestalt framework, described memory in terms of the capacity to form associations and to retain them free from interference over time. It was assumed that these general theories of memory were applicable at all ages, although the memory capacity of children was less than the capacity of adults.

However, there has been an increasing recognition that the development of memory cannot be described solely in terms of an increasing biological capacity for forming and retaining associations. There are also changes in the processes or strategies which are used by individuals at different ages to facilitate remembering. Information-processing theories of memory distinguish three major processes—acquisition, retention, and retrieval. Generally, acquisition or encoding involves the learning of new behaviors or the memorizing of new information. This information must then be retained or stored in such a way that it is available at a later time. Encoding and retention often involve the integration of new information with what is already known from earlier occasions. Finally, the individual must be able to retrieve the information. Retrieval can involve either the recognition of external events as familiar, or the recall of memories solely on the basis of stored information. These distinctions are useful, because they allow the specification of the developmental course of each separate process, and there is no reason to assume that the processes develop in parallel throughout the life span.

Research

In addition to this emphasis on processes or strategies for remembering, there have been other changes in the character of research on children's memory. First, there has been an increasing recognition that developmental changes in processes cannot be explained solely in terms of the increasing age of the individual, but rather must be expressed as a function of independent variables, such as the activities of the child, social, cultural, and educational influences, and other cognitive changes, which can act over several years to bring about certain changes in memory processes. Second, the recognition of developmental change as a key problem requiring explanation has made obvious the similarities among investigations of children's memory and investigations of memory changes in adulthood and old age. As a result, each of these areas is being enriched by familiarity with the theories and research methods being used to investigate other regions of the life span. Third, developmental research in memory is now being conducted in other cultures in order to isolate the environmental and cultural variables which may affect the rate or the sequence of developmental changes in memory. The necessity for attention to the appropriate historical context of memory development is illustrated by the observation that preschoolers tested after 1969 benefit more than those tested previously from the use of pictorial elaboration in learning paired associates (Reese, 1974).

Memory in Infants

The habituation of various behavioral and autonomic responses to the repeated presentation of auditory and visual stimuli is evidence that infants can acquire memory traces and so recognize these stimuli as familiar. Further evidence is provided if the presentation of new or slightly altered stimuli produces an increment in responding, indicating an ability to compare the new stimulus with the memory trace of previously presented stimuli. Long-term recognition memory has been demonstrated in infants as young as five to six months of age, who can recognize an abstract pattern seen 48 hours earlier and photographs of faces presented two weeks previously (Fagan, 1973). Nevertheless, there are a number of methodological problems associated with habituation research in infants, and the processes which might be involved in infant recognition memory have not yet been identified. For these reasons, recognition memory in infants is often not considered to be continuous with the memory processes that develop later in childhood.

Memory in Childhood and Adolescence

Recognition memory abilities continue to improve significantly from two to four years of age. During this time, children become able to remember many different stimuli and to discriminate previously presented stimuli from new stimuli which they have not seen before. In one such investigation, children were able to recognize approximately 90% of 18 previously viewed objects when these were presented along with 18 new objects (Perlmutter and Myers, 1974).

Recall abilities depend on the development of symbolic or representational abilities at the conclusion of the sensorimotor period, such that an object or event which is not immediately visible can be reconstructed or imagined in thought by the child. Thus, the retrieval of information in a recall procedure is considerably more difficult than is the recognition of stimuli as familiar. Recall abilities have been demonstrated for children as young as two years of age, who were shown pairs of objects, which were then hidden in a box. The children were able to recall a single item over 90% of the time and recalled 75% of all the items shown (Goldberg, Perlmutter, and Myers, 1974).

The major change in memory abilities during early childhood is an increase in the number of learning and memorizing processes or strategies which can facilitate later recognition and recall. As children grow older, they not only become more able and likely to use these strategies, but also have a better understanding of the circumstances which call for the use of particular strategies (Flavell, 1970; Meacham, 1972). This increasingly active, intentional, or deliberate use of strategies for remembering can be illustrated with examples from three widely used research paradigms: paired-associates learning, serial learning, and free recall.

Paired Associates. In a paired-associates learning procedure, a stimulus and a response item are presented together as a pair. The task is to indicate the response item when the stimulus item is presented alone. One way to facilitate paired-associates learning is to construct or elaborate upon an event which can provide a shared meaning for the two items. Older children are more able than younger children to use sentences with verbs and prepositions, rather than conjunctions, and to construct imaginative mediating events in their attempts to provide shared meanings. Older children are also more likely to spontaneously engage in such elaboration, and so the prompts which are required to elicit elaboration can be less explicit. For example, the instruction to generate a sentence relating the items is not sufficient to facilitate learning in five-year-olds but is sufficient for children seven years of age and older. A more explicit prompt, providing a sentence or a picture which relates the items to be remembered, can facilitate learning for four- and five-year-olds, but is even more effective for older children. Adolescents spontaneously engage in elaboration, so a minimal instruction

to learn the items as well as possible is sufficient to promote elaboration and successful learning (Rohwer, 1973).

A recurrent issue has been whether paired-associates learning at various ages is facilitated by verbal or pictorial presentation of prompts and items to be remembered. Research has supported a facilitative effect for both modes, as well as shown no differences as a function of modality; one implication is that the differences are due merely to procedural variations. The emphasis in such investigations is generally upon acquisition rather than retention over long intervals of time. However, when subjects have been tested one week after initial learning, retention has been better for items presented as pictures than for items presented as words (Calhoun, 1974).

Serial Recall. Further evidence for the increasingly active involvement of older children in memorizing is found in studies of serial recall. In the serial recall procedure, items of a list to be remembered are presented one at a time, and the task is to remember all of the items in the order presented. Between eight and ten years of age, children acquire the strategy of rehearsal, repeating items in a list over and over, which greatly facilitates performance on the serial recall task (Frank and Rabinovitch, 1974). A variety of behavioral data is observed with the development of rehearsal abilities: younger children are able to rehearse only two or three items, while older children can rehearse many more; rehearsal is accompanied by improved recall of the initial items in a series; and while a child is rehearsing, there are often accompanying lip movements (Flavell, 1970).

Serial rehearsal appears to be a relatively simple memory activity, and the benefits in improved recall are substantial, so efforts have been made to teach rehearsal to children before the age at which rehearsal normally occurs. Five-year-olds can engage in rehearsal following instructions to whisper aloud the names of the items as they are presented, and there is a corresponding improvement in serial recall. Nevertheless, when a free choice of memorizing activities is allowed, or when an additional serial recall test is administered the following week (Hagen, Hargrave, and Ross, 1973), children between five and eight years of age abandon the new rehearsal strategy. The failure to spontaneously engage in a memory activity demonstrated to be within their capability has been termed production deficiency (Flavell, 1970). Cross-cultural research indicates that certain aspects of formal schooling rather than the age of the child may be critical for the development of rehearsal abilities according to the ages outlined above (Wagner, 1974).

Free Recall. A free recall procedure, in contrast to the serial recall procedure, does not require that items be recalled in the order in which they were presented. A consistent finding in free recall is that a greater number of items can be recalled if they are categorized into many small groups, since the names of the appropriate categories can then assist in the recall of the various items within each category. For children as young as two years of age, the presentation of blocked or easily categorizable lists results in greater clustering during recall and a greater number of correctly recalled items, than does the presentation of a list of randomly arranged items. With increasing age, children become better able to take advantage of the initial organization within lists of items. However, in a recent investigation, which used categorized items that were not also highly associated, the availability of categories did not facilitate recall for five- and ten-year-old children (Lange, 1973).

Older children are more active than younger children in categorizing items for free recall. Evidence is obtained from investigations in which children are allowed a study period during which they can actively manipulate pictures of items that later must be recalled. The sorting of these items increases with age, with a substantial increase occurring at approximately ten years of age (Neimark, Slotnick, and Ulrich, 1971). The ability to categorize per se also undergoes a sequence of developmental changes, with the categories of younger children being more fragmented and involving different concepts than those of older children. Several attempts have been made to train children between six and ten years of age to sort items to be recalled into appropriate categories. Such training is generally successful, resulting in greater recall and greater clustering of items during recall. Cross-cultural research has shown that exposure to formal education and

modern living circumstances can alter the categories which are used to sort items in a free recall task (Scribner, 1974).

Attention to the organization of items can be important not only during acquisition, but also during the retrieval phase of the free recall procedure. When older children and adults are provided with names of the categories of items to be recalled, the number of items successfully retrieved is increased. Children under approximately nine years of age, however, continue to be less successful at recalling all of the items, unless they are also reminded of the number of items within each category (Kobasigawa, 1974). The value of retrieval cues in facilitating recall is not readily apparent to young children. For example, a strong suggestion by an adult is necessary for three- to five-year-old children to use pictures as retrieval cues in recalling the names of toys which are hidden (Ritter, Kaprove, Fitch, and Flavell, 1973).

Organization of Memory. A current conception of the organization of memory considers memory traces as lists of attributes. Various investigations, typically involving a false recognition procedure, indicate a developmental change in the attributes available for encoding. For example, seven-year-old children can encode items according to sounds or taxonomic categories, while eleven-year-olds become able to encode according to the evaluative dimension of the semantic differential. It is likely that encoding in terms of attributes is characteristic of memory at all ages, but with increasing age there is a greater flexibility in choosing appropriate attributes for remembering.

When items or words are presented within sentences, the semantic information which can be encoded is of course more complex than for single words. In investigations of semantic memory for sentences, adults confidently but incorrectly recognize as familiar new sentences based on premises found in sentences which were actually presented earlier. These instances of false recognition suggest that in comprehending sentences, semantic information is evaluated with respect to and integrated with the listener's previous understanding of the world. Remembering then depends upon the reconstruction of the original event from the semantic information, rather than the retrieval of the sentence as it was actually presented. In various investigations, children between the ages of five and ten also incorrectly recognized semantically correct but nonpresented sentences, thus indicating their ability to acquire and remember semantic information in the same manner as adults (Paris and Mahoney, 1974). This theory of semantic integration is consistent with Piaget's theory of memory, according to which recall and recognition are processes of interpretation or reconstruction based on the more general structures of intelligence. The emphasis in Piaget's theory is thus not upon the verbatim recall of information, but rather upon changes in the interpretation of that information as the structures of intelligence continue to develop (Piaget and Inhelder, 1973). Within either theory, it is not memory abilities per se which change with development, but rather the means by which the child is able to comprehend the material that is presented to him.

Self-Awareness of Memory Abilities. The development of memory abilities during childhood can thus be described as an increasingly deliberate use of such memorizing strategies as visual and verbal elaboration, labeling, serial rehearsal, self-testing, and categorizing. From the child's point of view, memorizing might be viewed as a matter of problem solving, in which he must choose the most appropriate strategy for the items to be remembered (Meacham, 1972). A characteristic and still unexplained feature of development during this period, however, is the occurrence of what Flavell (1970) has termed production deficiency, that is, points in the developmental sequence at which the child does not spontaneously use memory strategies which are, however, within his range of abilities. The case of production deficiency in serial rehearsal has already been mentioned, but similar data exist for categorizing during acquisition and the use of category names during retrieval. Although production deficiencies may simply reflect lack of experience and feedback regarding the efficiency of various memorizing strategies, the failure of children to spontaneously use such strategies following training argues against such an explanation.

A more plausible explanation is that a production deficiency occurs when a newly developing memorizing strategy still requires the guidance of an adult. At a latter point in development, the new strategy has been elaborated and practiced sufficiently so that it can be controlled by the child himself. In addition, the subordination of the strategy to the goal of remembering in a means-end relationship may be a necessary step (Meacham, 1972). A second, more general explanation is that production deficiencies reflect an inability to plan, that is, a failure to consider the relationship between memorizing activities and the goal of remembering, and to engage in some activity at the present time in order to facilitate future recall (Flavell, 1970).

This latter hypothesis regarding production deficiency has led to several investigations of children's metamemory, that is, knowledge of memory strategies and the ability to assess the state of one's own memory. In one such investigation, the ability of four-year-olds to recall names of pictures was tested following instructions to look at the pictures and also following instructions to remember the names of the pictures. The two conditions did not produce differences in the number of names recalled, nor in the observable study behaviors of the four-year-olds. Differences were found for seven- and ten-year-old children. It can be concluded from these data that four-year-olds do not understand that special activities other than merely looking are needed in order to effectively remember (Appel, Cooper, McCarrell, Sims-Knight, Yussen, and Flavell, 1972).

Additional evidence that younger children lack knowledge of their own memory abilities is obtained by asking children to estimate the number of pictures they can recall. Although seven- and nine-year-old children can make accurate estimates, a large percentage of four- and five-year-old children make unreasonably high estimates. In the same investigation, older children were found to be better able to assess and report their own readiness to be tested for recall (Flavell, Friedrichs, and Hoyt, 1970). In addition, eight-year-olds and college students are more able than six-year-olds to focus their study efforts on those items which had been missed in a preceding recall test (Masur, McIntyre, and Flavell, 1973). Together, these and other investigations indicate that what a child does when confronted with a memory task is closely related to his understanding of what it means to remember and his appraisal of his own remembering abilities.

Memory in Adulthood and Old Age

Whether or not there is considered to be a decline in memory abilities during old age depends upon the importance attributed to such methodological problems as the confounding of age and cohort experiences, such as amount of formal education, and the failure to equate levels of motivation during testing and to ensure equal familiarity and interest level of the items to be recalled. Explanations for the decline have focused upon the need for extra time during the acquisition phase in order to take advantage of organization in the items to be remembered or to engage in various memorizing activities, and upon the need for retrieval procedures which reduce the potential for interference between items being recalled and items still being remembered (Talland, 1968).

Conclusions

The study of developmental changes in memory will be pursued, both for reasons of application in education and also because of the close dependence of many areas of cognition and social interaction upon memory processes. Although the task of describing developmental changes is proceeding rapidly, there is a clear need for a theoretical model to provide an explanatory framework for the observed changes. Developmental psychologists are currently relying on an information-processing model (Reese, 1973); yet this model is not strongly developmental nor able to consistently explain changes over the entire life span. It is likely that a better understanding of memory development will come not from the study of memory alone, but rather from a consideration of the child's ability to organize and to control his entire repertoire of cognitive processes and strategies, only a limited number of which are specifically useful as memorizing strategies.

BIBLIOGRAPHY

APPEL, L. F.; COOPER, R. G.; McCARRELL, N.; SIMS-KNIGHT, J.; YUSSEN, S. R.; and FLAVELL, J. H. The development of the distinction between perceiving and memorizing. *Child Development,* 1972, *43,* 1365–1381.

FLAVELL, J. H. Developmental studies of mediated memory. In H. W. Reese and L. P. Lipsitt (Eds.), *Advances in child development and behavior* (Vol. 5). New York: Academic Press, 1970. Pp. 182–211.

FLAVELL, J. H.; FRIEDRICHS, A. G.; and HOYT, J. D. Developmental changes in memorization processes. *Cognitive Psychology,* 1970, *1,* 324–340.

GOLDBERG, S.; PERLMUTTER, N.; and MYERS, N. Recall of related and unrelated lists by 2-year-olds. *Journal of Experimental Child Psychology,* 1974, *18,* 1–8.

HAGEN, J. W.; JONGEWARD, R. H., JR.; and KAIL, R. V., JR. Cognitive perspectives on the development of memory. In H. W. Reese (Ed.), *Advances in child development and behavior* (Vol. 10). New York: Academic Press, 1975.

LANGE, G. The development of conceptual and rote recall skills among school age children. *Journal of Experimental Child Psychology,* 1973, *15,* 394–406.

MEACHAM, J. A. The development of memory abilities in the individual and society. *Human Development,* 1972, *15,* 205–228.

PARIS, S. G., and MAHONEY, G. J. Cognitive integration in children's memory for sentences and pictures. *Child Development,* 1974, *45,* 633–642.

PIAGET, J., and INHELDER, B. *Memory and intelligence.* New York: Basic Books, 1973.

REESE, H. W. Models of memory and models of development. *Human Development,* 1973, *16,* 397–416.

REESE, H. W. Cohort, age, and imagery in children's paired-associate learning. *Child Development,* 1974, *45,* 1176–1180.

ROHWER, W. D., JR. Elaboration and learning in childhood and adolescence. In H. W. Reese (Ed.), *Advances in child development and behavior* (Vol. 8). New York: Academic Press, 1973. Pp. 1–57.

WAGNER, D. A. The development of short-term and incidental memory: A cross-cultural study. *Child Development,* 1974, *45,* 389–396.

JOHN A. MEACHAM

MEMORY: EFFECTS OF BRAIN DAMAGE

Disturbances of memory due to brain trauma, disease, or degeneration have been a topic of discussion for some time, but it was not until the 1970s that an understanding of some of the factors contributing to this problem was reached. The primary reason for this rather dramatic increase in interest in amnesia has been the rapid development of techniques for assessing memory in normals. The large number of paradigms used to study memory that have been generated during this period provided the tools to allow the investigation of disorders of memory as well as normal memory. Furthermore, the emergence of various theories of memory allowed investigators the opportunity to propose alternative theories of the amnesic process.

Amnesias

Amnesia can be caused by a wide variety of factors, including psychological as well as organic disorders. Purely psychological disturbances, which are often manifestations of intense emotional fears, serve to keep the patient from recalling some events or, in some cases, any event at all. Organic amnesias, on the other hand, are manifestations of an injury to some portion of the cerebrum. These effects can be temporary or permanent depending upon the extent of injury and the particular area of the brain that has been affected. The most frequently studied amnesic patients are those who have suffered brain degeneration following chronic, long-term alcoholic abuse. These patients, known as alcoholic Korsakoff patients, are almost totally unable to learn any new information. This impairment will continue throughout their lifetime, since the brain damage they have suffered is irreversible. A second frequently studied group of patients consists of those who have recovered from encephalitis but have, as a residual disorder, an amnesic syndrome. This syndrome is not always a direct consequence of encephalitis, since many of the patients who survive show no evidence of amnesia. It is, however, occasionally a result of the high fever and anoxia experienced during an encephalitic attack. One other population that has come under careful scrutiny because of their amnesia for particular "types" of materials are temporal-lobe patients. Many of these patients have had one or more of their temporal lobes removed by surgery to alleviate the occurrence of epileptic seizures. One of the most famous of these cases, and one of the first upon which the new sophisticated techniques of memory theorists was applied, was Scoville and Milner's patient, H. M. (Milner, 1970):

H. M. is a patient who had suffered generalized epileptic seizures from the time he was 16. By 27 he could no longer function on a job or lead a normal existence. At this time a bilateral medial temporal-lobe resection was performed in order to reduce his seizure activity. Following the successful operation the patient's personality remained as it had been, his I.Q. actually increased, but his memory for events covering the year before his operation was poor and his ability to learn and retain new information was almost zero. In fact, his memory was so bad that he forgot whatever he was asked to remember just as soon as he was distracted from rehearsing the information.

Formal testing revealed that H. M. could retain verbal material for as long as even 15 minutes if he was allowed to rehearse the information. However, as soon as his short-term memory capacity was exceeded or he was distracted from this rehearsal, he forgot the material. His ability to retain nonverbal information was impaired whether or not he was distracted. Within 30 seconds he forgot even simple perceptual stimuli such as triangles, squares or circles.

Despite these enormous deficits, H. M. did have some residual abilities to learn, though the process was laborious. For instance, Milner found that H. M. could learn a very short visual maze that normally takes a person only a couple of trials to master. However, it took H. M. 155 trials before he could learn the maze. Amazingly, though, H. M. retained his learning a week later and even two years later he showed extensive savings. At this time it took him only 39 trials to relearn the maze, a savings of 116 trials.

Another instance in which H. M. was able to learn a task was when he was asked to trace a drawing of a star by looking only at a reflection of the drawing in a mirror. Not only did he do this as well as normals, but his improvement from trial to trial was also normal. In fact, his performance on the second day, and on the third, was as good on the first trial of each day as it had been on the last trial the day before. Evidently, this type of pure motor skill retention was not affected by his bilateral temporal removal.

Similar results have been obtained with a population of amnesics suffering from extensive diencephalic-limbic damage including damage to the n. medial dorsalis and the mammillary bodies as a direct, or perhaps indirect, consequence of many years of chronic alcoholism. These patients, alcoholic Korsakoff patients, were studied in great detail by Talland (1965) and Cermak and Butters (1973). Like H. M., these patients' IQs remained normal but they were unable to recall day-to-day and current events. They were sometimes disoriented in time and space and had retrograde amnesias of varying densities.

Formal testing of these patients revealed that they too forgot information at a much faster rate than do normals. Given only three words to try to remember, if rehearsal was prevented by a counting task, the patients could only remember 33% of the material 3 seconds later and only 5% after 9 seconds. Normals under the same conditions were correct 80% of the time after a 3-second retention interval and 60% of the time after 9 seconds. When the patients were allowed to rehearse during this interval they were as likely to remember the material as normals, but only when the to-be-remembered information was verbal material. When it was nonverbal (e.g., geometric patterns), the patients could not recognize the pattern above a chance level after only 20 seconds. Apparently, like H. M. their verbal rehearsal mechanism was intact but any form of even semipermanent storage was defective. On the other hand, their nonverbal rehearsal mechanism, which might rely on visual imagery for normals, was evidently impaired for Korsakoff patients. Consequently, they could not hold nonverbal information in store even when not distracted.

Korsakoff Syndrome

One question investigated regarding these patients was why they could not transfer verbal information from their rehearsal system to a permanent memory system. It was discovered that the primary reason for this difficulty was their extreme sensitivity to the effects of interference. Any increase in interference by massing the trials or increasing the similarity of the material affected the Korsakoff patients' retention more than the normals'. The reason for this increased sensitivity was in turn shown to be a deficit in the extent to which the patients analyzed the incoming information. Unlike normal subjects, Korsakoff patients tend to rely upon their acoustic analysis of the to-be-remembered verbal information, whereas normals automatically analyze some of the semantic features of the material—its meaning, associations, context, categorical inclusions, and so on. Korsakoff patients tend to try to retain verbal information solely on the basis of the "sound" of the word, which is sufficient provided no distraction occurs between the time the material is presented and the time the patient tries to recall it. This type of retention is similar to the way a normal tries to retain a telephone number he has just looked up in a telephone book. He cannot make meaning out of the number, or think of associates to the number, so he just keeps saying it over and over to himself. Even for normals the rate of decay of this type of informational analysis is very

rapid and the rehearsal mechanism easily disrupted.

Evidence that Korsakoff patients are probably trying to hold verbal information on the basis of its sound rather than its meaning came from two separate experiments. In the first experiment, interference between individual memory tasks was generated by drawing all the to-be-remembered words from the same category (e.g., animals). Then, without warning, the patient was asked to try to remember three words from an entirely different category (e.g., vegetables). When normals were asked to do this they found it very easy because they automatically analyzed the meaning of the words, realized that a different type of word had been presented, and consequently did not get this new category of word confused with the prior words. The Korsakoff patients, on the other hand, demonstrated absolutely no increase in recall when categories were switched and, in fact, did not even realize a switch had occurred. It could be pointed out to them that their words represented different categories, but they expressed surprise that this was so and said they had not realized it at the time they were asked to remember them. The second experiment, pointing to the hypothesis that Korsakoff patients tend to rely on acoustic encoding, involved the detection of repeated words in a long list of visually presented words. Some of the words were repeated, but in addition there were several homonyms within the list plus several highly associated words and even some synonyms. While the Korsakoff patients detected nearly as many repeated words as did the normals, they "falsely" recognized significantly more homonyms as being repeats than did the normals. However, they did not "falsely" recognize synonyms as repeats.

That the Korsakoff patient's dependence upon acoustic encoding might simply be a result of a slower rate of processing information is evidenced by the fact that these patients take longer to respond to the written question "Do the letters A and a have the same name?" than do normals, but are not slower in responding to the question "Are an A and A identical?" The first question requires a level of cognitive processing beyond the mere perception of a visual stimulus, and the patients' slower response indicates a slower processing of the information. It has also been discovered that these patients' identification threshold for real words is much higher than normals and that the interstimulus interval between a to-be-recognized stimulus and a masking stimulus has to be longer for these patients than for normals. All this evidence points to a slower rate of information processing, which may in turn be the basis for their dependence on acoustic encoding, their consequent sensitivity to interference, and their resultant inability to learn and retain new information.

Despite these impairments, Korsakoff patients can learn some new tasks in a manner similar to the way H. M. learns. For instance, they can learn and retain a pursuit-rotor task and, with extensive practice, a simple four-choice-point finger maze. In addition, their 24-hour savings of an overlearned verbal paired associate is quite good. However, they are severely limited in the number of paired associates they can learn at any one time, and their recall of these associates does eventually disappear. Their recall of the pursuit-rotor task and of the maze seems to last considerably longer. They still take less time to learn months after original learning even though they insist that they have never seen the test apparatus before each and every time they are retested.

Postencephalitic Amnesia

A number of reports have documented the amnesic syndrome following an encephalitic attack. These postencephalitics have probably suffered extensive cortical damage during their period of intensely high fever and because of the rather general encephalitic attack on the entire central nervous system. While the majority of these patients do not survive, those that do occasionally (but by no means always) display an amnesic syndrome highly similar to that found in bilateral temporal-lobe and alcoholic Korsakoff patients. However, there do seem to be some subtle differences in this syndrome that are not shared by other amnesic populations. For instance, several reports of individual postencephalitic patients have shown that their ability to retain verbal information over short periods of time (0–30 sec) is intact even when a distractor task fills the retention interval. Yet recall minutes later is as bad as it is for the Korsakoff patients. In addition, the retrograde amnesia for postencephalitics is

sometimes worse than it is for other amnesic patients. One of these patients (S. S.) was extensively studied by Cermak, who showed that his ability to retain verbal information over a short period of distraction was probably a result of his perfectly normal ability to process information on the basis of its meaning and his normal "rate" of processing as well. S. S. was also able to learn a series of 50 paired associates, all based upon current-information questions such as "Who is the President?" But it took several months of intensive therapy to build up this meagre repertoire. Even after all this therapy, S. S. was still not able to incorporate this new information into his basic body of stored knowledge. In other words, he could not make logical deductions from this information or carry out commands he had learned such as "What do you do when you enter your house"—"Put on my sweater." He never once put on his sweater after entering the house even though asked at that very time the question "What do you do when you enter your house?" Thus, his new learning was on a purely rote, not cognitive, level and it represented a childlike method of memorization such as might be used in learning a multiplication table.

Bilateral Hippocampal Damage

There are, then, three basic types of organically produced general states of amnesia: that produced by bilateral hippocampal damage, that produced by limbic system damage including the mammillary bodies and n. medial dorsalis, and that caused by diffuse cortical damage (which may of course include both temporal lobes plus the limbic system). In addition to the general amnesia states there are specific forms of amnesia created by damage to specific areas of the brain. For example, it has been discovered that the left temporal lobe is concerned with verbal memory, while the right temporal lobe is necessary for nonverbal memory (visual pattern recognition). In other words, a patient suffering unilateral left-temporal-lobe damage has greater difficulty remembering verbal material than a normal, but no abnormal difficulty with nonverbal material. Damage in the right temporal region produces the opposite deficit.

Milner (1970) demonstrated this localization

by means of two techniques, neither of which relies upon using patients with temporal-lobe damage. The first is performed by the injection of sodium amytal into one of the internal carotid arteries. This produces a transient hemiparesis of the opposite limbs plus an almost total depression of the other functions controlled by that hemisphere of the brain. Known as the Wada test, this injection can cause an otherwise intact person to become aphasic if the injection is in the left hemisphere. In addition, Milner has been able to show that verbal material presented to the patient while under the effects of the drug in the left hemisphere is less well remembered than is nonverbal material. Since the opposite result occurs when the injection is in the right hemisphere, it can be concluded that the left is dominant for verbal memory and the right for nonverbal. Damage or temporary suppression of either hemisphere will result in an impairment in the ability to remember the type of information processed by that hemisphere.

The second way that the same phenomenon has been studied is by using patients in whom the corpus callosum has been severed. In most cases this operation was performed to check the spread of epilepsy from one hemisphere to the other. The effect of such a split is to make the two hemispheres operate independently of one another. Through careful examination it can be demonstrated that verbal material projected to the right hemisphere is remembered less well than nonverbal material presented to that same hemisphere. Also, as might now be expected, nonverbal material is remembered at a lower level than verbal when all material is presented to the left hemisphere. Thus, it can again be concluded that the left hemisphere is responsible for retention of verbal material and the right hemisphere for nonverbal.

Temporal-Lobe Damage

Temporal-lobe patients have also been shown to have a modality-specific deficit as well as a material-specific deficit. It has been shown that their recall of aurally presented material is inferior to their recall of the same type of material presented visually. In other words, a left-temporal lobe patient's short-term recall of verbal material presented aurally is worse than his recall of the same material pre-sented visually, though even this latter material is recalled less well than normal. Precisely the opposite modality-specific effect is believed to exist for patients with damage to their parietal-lobe area, especially the right parietal lobe. These patients have greater difficulty retaining visually presented material than aurally presented material. In fact, some of these patients are totally unable to recognize faces of people they have seen on multiple occasions (prosopagnosia), although other types of memory remain intact.

BIBLIOGRAPHY

CERMAK, L. S., and BUTTERS, N. Information processing deficits of alcoholic Korsakoff patients. *Quarterly Journal of Studies on Alcohol*, 1973, *34*, 1110–1132.
MILNER, B. Memory and the medial temporal regions of the brain. In K. H. Pribram and D. E. Broadbent (Eds.), *Biology of memory.* New York: Academic Press, 1970. Pp. 29–50.
TALLAND, G. A. *Deranged memory.* New York: Academic Press, 1965.

LAIRD S. CERMAK

MEMORY: GENERAL CHARACTERISTICS OF RECOGNITION

There are many ways in which one can ask whether a given item of information has been stored in memory. The experimental study of recognition memory always involves a test in which information is presented which has been encountered earlier for study and asking whether or not this information was, in fact, studied earlier. Intuitively, it has seemed to layman and psychologist alike that recognition is not only easier than recall, but that it is also much more rapid, direct, and based on something like a feeling of familiarity. It shall be seen that many of these intuitions are in dispute.

Some simple contrasts between recall and recognition need to be clearly understood at the outset. A common comparison is between two kinds of examinations, a test of recall in which information must be written in a blank space set aside for the answer, and a multiple-choice test in which the student is supplied with the appropriate answer as well as inappropriate answers, and must indicate which of the alternatives is correct. It is a rare student who, given a choice, would elect the recall test. In electing the multiple-choice test, the student is choosing a recognition memory procedure. In fact, an earlier generation referred to the recall procedure as a test of reproductive memory, in that one is required to reproduce information stored earlier, rather than to identify what might be called a copy of previously stored information, as in recognition.

The theoretical question about recognition memory most intriguing to researchers is this: How, in fact, do subjects know that something is familiar when it is encountered at a later time? Closely related to the concern with this question is a theoretical attempt to distinguish between the processes occurring when people attempt to recall information and the processes occurring when they attempt to recognize information. As seen below, whether or not two different kinds of memory processes are at work in recall and recognition is an issue of considerable contemporary interest and controversy. The significance of accounting satisfactorily for the recognition process lies in the observation that the recognition of some event or piece of information as being familiar or appropriate is what might be termed the brute fact of memory. Even theorists attempting to account for recall usually incorporate a recognition step into their models. For example, when a subject attempts to recall the name of his third grade teacher, how does he know that the final answer is indeed correct and that the earlier names that came to mind were not correct? A recognition component seems to be involved in recall, it appears, and must be accounted for in any complete theory of memory.

Procedures

Theoretical issues will be returned to after a brief account of the procedures used in laboratory research on recognition memory and some of the main findings. In a standard recognition memory experiment, subjects are presented with a list or set of items to study after having been told that a test on the items will follow. The studied items may be digits, words, pictures, faces, sentences, or whatever else is of experimental interest, but by far the most research has been done using lists of ordinary English words. At some later point in time, a test is administered. The time interval between the end of the study period and the beginning of the test period defines the retention interval.

All recognition memory tests present the subject with two types of items: items which were actually studied, called old or *target items,* and items which were not studied but are of the same type as the target items. These are called new or *distractor items,* or occasionally, *lures.* There are two major types of recognition tests: the *yes-no* test and the *forced-choice* test. With the yes-no test, the subject indicates for each item on the test whether it is an item he believes he studied earlier *(yes)* or one which he did not study *(no).* With the forced-choice test, like the familiar multiple-choice test at school, one old item is presented along with one or more new items and the subject attempts to select the old item. With the yes-no test, two response proportions provide the basic measures of mnemonic performance: correct acceptances (the proportion of truly old items identified as old) and incorrect acceptances, or false alarms (the proportion of new items incorrectly identified as old). These two proportions are often used to derive a single measure of performance, but which measure is reported depends on certain theoretical considerations too detailed to go into here (Banks, 1970). A useful first approximation is simply the proportion of correct acceptances minus the proportion of incorrect acceptances.

Some reflection will make it obvious why both measures need to be taken into account in assessing recognition performance. One subject may, for various reasons, adopt a strategy of calling almost all items on the test old, lest he fail to recognize an old item. His more cautious friend of equal mnemonic ability may, for reasons of his own, hesitate to identify any item as old unless he is certain. More cautious observers will, of course, correctly identify fewer old items but, at the same time, will have considerably fewer false alarms. If only correct identifications of old items as old are considered, nonmnemonic factors may give a misleading picture. How uncertainty is resolved is a valid topic of psychological inquiry in its own right and constitutes the domain of decision theory, a topic which is only of peripheral concern here. The forced-choice procedure described above is less contaminated by these criterion or decision problems.

It may be noted that in real life one is usually

in the position of deciding about a single event and, therefore, false alarm rates, or the disposition of an observer to call things familiar in general, are not known. The line-up procedure used by police departments is an attempt to deal with this problem by using a variation of the forced-choice method.

Another important feature distinguishing experimental studies of recognition from everyday experience should be pointed out. In laboratory studies using words all of the items on the test set, including the new words, are familiar in that the subject has encountered them before at some point in his existence. The question addressed to the subject is not "Have you ever seen these words before?", but rather "Which of these words did you study in this particular experiment?" Recognition is being tested for events that occurred in a specific, clearly demarked context. While in real life this kind of context-specific question is sometimes asked, for example, "Was Henry at the party last night?" memory is also frequently tested with no particular context specified. Two examples of such context-free queries are: "Have you ever seen the name Xanthippe?" and "Do you know I. W. Dragon?" It is essential in experimental work to have control over the conditions occurring when information is registered into the memory system, hence all of the work discussed here concerns recognition memory for events occurring in a specific, known context. This is not to say that the more general, context-free recognition question is not important, but simply to acknowledge the limitations.

Findings

Perhaps the most commonly observed characteristic recognition memory is the high level of retention shown. Implicit in such observations is a reference to the presumably lower levels of recall to be found in comparable situations. For example, R. N. Shepard presented subjects with sets of 540 or 612 items to study one at a time. The sets of items were made up of either words, sentences, or pictures. After the series of items had been studied, recognition was tested by presenting each subject with about 60 test pairs, each pair consisting of a target item from the study set and a distractor item of the same type. Correct performance immediately after presentation of the study list was 90% for the words, 88% for the sentences and 98% for the pictures. Further testimony to the enormous capacity for storing information comes from studies of recognition for pictures done by R. N. Haber in which subjects studied thousands of pictures and showed forced-choice recognition performance of about 90%. The type of material being studied turns out to be a potent determiner of recognition performance with pictorial material superior to other kinds of material tested so far. It is difficult to pinpoint the reasons for this remarkable capacity to store visual information.

A puzzling finding has been that, whereas words of high frequency of usage in English tend to be more readily recalled than words of low frequency, in recognition testing it is the less common words which lead to superior performance. This finding is interesting both as a recognition phenomenon needing explication and because it is difficult to reconcile with simple models suggesting that recognition is simply a more sensitive measure of the memory trace than recall. If traces only differ in strength, it would have to be the case that high and low frequency words differ in strength depending on which measure of memory is being employed, an impossible situation.

Evidence for forgetting is not absent when memory is assessed by recognition. With poorly integrated material such as three-digit numbers, recognition declines rapidly as other numbers are studied and tested. With ordinary words, recognition has been shown to decline over retention intervals measured in hours. In the study by Shepard recognition of pictures after 120 days had declined to a median score of 57% correct, barely above chance.

Two important determinants of recognition performance are the number of *distractors* or new items on the test and the similarity of the distractors to the studied material. In fact, some psychologists have demonstrated that the usual superiority of recognition scores over recall scores can be eliminated by either equating the number of alternatives in the two cases, or by making the new items very similar to the old items on the test. In particular, the similarity between old and new items with certain kinds of learning materials may be manipulated across a wide range with corresponding changes in recognition performance.

As in all research on human memory since Ebbinghaus, the effects of repetition have been investigated with recognition memory and the usual facilitation of performance by repetition has been found. An interesting effect of repetition on both recognition and recall is that when repetitions of a study item are separated or spaced, rather than being adjacent, performance is facilitated. Agreement on why this should be the case or what it tells us about memory is yet to be reached.

Theory and Applications

It is customary to analyze memory into three temporal stages. Events occurring at the time of study, when information is put into the system, are usually considered as having to do with the *encoding* process; possible changes in the nature of stored information occurring after encoding but before retrieval, including information loss, concern the *storage* phase; events obtaining at the time that information is demanded of the memory system are said to concern *retrieval*. These stages are mainly differentiated, then, by when they occur in the temporal chain of events which, in their totality, constitute remembering. Within this framework, the question of which phase is implicated when memory fails or forgetting is observed, may be considered. In recognition, forgetting takes the form of failure to recognize a target item as old. In recall, it takes the form of failure to reproduce information put into the system earlier. One possibility, of course, is that the item was never encoded in the first place, perhaps due to attentional factors. This is not a trivial matter. Inadequate registration probably accounts for the "forgetting" of names at a party. Fortunately, in experiments encoding can be ensured. Assuming, then, that encoding has occurred, there remain two possibilities. First, the information has been lost while in storage through decay or interference; secondly, the information has been conserved but is not being retrieved for various reasons. Distinguishing between these two states is exceedingly difficult. Many theorists attempt to meet this problem by assuming that recognition memory does not involve retrieval processes to

any significant extent and, therefore, it directly assesses whether the queried information is in the memory store. This is not, however, the only assumption possible.

For example, if the word *orange* was on the list the subject studied ten minutes ago, and he now indicates on a recognition test that orange was *not* on the list, it might be concluded that the stored information about the item is simply not there any more. If, on the other hand, it is admitted that the recognition procedure does involve retrieval processes, then it remains possible that the stored information is intact but is not accessible under the prevailing retrieval conditions. In certain kinds of memory deficiencies, such as the amnesias or in aging, much research has been generated by the question of whether these deficiencies should be characterized as primarily deficiencies of storage or deficiencies of the retrieval mechanisms. Researchers in these areas have tended to assume that, by using a recognition memory test, they were avoiding retrieval problems and therefore could directly assess what information is in storage. This, however, is not a necessary assumption.

Proponents of a direct access view of recognition memory assume what computer scientists call a content-addressable memory system. Many contemporary theories of recognition memory, particularly the more quantitative theories (Murdock, 1974) have assumed direct access of the memory trace. The trace corresponding to the input being queried is examined with the judgment of old or new depending on the *familiarity* or *strength* of the accessed memory trace. This theory has the advantage of lending itself to mathematical modeling by virtue of its simplicity and a priori ruling out of retrieval processes. On the other hand, to many other theorists, this approach to recognition seems to beg the question. How the subject gets from the test item in the environment to its representation, if any, in memory seems to these theorists too important a question to be bypassed by assumptions of "direct access" to a trace containing the information needed to accomplish the task.

Some recent findings which question the simplifying assumption of direct access in recognition will be mentioned here. While *retrieval processes* remain perhaps the most intractable area of memory theory, it is generally agreed that one aspect of any search process must be that it takes time. Thus, R. C. Atkinson and his associates have shown that the time taken to recognize a previously studied target word on a test increases linearly with the length of the list studied. It takes longer to recognize *orange* as an old word if it was one of 32 words studied than if it was one of 8 words studied. If the subject directly accessed the stored representation of *orange* to see whether it had occurred on the target list, the time to do so should be independent of set size. But it is not.

A related finding concerns the effects of the organization of the material learned on memory. One way in which organization is manipulated is by presenting subjects with lists of words which fall into readily identifiable taxonomic categories such as animals, flowers, occupations.

This type of categorization has been shown to facilitate recall. It is argued that this facilitation is due to a reduction in the difficulty of retrieval, in much the same way that orderly classification in libraries facilitates the retrieval of stored books. The point here is that organization in the form of categorized lists has been shown to affect recognition as well as recall, both in terms of error reduction and speed of response. Again, these data are consistent with the hypothesis that recognition memory involves some retrieval demands.

It should be emphasized that to say that both recall and recognition involve retrieval processes is not the same thing as saying that there are no process differences between recall and recognition. The term *retrieval* involves a number of sub-processes which are not as yet understood. It is likely that when these sub-processes have been elucidated the ways in which recall and recognition differ and the ways in which they are alike will also be made clearer.

J. A. Anderson and G. H. Bower have offered an influential model in which recognition is achieved by retrieving contextual information associated with the target item. According to this view, associations between a target item and various contextual elements active at the time of its occurrence are stored in memory. At the time of test, when the subject must decide whether a test item is old, he bases this judgment on whether or not he retrieves appropriate contextual information. For example, the subject might recognize *orange* as a familiar word because he remembers that it came after the word *trend* and that both words were near the beginning of the list. This theory does not assign a major role to a hypothetical strength or familiarity of a directly accessed trace of the target item but instead emphasizes the role of retrieved information associated with the target. Anderson and Bower discussed how subjects certify their recognitions, that is, how they answer the question of "How do you know that *orange* was on the list?" This is a different question from "Was *orange* on the list?" Indeed, it does happen that an event seems familiar and one tries very hard to remember where or when it was encountered before. In so doing, one may be said to be straining after context. Until some part of the context is retrieved the validity of the recognition cannot be ascertained. Perhaps the term *partial recognition* should be used in such a case.

A similar point of view in comparing recall and recognition was presented by H. L. Hollingworth in 1913 and deserves attention. Hollingworth argued that recognition and recall are essentially the inverse of one another. In recall, a context is specified and some specific information is demanded. All recall tests specify something about the information demanded, for example, "Who was that lady I saw you with last night?, "What were the words on the list you learned yesterday in this room?" In recognition, however, the situation is turned around. The target item is presented to the subject and he must recall some features or aspects of the context in which it occurred in order to adequately recognize it. According to this view, then, recall and recognition differ mainly in what is being remembered: In recall, the effort is to retrieve the target item; in the case of recognition, the effort is directed toward retrieving information about the psychological setting, mainly physical and temporal, in which the target item occurred. It was pointed out earlier that laboratory experiments have a special characteristic in that the context is clearly known in advance, that is, the subject is told that the word on *that* list, in *this* room, at *that* time is wanted. This feature, it now appears, has led theorists to perhaps overgeneralize the role of feelings of familiarity divorced from the retrieval of contextual information in accounting for recognition memory.

BIBLIOGRAPHY

BANKS, W. P. Signal detection theory and human memory. *Psychological Bulletin*, 1970, 74, 81–99.
MURDOCK, B. B., JR. *Human memory: Theory and data.* Potomac, Md.: Erlbaum Associates, 1974.

EUGENE WINOGRAD

MEMORY: INTERFERENCE THEORIES

Retroactive Inhibition

Interference will be defined as the negative effect one set of learned materials has on the learning or recall of another set. The first clear demonstration of interference was by Müller and Pilzecker in 1900, who showed that the interpolation of a second set of material to be learned between the learning and recall of an original set would impair recall of the original set. The then prevailing idea, that forgetting was due to spontaneous decay of the memory trace, did not fit this finding. Rather, the forgetting was obviously due to interpolated learning. The major task of memory research since Müller and Pilzecker has been to further investigate and find an explanation for the interference phenomenon.

Müller and Pilzecker postulated that there is perseveration of neural activity beyond the learning period, and that the disruption of this activity would result in a failure of consolidation of the memory trace. It was the interpolated learning which inhibited the perseveration of the prior list; thus the name, *Rückwerkende Hemmung,* or *retroactive inhibition* (RI), which is still used.

The idea that memory has two phases, an active perseverating phase, and a more stable, consolidated phase, is analogous to the current conception of a short- and long-term memory. In a typical interference experiment, however, it is likely that at the beginning of interpolated learning the original list is already in long-term memory, at which point it would be too late for anticonsolidation to occur. It seems then that Müller and Pilzecker discovered an

important phenomenon, and developed an interesting theory, but one had nothing to do with the other.

At any rate, the earliest interference experiments soon revealed the difficulties of an anticonsolidation theory. Heine, Müller's student, showed that an RI effect was not obtained when a recognition test of recall was used. Surely, if the neural substrate of memory had failed to consolidate, then performance should be poor even on a recognition test.

The most important difficulty, however, involved the finding that similarity of original and interpolated tasks was a critical factor in producing interference. DeCamp reported a series of studies in 1915 in which nonsense syllables were first learned, followed by a different activity (e.g., multiplication or addition) or by a period of rest. DeCamp's main finding was that almost no RI was produced in his experiments. Noting that Müller and Pilzecker had used nonsense syllables for both original and interpolated learning, he theorized that RI involved transfer between similar tasks, rather than the disruption of a perseverating trace by a new activity.

Webb, in 1917, published studies in which he further developed the idea of transfer. He used mazes for both original and interpolated learning, and had both rats and humans learn the same mazes (the people performed a little bit better than the rats). Webb was interested in both the transfer of learning (i.e., how the learning of one maze affected the learning of a second maze), and in RI (i.e., how the learning of the second maze affected the recall of the first maze). Webb's major finding was that transfer of learning and RI were related such that the more positive was the transfer, the smaller was the RI. He thought that RI could be accounted for in two ways. First, one could imagine that elements of the original learning would transfer to the interpolated learning. If these transferred elements were congruent with what was required in the interpolated task then there would be facilitation; if these elements were incongruent, then they would be disruptive, and would themselves become disrupted. Disruption of the first list elements would result in RI. This is an interesting notion since it anticipates the concept of unlearning postulated by Melton some time later. Second,

Webb stated that elements of the learned second task could transfer to the recall situation and disrupt the recall of the first task material. This idea anticipates the theory of competition of response, which will be discussed in connection with McGeoch.

Following the work of DeCamp and Webb it remained for Robinson to include both similar and dissimilar interpolated lists in the same experiment. His findings supported the conclusions of the earlier investigators; similarity between original and interpolated lists resulted in RI, dissimilarity resulted in little or no RI. In addition, Robinson varied the time interval between the end of original learning and the onset of interpolated learning. Anticonsolidation theory should predict more RI the shorter that interval was, but no such effect was obtained.

Proactive Inhibition

Most studies of interference have been concerned with RI, but there is a related phenomenon, *proactive inhibition* (PI), which according to Underwood may be of more consequence as a source of forgetting. PI refers to a decrement in the recall of a second list attributable to the learning of a prior list. This phenomenon is very difficult for the anticonsolidation theory to deal with since the disruptive list comes before and not after the list to be recalled. An interesting, and theoretically challenging aspect of PI is that it develops over time. In this respect it resembles forgetting in everyday life, where memories seem to fade over time.

The research discussed so far made the transfer theory a more attractive hypothesis than anticonsolidation, and it soon became dominant. Research and theory were then directed toward a more precise specification of the mechanisms of transfer. The guiding ideas for much of this work derived from associationism and behaviorism. From associationism came the notion of transfer of identical elements. Learning consisted of the formation of associations between elements; transfer would then be beneficial or harmful depending on how the elements of an old task related to the elements required to be learned in a new task. Behaviorism contributed the distinction between stimulus and response, so that the association was no longer between elements of equal status, but between some cue event and

some action by the organism. The S-R association theory has great power since the same constructs describe both learning and recall. Learning refers to the formation of S-R associations, while recall refers to the activation of R by S to which it was previously associated. This source of strength is also a weakness, since by tying recall to the same cue involved in learning all recall becomes reproductive, and novel responses become difficult to explain.

Competition of Response

In the 1930s McGeoch consolidated much of the previous theory and research with his notion of competition of response. Two principles were involved: (1) responses will be evoked to stimuli similar or identical to the ones to which they were learned; (2) if more than one response is potentially evokable by a stimulus then they will compete such that the probability of each occurring will be diminished. With these simple ideas many of the basic laboratory findings concerning transfer and interference could be explained. For example, given that the subject *(S)* has learned to respond to stimulus *A* with response *B,* if *A-C* has now to be learned negative transfer would be expected since the *B* response would compete with the correct *C* response. Similarly, if after *A-C* has been learned *A-B* has now to be recalled RI will occur because *C* will compete with the correct *B* response. It should be obvious that this mechanism would explain PI as well. Positive transfer effects can also be explained. If *A-B* has been learned *C-B* could be easy to learn if there is some similarity between *A* and *C,* since then *C* will tend to evoke *B* directly, and also indirectly through its similarity to *A,* thus increasing the probability of *B* occurring.

Two aspects of McGeoch's theory are of great importance. First, the analysis of interference phenomenon in terms of stimulus and response properties proved very fruitful and generated an enormous amount of research. Second, McGeoch saw interference occurring at the point of recall where responses compete. Interference was not a special mechanism, but was an aspect of the recall process itself.

While competition of response has been a useful theory it is probably too imprecise to guide further research. For one thing, the mechanism by which one response blocks another is not at all clear. The basic assumption of the theory seems to be that there is a limit of one to the number of responses which can be evoked by a stimulus. The strongest, or at least the first to occur of two competing responses, will block the occurrence of the other, or if two responses are evoked simultaneously neither will occur, as if they were two people trying to squeeze through a narrow door. But this assumption is false, two responses are often given to a stimulus. Furthermore, there is evidence that interference is generated by an entire list and not by a specific item or response. Runquist has shown that recall of a given *A-B* pair is not related to the learning strength of its corresponding *A-C* pair, and DaPolito has shown that the probability of recall of *A-B* is independent of whether *A-C* is recalled or not. In addition, Ceraso and Tendler have shown that recall of an *A-B* pair is independent of whether the corresponding *A-C* pair is present in the interfering list or not. All that is necessary is that some *A-C* pairs be present in the competing list. The last study is significant because it concerns PI, which according to theory should be wholly produced by competition of response. Thus, while there may be interference produced at the point of recall, the mechanism of response competition seems to be an inadequate explanation for it.

An earlier criticism of competition comes from Melton who argued that in addition to competition at recall, interference also occurred as an unlearning, or weakening of the first list during second list learning, and before recall. Melton suggested that the cause of unlearning was the extinction of the first list responses, which were incorrect, and therefore not reinforced in the context of second list learning.

There seems to be sufficient evidence to support the distinction between interference during second list learning, and interference at the point of recall. The most important line of evidence was first developed by Melton in showing an asymmetry between first and second list recall. If interference was simply a matter of recall interference after both lists are learned, then one should expect the lists to suffer the same amount of interference. In their studies, Melton and Von Lackum found that more RI was produced than PI. This is intelligible if it is assumed that the first list suffers unlearning plus recall interference, while the second list suffers only recall interference.

Subsequent research showed that the pattern of first and second list recall was somewhat more complex. Relative to a control list baseline, the first list shows a large recall decrement if tested immediately after second list learning, and remains relatively stable if tested after that. The second list, on the other hand, is recalled well at first, and shows increasingly poor recall over time, ultimately dropping to the level of first list recall. Again, this asymmetrical pattern leads to the idea that different factors are affecting first and second lists.

Two-Factor Theory

Theoretical analysis of the temporal pattern described above has been presented by Underwood. He notes that if unlearning is indeed an extinction-like process, then one should expect spontaneous recovery to follow unlearning. The increase in PI over time could be attributed to the increasing competition met by the second list from the recovering first list. There have been enough reports of recovery in the literature to make it probable that the phenomenon exists. However, since most often one finds a drop in second list recall without first list recovery it is not clear that that drop in recall can be attributed to recovery.

At any rate, the distinction between unlearning and recall interference while not conclusively demonstrated has enough face validity to have been widely accepted. What is questionable, however, is that extinction is an adequate explanation for unlearning. For one thing extinction is itself a phenomenon which has been explained in various ways. What we have then is an analogy between two phenomena. Furthermore, there are operational differences between the two. Unlearning is more like counterconditioning, where a new response is learned, rather than an old one nonreinforced as in extinction. In addition, in extinction studies it is one response which is learned and then extinguished, while interference studies involve many pairs. It seems unlikely that a first and second list of one pair each could produce interference (of long-term memory). Finally, extinction affects performance (i.e., what a person or animal does), while unlearning affects what a person can remember, and these cannot be equated in any simple way. It would seem then that despite superficial similarities, the two are quite different phenomena, and that not much is gained by describing one in terms of the other. In fact, one might wonder why such diverse phenomena are seemingly both associated with recovery over time.

Together the competition and extinction theories comprised the two-factor theory of interference, and were for some years the dominant concepts used to explain recall interference and unlearning respectively. Despite their theoretical shortcomings, these concepts have features which still command attention. These include:

1. The distinction between unlearning and recall interference. Certain current theories, for example, response set suppression, or stimulus encoding would qualify as unlearning theories since they attempt to specify events taking place at interpolated learning which effect subsequent recall. Theories based on search difficulties in recall might be thought of as recall interference theories since they are based primarily on characteristics of the recall process itself.

2. The distinction between stimulus and response; which is of interest in a number of ways. First, many current theorists make the distinction between a retrieval cue and the item to be retrieved. These terms are related to stimulus and response, but have a different conceptual base. One challenge to such theorists will be to deal with the empirical laws concerning interference, which have been by and large successfully dealt with by S-R theorists. A second point of interest concerns the locus of interference. While traditional theory has placed the difficulty on the response side, some theorists locate the difficulty in trace location or in stimulus recognition.

Response Set Suppression

An example of current theorizing is the response set suppression mechanism, postulated by Postman (1972; 1973) to account for unlearning. Earlier, Newton, and Wickens had shown that more RI was produced as the interpolated list was learned closer to the point of recall. They interpreted their data to mean that learning a second list induced a set to give second list responses, which set would persevere into the first list recall period, and thus produce RI. Similarly, Underwood and Schulz had pointed out that during the learning of a second list, Ss quickly came to confine their responses to the appropriate ones, and not to emit (even as guesses) first list responses. They postulated a list selector mechanism which limits responses to the appropriate set. The opposite face of list selection is the suppression of inappropriate responses, and, as Postman states, if this suppression lasts beyond second list learning it could account for RI.

In many ways this theory is similar to the extinction theory; the inhibiting effect is on the response side, it is presumed that the inhibition will dissipate over time, and PI would be explained by the increasing competition from the recovering first list. The chief difference from extinction theory is that the suppression operates on the entire list of responses, rather than on the associative bond between each stimulus and response.

Evidence for the theory comes from studies which show that RI is greatly reduced when a test of associative matching is used, indicating that the association itself is not the locus of the interference. Evidence showing that interference is not item specific, but of the entire list is only sometimes obtained for RI. This may suggest that in addition to response suppression other factors are at work and produce item specific interference.

Stimulus Encoding

A more radical departure from traditional theories is that of Martin in postulating that interference is related to stimulus encoding rather than response production. The notion of coding is based on the observation that the same event may be identified in different ways by the observer. For example, in Rubin's reversible figure one may see either two faces or a vase. Köhler and, before him, Höffding had pointed out that associative recall could not occur if the A term in an A-B association is not properly identified or encoded. Applied to the A-B, A-C interference paradigm, Martin points out that A may be encoded in one way (A_1) when paired with B, and another way (A_2)

when paired with C, or it may be encoded in the same way in both contexts. Negative transfer would only occur to the extent that A is encoded in the same way in both lists. Note that while encoding would determine whether or not transfer takes place, the mechanism of interference would remain as some sort of competition between B and C responses. The situation is somewhat different with respect to RI. RI could be attributed to the encoding of the recall stimulus as A_2 rather than as A_1. PI could be accounted for by the development of a tendency over time to stop coding the A stimulus as A_2, although it is not clear why this should occur.

One difficulty with the encoding hypothesis is that it predicts negative transfer under conditions where A is encoded in the same way in A-B and A-C, and predicts RI where the coding is different in the two lists. The usual finding, however, is that negative transfer and RI tend to occur under the same conditions.

At present, there are many details of the encoding process which are unclear, and there is not substantial evidence for the hypothesized role of encoding in RI or PI. However, there is already sufficient evidence that stimuli can be encoded in different ways, and that failure to properly encode a stimulus can lead to failure to recall an item associated with that stimulus. It would seem that the right conditions could be found to produce interference due to stimulus encoding.

Response set suppression and *stimulus encoding* hypotheses are alternative explanations for unlearning. It is also possible that either or both processes may occur under certain conditions. For example, it would seem reasonable that stimuli which lend themselves easily to multiple encoding would result in RI due to encoding, while stimuli which tend to a single encoding would result in response suppression. What is needed is some measure or index of these different sorts of hypothesized processes.

Recall Interference

While the above mentioned theories are concerned with unlearning, Ceraso has presented a theory which concentrates on the mechanism of recall interference. A trend in contemporary psychology is to view recall as a process of search guided by the information presented at

recall, and the requirements of the particular task. Rather than competition of response, the phenomenon of recall interference is postulated to be due to the difficulty in retrieval of a given item as the search field increases in size (i.e., contains more items). Ceraso has presented evidence that recall of an item is poorer when it is embedded in a long as against a shorter list. Recall interference is seen to be an instance of this same phenomenon, and is held to operate in the following way: Immediately following the learning of two lists, search for an item is over the field which represents the list in which the item was learned. Since some sort of unlearning has occurred, first list recall will be poor. Over time there is a merging of the lists in memory, so that search is now over the combined lists, which should result in lowered recall for both lists. In point of fact, only the second list typically falls in recall over time, so Ceraso has postulated that there is indeed a spontaneous recovery of the first list which counters its loss due to list merging. One piece of evidence for list merging is the evidence, cited earlier, which showed that PI was characterized by list interference rather than specific item interference.

There is no doubt that the search theory is oversimplified. For example, if recall is just a matter of search why cannot all items be retrieved if sufficient search time is allowed? Also the notion of merging over time suggests a process whereby memories are spontaneously grouped into larger units over time. Recently, however, Houston has shown that PI (which should be an index of list merging) occurs only when Ss are led to anticipate that they will be tested for recall over time. This could indicate that there is a more active process occurring over time, perhaps a reorganization of the contents of memory, which results in forgetting. Thus, a search theory of interference is likely to be more satisfactorily stated as the nature of the organization of memory and of the search process becomes better developed.

In summary, recent theories of interference have suggested new mechanisms by which unlearning and recall interference might be explained. None of these has amassed sufficient evidence to be widely accepted, nor perhaps are they even sufficiently clearly stated to be tested. They form, instead, part of the continuous process whereby our ideas about human memory are sharpened and enriched.

BIBLIOGRAPHY

BRITT, S. H.   Retroactive inhibition: A review of the literature. *Psychological Bulletin,* 1936, *32,* 381–440.

CERASO, J.   The interference theory of forgetting. *Scientific American,* 1967, *217,* 117–124.

MARTIN, E.   Memory codes and negative transfer. *Memory and Cognition,* 1973, *1,* 495–498.

MURDOCK, B. B.   Remembering and forgetting. In B. B. Wolman (Ed.), *Handbook of General Psychology.* Englewood Cliffs, N.J.: Prentice-Hall, 1972. Pp. 530–543.

OSGOOD, C. E.   The similarity paradox in human learning: A resolution. *Psychological Review,* 1949, *56,* 132–143.

POSTMAN, L.   Transfer, interference and forgetting. In W. Kling, and L. A. Riggs (Eds.), *Experimental psychology* (Vol. 2). New York: Holt, Rinehart and Winston, 1972. Pp. 1019–1132.

POSTMAN, L., and UNDERWOOD, B. J.   Critical issues in interference theory. *Memory and Cognition,* 1973, *1,* 19–40.

UNDERWOOD, B. J.   "Spontaneous recovery" of verbal associations. *Journal of Experimental Psychology,* 1948, *38,* 29–38.

UNDERWOOD, B. J.   Interference and forgetting. *Psychological Review,* 1957, *64,* 49–60.

JOHN CERASO

MEMORY: PHYSIOLOGICAL BASIS

A major obstacle in studying complex behavioral functions such as memory is that the bioscientist cannot yet identify functional brain components which mediate the alteration of behavior as a result of prior learning and experience. Although molecular concomitants of behavior are reported, their specificity remains uncertain. For the present, we must rely on various measures of overt behavior as well as of autonomic function (e.g., cardiovascular changes and gastrointestinal motility), and examine variables that alter them. Another major problem is that it is often necessary to use animal models to learn about human behavior.

Interventive techniques that impair or facilitate memory are commonly used to probe the neurobiological phenomena underlying long-term memory formation. Impairment of memory may be induced for information acquired before the administration of an amnestic agent (retrograde amnesia), or for learning which occurs subsequent to its application (anterograde amnesia). These terms both refer to a block of recently acquired information, since more remote memories remain intact. Progressively less amnesia is observed as an amnestic treatment is removed in time from the learning experience. In the case of retrograde amnesia this suggests a time-dependent alteration in the susceptibility of memory following learning, and is consistent with the assumption that memories undergo a transition with time from a labile form to a stable form which resists disruption, that is, memories are *fixed* or *consolidated.* Time-dependent treatment effects which purportedly enhance consolidation have also been reported; greater facilitation is claimed when the agent is given closer in time to learning. Although a given treatment might appear either to impair or enhance memory formation, alternative interpretations are possible even in the presence of seemingly adequate control procedures. A treatment may alter performance without directly involving memory by affecting emotionality, attention, motivational level, motility or sensory thresholds (Agranoff et al., 1975).

Antibiotic Blockers of Macromolecular Synthesis

That long-term memory resides in some stable chemical form rather than in labile electrical circuits was inferred 20 years ago, from the survival of memory in the rat under conditions which produced electrical silence of the brain. A more dramatic demonstration of the chemical mediation of memory is the finding that memory formation is impaired in various species by antibiotics which have little effect on general brain metabolism, but selectively inhibit protein synthesis (e.g., puromycin, cycloheximide) or RNA synthesis (e.g., actinomycin D, camptothecin). Blocking of DNA synthesis does not disrupt memory (Agranoff, 1971).

Memory is not lost immediately following injection of antibiotics, but over a period of hours to days, suggesting that the injection leads to production of a faulty structural memory which is degraded more rapidly than usual, or alternatively, that the agent blocks formation of macromolecules that mediate the conversion of a transient memory form to a more permanent one. The process of memory fixation of avoidance conditioning in both goldfish and mice has been shown to begin subsequent to the animal's removal from the experimental apparatus, suggesting that a change in the environment triggers its onset (Agranoff, 1975).

To our knowledge, no specific memory disturbances have been reported in human patients treated with various antibiotics, probably because the agents do not penetrate the blood-brain barrier. However, patients who were deprived of the amino acids phenylalanine and tyrosine in an effort to starve rapidly growing tumors reportedly developed a memory disturbance characterized primarily by anterograde amnesia. The amnestic syndrome, which resembled the Scoville-Milner syndrome, the effects of bilateral destruction of the medial temporal lobes, was reportedly reversed upon reinstatement of a full amino acid diet (Agranoff et al., 1975).

Electroshock

Electroconvulsive shock (ECS) has been used to assess the time course of memory consolidation in animals. Differences in consolidation time estimates which have ranged from seconds to days have been attributed to various experimental parameters, such as complexity of the training task, method of ECS delivery, ECS current parameters, as well as the species of animal used. Similarly, the presence or absence of amnesia, as well as the time course of consolidation following ECS, has been reported to vary as a function of whether autonomic or behavioral indexes of memory were used.

The efficacy of ECS in inducing amnesia is independent of overt convulsions, since elimination of the latter with anesthetics does not attenuate amnesia. Nevertheless, the amount of seizure activity resulting from the passage of current through the brain has been correlated quantitatively with degree of measured amnesia. ECS reportedly alters brain acetylcholine, serotonin, calcium, protein, and monoamine oxidase levels; however, as yet, these effects have not been successfully related to the mechanism by which ECS interferes with memory (Jarvik, 1972).

Electroconvulsive therapy (ECT) administered to humans can produce both anterograde and retrograde amnesia. However, the permanence of both types of amnesia remains to be explored. ECT-induced anterograde amnesia may not be evident if tests are made soon after learning, but may develop later. Bilateral ECT is claimed to disrupt retention of verbal auditory material more than unilateral ECT to the nondominant hemisphere, suggesting that the dominant hemisphere is critical to verbal memory fixation (Fink et al., 1974).

Temperature

Reduction of body temperature causes time-dependent, retrograde retention deficits in rodents. Anesthetics are reported to attenuate both hypothermia-induced amnesia and concomitant paroxysmal spike discharges in the cortical EEG. The mechanism of the memory-disrupting effects of hypothermia and ECS may therefore be related, in that brain seizures are implicated in both phenomena. Cooling of goldfish extends the interval during which memory is susceptible to ECS-induced amnesia, while increased temperature accelerates the development of insusceptibility to puromycin- or ECS-induced amnesia. Raising body temperature of fish to the point of heat narcosis produces retrograde amnesia. Little is known regarding temperature effects on memory in man (Agranoff, 1975).

Anesthetics and Sedatives

Thiopental, pentobarbital, secobarbital, and amobarbital have all been reported to impair memory in animals. Degree of human memory disruption has been related to the blood thiopental concentration. Spinal anesthesia has occasionally been reported to result in transient global amnesia. Anterograde and retrograde amnesia have been observed after intracarotid injection of sodium amytal contralateral to the side of a preexisting temporal lobe abnormality. These findings suggest that the mechanism of action may in this case be site-dependent, since bilateral medial temporal lobectomy produces similar results.

Non-hydrogen-bonding anesthetics such as nitrous oxide, ether, carbon dioxide, and halothane are reported to produce amnesia in animals. Several of these drugs are reportedly effective in inducing amnesia in humans. The type of memory loss in humans may be correlated with the depth of anesthesia. Nonverbal acoustic memories are impaired at very low nitrous oxide concentrations, while memory for verbal material is reportedly disrupted by higher dosages (Jarvik, 1972).

Cholinergic Drugs

Two anticholinesterases, diisopropyl fluorophosphate (DFP) and physostigmine, impair long-term memory formation in rodents. Paradoxically, injection of DFP into rats following "physiological forgetting" has been reported to lead to apparent recovery of memory. Scopolamine disrupts memory formation in rodents, and its apparent amnesic action when used as a preanesthetic in human obstetrical cases is well-known. As with other agents possessing anterograde effects, its action on memory cannot easily be separated from confusional effects. The mechanism by which scopolamine affects memory was clarified in a controlled study on human subjects comparing the effects of scopolamine, methyl scopolamine, and physostigmine. Scopolamine is known to act both centrally and peripherally, blocking synaptic acetylcholine receptors. Methyl scopolamine acts like scopolamine but cannot cross the blood-brain barrier in significant amounts. Physostigmine prolongs the effectiveness of acetylcholine by interfering with the action of the degradative enzyme, cholinesterase, and acts both centrally and peripherally. Only scopolamine affected memory in the dosages used, suggesting that interferences with cholinergic transmission in the brain impairs memory. Short-term memory was reportedly unaffected, while long-term storage was significantly impaired. It has been postulated that there are similarities between the type of memory defect produced by scopolamine in normal subjects and that seen in aging subjects in whom long-term memory storage and general cognition are similarly impaired with sparing of immediate memory. Interference with the human cholinergic system could therefore be one source of memory deficits seen in old age (Agranoff et al., 1975).

Other Substances and Treatments

Carbon dioxide has been reported to induce time-dependent amnesia in such diverse species as insects and mammals. It has been suggested that carbon dioxide may induce amnesia by altering 5-HT (serotonin) levels in the hippocampus, since trained rats evidence a rise in 5-HT levels, while animals that are both trained and treated with CO_2 do not evidence a comparable change. Hypoxia has been found to produce amnesia in rodents; however, its effect on human memory is unclear.

Diets deficient in vitamin E have been reported to lead to accumulation of lipofuscin in the central nervous system (CNS) and to impair memory in rats. This is of possible interest in that centrophenoxine, which is reported to deplete brain lipofuscin, has also been reported to facilitate human memory. These claims have not yet been fully documented.

Retrograde and anterograde amnesia resulted from an inadvertent large dose of enterovioform in a human patient. Since the drug produces distinct hippocampal and amygdala lesions in mice, the effect in man may be mediated by a site-specific mechanism (Agranoff et al., 1975).

Korsakoff's Syndrome

Korsakoff's syndrome is seen in chronic alcoholics who, in replacing food with ethanol, acquire a thiamine deficiency. Administration of thiamine to acutely ill patients with only ocular and cerebellar but not amnestic symptoms is reported to prevent the development of permanent sequelae, which include anterograde and retrograde amnesia. A traditional opinion has been that amnesia is caused by lesions in the mammillary bodies; however, patients without a known memory defect during life have shown mammillary body pathology on autopsy. More recently, the amnestic defect has been attributed to lesions in the medial dorsal nuclei, and perhaps in the medial pulvinar. In any event, it appears that thiamine deprivation in man in association with alcoholism may cause amnesia by creating lesions in sites requisite for memory fixation (Agranoff et al., 1975).

Posttraumatic Amnesia

Human amnesia associated with head injuries includes both anterograde and retrograde aspects. Apparent inability to consolidate new memories (i.e., anterograde amnesia) may last for weeks following the trauma, and is correlated with severe brain damage and with some permanent cognitive loss when it extends beyond 24 hours. Retrograde amnesia of traumatic etiology is always accompanied by some anterograde amnesia. Moreover, the more severe the anterograde component, the greater the time encompassed by the retrograde amnesia. The onset of amnesia can be delayed some time after the blow to the skull, suggesting that the cause of the amnesia is not the blow itself nor its immediate effects on the brain, but subsequent events, such as changes in the permeability of the blood-brain barrier, or cerebral edema. Alterations in the blood-barrier have been reported following convulsions, as well as following physical trauma (Barbizet, 1970; Whitty and Zangwill, 1966).

Memory Loss with Aging

Disorders of cognitive function that occur with age fall into two major categories: chronic organic brain syndrome associated with senile brain disease, and disorders associated with cerebral arteriosclerosis. The major cognitive symptom in senile brain disease is loss of memory for recent events. In more advanced stages of the disease, memories for remote events are disrupted as well. In contrast, arteriosclerotic memory disorders are sporadic, often arising suddenly as a consequence of circulatory changes in the brain.

Senile brain disease can be identified postmortem by the shrinking of the cerebral cortex and the presence of neurofibrillary tangles and plaques in atrophied areas of the brain. A positive correlation has been reported between the number of plaques in the cerebral grey matter on autopsy and the severity of the previously assessed dementia. It has been speculated that overproduction of fibrous protein causes neuronal degeneration by the displacement of cellular organelles. Alternatively, a qualitative change in fibrous proteins could result in neurofibrillary tangles, as well as other disruptions in cellular function.

Both cerebral oxygen consumption and cerebral blood flow tend to decline in old age. Whether these changes are related to the memory deficits seen in old age remains unclear, although studies have reported attempts to facilitate memory in the aged by increasing blood oxygen levels (Jarvik et al., 1972).

Storage or Retrieval

Both spontaneous and induced recovery from apparent amnesia have been reported in animals, implicating retrieval deficits rather than storage failure as the mechanism underlying the original performance decrement in these studies. For example, recovery of memory has been reported following amnesia by ECS. In a number of experimental paradigms, recovery is not demonstrable.

ECT-induced anterograde amnesia in humans is reported to be greater for recall than for recognition. These results suggest the underlying factor might be a retrieval deficit. The gradual, partial recovery from retrograde posttraumatic amnesia suggests that at least part of that deficit is one of retrieval. In studies with thiopental, however, equivalent memory loss is found using both recognition and recall tests. Furthermore, the deficit observed is not state-dependent, since subjects under sedation remember material acquired in a nonsedated state, and recall of material learned under sedation is not recalled more easily upon subsequent reinstatement of sedation. In this instance, storage, not retrieval would appear to be affected by the drug.

Facilitation of Memory

Subconvulsive doses of a variety of central nervous system stimulants have been reported to facilitate memory in animals: strychnine, diazadamantan, pentylenetetrazol, picrotoxin, bemegride, caffeine, and flurothyl. It is noteworthy, however, that several of the same drugs reportedly produce memory impairment when given in larger doses. There have been reports of memory facilitation by agents believed to stimulate protein synthesis, for example, ribaminol, and RNA synthesis (e.g., magnesium pemoline), as well as RNA itself, but both biochemical and behavioral aspects of these claims have been questioned. Numerous laboratories have reported facilitation of learning and memory in rodents by the administration of amphetamine, a drug known to alter biogenic amine metabolism.

Various drugs have been administered to human geriatric patients in attempts to improve memory. Most of these agents may be categorized as follows: (a) putative RNA and protein synthesis stimulators; (b) CNS stimulants; (c) antidepressants; (d) anticonvulsants; (e) vasodilators; and (f) β-adrenergic blockers. To our knowledge, none of the purported instances of memory facilitation in humans can survive critical evaluation. Many studies do not include adequate control groups to rule out potential treatment effects on performance which might be misinterpreted as true changes in cognitive function. Moreover, dose response curves are rarely reported, parametric determinations of optimal drug administration-test intervals are seldom made, and comprehensive comparative studies assessing the relative efficacy of the treatments are usually lacking. It should be noted that numerous failures to replicate claims of success with specific agents have been reported (McGaugh, 1973).

Concomitants of Memory Formation

Alterations in the composition of components of brain regions or brain cells have been reported in animals trained at particular tasks. Studies on rat motor-skill learning indicate that neurons and glia evidenced reciprocal increases and decreases in nucleic acid bases. Studies with labeled uridine in the mouse indicate an increase in labeling of RNA over the entire brain, but particularly in the diencephalon, as a result of training in a jump-up avoidance task. While such studies are suggestive, there has not been a clear-cut demonstration of a stimulation of *de novo* RNA synthesis that is linked to behavioral experience. From the biochemical standpoint, many of the reported labeling effects may simply reflect experimentally-produced regional attentions of endogenous unlabeled precursor pools rather than a change in RNA synthesis concomitant with specific learning. This possibility cannot be readily excluded experimentally since in vivo labeling experiments do not readily permit precursor pool measurement. Human studies on concomitants of memory function are lacking. More recent progress in noninvasive diagnostic neurological techniques may eventually prove useful for this purpose (Ansel and Bradley, 1973).

BIBLIOGRAPHY

AGRANOFF, B. W.   Effects of antibiotics on long-term memory formation in the goldfish. In W. K. Honig and P. H. R. James (Eds.), *Animal memory.* New York: Academic Press, 1971. Pp. 243–258.

AGRANOFF, B. W.   Biochemical concomitants of the storage of behavioral information. In L. Jaenicke (Ed.), *The 25th Mosbacher colloquium.* New York: Springer-Verlag, 1975.

AGRANOFF, B. W.; SPRINGER, A. D.; and QUARTON, G. C.   Biochemistry of memory and learning. In P. J. Vinken and G. W. Bruyn (Eds.), *Handbook of clinical neurology* Vol. 29. Amsterdam: North-Holland, 1975. Chap. 16.

ANSEL, G. B., and BRADLEY, P. B. (Eds.).   *Macromolecules and behavior.* London: Macmillan, 1973.

BARBIZET, J.   *Human memory and its pathology.* San Francisco, Calif.: Freeman, 1970.

FINK, M.; KETY, S.; McGAUGH, J.; and WILLIAMS, T. A.   (Eds.). *Psychobiology of convulsive therapy.* Washington, D.C.: Winston, 1974.

JARVIK, M. E.   Effects of chemical and physical treatments on learning and memory. *Annual Review of Psychology,* 1972, *23,* 457–486.

JARVIK, M. E.; GRITZ, E. R.; and SCHNEIDER, N. G.   Drugs and memory disorders in human aging. *Behavioral Biology,* 1972, *7,* 643–668.

McGAUGH, J. L.   Drug facilitation of learning and memory. *Annual Review of Pharmacology,* 1973, *13,* 229–241.

WHITTY, C. W. M., and ZANGWILL, O. L. (Eds.).   *Amnesia.* London: Butterworth, 1966.

ALAN D. SPRINGER
LINDA M. SPRINGER
BERNARD W. AGRANOFF

MEMORY: PSYCHOANALYTIC THEORY

There is no psychoanalytic theory of memory in the sense of a coherent and comprehensive explanatory and predictive system. Rather, scattered over a wide range of works, there are speculations, ideas, and hypotheses, and often loosely formulated, concerning remembering, forgetting, and related phenomena. In their common concern with the motivational aspects of memory, however, these scattered ideas are conceptually unified.

What is distinctive about the way psychoanalytic theory looks at memory is its strong emphasis on motivational factors, its dynamic view of memory. The term *dynamic* is intended to convey, not only the motivated nature of specific instances of forgetting and remembering, but the central role memory plays in the general process of gratification of needs and instinctual drives, and in the processes of symptom formation, on the one hand, and therapeutic change on the other.

The term *instinctual drive* is a translation of the German word *Trieb* used by Freud. The proper translation for *Trieb* has been debated— should it be "instinct" or "drive" or perhaps some other term? This paper follows Waelder's (1960) suggestion and uses the term instinctual drive.

For present purposes, instinctual drive will be, again following Waelder (1960), broadly defined as "powerful strivings . . . which are rooted in [our] physical nature," are goal directed, exert constant pressure for gratification, have psychological consequences when not gratified, and are capable, by various psychological maneuvers, of being inhibited, renounced, and under appropriate conditions, revived.

Repression and Motivated Forgetting

The most obvious expression of the psychoanalytic theory of memory is found in its attempt to explain, not the *adequate* activity of remembering, but the *inadequate* activity of forgetting as a manifestation of repression. Repression, certainly basic both historically and conceptually in psychoanalytic theory, can be viewed, in part, as motivated forgetting. According to Jones (1911), Freud regarded "repression as a biological defense mechanism, the purpose of which is to guard the mind from painful experiences" and which is expressed as a tendency to forget painful or disagreeable memories.

As Wolitzky, Klein, and Dworkin (1975) have pointed out, the essence of repression is the unconscious inhibition of awareness of a prohibited wish or impulse and derivative ideas and memories consequent to their disavowal. Such inhibition and disavowal is manifested in the avoidance of ideas, thoughts, actions, and memories that would "open a way toward the gratifying but pain-associated fulfillment" or in the failure to comprehend the "meaning of behaviors that do accomplish the gratification in substitutive manner." Thus, repression may be manifested not only in the forgetting of a memory or idea connected to a prohibited wish, but also in the failure to comprehend the connection between the memory or idea and the wish.

The effects of repressed ideas and memories are seen not only in regard to the originally repressed material and in the dramatic forms of hysterical symptoms, but in regard to even indirectly related material and in the everyday form of *faulty actions,* such as slips of the tongue, forgetting of proper names, misreadings. The German words for the many examples of "shortcomings in our psychical functioning," cited by Freud in his *The Psychopathology of Everyday Life,* reveal more clearly than the English words their internal similarity. They all contain the prefix *ver-* (which roughly corresponds to the English *mis-,* as in *mis*understand, *mis*read). Thus, the examples include *vergessen* (forgetting), *versprechen* (slips of the tongue or misspeaking), *verlesen* (misreading), *verschreiben* (slips of the pen or literally, miswriting), and *vergreifen* (bungled actions). For Freud, then, forgetting was but one example of faulty functioning.

Freud claimed that quite often what one forgets turns out to be linked in some way, directly or indirectly, to unconscious ideas significant and painful to oneself. He explained such forgetting as a result of the tendency "to avoid the awakening of pain" through memory. He makes clear that the pain to which he refers is that psychic pain which would be aroused if the unconscious wishes and impulses to which the forgotten idea is related were to gain access to consciousness and thereby succeed in provoking anxiety and conflict. In short, such forgetting is motivated by unconscious factors and occurs as a means of dealing with the repressed ideas to which the forgotten material has become linked.

Thus, although the forgotten material may, in itself, be quite neutral in content, its associative link to repressed ideas is critical in understanding why it is forgotten. Slips of the tongue and other parapraxes (Jones's term for *Fehlleistung* or "faulty function") are also attributed to unconscious motives and are explained in essentially the same way as forgetting. Both forgetting and other parapraxes are occasioned by a link between current activity and repressed ideas.

Why the faulty action follows contact with repressed ideas is critical to understanding psychoanalytic theory. If it were simply hypothesized that anxiety is aroused by contact with repressed material and that such anxiety has a disruptive effect on subsequent behavior, as manifested by forgetting, slips of the tongue, or the like, there would be no theory of *motivated* forgetting and parapraxes. That is, there would be no theory dealing with unconscious purposes and motives. And it is precisely with such purposes and motives that psychoanalytic theory deals. Therefore, it is important to add that in both forgetting and other parapraxes, the faulty action reflects both the prohibited wish and an attempt to deal with the anxiety aroused by the threatened emergence of the prohibited wish into consciousness. In forgetting, the method of dealing with such material is its removal from conscious awareness and expression. In other parapraxes, such as slips of the tongue, the prohibited striving asserts itself indirectly by distorting the word or idea in associative connection with it. And the content that does emerge into behavior or consciousness (the slip of the tongue spoken, the incorrect word read, the bungled action carried out) reflects neither complete repression nor complete expression of the prohibited material, but rather a compromise between the two.

One question that arises is whether all forgetting is motivated by unconscious factors or, indeed, motivated at all. It is clear from Freud's writings that he was reluctant to claim that all forgetting was the result of unconscious motivation and recognized the operation of nonmotivational factors in forgetting. But the kind of forgetting that was of interest to Freud was that motivated by unconscious factors.

Another question that is of interest is the seeming paradoxical relationship between repression and forgetting. Insofar as repression includes the unavailability of memories, ideas, and so forth, to consciousness, it seems, by definition, to involve forgetting. But, as Schlesinger (1964) has pointed out, repression is a form of *permanent memory* insofar as repressed ideas and memories continue to remain active, continue to have long-term effects on behavior, and continue to be preserved in their original form and with their original intensity. Indeed, given the "timelessness of the unconscious," the best way to preserve a memory or idea is to repress it. In fact, Freud points out that often the task of psychotherapy is to help bring repressed material to consciousness, aid in its being worked

through, and thus enable the patient to finally "forget." The paradox is largely resolved when one considers that remembering and forgetting are being used in two senses: (1) from the commonsense point of view of availability versus unavailability to consciousness, and (2) in the sense of exerting usually undesirable effects on functioning. The idea that repression serves to preserve memories, however, would still seem to hold.

Also of great interest is the question of systematic empirical support for the concept of repression defined as motivated forgetting. From about the late 1920s periodic interest has been expressed in experimental investigation of repression. As Rapaport (1950) and Mackinnon and Dukes (1962), among others, have pointed out, most of the studies "failed in their specific goal of bringing repression as conceived by the psychoanalysts into the laboratory for experimental study." Studies on the relationship between memory and hedonic tone, task incompletion, induced experiences of failure and associated external pain or threat have been carried out as presumed laboratory analogues of repression. Unfortunately, none of these has very much to do with repression as it is defined in psychoanalytic theory.

For laboratory studies to be relevant to repression, as it is defined and used by psychoanalytic theory, they must include material relevant to unconscious wishes or impulses and "a conflict which stimulated inhibition of an activated unconscious wish, tendency, or impulse" (Wolitzky, Klein, and Dworkin, 1975). There are only a few studies which meet these criteria.

One study that demonstrated parapraxes in a laboratory situation was an early one carried out by Erickson (1939). His basic technique was to present hypnotic suggestions that in their waking state subjects recall as their own an experience suggested by the hypnotist and of which they were to be ashamed. According to Erickson, the subjects behaved as though the suggested experience was out of their own past. Most important, they showed slips of the tongue and bungled actions.

Luborsky (1964, 1973) used the psychoanalytic situation to collect systematic data on the particular phenomenon momentary forgetting, in which one is about to say something, forgets what it is, and then recovers the thought. He reported that, as compared to control segments, segments of the patients' verbalizations preceding instances of momentary forgetting consistently contained evidence of buildup of cognitive disturbance and presence of emotionally-laden and conflictful themes, for example, lack of control and competence; transference references. He interprets these results as suggesting that prior to momentary forgetting, the patients' associations have made contact with repressed ideas and memories threatening to intrude into awareness, with the result that cognitive disturbance and defensive momentary forgetting occur.

In a laboratory study that was designed to correct the aforementioned defects of other experiments and to create an analogue faithful to the clinical meaning of repression, Wolitzky, Klein, and Dworkin (1975) presented to an experimental group of subjects, under conditions of hypnosis, a fantasy containing eight critical words. The fantasy was designed to elicit feelings of rejection and reactions of regression, the contemplation of pleasurable infantile wish fulfillment, and a conflict over seeking or desiring such wish fulfillment in the present. A control group was given a fantasy similar in length and structure, that contained the same eight critical words, but that did not elicit the conflict. They found that the experimental subjects recalled and recognized fewer of the critical words than the control subjects.

To this point, forgetting and the conditions and motives for forgetting have been discussed, rather than a general psychoanalytic theory of memory. The fact is, however, that the psychoanalytic explanation of forgetting, with the central role given to instinctual strivings and their repression, is based on an implicit theory of memory, in particular, on an implicit idea of the relationship between instinctual strivings and memory.

Memory Traces, Repression, and Wish Fulfillment

If forgetting, slips of the tongue, bungled actions, and other parapraxes must be employed to keep repressed ideas and material associatively linked with repressed ideas from overt expression and from gaining access to consciousness, it is only a testimony to the strength and persistence of these repressed ideas. And, indeed, the strength and persistence of repressed instinctual strivings in organizing and utilizing memory are essential features of the psychoanalytic theory of memory.

According to Freud, momentary excitations of the perceptual system are transformed into lasting traces by the memory system. Although stored memories can become conscious, as a rule, they remain unconscious. Some memories, of course, while not in consciousness, are readily accessible. They are preconscious and not dynamically repressed. Repressed ideas, memories, and wishes, are represented in memory traces which are unavailable to consciousness, that is, they are forgotten. However, the forgetting is dynamic since a counterforce is necessary to maintain it. The repressed material is continually striving to force its way into consciousness, "to carry the important memory-traces into consciousness."

Freud (1937) was not merely being metaphorical, but really proposing that repressed material could have palpable effects on experience and behavior. This is seen in his explanations of hallucinations and delusions as the result of the "upward drive of the repressed . . . [forcing] its content into consciousness" and in his belief that the "ultra-clear" (*überdeutlich*), almost hallucinatory recollections that sometimes follow the analyst's presentation of a construction of some aspect of the patient's childhood are due to the fact that the "upward drive of the repressed, stirred into activity by the putting forward of the construction, has striven to carry the important memory-traces into consciousness" (p. 266).

Indirect manifestations of this *upward drive* for expression and the struggle against overt and patent expression are the parapraxes already discussed. More serious manifestations are the "symptoms and inhibitions [which] are the consequences of repressions . . . [and] are a substitute for these things forgotten" (pp. 257–258). Like parapraxes, symptoms are partial, disguised, and compromise expressions of repressed wishes and thus entail partial drive gratification. And like parapraxes, they are unsuccessful attempts at forgetting—insofar as the forgotten material is not finally resolved and fully forgotten, but intrudes into behavior, with symptoms as a particularly troublesome intrusion.

The task of psychoanalysis "aims at inducing the patient to give up the repression"; "to recollect certain experiences and the affective impulses called up by them which he has for the time being forgotten" (1937, pp. 257–258). After the repressed material is brought to consciousness, experienced, understood, and worked through, it can finally be laid to rest and fully "forgotten."

Some comments are in order regarding Freud's concept of memory trace and the task of psychoanalysis as stated above. Freud's memory trace concept appears to be based on a model of memory belonging to what Neisser (1966) has called the *reappearance hypothesis.* The memory trace is viewed as a faithful record, almost an exact copy, of past experience which, if activated, can result in recovering the past experience with perceptual vividness. The alternative view is that what is stored in memory are, not copies of experiences, but constructions of events, and what is involved in recall are imaginative reconstructions in the light of present attitudes and needs. Despite his basic conception of memory trace as replica, Freud (1937) recognized that in the psychoanalytic situation, what often emerges is "an assured conviction of the truth of the [analyst's] construction" rather than reappearances of childhood material.

There are many questions left unanswered by the capsule account above. But what is clear is the central role memory plays in psychoanalytic theory. It is an essential aspect of drive gratification, critical to an understanding of repression, and critically involved in symptom formation and pathology on the one hand and in therapy, on the other. Indeed, psychoanalytic theory is probably the only theory which proposes that "forgetting" (or repression) can help make one ill and remembering can help make one well.

According to Freud, the press for satisfaction of instinctual drives sets up constant pressure for cathecting the memory image of an experience of satisfaction. Cathexis can be defined as referring to an idea or memory or representation of a person or object being intensified or emotionally charged by virtue of one's emotional and libidinal involvement with that idea or representation. The primitive tendency of the psychic apparatus, upon confronting the press of internal need, is to recathect the mnemic image of past experiences of satisfaction. Freud speculates, for example, that the infant, when experiencing hunger, recathects the mnemic image of past experiences of satisfaction and reexperiences the breast and the feeding situation with hallucinatory vividness. This response, however, does not succeed in eliminating internal stimuli and in satisfying drive. The very beginnings of thinking and reality testing are rooted in this failure of hallucinatory wish fulfillment. But, as Freud pointed out in a number of his writings, he viewed thinking only as a circuitous route to gratification. "All [this] activity of thought," he proposed, "merely constitutes a roundabout path to wish fulfillment which has been made necessary by experience. Thought is after all nothing but a substitute for a hallucinatory wish" (1900, p. 606).

In a sense, then, memory, along with other cognitive functions, is always organized by drive. The push to recathect a mnemic image comes from the urge to reexperience satisfaction. This is true even for reality-oriented cognition which, as noted, develops as a necessarily circuitous means of experiencing satisfaction because the more direct path does not work. It is in this sense that memory, even when reality-oriented, and conceptually organized, is always also *drive organized.* It is always, according to Freud, directly or indirectly in the service of, and organized for, fulfillment of wishes stemming from drives.

Ego Psychology and Drive versus Conceptual Organization

It is important to note that a somewhat different conception of thinking emerges from more recent formulations in psychoanalytic ego psychology which stress the aspects of thought and of other ego functions that develop and function autonomously and independent of instinctual drive (e.g., Hartmann, 1950, 1958; Hartmann, Kris, and Lowenstein, 1946). Thus, while they do not dispute Freud's idea that the failure of hallucinatory wish fulfillment can be an impetus to the development of thought; the capacity for thought and the development of thought, they would point out, have bases independent of instinctual drive. With regard to memory, Hartmann (1958) notes that

memory, associations, and so on are functions which cannot possibly be derived from the ego's relationships to instinctual drives or love-objects, but are rather *prerequisites* for our conception of these and of their development. (p. 15)

Freud's emphasis on the drive-serving aspects of memory and other ego functions can perhaps be reconciled with Hartmann's emphasis on their maturational autonomy by distinguishing between adaptive function and structural characteristics. From the point of view of adaptive function, memory, along with other ego functions, in order to be adaptive, must be organized "for the purpose of" fulfilling needs and gratifying drives. From the point of view of structural characteristics, memory can be conceptually organized or drive organized, that is, it can be organized according to objective characteristics of events, consensually validated dimensions, and the logic of reality or it can be organized along drive-relevant, idiosyncratic dimensions and the logic of peremptory urges. Here, language plays tricks. For the means of organization most adaptive for drive gratification is not drive but conceptual organization. The latter, because of its reality orientation, is more likely to be adaptive in fulfilling needs and gratifying drive, while drive organization is less likely to be capable of need fulfillment and drive gratification. For example, an hallucinating psychotic individual whose cognitive behavior, according to psychoanalytic theory, is dominated by drive organization is, by virtue of such organization, less likely to be able to take actions in reality which will lead to an "experience of satisfaction."

The issue of drive versus conceptual organization of memory (Rapaport, 1951, 1960), if taken beyond the specific question of the relation between drive and memory, raises the general question of how events are stored, organized, and retrieved in memory. Posing the question in these general terms opens the door to considering a wide range of factors. The broad psychoanalytic contribution to a study of memory may lie, not in its specific stress on drive factors in memory, but in the importance it gives to the investigation of emotional and motivational factors in memory organization, particularly if "emotional" and "motivational" are broadly conceived to include attitudes, interests, and subtle affective and evaluational responses.

BIBLIOGRAPHY

FREUD, S. (1900). *The interpretation of dreams.* New York: Avon Books, 1965.

FREUD, S. (1901). The psychopathology of everyday life. *Standard Edition.* London: Hogarth Press, 1969, *6.*

FREUD, S. (1937). Constructions in analysis. *Standard Edition,* 1964, *23.*

HARTMANN, H.; KRIS, E.; and LOWENSTEIN, R. Comments on the formation of psychic structure. *Psychoanalytic Study of the Child,* 1946, *2,* 11–38.

HARTMANN, H. Comments on the psychoanalytic theory of the ego. *Psychoanalytic Study of the Child,* 1950, *5,* 74–96.

HARTMANN, H. *Ego psychology and the problem of adaptation.* New York: International Universities Press, 1958.

JONES, E. The psychopathology of everyday life. *American Journal of Psychology,* 1911, *22,* 479–480.

LUBORSKY, L. Forgetting and remembering (momentary forgetting) during psychotherapy: A new sample. *Psychological Issues,* 1973, *8* (Monograph 30), 29–55.

MACKINNON, D. W., and DUKES, W. F. Repression. In L. Postman (Ed.), *Psychology in the making.* New York: Knopf, 1962.

NEISSER, U. *Cognitive psychology.* New York: Appleton-Century-Crofts, 1966.

RAPAPORT, D. *Emotions and memory.* New York: International Universities Press, 1950.

RAPAPORT, D. Comment on Freud's formulations regarding the two principles in mental functioning. In D. Rapaport (Ed.), *Organization and pathology of thought.* New York: Columbia University Press, 1951.

RAPAPORT, D. The structure of psychoanalytic theory. *Psychological Issues,* 1960, *2* (Monograph 6).

WAELDER, R. *Basic theory of psychoanalysis.* New York: International Universities Press, 1960.

WOLITZKY, D. L.; KLEIN, G. S.; and DWORKIN, S. F. An experimental approach to the study of repression: Effects of an hypnotically induced fantasy. In D. P. Spence (Ed.), *Psychoanalysis and contemporary science* (Vol. 4). New York: International Universities Press, 1975.

MORRIS EAGLE

MEMORY: QUANTITATIVE APPROACHES

Quantitative analysis of human memory is as old as the experimental study of human memory. In his pioneer investigation, Herman Ebbinghaus not only reported extensive experimental studies of memory but also suggested a quantitative formulation of the forgetting curve which generally characterized his data. Subsequent work early in this century had as one of its aims the determination of the curve of forgetting, and Strong found an exponential decay curve for recognition memory which differed from the inverse logarithmic function reported by Ebbinghaus. Early theoretical approaches to memory and learning were modeled after those popular and successful in physics; initial assumptions were stated in the form of differential equations and deductions of the theory required their solution. Perhaps the most successful of such attempts was the rational learning curve of Thurstone, where initial assumptions about the rate of error elimination and the rate of growth of response strength with reinforcement resulted in an ogival or S-shaped learning curve.

In the 1950s, Markov models began to appear, and this was a natural concomitant of advances in probability theory and stochastic processes. Early work focused on associative learning, probability learning, generalization, discrimination, and choice. The theoretical superstructure for much of this work was the stimulus sampling theory of Estes, and much of this research has been reviewed by Atkinson, Bower, and Crothers (1965). At the same time, there were important developments in choice theory, measurement theory, and computer simulation. Since the mid-1960s, quantitative analyses of memory have probably had their biggest impact on process models, where the attempt is made to describe and understand the underlying processes involved in the encoding, storage, and retrieval of information in human memory.

Most of the process models have dealt either with item information, associative information, order information, or free recall. Item information refers to whatever information is stored in memory to make possible recognition of events, objects, or experiences one has encountered before. Associative information underlies associations, and order information underlies memory for sequences such as the days of the week, the months of the year, or how to spell words. Free recall by contrast is an experimental paradigm involving order-free recall of a set of related or unrelated items. Free recall

has received considerable experimental and theoretical attention. The remainder of this article considers each in turn.

Item Information

The dominant theoretical approach to the encoding, storage, and retrieval of item information has long been strength theory which, informally, probably represents the intuitions about memory of the man in the street and, more formally, has been developed in the work of Norman and Wickelgren. This theory says that a memory trace has a representation in memory to which a unidimensional measure of strength can be assigned. The outcome of the encoding process can be described by parameter α and subsequent interference (e.g., the presentation of other items) decreases this strength by some fraction ϕ. With exponential forgetting the time course of memory-trace strength is given by the equation

$$d'(i) = \alpha \phi^i \qquad (1)$$

where $d'(i)$ is the strength of the memory trace d' after i units of interference. The measure d' comes from the theory of signal detection, which has had considerable application to human memory.

With a signal-detection analysis, strength theory assumes that old items have one distribution, new items have a second distribution and that, in responding to a test item, one is sampling from these two distributions and trying to reach a decision. If the observation exceeds a cutoff or criterion, the response will be "yes," if it does not, the response will be "no," and a maximum-likelihood principle is used to determine the location of this yes-no cutoff. The d' value simply characterizes the mean strength of old items relative to new, and β (the ratio of the two ordinates at the point of intersection) locates the criterion. These relationships are illustrated in Figure 1, where x is the strength axis, $f_o(x)$ and $f_n(x)$ the old-and new-item distributions, and x_c is the criterion.

Strength theory predicts not only the exponential forgetting described by Equation (1) but also many detailed features of the data obtained from recognition-memory experiments. Hits and false alarms (Fig. 1) should be sensitive to the prior probabilities of old and new

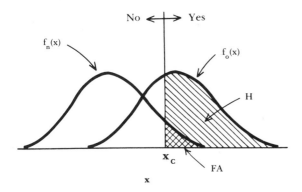

Fig. 1. Overlapping new-item and old-item distributions. The horizontal *x* axis represents memory-trace strength, and the location of a sample relative to the criterion (x_c) determines whether the ensuing response will be "no" or "yes." In the figure, *H* denotes hits and *FA* denotes false alarms. (From B. B. Murdock, Jr., 1974, p. 29; reprinted with permission of publisher.)

items and costs and payoffs (payoff for correct responses, costs of errors). A confidence-judgment procedure can be used to obtain the equivalent of multiple decision cuts on the strength axis, and an ROC or receiver operating characteristic curve (a plot of cumulative hit rate as a function of cumulative false alarm rate) should be linear on normal-normal coordinates if the theory is correct. With a forced-choice procedure, one can predict percent correct by assuming that it is the probability that one observation drawn at random for $f_o(x)$ will exceed all remaining observations drawn at random from $f_n(x)$.

Strength theory generally does a fine job of accounting for the detailed features of data from recognition-memory experiments, and tests of the basic assumptions show them to be reasonable. However, it seems unable to account for list-discrimination effects (e.g., one's own name would be a "strong" item yet it would be unlikely to elicit a false alarm). Also, work on high-speed scanning suggests that the direct-access view of retrieval implicitly assumed by strength theory may not be correct. An alternative to strength theory is an attribute view, several versions of which have been proposed.

Associative Information

The one-element model of Bower was a particularly successful application of stimulus-sampling theory to a specific problem. It assumed that, in paired-associate learning, an association was either formed or not, and the probability that an association was formed did not increase with repetition. With binary responses, a correct response could come about either because an association was in the learned state or through guessing. With only a single parameter, the transition parameter *c*, the model was capable of describing in detail the experimental data from paired-associate learning experiments with binary responses. However, subsequent studies soon showed that binary responses seemed to be a special case and, in particular, the stationarity assumption was contradicted when the size of the response ensemble exceeded two.

Increasing interest in short-term memory led to a natural extension of the Bower model wherein three states were proposed. An association could either be in a null (unlearned) state, a transient or short-term state, or a more permanent long-term state. While the long-term state was absorbing, the short-term state was not, and the effect of repeated presentations would depend upon whether a particular association had been forgotten, dropped from the short-term to the null state. Various versions of such a three-state Markov model were proposed, and as further information about the spacing effect became known, detailed assumptions of the models were modified to account for it. The spacing effect refers to the fact that the benefits of repetition are curvilinear, being greatest, for paired associates, at intermediate spacings or lags. Also, these three-state models were able to account for the nonstationarity effects commonly reported in list-learning experiments.

With active research in short-term memory starting in the 1960s, a number of detailed findings became available which required further explanation. Currently, a fluctuation model seems best able to encompass the known facts about association, at least in the short-term area. This model, like the Bower model, assumes that associations are all-or-none, but unlike the Bower model, recovery from the null state is possible. The presumed fluctuation is between these two states, and the experimental asymptote and recency effects so characteristic of experimental data are a consequence of this fluctuation process going to equilibrium. List-learning effects can be explained by changes in the transition probabilities with repetition. Recognition tasks can be explained on the basis of independent forward and backward associations plus a rational guessing scheme. So far, at least, the fluctuation model is able to fit the experimental data fairly well with only a few free parameters.

Order Information

The discussion has centered up to now on mathematical models, where explicit expressions can be stated or derived. Another type of quantitative approach to human memory is through computer-simulation models, where the assumptions of the model are stated in a computer program. The predictions of the model are not derived analytically but instead by running the program on the computer with the computer as subject. In fact, the computer functions in three capacities; it compiles the program (the model) into a form which can be run as an experiment on the computer; it serves both as experimenter and subject in collecting the data; and it often does the data reduction and analysis as it would for any experiment which collected a substantial amount of data.

One of the early and still popular models for order information is EPAM, an acronym for *Elementary Perceiver and Memorizer*. This is a computer-simulation model which incorporates three memory structures: a short-term memory, a working or acquisition memory, and a long-term store. Short-term memory is a buffer store of very limited size, working memory contains the internal representations of stimulus objects being learned, having a tree structure called the discrimination net, while long-term memory contains a relative permanent repository of the images. The underlying processes involving learning and memory are assumed to be serial (one at a time), and each unitary process is assumed to require a finite amount of time to perform. Observable behavioral consequences are the result of many such molecular processes, and the total time is then seen as the sum of the components.

The model is capable of making quantitative predictions about serial learning, and in particular, the ubiquitous serial-position curve. In most serial tasks, the point of maximum difficulty is toward the latter-middle part of the list, with beginning and end the easiest. EPAM

is also capable of making accurate predictions about a number of other phenomena characteristic of both serial and paired-associate learning. In the model, slowly developing effects are manifestations of the concatenation of the underlying processes which, while individually quite fast, are slow in the aggregate. Therein lies one of the problems with EPAM, as many of the same effects (and, in particular, serial-position effects) can be obtained after a single presentation of a short list of items. It is not clear how the model would explain that. Another problem with computer-simulation models such as EPAM is that they are not easy to use. They require not only familiarity with the particular programming language but also access to a large computer and funds to pay for it in order to discover what predictions the models make. Finally, the "predictions" are in reality data though obtained from a rather different subject than ones usually tested. These data have all the variability of data characteristic of human memory performance. As a consequence, the same problems are often encountered in interpreting the "theory" as in interpreting experimental data.

Free Recall

Models of free recall epitomize the process models which are now so popular in the analysis of human memory. A progenitor of current models was the filter theory of Broadbent, which was the first systematic and detailed information-processing model of memory and attention. As in EPAM, it assumed discrete storage systems and a limited-capacity channel through which processed information must flow. Glanzer and Waugh and Norman elaborated on the importance of separate and independent short-term (primary memory) and long-term (secondary memory) stores, and showed how experimental data could be analyzed into the two components. Probably the most elaborate and detailed model of this sort is the buffer model of Atkinson and Shiffrin which, though originally designed for paired associates, has come to have greater significance for free recall.

The main feature of the model is the rehearsal buffer, which can only hold a limited number (*r*) of items and from which loss occurs only by displacement. This latter view has, however, been modified since its original formulation. When an item is presented, there is some probability α that it enters the buffer. Transfer of information to long-term memory continues as long as the item stays in the buffer, and the transfer rate is θ. Once displaced from the buffer, decay of information from long-term memory occurs at a rate determined by the decay parameter Υ. Recall probability is then determined jointly by the probability that an item is in the buffer, or short-term memory, and its current strength in long-term memory. Standard parameter-estimation techniques exist for obtaining best-fitting values for a given set of data, and early application of the equations to experimental data obtained from a continuous paired-associate task gave quite promising results.

Conclusion

A variety of quantitative approaches to human memory have been suggested, a few of which were briefly discussed here. More ambitious and more successful attempts are bound to occur as our knowledge increases in breadth and depth. Quantitative approaches are an attempt to help us understand the complex processes involved in the encoding, storage, and retrieval of information from human memory. Ultimately, we will only be able to say we really understand human memory when physiological mechanisms, behavioral data, and quantitative models converge.

BIBLIOGRAPHY

ATKINSON, R. C.; BOWER, G. H.; and CROTHERS, E. J. *An introduction to mathematical learning theory.* New York: Wiley, 1965.

COOMBS, C. H. *A theory of data.* New York: Wiley, 1964.

COOMBS, C. H.; DAWES, R. M.; and TVERSKY, A. *Mathematical psychology: An elementary introduction.* Englewood Cliffs, N.J.: Prentice-Hall, 1970.

FEIGENBAUM, E. A., and FELDMAN, J. (Eds.). *Computers and thought.* New York: McGraw-Hill, 1963.

LUCE, R. D. *Individual choice behavior.* New York: Wiley, 1959.

MILLER, G. A. (Ed.). *Mathematics and psychology.* New York: Wiley, 1964.

MURDOCK, B. B., JR. *Human memory: Theory and data.* Potomac, Md.: Erlbaum, 1974.

NEIMARK, E. D., and ESTES, W. K. (Eds.). *Stimulus sampling theory.* San Francisco: Holden-Day, 1967.

NORMAN, D. A. (Ed.). *Models of human memory.* New York: Academic Press, 1970.

RESTLE, F. *The psychology of judgment and choice.* New York: Wiley, 1961.

RESTLE, F., and GREENO, J. G. *Introduction to mathematical psychology.* Reading, Mass.: Addison-Wesley, 1970.

See also MEMORY: COMPUTER SIMULATION

BENNET B. MURDOCK, JR.

MEMORY: RETRIEVAL FROM LONG-TERM STORAGE

Retrieval from long-term memory is a central problem in human verbal memory and learning. The familiar difficulty in retrieving even well-known information from long-term memory has been documented by studies of the "tip-of-the-tongue" phenomenon (Brown and McNeill, 1966), and the incompleteness of retrieval from long-term memory in verbal learning has been demonstrated by the use of cues to increase retrieval (Tulving and Pearlstone, 1966). Spontaneous retrieval without further presentation has shown that most recall failure during verbal learning is due to retrieval failure rather than retention failure (Buschke, 1974).

Retrieval from long-term memory has been considered in two different ways in experimental psychology: in studies of verbal learning and in studies of category recall. In studies of verbal learning, both Glanzer (1966, 1972) and Craik (1968), employing free recall, have shown that true retrieval from long-term storage is demonstrated by recall after appropriate verbal interference. The verbal interference prevents the immediate recall of items just presented, that is from short-term storage. In studies of category recall by spontaneous naming of all items included in some well-known category (Brown, 1923; Bousfield and Sedgewick, 1944; and Buschke, Goldberg, and Lazer, 1973), retrieval from long-term memory means exhaustive retrieval directly from permanent storage. In verbal learning, long-term memory refers to the retention of information about items presented for learning, information that facilitates the selective retrieval of those items from permanent storage. In category retrieval, long-term memory means permanent memory. Learning to recall a restricted set of particular items and recalling all items from a particular category both involve retrieval of information about items already retained in permanent memory. Learning to recall a specific list of already familiar items, however, requires *selective* retrieval of only those specific items from permanent storage. Recall of a category requires *exhaustive* retrieval from permanent storage of every item so categorized in permanent memory.

Exhaustive Retrieval

Studies of exhaustive retrieval from long-term memory that require retrieval of all items from a category have shown that while it is possible to retrieve items from a particular category without thinking of other items that do not belong to the category, it is surprisingly difficult. The rate of such retrieval decreases rapidly long before most items in the category have been retrieved. Such retrieval, moreover, improves spontaneously on repeated attempts to recall items from that category even though there is no further presentation of additional items to the subject. About 85% of previously retrieved items are retrieved again on a second retrieval attempt, and about twice as many new items are gained on the second retrieval as are lost from the preceding retrieval. Such retrieval is quite idiosyncratic. It is not necessarily restricted to more common items.

Spontaneous retrieval of all items in a category can be improved by reminding, that is, by allowing the subject to review an extensive list of items in that category. Such reminding is most effective when it occurs after the subject has already attempted at least one spontaneous retrieval (Buschke, Goldberg, and Lazar, 1973), so that the retrieval of additional items can be integrated with the retrieval of items already recalled.

The clustering of closely related items found in spontaneous retrieval of items from a category in permanent memory indicates that such retrieval may be useful for investigating the organization of information in permanent storage, as well as for investigation of retrieval from permanent storage. A better understanding of the organization of permanent storage should also be relevant for analysis of retrieval from long-term memory in verbal list learning. The latter usually involves the selective retrieval of already well-known items from permanent storage.

Selective Retrieval

Most studies of free recall list learning have not permitted the evaluation of storage, retention, and retrieval from long-term memory during learning. The presentation of all items in the list before each recall attempt results in retrieval from both long-term memory and short-term memory. Since an accurate estimate of what is retrieved from long-term memory alone is necessary to evaluate the amount of previous storage and continuing retention in long-term memory, storage and retention cannot be measured under those conditions. Tulving has shown how retrieval from long-term memory may be estimated even with continuing presentation of all items throughout learning. This is done by identifying retrieval from long-term storage with the recall of items after the inference provided by the presentation and recall of at least seven other items (Tulving and Colotla, 1970; Craik and Birdwhistell, 1971). This analysis of retrieval from long-term memory is justified by Glanzer's demonstration that such interference will prevent the immediate recall of items from short-term storage, leaving only items retrieved from long-term memory.

Retrieval from long-term memory during verbal learning is, however, shown most directly by spontaneous retrieval without further presentation. This type of retrieval also permits straightforward evaluation of storage and retention in long-term memory. A more direct method for showing true retrieval from long-term memory, without contamination by immediate recall from short-term storage, is simply to restrict the presentations so that retrieval from long-term memory is shown by spontaneous recall over prolonged testing without further presentation. This can be carried out by use of learning paradigms such as *selective reminding*, or *restricted reminding*, in which any further presentation after the initial presentation of the list is limited appropriately to allow the subject to show learning by recall without further presentation (Buschke, 1973, 1974).

In the more general *selective reminding*, after the initial presentation of the entire list the only items presented on each trial are those items that were not recalled on the immediately preceding trial. Since any item that was recalled on the immediately preceding trial is not presented on the next trial, the subject can show its retrieval from long-term storage by recall without presentation on the next trial. In *restricted reminding* each item is presented only until it has been recalled just once. Since an item is never presented again after it has been recalled once, the subject can show its retrieval from long-term storage by recall without presentation on any subsequent recall attempt after its last presentation (when it was first recalled). Similarly, the use of only a *single presentation* of the list before repeated attempts at spontaneous retrieval also allows the subject to show retrieval from long-term storage by spontaneous recall without further presentation.

Such spontaneous retrieval of an item without further presentation also demonstrates its *storage* or initial encoding on or before its last presentation, and shows its continuing *retention* in long-term storage despite any recall failures. Although even a single presentation of the list may be sufficient for initial encoding and storage of much of the list under some circumstances, the additional presentation in restricted reminding of each item until it has been recalled at least once provides more opportunity to store all items and to revise storage or retrieval for reliable retrieval of all items together. While such additional presentation of each item until it has been recalled once appears to be sufficient for initial storage of nearly all of a 20 item list by normal young adults, the further presentation in selective reminding of any items not recalled on the immediately preceding trial should result in eventual storage of all items. Such selective presentation of items not recalled on the preceding trial may also maximize learning by drawing the subject's attention to items that may not have been learned yet; this may also occur to some extent in learning by restricted reminding. When storage and retrieval in such verbal learning are good, selective reminding becomes equivalent to restricted reminding, since no more presentations will be needed in selective reminding when an item is stored by the time of its initial recall and is consistently retrieved thereafter.

Storage and subsequent retention in verbal learning can be demonstrated only by spontaneous retrieval from long-term storage without further presentation. Restricted reminding

provides the most accurate evaluation of storage, especially when retrieval itself is not very effective, since spontaneous retrieval of an item an *any* subsequent recall attempt will demonstrate its storage on or before the trial when that item was last presented. Although the additional presentation of some items after recall failure in selective reminding may interfere with accurate evaluation of storage and retention, it appears that additional presentations after the initial retrieval of an item from long-term storage by recall without presentation usually serve only as reminders. This is so since the probability of recall with such reminding is very great while the probability of recall with presentation before the initial retrieval of an item from long-term storage is much lower. While selective reminding provides maximal storage, restricted reminding provides the most accurate evaluation of storage, retention, and retrieval, without confounding by any additional presentation after initial recall.

Analysis of Verbal Learning

The evaluation of storage, retention, and retrieval in free recall verbal learning by restricted reminding is illustrated by the following analysis. Ten young adults learned a random list of 20 unrelated words by restricted reminding. Each subject was tested individually. The list was read aloud to each subject, who then recalled the items in any order after an additional verbal task, used to prevent rehearsal and recall from short-term storage. Although each of the items in the list was presented only until it was recalled once, the subjects tried to retrieve all of the items on each recall attempt. In order to obtain the maximum recall on each trial necessary for accurate evaluation of storage, retention, and retrieval from long-term memory, these subjects also used extended recall: They were given enough time and encouragement on each trial to recall some more items even after additional retrieval seemed impossible.

The left panel of Figure 1 shows the analysis of free recall learning by restricted reminding. *Initial recall* shows the cumulative number of items recalled at least once. Since the items were never presented again after their initial recall, the curve for initial recall also indicates

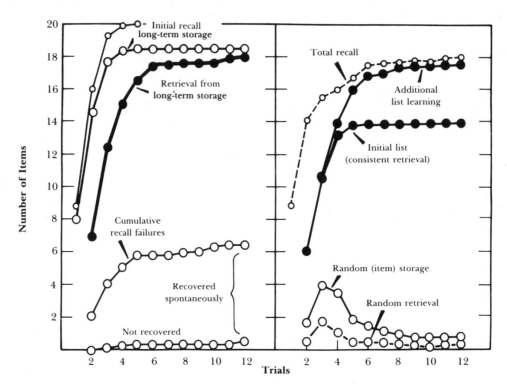

Fig. 1. Analysis of retrieval from long-term memory in free recall verbal learning by restricted reminding, without any further presentation of each item after it is recalled once. Left: analysis in terms of storage, retention, and retrieval from long-term storage. Right: analysis of total recall in terms of retrieval from the two stages of (item and list) learning shown by random and consistent retrieval from long-term storage. (From Buschke, H., Retrieval in Verbal Learning. *Transactions N.Y. Academy of Sciences,* 1974, *36* (8), 721–729. Reprinted by permission.)

that there were practically no more presentations after trial 3. *Long-term storage* shows the cumulative number of items in long-term storage, when storage on initial recall (last presentation) was verified by subsequent spontaneous recall without further presentation. The relatively close correspondence between initial recall and long-term storage indicates that initial recall may provide a reasonable indication of long-term storage, since almost all items were stored on if not before the trial on which they were first recalled.

Retention is shown by the difference between the lower two curves which show the cumulative number of recall failures and the number of such items that were not recovered again. The lower two curves together show good retention despite recall failure, since very few items were permanently lost after a recall failure. Most of the recall failures were recovered again spontaneously, without any further presentation. This shows that such recall fail-

ures represent retrieval failure rather than retention failure, and justifies the assumption that items remain in long-term storage after their initial encoding (Buschke, 1974).

Retrieval from long-term storage shows the number of items retrieved from long-term storage by recall without presentation on each trial. Retrieval from long-term storage increased spontaneously without any further presentation. Retrieval was fairly complete at first, when there were relatively few items in long-term storage. Although spontaneous retrieval increased rapidly during the early trials, retrieval was less complete when the number of items in long-term storage increased, and then slowly became more complete again in the later trials. Spontaneous retrieval from long-term memory without further presentation can increase only if the recall of items is maintained after their spontaneous recovery. Since reliable retrieval of items is almost always maintained after an item has been recovered spontaneously from long-term memory, it appears that the very slow increase in total retrieval on later trials was due principally to difficulty in finding the remaining items for spontaneous retrieval from long-term memory. This is consistent with findings that forced recall, requiring as many responses as items in the list, can increase retrieval without increasing intrusions (Ritter and Buschke, 1974) and that subjects can discriminate list items from intrusions without feedback (Buschke, 1975).

This analysis of storage, retention, and retrieval from long-term memory shows that verbal learning is limited more by retrieval than by storage or retention, and that continuing presentation of all items throughout learning is not necessary. Continuing presentation of all items may even interfere with organized retrieval. Disruption of retrieval by presentation before recall is indicated by the curve showing cumulative recall failures. Most of these recall failures occurred during the early trials when the continuing presentation of any items not yet recalled interfered with the retrieval of other items already stored. While some presentation is necessary for initial storage, further presentation does not appear to be necessary either for continuing retention or for increasing retrieval from long-term memory. When verbal learning involves the selective retrieval of already familiar items from permanent memory, it may be most useful to regard presentations simply as instructions that specify which items are to be retrieved selectively from permanent memory, or as reminders that tell a subject which items he forgot to retrieve from long-term memory.

Although analysis of verbal learning in terms of storage, retention, and retrieval does increase understanding of verbal learning, it does not explain why retrieval from long-term memory increases during verbal learning. Moreover, it does not tell us whether lower retrieval is due to ineffective retrieval or to inadequate storage, and whether lower storage is due to inadequate storage or ineffective retrieval. However, it is possible to analyze learning in another way that does not depend on the distinction between storage and retrieval. Verbal learning can be analyzed in terms of stages of learning that are indicated by empirically obvious stages of retrieval in the recall of each item.

Stages of Learning

The retrieval of each item from long-term storage can be characterized as either random or consistent. At first retrieval may be inconsistent or random, varying from one recall attempt to the next. Eventually consistent retrieval on every recall attempt is achieved. Random retrieval and consistent retrieval appear to represent distinct stages of learning, since random retrieval from long-term storage does not improve prior to the abrupt onset of consistent retrieval (Kintsch and Morris, 1965; Buschke, 1974). This is illustrated by the lower two curves in the right panel of Figure 1. The curve labeled "random storage" shows the number of items in long-term storage that are not consistently retrieved on all recall attempts, that is, that can only be retrieved inconsistently. Their retention in long-term storage was demonstrated by recall without presentation. The curve labeled "random retrieval" shows the number of such items that were retrieved on each trial. Such random retrieval does not improve over trials. Retrieval does not improve gradually until consistent retrieval is achieved, but remains relatively constant prior to the abrupt onset of consistent retrieval. This justifies analysis of retrieval during verbal learning in terms of the relative contributions to total recall by random and consistent retrieval of items in different stages of learning. Since total recall is composed of varying amounts of random and consistent retrieval, it seems necessary to specify the respective contributions of random and consistent retrieval during the course of learning.

This analysis of verbal learning in terms of the stages of retrieval accounts for total recall during learning in terms of the following components: The number of items in the first stage of learning, retained in long-term storage for inconsistent or random retrieval (random storage); the number of such items randomly retrieved on each trial (random retrieval); the number of items that are consistently retrieved from their first recall, that is, the number of items going directly to the second stage of learning (initial list/consistent retrieval); the number of items transferred from the first stage to the second stage of consistent retrieval (additional list learning).

The two components of consistent retrieval

shown in the right panel of Figure 1 are labeled "initial list" and "additional list learning" because consistent retrieval of an item on all recall attempts, without any further presentation indicates that the item has been learned as part of the list; that is, the retrieval of that item has been integrated with the retrieval of other items so that it can always be retrieved, without any further interference due to the prior recall of other items (Roediger, 1974). Since recall of all items in a list on every recall attempt without further presentation indicates that the entire list has been learned, the consistent retrieval of some items on all recall attempts without further presentation should indicate that those items have been learned as a list. Therefore, it is possible to estimate the amount of list learning during verbal learning by counting the cumulative number of items that are consistently retrieved as learning progresses. This simple and easily calculated measure of list learning does not require the incorrect assumption that the organization of retrieval implicit in list learning must necessarily be reflected by an increasingly consistent order of recall. Better organization of the information in storage may permit more flexibility in retrieval, resulting in more, not less, variability of output order. Thus it seems reasonable to identify the second stage of consistent retrieval with list learning. The first stage of random retrieval can reasonably be regarded as a stage of item learning, in which the information about that item retained in long-term storage only allows inconsistent retrieval of that item by itself, but not integrated with the retrieval of other items.

The right panel of Figure 1 shows that a large part of total recall is due to initial list learning, shown by consistent retrieval from the very first recall of an item onward. Only a small part of total recall is due to random retrieval of items in the first stage of learning. As learning proceeds, the number of items in the first stage of learning (random item storage) decreases and the number of items in the second stage of list learning increases (additional list learning), as more items are transferred from the first stage of item learning to the second stage of list learning. This analysis indicates that retrieval from long-term storage increases during verbal learning because of an increase in the number of items that are always retrieved,

and not because of any improvement in the random retrieval of those items that are not yet consistently retrieved.

Random and Directed Search

The results of this kind of analysis of retrieval from long-term memory in terms of stages of retrieval appear to support the theoretical analysis of storage and retrieval processes in long-term memory formulated by Shiffrin and Atkinson (1969), who have elaborated the role of random and directed search, recovery, and response generation in retrieval from long-term memory. It seems reasonable to suppose that the selective retrieval of a specific set of already familiar items from permanent memory in verbal learning may initially involve relatively random search in permanent storage for inconsistent retrieval, followed by progressive elaboration of more directed searching for consistent retrieval as learning progresses. These methods of investigation and analysis of *selective retrieval* from permanent memory (verbal learning or episodic memory) and of *exhaustive retrieval* from permanent memory (category retrieval of semantic memory) have significant applications in the evaluation of children with learning disorders and neurological patients with disturbed memory and learning, and in investigation of the development of memory and learning and its decline in aging. They also increase our understanding of verbal memory and learning.

BIBLIOGRAPHY

BROWN, W. To what extent is memory measured by a single recall? *Journal of Experimental Psychology,* 1923, *6,* 377–382.

BUSCHKE, H. Selective reminding for analysis of memory and learning. *Journal of Verbal Learning and Verbal Behavior,* 1973, *12,* 543–550.

BUSCHKE, H. Spontaneous remembering after recall failure. *Science,* 1974, *184,* 579–581.

BUSCHKE, H.; GOLDBERG, P.; and LAZAR, G. Reminding and retrieval from permanent storage. *Journal of Experimental Psychology,* 1973, *101,* 132–138.

CRAIK, F. I. M. Two components in free recall. *Journal of Verbal Learning and Verbal Behavior,* 1968, *7,* 996–1004.

GLANZER, M. Storage mechanisms in recall. In G. H. Bower (Ed.), *Psychology of learning and motivation* (vol. 5). New York: Academic Press, 1972. Pp. 129–193.

KINTSCH, W., and MORRIS, C. J. Application of a Markov model to free recall and recognition. *Journal of Experimental Psychology,* 1965, *69,* 200–206.

Ritter, W., and Buschke, H.   Free, forced, and restricted recall in verbal learning. *Journal of Experimental Psychology,* 1974, *103,* 1204–1207.

Shiffrin, R. M., and Atkinson, R. C.   Storage and retrieval processes in long-term memory. *Psychological Review,* 1969, *76,* 179–193.

Tulving, E., and Pearlstone, Z.   Availability versus accessibility of information in memory for words. *Journal of Verbal Learning and Verbal Behavior,* 1966, *5,* 381–391.

HERMAN BUSCHKE

MEMORY: RETRIEVAL FROM SHORT-TERM STORAGE

Short-term memory has been studied by experiment for nearly a century, but never so intensively as in recent years. The current interest dates from the late 1950s, and is largely a product of the information-processing approach to psychology—an approach rooted in earlier developments in cybernetics and information theory. The view of man as a processor of information prompted the question of whether there is a functionally distinct short-term memory store. A debate of this question helped generate a wealth of short-term memory research. The question itself, however, has not yielded any simple answer, which means that the definition of short-term memory must remain arbitrary. For the present purposes, short-term memory will be used, rather loosely, to refer to the subject-matter of a variety of experimental procedures in which information is retained over intervals of up to one or two minutes; in almost all of the research to be considered, the to-be-remembered material was verbal (usually digits, letters, or words) and was presented for study on just a single occasion.

By retrieval in short-term memory is meant the recollection, or bringing to consciousness, of a recent event. Before the advent of the information-processing school, short-term memory was usually conceptualized within an associative framework, and was studied with procedures involving near-optimal retrieval conditions. Recall failure was taken to mean that an association had either never been formed, or else was no longer intact. With the information-processing approach, and an orientation toward memory *stores,* it became meaningful to inquire just how access might be gained to the stored information. It happened that during its early days, the information processing school largely ignored the question of how stored information is retrieved, and instead focused on the conditions under which various kinds of information are registered in, and lost from, the various hypothetical stores. During the 1960s, however, retrieval began to emerge as a significant issue in the understanding of short-term memory. To some extent, the issue was raised within the context of the debate of the qualitative distinction between short- and long-term memory. Thus, in his opposition to the distinction, Melton (1963) claimed that the retrieval environment—a well-established determinant of long-term memory performance—can be an important factor in short-term memory. A variety of subsequent developments have emphasized and established the significance of the retrieval component of short-term memory. The next section considers some of these developments.

Emergence of Retrieval as a Significant Issue

Retrieval and the Organization of Memory. One aspect of the current interest in short-term memory has been the development of the organizational school (e.g., Tulving, 1962). This school emphasizes the importance of organizing the to-be-remembered material, and there are now numerous demonstrations that recall can be considerably increased if the subject actively organizes the to-be-remembered items into groups or chunks. Alternatively, items are well recalled if they have been fitted into some previously learned organizational structure. A well-known example of such a "mnemonic technique" is the one-bun method. This entails learning number-word rhymes—one-bun, two-shoe, three-tree, and so on. To remember a list of items, such as the words *boat, horse, piano,* each item is associated in turn with one of the rhyme words. Thus a series of images might be formed—first of a boat sinking under the weight of a gigantic bun, next a horse proudly wearing fancy shoes, then a piano sprouting a tree. The list items can then be recalled with relatively little effort by using the rhyme words as reminders or "retrieval cues." Despite considerable problems in separating retrieval from storage effects, the view that active organization and the use of mnemonic techniques enhances retrieval efficiency is at least intuitively plausible. Consequently, the research of organizational factors in memory has done much to focus attention on the retrieval aspect of memory.

The research of memory organization has also helped promote the free-recall procedure, since the freedom to recall items without regard to order should permit expression of their organization in memory. Characteristic of free-recall performance is the temporal irregularity with which the list items are produced; pauses of several seconds are frequently terminated by the retrieval of two or three items in quick succession, suggesting that access to a chunk has been achieved. More basic than temporal chunking in recall is the very fact of the pauses themselves: an item recalled after a pause must have been in memory during the pause, and hence the pause itself suggests that the retrieval process is a significant determinant of memory performance.

Subjective Reports. Introspection has not proven a particularly fruitful approach to short-term memory. It seems that a subject can tell us very little about *how* he retrieved a particular item, nor can he say much about an item he is still trying to retrieve. On the other hand, in certain areas of short-term memory research, subjective data have stimulated some interest in the retrieval process. A case in point is the *feeling-of-knowing* phenomenon: the subject studies a list of paired items, and then tries to recall the right-hand or "response" term of each pair as the left-hand or "stimulus" terms are re-presented. Next he considers each stimulus term to which he failed to recall the response term and states whether he really knows the correct answer even though he cannot recall it. Finally, the subject is shown the unrecalled response terms and tries to match them against their respective stimulus terms. The finding of interest is that the stimulus terms about which the subject claimed a feeling of knowledge are more successfully paired (Blake, 1973). Although its theoretical implications have still to be worked out, the feeling-of-knowing phenomenon does suggest that the retrieval process is rather more complex than has often been assumed.

Primary Memory. Primary memory refers to those very recent perceptual encounters or thoughts that are still in consciousness or the "psychological present" (James, 1890). The 1960s saw a resurgence of interest in primary memory, an interest attributable in general to the vast increase in short-term memory research, and specifically to the application of the concept to a particular phenomenon—the recency effect in free recall. The recency effect refers to the comparatively high level of recall of items presented near the end of the list. Recent research has shown that if a free-recall task is made more difficult, for example, by increasing presentation speed from a leisurely to a fast pace, or by using rare as opposed to familiar words, then recall is typically reduced for all except the last few list items (Glanzer, 1972). This result has usually been taken as indicating that free recall is mediated by two distinct memory systems. That is, recency items derive from a limited-capacity primary memory system, whereas prerecency items are retrieved from a large and more permanent system with a probability that varies with a wide variety of factors. Although primary memory is conceptualized in a number of ways, it is generally agreed that primary memory items are in a state of high retrievability.

The fact that there may be little or no difficulty in reporting primary memory items has not prevented the study of the mechanism by which primary memory information is utilized. Such research clearly requires an index of performance other than probability of recall. The most commonly adopted index is recognition reaction time. Thus, a person might receive a list of from one to six items followed by a test item, and his task is to indicate as quickly as he can whether or not the test item appeared in the list. Experiments of this sort have investigated how reaction time changes with the number of list items, the modalities of the list- and test-items, the size of the vocabulary from which the items are selected, and so on. A finding of particular interest is that, under a fairly wide range of conditions, reaction time increases by about 35 or 40 milliseconds for each increment in list length; moreover, although negative responses have usually been found to take longer than positive responses, this difference is independent of list length. This pattern of results has suggested a model of primary memory scanning, according to which the test item is compared to all of the list items in turn, and only after this exhaustive search is completed is the response made (Sternberg, 1969).

The recognition reaction time procedure has also been applied to considerably longer presentation lists. This research has yielded a pattern of results which differs substantially from the pattern obtained with short lists—a fact that accords well with the notion that different types of processes are involved in using stored information, depending on whether or not the information is still represented in primary memory (Burrows and Okada, 1975).

Recall-Recognition Comparisons. It has long been known that previously encountered things can be recognized more readily than they can be recalled. Until quite recently this fact was usually attributed to a difference in response threshold in the recall and recognition procedures; the trace must be strong or intact for recall, whereas a weak or partially faded trace will suffice for recognition. This threshold theory did not stimulate very much research or thought about the nature of retrieval. The 1960s, however, saw a good deal of interest in the relation between the recall and recognition processes. This interest was prompted largely by findings of an interaction between experimental conditions and performance on recall and recognition tests (McCormack, 1972). For example, older adults were found to recall lists of unrelated items less well than younger adults, though in recognition the two groups perform about equally well. Item familiarity affects both recall and recognition, although in opposite directions: recall is higher and recognition lower for familiar than unfamiliar items. As a general rule, recall appears to be more vulnerable than recognition to changes in experimental condition, particularly if the changes are likely to be relevant to the organization of the to-be-remembered items. Thus, recall is better, and recognition much the same, after intentional than after incidental learning.

That variables can have different, even opposite, effects on recall and recognition is clearly incompatible with simple threshold theory: if recall and recognition differ merely because of a difference in response or retrieval threshold, then any manipulation that, say, increases recall should also increase recognition. The principal response to this difficulty has been the

revival of the two-stage theory of recall. This theory will be considered below.

Effects of Recall on Subsequent Recall. It was long assumed, at least implicitly, that registration of to-be-remembered material occurred only during experimenter-designated "study trials." Recent research, however, has shown effects of a recall test on subsequent recall performance. Thus, a single free recall test of a once-presented list, for example, is about as effective in increasing subsequent recall as a second list presentation. Findings of this sort have, not surprisingly, helped focus attention on the recall test. More particularly, they have often been attributed to the effects of retrieval on subsequent retrieval.

A related finding is the *inhibition* in recall when some of the to-be-remembered items are supplied to the subject "free." Specifically, if a list of random items is studied for free recall, and a sample of these items is given as "free" items in a recall test, then the proportion of remaining items recalled is slightly lower than it would have been if no free items had been given. This finding is not well understood, standing as it does in stark contradiction to the basic tenets of the organizational theory of memory. Nonetheless, the finding has fostered an interest in retrieval—the most familiar interpretation being that implicit retrieval is involved in recognizing the free words, and this has the effect of inhibiting the retrieval of further items.

The Method of Retrieval Cueing

Although each of the developments considered in the last section helped focus attention on the retrieval aspect of short-term memory, none provided a completely satisfactory method for the systematic study of retrieval independently of prior memory processes. It is, however, a relatively simple matter to manipulate the retrieval environment without affecting conditions of registration or retention. The effectiveness of a given retrieval cue tells something about the nature of the retrieval process, namely, the extent to which it can utilize the information inherent in the cue. Some insight of how the retrieval process functions can therefore be gained by determining the effectiveness of various types of retrieval cues. Further, by successively cueing a given set of items with two or more types of retrieval cues, it is possible to work out the functional relationship between different types of cues.

The types of cues most frequently used are semantic associates (for instance, *priest* for the target word *church*), rhymes *(birch),* category names *(religious building),* and initial letters (*c, ch, chu, chur,* etc.). The relative effectiveness of such cues is currently being investigated as a function of study (registration) conditions and of retention interval. Different study conditions can be obtained by varying the speed or the context of item presentation. Presentation context will depend on whether the to-be-remembered items are related, but can often be varied more conveniently by placing each to-be-remembered item in a particular type of sentence, or alongside a word to which it is related in some way. An important finding is that the effectiveness of a given retrieval cue will vary, often quite drastically, with the presentation context of the cued item.

Retrieval in Short-Term Memory: Two Theories

The rising interest in the retrieval component of short-term memory led inevitably to the development of general theories of retrieval. Two such theories—two-process theory (McCormack, 1972), and episodic theory (Tulving, 1975), are outlined here.

Two-Process Theory. Retrieval is often conceptualized within the framework of an associative theory of memory, according to which memory for a list of words is carried on a permanent associative network. Specifically, each word corresponds to a particular node, and the encoding of a word as a member of a list entails appending an occurrence tag to its node. In a recall test, retrieval involves a search for potential target nodes, and then a decision of whether these nodes are appropriately tagged. A positive decision causes a word to be recalled. In free recall, the search may be guided by general properties of some or all of the list items, while in cued recall, the search is concentrated in the associative vicinity of the cue nodes. In recognition, the test and target items share the same node, so that the search phase of retrieval is effectively bypassed.

By assuming that a variable can affect the two components of retrieval in different ways, or to a different extent, two-process theory can account for an interaction of the variable with recall and recognition performance. The notion that recognition involves only a decision of whether there exists an appropriate tag, however, is difficult to reconcile with findings that recognition does vary, in some cases, with the context of the test items, and that recallable words may not be recognized (Watkins and Tulving, 1975).

Episodic Theory. According to episodic theory, each item in a study list is encoded into a unique trace. Although the general knowledge concerning the words or their referents is a significant determinant of the type of trace formed, the traces are retained independently of this knowledge. The theory therefore draws no qualitative distinction between recognition and recall; the term recognition is used when a nominal copy of the target item is presented as a retrieval cue. The effectiveness of a retrieval cue depends on whether it is encoded in a way sufficiently compatible with the trace. Since a particular item tends to be encoded in similar fashion on successive occasions, the "copy cues" of a recognition test are often relatively effective; on the other hand, since successive encodings are not identical, recognition may fail even though the required trace is available in memory. Unfortunately, the mechanism of retrieval in episodic theory is less explicitly formulated than in two-stage theory.

Conclusion

Although students of short-term memory have always sanctioned the conceptual distinction between registration, retention, and retrieval, they have only recently given much attention to retrieval. If this three-stage analysis is to provide a viable basis for a general theory of short-term memory, then there arises the question of the best research strategy for describing the individual stages. It is tempting to focus first on the early stages, and to leave retrieval for later research; indeed, a chronological approach has been widely adopted, especially by the information-processing school. A case can be made, however, for reversing this strategy and working backwards in time.

Manipulating the encoding conditions may affect not only trace formation, but also, indirectly, the way the traces change during storage, as well as the effectiveness of a given retrieval environment. On the other hand, the retrieval stage can be manipulated independently of the earlier stages by simply imposing different retrieval conditions on specified conditions of registration and retention. It is possible, therefore, that future research in short-term memory will continue to pay more attention to retrieval.

BIBLIOGRAPHY

BLAKE, M.   Prediction of recognition when recall fails: Exploring the feeling-of-knowing phenomenon. *Journal of Verbal Learning and Verbal Behavior,* 1973, *12,* 311–319.

BURROWS, D., and OKADA, R.   Memory retrieval for long and short lists. *Science,* 1975, 181, 1031–1033.

GLANZER, M.   Storage mechanisms in recall. In G. H. Bower (Ed.), *The psychology of learning and motivation: Advances in research and theory* (Vol. 5). New York: Academic Press, 1972.

JAMES, W.   *Principles of psychology.* New York: Holt, 1890.

McCORMACK, P. D.   Recognition memory: How complex a retrieval system? *Canadian Journal of Psychology,* 1972, *26,* 19–41.

MELTON, A. W.   Implications of short-term memory for a general theory of memory *Journal of Verbal Learning and Verbal Behavior,* 1963, *2,* 1–21.

STERNBERG, S.   Memory scanning: Mental processes revealed by reaction-time experiments. *American Scientist,* 1969, *57,* 421–457.

TULVING, E.   Subjective organization in free recall of "unrelated" words. *Psychological Review,* 1962, *69,* 344–354.

TULVING, E.   Ecphoric processes in recall and recognition. In J. Brown (Ed.), *Recall and recognition.* London: Wiley, 1975.

WATKINS, M. J., and TULVING, E.   Episodic memory: When recognition fails. *Journal of Experimental Psychology: General,* 1975, *104,* 5–29.

MICHAEL J. WATKINS

MEMORY: THE ROLE OF ENCODING

Human memory is composed of three fundamental processes: encoding, storage, and retrieval. *Encoding* refers to the process by which an event or object is transformed into some representation so that it may be placed in memory. When a stimulus such as a word, sentence, picture, or musical composition is presented to a person, the stimulus event as such is simply physical energy impinging upon his senses and nervous system; this energy is transformed into some representation which is then stored in memory. This representation in memory is the encoded version of the nominal (physical) stimulus event. For example, if presented the scrambled letters *eocd,* one might rearrange them into the meaningful word *code,* and thus remember the new arrangement rather than the letters as presented. Similarly, if asked to remember the geometric figures ○, □, and △, humans can readily code these events verbally as "circle," "square," and "triangle."

Memory *storage* refers to the maintenance of encoded information over time. Storage can be understood by a simple analogy in which memory is viewed as a process of placing things in a filing cabinet, storing them until needed, and taking them out of the cabinet when necessary. Information placed in the filing cabinet is said to be stored; presumably if it is in storage it is permanent, and some models of memory make the explicit assumption of the permanence of storage. Information may be stored but it may not be possible to locate or retrieve the information. Presence of the information in the file is no guarantee that it can be located; similarly, presence of information in memory is no assurance that it is retrievable. Thus, information may be available in memory but not accessible. *Availability* refers to the fact that information is stored, whereas *accessibility* refers to the fact that it can be located or retrieved. *Retrieval* thus refers to the matter of getting information out of storage.

The concept of encoding emphasizes the active, organizing nature of human learning and memory and presumes that the prepresentation of events in memory does not mirror events simply as they appear in the external physical world. Adherents of encoding reject the view of man as an empty organism and reject the assumption that psychology studies the correlation of external stimulus and response events alone. Rather, the assumption of encoding carries with it the acceptance that behavior is mediated by a person's cognitive state, which interprets and provides meaning to stimulus events. Thus, the important stimulus for behavior is not the nominal or external stimulus but the stimulus as coded by the organism.

Coding

The concept of coding is related to mediational concepts stemming from classical stimulus-response (S-R) theory. Historically, S-R mediating responses have been tied in a fairly direct manner to nominal stimulation. This is seen, for example, in the concept of response-produced cues as used in Hullian theory. Perhaps the fundamental distinction between mediation and coding is that mediating responses are stimulus-determined whereas coding responses are determined by both sensory states and cognitive states of the organism, the latter being influenced by instructional sets, attitudes, and strategies. In turn, coding and mediation serve a similar conceptual function in that they both allow for more flexible behavior than that encompassed by single-stage theories of behavior.

The concept of coding is related to organizational concepts of Gestalt theory. As noted, it is not events in the physical world that are remembered but the encoding or interpretation of these events. The encoding of stimulus events is dependent not only on the stimulus itself, but on sets, attitudes, and cognitive states. This point was made by Gestalt theorists, who emphasized that the important stimulus for an organism's behavior was the stimulus as perceived as distinct from the physical stimulus itself. Moreover, Gestalt theorists contended that the interpretation of events resulted from certain organizational processes operating on sensory input. These organizational processes relate to the laws of grouping in perception and memory such as temporal or spatial proximity of elements, similarity, and good figure. These Gestalt principles of grouping determine the way humans organize or encode information, and in turn, determine the characteristics of their recall.

The more general significance of encoding is the recognition that prediction and interpretation of human performance is dependent upon knowledge of the representation of events in memory. For example, the representation of an event in memory, such as the word *jam,* will depend upon the way in which it is encoded. The verbal context in which the word *jam* is learned (e.g., *strawberry . . . , traffic . . .*) will determine the kind of features encoded in memory. Similarly, the way in which a stimulus is encoded may conceivably affect its function in tests of transfer or concept identification. Thus, it is important to know the features or attributes of an event which are represented in an encoding since it is these features which can govern performance in memory, transfer, and conceptual behavior.

The Encoding Concept

The concept of encoding has been used by psychologists in several ways. At the most general and inclusive level, *encoding* refers to the transformation of a stimulus into some representation. Within this general definition, several uses can be identified. Psychologists occasionally use *coding* to refer, at the simplest level, to *stimulus selection.* Used in this fashion, coding becomes a rather directly measurable process which refers to the selection of some part or fraction of a compound stimulus. For example, if a subject is asked to learn the association *xug-table,* where *xug* functions as a stimulus for the response *table,* he may in fact select only the first letter of the trigram to cue the response. A particular element of the compound is selected presumably if it can be distinguished from other stimuli to be learned in a list. Used in this fashion, coding and selection are identical processes. This usage, however, does not reflect the more general usage of the coding concept. Indeed, coding is generally regarded as a process one stage beyond that of stimulus selection.

Coding is frequently viewed as an *elaborative* or reconstructive process involving either rearrangement of the nominal stimulus or complete transformation to a new state. In this instance, coding is essentially an additive process involving either partial or full replacement of the stimulus with some new representation or an enhancement of the stimulus by adding additional information with the unit to be remembered. An example is seen in the use of natural-language mediators for the learning of nonsense syllables. In this case, a CVC (a consonant-vowel-consonant) stimulus is altered in some way to make a stimulus-response pair more easily learned. For example, if presented the pair of items *IGW-MAN,* the subject might transform *IGW* into *IGnorant,* thus enabling the association *IGnorant-MAN.* Similarly, the pair *KHQ-FAN* might involve changing *KHQ* to *RADIO,* thus facilitating the association *RADIO-FAN.*

A similar use of coding is seen in coding as *rewriting.* For example, subjects may be shown a series of black or white patterns which can be coded as B, B, B, B, W, W, W, W. In this case the first four patterns are black and the second four are white, so that all that need be remembered to recall the sequence is "four black, four white." Another sequence which is more complex might be W, B, B, W, B, W, W, B, which would be more difficult to remember. Similarly, subjects can recode a series of binary digits by rewriting each group of digits as follows: a sequence of 000 is coded as 0, 001 as 1, 010 as 2, 011 as 3, a procedure familiar to users of digital computers. In this manner, a series of 21 digits could be rewritten as only 7 digits, well within the human memory span. The obvious significance of such coding is that it enables humans to place much more information in memory than would otherwise be the case.

Another view of coding emphasizes the features or *attributes* that are stored. The memory of an event might be coded in terms of multiple attributes such as temporal characteristics, spatial characteristics, frequency characteristics, and so forth.

Some Phenomena of Coding

Context Effects.   The role of coding is seen in a variety of ways in studies of learning, memory, transfer, discrimination, and conceptual behavior. One of the most pronounced effects of coding is seen in context effects in recognition memory, in which it is shown that the verbal context accompanying a to-be-remembered word or other verbal unit affects the subsequent recognition of that word or unit. The general procedure of context studies has been to present an item embedded in some specific verbal context during training; this context typically consists of an adjective, phrase, or sentence. Moreover, different adjectives can be used in training so as to bias the semantic interpretation of the word—for example, *strawberry jam* versus *traffic jam, spiked punch* versus *hefty punch.* At testing, the target word can be presented with the same context as during training, with new context, or with no context (i.e., the word alone). In general, the result of changing the context to a new adjective is to produce poorer recognition performance relative to conditions in which the context remains the same. This is particularly the case if the new context biases a meaning which is different from the initial encoding. Deletion of all context in testing can result in recognition performance intermediate between that produced by no change in context and context changes which alter the meaning of the word. Context effects clearly show how the prevailing context may bias the encoding of an item; moreover, context effects have led some psychologists to argue for retrieval process in recognition memory.

Context effects have been observed in studies of perceptual memory using both recall and recognition tasks. In studies of perceptual recall, subjects have been shown ambiguous visual patterns which are assigned verbal labels. For example, a pattern consisting of two circles connected by a straight line is labeled *eyeglasses* in one condition and *barbells* in another. Subjects are given a list of such visual forms and assigned one of two possible labels. The basic question is: Does the label influence the way in which the form is perceived and remembered? In tests of reproduction, subjects are asked to draw the forms; in general, the reproductions tend to appear like those suggested by the label. Clearly, the label affects the reproduction, but the result may be attributed to the way the label influences encoding and to effects at retrieval as well.

Similar context effects are seen in recognition memory of visual forms and letter strings. Recognition memory of visual forms is enhanced if subjects are given training in associating the forms with words "representative" of the forms. The effect of labeling with "unrelated" words or nonsense syllables is slight but discernible. For labels to be maximally effective they should be conceptually related or "representative" of the visual patterns. The advantage of verbal labels or context increases as shape and letter-string stimuli become less codeable or meaningful, or more ambiguous. As a stimulus is more difficult to integrate as a unit or chunk, the effects of labeling context become greater. These findings have been interpreted in terms of a conceptual coding hypothesis.

Chunking.   Another class of findings related to coding is *chunking* in memory. Since short-term memory is a limited-capacity system, one way of reducing these limitations and thus increasing the amount of information retained is by chunking. One type of chunking is regrouping of elements; for example, the three-chunk letter sequence *r umw ig* may be regrouped into the pronounceable sequence *rumwig.* Another type of chunking is seen in recoding, in which a binary series such as 001100010011, broken up into groups of three, can be translated into 1423. In this fashion, as noted earlier, humans can increase their immediate memory for binary strings. The principle of chunking by recoding can be applied to other sequences. More generally, the significance of chunking is that memory is apparently more dependent upon the number of chunks of information than upon the bits or units of information and that chunking can enable humans to overcome some of the constraints of short-term memory.

Clustering. Clustering in free recall is another finding which reflects the organizational (encoding) structure of human memory. *Clustering in free recall* refers simply to the finding that output in recall is governed by semantic or other relations among the items. Clustering may be of two types: associative and categorical. *Associative clustering* refers to situations in which associatively related words such as *needle-thread* would be recalled adjacently even though presented in random order. Thus, associated word pairs tend to be recalled together. *Categorical clustering* refers to situations in which the recall of items is related to conceptually related or meaningfully related items in a list. For example, words belonging to a particular category such as vegetables or minerals would be recalled together. The finding of clustering reflects both the operation of encoding and retrieval processes.

Release from Proactive Interference. The memory of a word may be regarded in terms of a class of attributes or features that are stored; these attributes may be semantic, acoustic, temporal, spatial, and so forth. One way of studying the attributes in terms of which memories are stored is by a procedure known as *release from proactive inhibition.* It is known that recall becomes progressively poorer with successive tests. This deterioration in performance reflects the accumulation of proactive interference—that is, interference associated with prior learning. Proactive inter-

ference (PI) accumulates only if the material is of the same class; if the test material is changed to a new class of items, then memory will improve. This improvement is referred to as release from PI. In the typical study of release from PI, subjects are given four trials in a short-term-memory experiment. On each trial the subject is briefly presented three words to remember. On the first three trials the words all belong to the same category, such as foods; on the fourth test trial, a new category is introduced, while a control subject continues to receive words of the same category. As noted, when switched to a new category recall typically shows a pronounced improvement. Such findings are explained by assuming that the subject encodes the particular category as part of his memory for each word. More generally, this technique enables psychologists to study the memory representation by switching from one class of materials to another.

Repetition-Variation Effects. Another finding attributable to encoding processes concerns the role of repetition in memory. In one situation, within the single presentation of a long list of items the more widely spaced the two presentations of a particular item the better is the recall of that item. For example, in one study the probability of recall was compared for repeated items with a lag of 40 (i.e., 40 intervening items) and for repeated items with a lag of zero. The probability of recall at the longer lag was twice that of the shorter lag. This effect has been explained by assuming that the prevailing context is more likely to be different with greater lags and that the more varied the context the greater the number of retrieval cues.

The study of varied input versus repetition in memory has been approached in two additional ways. In one case, variation in only contextual stimuli present during training is introduced and subjects are tested for memory of consistently associated responses. For example, subjects may be shown photographs of a particular person in different poses or dress and learn an arbitrary name for each person. When the photographs are varied—for example, same people but different poses and dress—during training, varied training led to superior cued recall when cued with either old or new photos. Thus, seeing events in varying context rather than repeated context augments memory.

Alternatively, a second approach to the study of variability versus repetition is to vary directly the structural properties of the entire stimulus to be placed in memory as distinct from varying only the contextual elements. In such studies, groupings of digit or letter strings have typically been used. If the letter or digit grouping is one which contains an inherent structure which can be encoded as an intact chunk, then variable input characteristically facilitates recall. For example, if letter groupings such as *b anc ow* are presented variably on successive presentations, recall is substantially higher than if the sequences are consistently presented. Similarly, if a digit series has a detectable structure (e.g., 2 46 35 7), variable input facilitates recall. These findings are interpreted in terms of a perceptual regrouping hypothesis, whose principal assumption is that variation in the experimenter-imposed grouping rule or structure increases the probability that humans will discover the underlying structure. The spatial grouping of the letter sequence, which is irrelevant to the subsequent recall test, changes on successive presentations. It is therefore assumed that subjects are more likely to recognize the irrelevance of the experimenter-defined grouping and will attempt to encode the letter sequence in a unitary fashion which will enhance recall.

Mnemonics. A variety of mnemonic aids, which enable humans to learn more effectively, are all instances of coding operations. The process of recoding information in immediate memory is one instance. Similarly, the use of natural-language mediators is another; natural-language mediators reduce the memory load of learners by incorporating task materials such as nonsense syllables into words, phrases, or sentences. For instance, if subjects are presented the pair of items *riv-saf* as part of a list of paired associates, they may elaborate this as a phrase, such as *at the bottom of the RIVER they found the SAFE.* Similarly, imagery serves as a very powerful mnemonic in enabling humans to remember information.

Theoretical Issues

One issue of theoretical concern is the nature of the event encoded. Theorists are in general agreement that the encoding of words is multidimensional in that several features or attributes can be simultaneously encoded. The process of encoding may be very rapid and essentially automatic, as reflected in the release from PI paradigm. It may also be considerably slower in situations involving chunking or recoding. Moreover, the process of decoding, which is returning information to its initial state, may place serious constraints on recall and thus on the efficiency of coding operations.

Coding theorists differ in their conception of coding itself. Some view coding as tied to attentional or perceptual activity, in which coding responses are treated theoretically as implicit perceptual responses. Others view coding as the development of rules, strategies, or other higher-order events.

Coding theorists have emphasized the variability of encoding, and several versions of encoding variability theory have emerged. One version of encoding variability theory has been applied primarily to the analysis of transfer. It is argued that in transfer paradigms in which the stimuli remain identical in the two lists, nominally identical stimuli may be recoded such that the usual interference is minimized. Although it is evident that nominally identical stimuli may be perceived differently in successive lists, recoding does not appear to improve transfer performance.

The encoding variability theory has been formalized by Bower (1972) within the framework of *stimulus-sampling theory* to account for a number of phenomena in recognition memory. The basic assumptions of this stimulus-sampling theory of encoding variability include (1) each nominal stimulus in a learning situation may give rise to a number of possible stimulus elements; (2) for each nominal stimulus, there is a corresponding set of stimulus elements; (3) each stimulus element may be associated in an all-or-none fashion to one or more cognitive elements or responses; (4) performance to a given nominal stimulus is dependent upon the associative connections of the elements of the active sample. Using these assumptions, Bower developed a formal model which can account for a wide range of effects, including context effects, lag effects, list differentiation, and conditional relationships in paired-associate learning.

Another theoretical issue pertinent to retrieval mechanisms is the principle of encoding specificity. The principle emphasizes that if retrieval cues are to be effective, they must be stored with the information to be remembered at input. If they are not stored at input, then they cannot operate as effective retrieval cues. The evidence relevant to this principle appears contradictory at present.

BIBLIOGRAPHY

BOWER, G. H.   Stimulus-sampling theory of encoding variability. In A. W. Melton and E. Martin (Eds.), *Coding processes in human memory.* Washington, D.C.: Winston, 1972. Pp. 85–123.

ELLIS, H. C.   Stimulus encoding processes in human learning and memory. In G. H. Bower (Ed.), *The psychology of learning and motivation* (Vol. 7). New York: Academic Press, 1973. Pp. 123–182.

ELLIS, H. C.; PARENTE, F. J.; GRAH, C. R.; and SPIERING, K.   Coding strategies, perceptual grouping, and the "variability effect" in free recall. *Memory and Cognition,* 1975, *3,* 226–232.

JOHNSON, N. F.   Chunking and organization in the process of recall. In G. H. Bower (Ed.), *The psychology of learning and motivation* (Vol. 4). New York: Academic Press, 1970. Pp. 171–247.

MARTIN, E.   Stimulus meaningfulness and paired-associate transfer: An encoding variability hypothesis. *Psychological Review,* 1968, *75,* 421–441.

MELTON, A. W.   The concept of coding in learning-memory theory. *Memory and Cognition,* 1973, *1,* 508–512.

MELTON, A. W., and MARTIN, E. (Eds.).   *Coding processes in human memory.* Washington, D.C.: Winston, 1972.

TULVING, E., and THOMSON, D. M.   Encoding specificity and retrieval processes in episodic memory. *Psychological Review,* 1973, *80,* 352–373.

UNDERWOOD, B. J.   Are we overloading memory? In A. W. Melton and E. Martin (Eds.), *Coding processes in human memory.* Washington, D.C.: Winston, 1972.

WICKENS, D. D.   Encoding categories of words: An empirical approach to meaning. *Psychological Review,* 1970, *76,* 559–573.

See also MEMORY; MEMORY: RETRIEVAL FROM LONG-TERM STORAGE; MEMORY AND IMAGERY; MNEMONICS

HENRY C. ELLIS

MEMORY: THE ROLE OF MODALITIES

In the nineteenth and early twentieth century many philosophers and psychologists viewed memory as a record of basic sensory experiences or elements and of associations between those elements. However, Gestalt psychologists and behaviorists criticized this approach, and subsequently, the study of memory turned from efforts to describe introspectively the elements and associations of memory, and turned instead to attempts to formulate general empirical laws of learning. Studies of human learning focused primarily on the acquisition and retention of verbal or symbolic material, and it was often assumed that the mnemonic representation of this type of material was independent of sensory modality; that is, the way in which a person remembered a list of words, nonsense syllables, or other symbols, e.g., digits or letters, was independent of whether they were learned from a visual or an auditory presentation. In general, the data appeared to support this assumption because many qualitative characteristics of learning were unaffected by the presentation modality. For example, superior recall of the ends rather than the middle of a memory list, the so called "primacy" and "recency" effects, held true whether the person heard or saw the list.

In the last 20 years, however, psychologists have again become concerned with the effects of input modality upon memory for symbolic or linguistic material. There is now also increasing concern with detailed comparisons between sensory modalities, including kinesthetic, tactile, olfactory, and picture memory, one aim of this work is to generalize theories of memory for linguistic information to memory for nonsymbolic information.

Active Verbal Memory

In the early 1960s, Conrad (1964) and Sperling (1960) made observations suggesting that subjects remembered visually presented symbols by translating them into covert or subvocal speech. Subsequent recall was then based on a memory of this translation. The principal basis for this hypothesis was that subjects often made "acoustic confusion errors" in written recall of visually presented symbols. For example, if the letter *D* were presented visually, recall errors tended to be letters that were similar in sound to it, e.g., *B, C, P* or *T.* These errors were similar to the errors made in identifying spoken letters that are degraded by noise. Thus recall errors may have occurred because the subject "misperceived" what he had said to himself. Other investigators noted that a subject's verbal description of visual displays could be used to predict accuracy in recalling the displays in tasks requiring no overt verbal recall, either written or spoken. Observations of this sort supported the hypothesis that remembering both visual and auditory symbols involved implicitly speaking the symbols. This simple theory was immensely successful because it seemed to account for a great deal of empirical and introspective data.

Iconic Memory

It was also clear that this hypothesis needed elaboration to account for the data in detail. For example, it had been observed in Helmholtz's laboratory that subjects could report several letters from a visual display that was illuminated by a spark lasting only microseconds. It was implausible that translation of the visual letters into inner speech occurred during such brief display periods. However, the resolution of this problem seemed straightforward. A brief flash can produce positive and negative afterimages that persist beyond the offset of the physical stimulus. Subjects might continue translating or encoding visual information from the afterimage even though the physical stimulus had ended. Support for this hypothesis came from the work of Sperling (1960). His "partial report" technique involved a brief (50 msec) display of an array of random letters, e.g., three rows of four letters each. If a subject tried to report the entire array, typically he could report only about four of the twelve display letters correctly. However, for a brief period after the display, the subject appeared to have an image of the entire display. If the experimenter specified a row immediately after presenting the display, a subject could report any one of the three rows of letters with about 75% accuracy. This indicated that he had about nine of the twelve display letters available. As the signal was delayed, however, accuracy in reporting the specified row rapidly dropped, apparently due to the fading of the image. Sperling and others have firmly established the role of visual images in experiments of this sort. This type of memory has been called "visual information storage," "iconic memory," and "preperceptual visual memory." The characteristics of this type of memory are that

1. it decays rapidly with time, the typical useful duration being about 100 to 500 msec
2. its duration is affected by display condi-

tions such as display contrast and luminance, and the postdisplay conditions
3. the information retained in the image is preperceptual in that the display symbols have not yet been identified
4. the duration of the image is unaffected by whether the subject is paying attention to the display or trying to remember other nonvisual information
5. information that is not translated from the image before it fades is permanently lost.

Echoic Memory

Despite the addition of iconic memory, there remained unexplained modality differences in memory experiments. For example, if a list of words is presented serially at about two words per second, immediate recall is often better if the list is presented auditorily than if it is presented visually. The superiority of auditory presentation occurs primarily in the recall of the last few items of the list. Phenomenologically, it seems as if these last few items are retained in a kind of preperceptual auditory memory, somewhat analogous to iconic memory. This preperceptual, "precategorical acoustic store" (Crowder and Morton, 1969) or "echoic memory" appears to persist for at least several seconds, thus making it much more useful than the short-lived iconic memory.

Evidence for echoic memory comes from several types of studies, but primarily from the so-called "suffix experiment." In this paradigm, an auditory list of symbols (e.g., digits) is presented, and in some conditions, the last item in the list is followed by a "suffix" which might be any stimulus event, such as a sound, light, or word. Subjects are generally told to ignore the suffix or to regard it as a recall signal. In a series of experiments, Crowder has shown that the occurrence of a completely predictable speech sound (such as "zero" or "go") selectively impairs recall of the last few items on the list. On the other hand, an auditory suffix of this type has no such selective effect on recall if the same list of items is presented visually. With an auditory suffix, recall of an auditory list is about the same as recall of a visual list presented with or without a suffix. Furthermore, it does not seem to matter what the suffix is, so long as it is a speech-like sound. Thus, the suffix might equally well be a digit that is not used in the stimulus list, or a digit played backwards on a tape recorder, making it unintelligible.

Several characteristics of echoic memory suggest that it may be considerably more complex than iconic memory. First, the duration of echoic memory has been estimated to be from two to five seconds, ruling out simple explanations in terms of peripheral neural persistence. Second, only a speech-like suffix disrupts echoic memory. Third, echoic memory appears to be selective with respect to the type of auditory information that is retained. That is, apparently only relatively steady state speech sounds such as vowels are preserved in echoic memory. Transient speech phenomena, such as the stop consonants /b/, /d/, /g/, and so on, do not appear to be retained in echoic memory. This is inferred from the fact that with a list of syllables that differ only in the initial consonant (e.g., pah, bah, hag), recall of the syllables at the end of the list is not selectively impaired by the presentation of an auditory suffix. This last observation appears to converge with research on speech perception indicating that stop consonants, but not vowels, are perceived categorically. That is, subjects are generally unable to notice acoustic differences between various presentations of a particular consonant, but acoustic differences between presentations of a particular vowel are more readily noticed.

The above represents a commonly held view of the basic components of immediate memory for symbolic or linguistic information, and it resembles the view of memory outlined by Neisser (1967). However, several current issues are broadening, and may modify substantially, this view of memory. These issues involve

1. the influence of presentation modality on the retention of symbolic stimuli beyond the iconic or echoic level
2. the characteristics of memory for nonsymbolic material (e.g., tones, melodies, and pictures)
3. an interest in how the various forms of memory are coordinated and controlled.

Post-Iconic Visual Memory

The idea that visually presented symbolic material is retained only if it is translated into an active verbal memory is incorrect in light of recent data. It appears that a richer conception of active memory is needed, one that can represent visual and conceptual information as well as speech. Indeed, it seems that these different representations or codes may be active simultaneously, sometimes with minimal interaction. Four experimental approaches have demonstrated the existence of post-iconic visual memory. One approach has been to show that subjects can remember two sets of information, each presented to a different modality (e.g., auditory plus visual presentation), better than if both sets of information are presented to the same modality. Under some conditions, there is little interference between the two sensory modalities. For example, subjects can remember for 20 seconds or so several visually presented letters that are shown while the subjects shadow (repeat aloud) a different tape-recorded sequence of letters. In contrast, if the letters to be retained are presented auditorily as a part of the tape-recorded sequence that is being shadowed (the letters to be retained being recorded in a different voice), memory is quite poor. A second approach demonstrating the existence of post-iconic visual memory has been to probe a subject's memory some time after a stimulus presentation for the presence of modality specific information; for example, the position or color of a particular word in a display. A third approach has been to use a "release from proactive interference" paradigm. In this paradigm, subjects are given a series of short-term memory trials on a particular type of material, e.g., visually presented words. On each trial, the stimulus is presented and then the subject spends about 15 seconds on an interfering distractor task (e.g., counting backwards) before attempting recall. Performance typically declines with successive trials because material learned on earlier trials interferes with the retention of information on the current trial (proactive interference). However, if some characteristic of the material to be remembered is changed (e.g., presentation modality) so that the new information is now encoded differently, proactive interference is diminished and recall improves. A fourth approach has been to study characteristics of free recall. Several investigators have noted that recall of mixed modality word lists tends to be organized in terms of presentation modality (e.g., visually presented words being recalled first). Another observer noted that recall of the names of drawings of objects was organized in terms of the orientations of the drawings.

In the experiments just described, it is theoretically possible that modality specific information could be retained in memory in a relatively abstract way. For example, a subject might note the presentation modality of a word by adding a tag or label to the memory of the word. However, it appears that visual presentation actually produces a representation of the stimulus in memory that has some of the properties of the perceived stimulus; that is, the memory appears to have some of the characteristics of a visual image. Evidence for this view comes from several experiments that have demonstrated poorer accuracy and slower recognition of letters or words if the display is changed in ways that leave the symbolic content unaltered, such as a change in the color of the background of the display letters between the initial presentation and a subsequent recognition test.

One interesting aspect of this concern with modality specific information has been the realization that when a subject responds in these tasks, his recall may interfere with the memory that he is trying to report. For example, if a subject tries to report information retained in some sort of visual code, spoken recall is better than written recall, because the visual processing required for written recall interferes with the remaining visually coded information. Conversely, written recall is superior to spoken recall if the subject has coded the information auditorily.

Memory for Nonsymbolic Stimuli

Most memory experiments have used symbolic or linguistic stimuli. Therefore, research with nonsymbolic stimuli has typically focused on the similarities and differences between symbolic and nonsymbolic material, particularly with respect to questions of memory capacity, verbal mediation, and forgetting. Classical psychophysical research on the discriminability of stimuli in various modalities provides a background here, because these were, in fact, experiments in memory, inasmuch as the typical procedure involved sequential presentation of two stimuli, requiring the subject to remember the first stimulus in order to compare it with the second. Some con-

temporary investigators have returned to this task in order to study the characteristics of memory and forgetting of nonrepresentational stimuli (e.g., tones and sounds, tactile stimuli, motor movements, and odors) over relatively short periods of time. Although the available data are incomplete, and sometimes inconsistent, it appears that there are some generalizations emerging. First, even if a subject is not required to respond to a distracting interpolated task in the retention interval, the evidence suggests that there is usually increased forgetting as the retention interval is lengthened. This is in contrast to data for verbal retention where there is generally no forgetting of short stimulus lists in the absence of a distractor task in the retention interval. Also, for nonverbal stimuli, forgetting typically occurs rapidly during the first few seconds and is considerably slower thereafter. The rapid forgetting of nonverbal stimuli suggests that there may be no mechanisms for sustaining the memory of nonsymbolic stimuli akin to the rehearsal mechanism proposed for verbal stimuli.

Rapid forgetting of verbal stimuli is often observed if the retention interval is filled with another distracting verbal task, such as counting backwards. In contrast, however, the rate of forgetting for nonverbal stimuli often shows little or no effect of the distracting tasks typically used to produce forgetting in verbal memory experiments, although the rate of forgetting is affected if the distracting task involves processing additional stimuli in the modality of the stimuli to be retained.

Experiments with nonsymbolic stimuli can almost always be structured so that subjects will introduce verbal mediation. That is, if a sound is presented, a subject may try to guess what might have made the sound. If a visual pattern is presented, the subject may try to think of an object that could be represented by the pattern. As a result, what the subject retains may not be a direct representation of the stimulus information, but rather his associations or verbal labels for the stimulus. Consequently, how a subject describes or labels a stimulus often predicts subsequent recognition or recall performance. If the label or description incorporates the salient features of the stimulus, it will be subsequently recognized or accurately recalled. However, it is also clear that there is often a substantial nonlinguistic memory component. Some evidence supporting this notion has been discussed above. Other evidence comes from studies of memory for colors, pictures, voices, and sounds, where the accuracy of recognition memory seems to exceed the ability of subjects to describe the stimuli in unique, repeatable ways. For example, cultures differ substantially in the way they label colors. In a few extreme cases, a culture may have only two basic color names, yet the errors that people from these cultures make in recognition memory for colors are very similar to the errors found in cultures with completely different ways of labeling colors.

Superficially, there seem to be marked capacity differences across various modalities. For example, the ability of a subject to remember that a specific word or phrase occurred in a particular context seems poor by comparison with the ability to recognize previously seen pictures. Shepard (1967) compared the retention of words, sentences, and pictures, and found that recognition of previously seen pictures substantially exceeded performance for words and sentences. In contrast, recognition memory in other modalities, such as for sounds and odors, often seems inferior to both verbal and visual memory. However, comparisons of this sort are often questionable because it is difficult to equate the distinctiveness and discriminability of stimuli across modalities.

Several investigators have also attempted to make qualitative comparisons of memory in different sensory modalities. For example, it appears that the primacy and recency effects that are generally found with symbolic material may be lacking with pictorial material. Also, the retention of the sequential order may be poorer for pictorial than for symbolic stimuli. On the other hand, memory for nonverbal auditory stimuli (sounds or tones) may be similar to verbal memory with respect to primacy and recency effects and the preservation of temporal order.

Although in many situations subjects can control the way in which they store information, it seems that encoding the presentation modality of symbolic stimuli may occur automatically. For example, if a list of words is presented, some visually and some auditorily, subjects frequently remember the modality in which each word was presented, and subjects who are specifically instructed to remember presentation modality do so no better than uninstructed subjects. In addition, a single stimulus may potentially be represented in several ways, e.g., by a visual representation and by the name of the stimulus. Current research involves the question of what types of memory codes occur automatically, and what types of codes are under the control of a subject, and the question of what types of codes can be concurrently active (Posner, 1973).

In summary, where memory was once viewed as a relatively homogeneous entity, current theorists see a multiplicity of memory codes, both within and across sensory modalities. A start has been made at delineating the characteristics of these modality dependent codes, but a great deal is still unknown.

BIBLIOGRAPHY

CONRAD, R. Acoustic confusions in immediate memory. *British Journal of Psychology,* 1964, *55,* 75–84.

CROWDER, R. G., and MORTON, J. Precategorical acoustic storage (PAS). *Perception and Psychophysics,* 1969, *5,* 365–373.

NEISSER, U. *Cognitive psychology.* New York: Appleton-Century-Crofts, 1967.

POSNER, M. I. Coordination of internal codes. In W. G. Chase (Ed.), *Visual information processing.* New York: Academic Press, 1973. Pp. 35–73.

SHEPARD, R. N. Recognition memory for words, sentences and pictures. *Journal of Verbal Learning and Verbal Behavior,* 1967, *6,* 156–163.

SPERLING, G. The information available in brief visual presentations. *Psychological Monographs,* 1960, *74*(11, Whole No. 498).

SPERLING, G. A model for visual memory tasks. *Human Factors,* 1963, *5,* 19–31.

DON L. SCARBOROUGH

MEMORY: THE ROLE OF ORGANIZATION

The empirical study of memory began with the work of Herman Ebbinghaus in the middle to late 1800s (Ebbinghaus, 1913). Most of the early work involved tracing out relatively simple processes, such as rate of learning and rate of forgetting, but toward the end of the 1800s there was an increasing interest in the way certain situational and task variables influenced learning and retention. While this type of empirical exploration allowed investigators to develop preliminary laws for describing the learning process, much of this early work was non-theoretical.

This nontheoretical attitude was also evident in the work on organization and learning during the late 1800s and into the early 1900s. There was research on the effects of rhythm on memory, but it was confined to demonstrating and describing the effects rather than trying to explain them. The studies on prose learning also seem to be aimed primarily at demonstration and description rather than explanation. In terms of these issues, the emphasis on description is particularly interesting, because some rather difficult-to-understand phenomena were uncovered as a result of that work.

The Initial Data and the Concept of Meaningfulness

The first descriptions of the influence of organizational variables on learning were focused on the role of meaningfulness in the learning process (Johnson in Dixon and Horton, 1968). These descriptions were a natural outgrowth of the studies themselves, which involved a comparison between the learning of textual and nonsense materials. For example, some of the earliest work was a simple demonstration that prose was learned more rapidly than nonsense material and that poetry could be learned even faster than prose. In addition, there was evidence that some nonsense syllables were more meaningful than others and that learning was related to the degree of meaningfulness. Finally, in the middle 1950s, there were a number of studies in which subjects were asked to learn word sequences that varied in their approximation to English. Although the relationship was not perfect, there did seem to be a positive correlation between learning rate and approximation to English.

The initial explanation given for these effects was in terms of meaningfulness. Meaningful material was easier to learn than meaningless material, and the assumed mechanism was positive transfer coming from interitem associations that had been established through previous experience with the material. That explanation not only handled the early data but allowed psychologists to explain this phenomenon with the same concepts and mechanisms used to explain other learning phenomena.

While that explanation was parsimonious, it did tend to confuse what now appears to be two separate dimensions of meaningfulness and structure. Although there does appear to be an increase in meaningfulness as approximation to English increases, there is also an increase in the degree to which the sequence approximates the structure of English. That also is true of increasing degrees of meaningfulness for nonsense syllables. While some developments, such as case grammar, suggest that the dimensions of meaningfulness and structure may be intimately related, it also seems clear that they must be viewed as separate dimensions.

Organization as an Independent Process

In the early 1960s, there were a number of different research endeavors that began to raise questions regarding these simple descriptions of organizational effects. One of the first, and possibly the most basic, was a demonstration that the effect on learning of the meaningfulness of nonsense syllables could not be explained in terms of associations among the letters, because such measures did not correlate with learning rate. Only those measures that treated the nonsense syllable as a single unit had predictive value. For example, one of the best predictors was the pronounceability of the nonsense syllable. In addition, some studies indicated that if nonsense syllables could be recoded (e.g., change UBS into SUB or BUS), learning would be more rapid. Again, it seems most meaningful to treat the nonsense item as a unit rather than as a set of interassociated letters.

The work on sequence learning also raised questions regarding the role of organization in learning. For example, it began to appear that one of the major influences of varying approximation to English was on the length of sequence that could be recalled without error, rather than on the total amount of information that was remembered. Similarly, there were very strong grouping effects when subjects learned organized sequences. Subjects would report using such groups, and there would be a definite rhythm or pauses in their recall, even though the sequences were not presented with such a rhythm. Furthermore, the rhythm-defined units conformed to the groups they reported using.

A related effect is the fact that not all subjects who learned a highly structured sequence showed evidence of a benefit from the structure. If the subjects did not show a tendency to group in terms of the structure-defined units, they behaved as if they were learning a random sequence. Similarly, if an experimenter pointed out the boundaries of structure-defined units, the learning performance would show a very marked facilitation. All these studies on sequence learning seem to suggest that a critical issue regarding the use of organization in learning concerns the way in which subjects identify and use units or groups.

The final area of research that casts doubt on traditional accounts of organization is the work on category clustering in free recall. In these studies, subjects are presented with a long list of words that represent several instances of each of several categories (e.g., birds, flowers, trees). The words are not presented in category groups, but in random order, and the subjects are allowed to recall them in any order they choose. The results of these studies indicate that while subjects do tend to recall the words in category clusters, not all of the clustering can be explained in terms of interitem associations. Furthermore, the way subjects make a transition from one category to another during recall cannot be explained in terms of associations between items in the two categories. Again, the results seem to suggest that a unitization or grouping process occurs during learning, but that the process cannot be explained entirely in terms of interitem associations.

Organization and the Concept of Chunking

A common theme touched on above is that whenever learners use organization, a fundamental process is one of grouping or unitization. In 1956, George Miller published a classic paper in which he pointed out that memory span can be increased, and the amount of information held in memory increased, if the information can be grouped into large units or chunks. For example, if a subject is asked to recall a string of random letters immediately after presentation, he can produce about seven, but if the letters are organized into familiar words, the number of letters retained goes up dramatically. In fact, subjects can retain about as many unrelated words as unrelated letters.

Memory span seems to be relatively unlimited in terms of the amount of information retained, but it does seem to be severely limited in terms of the number of chunks of information retained (about seven).

At a superficial level, a *chunk* can be defined as a set of items or information that a person treats as a single unit within memory. The process whereby the item set is so unitized is termed *recoding*. Recoding usually occurs because the learner applied some prelearned grouping principle, although there are times when the learner must acquire the grouping rule during learning. For example, *cow man* might be treated as two memory chunks rather than six letters, because through prior learning the words had already been unitized. Furthermore, *cow boy* might be remembered as a single unit because through prior experience not only had the words *cow* and *boy* been unitized, but at a higher level the word *cowboy* also had been unitized. On the other hand, if the learner was presented with SBJ FQL, there would be a cue supplied for grouping (i.e., the blank space), but there would be no prelearned grouping principle that would allow the learner to integrate the groups into a single informational unit. Consequently, that sequence would be treated initially as six chunks, with one corresponding to each letter. However, with repeated trials, a learner might devise and acquire a recoding plan for SBJ and FQL so that the sequence could be retained as two chunks, rather than as a sequence of six letters.

The influence of learning a recoding scheme has been illustrated by asking learners to retain a sequence of binary digits (e.g., 01110010) after a single presentation. Normally, after a single presentation, subjects can retain sequences of about seven such binary digits. However, performance would be much higher if the subjects had previously learned a simple recoding scheme in which they grouped the digits into pairs, with a 00 pattern retained as a 1, a 01 pattern as a 2, a 10 pattern as a 3, and a 11 pattern as a 4. The above sequence of eight binary digits could then be retained as a sequence of 4 decimal digits (2413).

These relatively intuitive conceptions of a chunk have been operationally defined in terms of item sets that tend to be: (1) remembered and forgotten in an all-or-none manner; (2) recalled together when the learners can recall the items in any order they choose; or (3) within the same rhythm pattern in a learner's oral recall. In situations where it is possible to apply all three criteria to the same learning performance, the operations consistently identify the same item sets as chunks.

Conceptually, chunks have been viewed as item sets that are stored together in memory. Theoretically, that is the reason the items tend to be recalled in an all-or-none manner and together, and it is the basis for the operational definitions given above. A common view is that the items are represented in memory by a code of some type, and specific theories differ both in terms of the nature of the hypothesized code and the nature of the relationship between the code and the information. Some theories view the codes as abstract entities and others view them as being simple labels or names. The important point, however, is that it is generally assumed that there is a common memorial representation for all the information in the chunk, and retrieval of the representation entails retrieval of all the information it currently represents.

Chunking and Free Recall Learning

One of the first areas in which clear chunking effects were demonstrated was in *free-recall*. During recall, the subjects' output tends to occur in bursts of several items. If the list consisted of items from several categories, these items are recalled together even though they were not presented in that way. This effect is known as category clustering and it is related to both the degree and rate of learning (Wood in Tulving and Donaldson, 1972).

There are several sources of data which support the idea that categories represent chunks in a learner's memory. The first is that the categories tend to be recalled in an all-or-none manner. In addition, variables that influence the recall of categories may or may not have an influence on the recall of items from within a category, and vice versa. For example, some factor might result in subjects tending to forget the categories in a list, but for any remembered category there may be no reduction in the number of instances recalled.

The final bit of data indicating that categories function as chunks comes from experiments which demonstrate that subjects do not use associations between items from different categories as a way of moving from one category to another in recall. If category A and category B are related to one another, they will appear adjacently in recall, but that relationship does not arise because the items in the two categories are interassociated. It seems that the relevant relationship is between the categories and not between the instances of the categories.

There has also been work on organization in the free recall of lists of unrelated words, that is, no experimenter-provided organization. In these cases, organization is measured by determining the extent to which the order of a learner's recall becomes more stereotyped as learning progresses. The phenomenon is called subjective organization, and such stereotyping does seem to increase as learning increases. In addition, for an individual learner, the effect is highly related to rate of learning.

Chunking and Serial Learning

A large variety of grouping arrangements can be used with ordered series. The groups can be color coded, blank spaces can be left between certain items to suggest a grouping strategy, rhythm or pauses can be used with auditory presentation, or rules might be used. An example of rule-defined chunks might be a sequence such as 4 3 2 1 10 12 14 16 7 5 3 1 14 13 12 11.

Regardless of how chunks are induced, however, there is always a clear tendency for the chunks to be recalled in an all-or-none manner (Johnson in Melton and Martin, 1972). A common measure is to compute the likelihood that each item in the sequence was not recalled given that the immediately preceding item was recalled (transitional-error probability or TEP). The TEP is a measure of the independence of the two items involved. At the transition between two chunks, it is always very high relative to the TEP between items within the chunks. Such TEP spikes can be used to identify the chunking pattern used by a subject while learning a sequence.

Regardless of the method used to induce subjects to chunk in a particular manner, the TEP patterns obtained during learning invariably conform to the expected chunks. Furthermore, there is clear evidence that when subjects forget items, they tend to forget an entire chunk.

Finally, the rhythm patterns in recall match the chunking pattern quite closely.

As with categories in free recall, the relationships among chunks seem to be at the chunk level rather than relations between the items themselves. If, before learning the sequence, subjects form an association between two letters within the sequence, that prior association helps the sequence learning only if it is a within-chunk transition. If the association is between the last letter from one chunk and the first letter from the next, there is no benefit from the prior learning. Also, if after learning the sequence, subjects are given an item and asked to recall the next item in the sequence, they have a great deal of difficulty if they have to go from the last element of one chunk to the first element of the next, but they have little trouble if both items are from the same chunk. On the other hand, if they are probed with an entire chunk, they can produce the first item of the next chunk with very little difficulty. These results seem to indicate that it is knowledge about the relationships between chunks as units that allows us to go from one chunk to another in recall, rather than knowledge of interrelationships between the specific items.

Organization as a Hierarchical Arrangement of Chunks

While it seems clear that items can be coded into chunks, it also seems reasonable that the codes for chunks could themselves be recoded at a higher level into higher-order chunks. Within that framework, one can consider the organization of a sequence as being the hierarchical arrangement of chunks. For example, the sequence 9 3 4 6 U O L S can be viewed as eight items at the lowest level, but they can be grouped at the next level into "two odd numbers, two even numbers, two vowels, and two consonants." At the next level in the hierarchy those chunk codes can be reorganized into "four numbers followed by four letters," and at the highest level it can be construed as "sequence of items." Such higher-order chunking is termed recoding, and the organization for a set of items can be defined in terms of the pattern of recoding (Bower in Tulving and Donaldson, 1972).

One of the clearest examples of a hierarchical organization of serially ordered material is the organization of written language. The base elements are letters, which are grouped into syllables, which are grouped into words, which are grouped into clauses, and so on. Many studies indicate that sentence learning is a direct function of the extent to which subjects use such a structure. There is also evidence that subjects use a hierarchical structure when they learn to free recall categorized lists. If a list consisted of the categories *birds, mammals, flowers,* and *trees,* it could be reorganized at a higher level into *animals* and *plants,* and those two higher-order chunks could be reorganized at a yet higher level into *living things.* That would allow subjects to retain the entire list in terms of a single code that could be decoded into a hierarchical organization that represented the entire list. Studies that have used such lists have demonstrated both clustering of items into chunks and clustering of the higher-order chunks. In addition, such a hierarchical organization facilitates learning when performance is compared to that of lists consisting of an equal number of unrelated categories.

Given this view of organization, one organization might differ from another in terms of the pattern of recoding. It might also differ in the extent to which the recoding pattern conforms to a simple rule structure or to one previously learned. For example, if a letter sequence is viewed as having three levels—letters, chunks, and sequence—then the sequence SB JFQ and SBJ FQ differ only in the pattern of recoding. On the other hand, IB MFM differs from IBM FM in terms of both the organizational pattern and the extent to which prior knowledge can be used for the recoding. Numerous studies have indicated that both of these factors have a marked influence on learning rate. Some recoding patterns are easier to learn than others, and having prior knowledge regarding the recoding rule has a marked facilitating effect on learning. Finally, simply pointing out chunk boundaries to a learner has a very profound influence on his performance.

Taken together, these studies suggest that higher-order chunking does occur, and it does appear reasonable to view organization in terms of the pattern of recoding. In addition, any cues that can be given to help the learner quickly detect the hierarchical structure for a set of materials also has a facilitating effect on learning.

Organization as a Retrieval Plan

Some of the research on organization and memory has raised a question regarding *why* learners organize. While it is clear that there might be a reason for grouping IBMFM as IBM and FM, rather than grouping it as IB and MFM or not grouping it at all, it is less clear why learners should show the same tendency to group a sequence such as SBJFQ. Although subjects may not show any particular preference for grouping it as SBJ FQ as opposed to SB JFQ, almost every subject will use one of those two grouping strategies even when no grouping cues are provided.

One possibility is that an organizational network can be used as a scheme for searching our memory, or as a generative plan for the overt production of a complex response. If the role of organization is viewed in this manner, it would suggest that a distinction might be drawn between the role of the organization in the integration of a previously unknown information set, and the role of organization for establishing an organized network for the contents of our long-term memory (i.e., all our knowledge). Once a new information set has been organized into a unit, the long-term retention and availability of that unit might depend upon its then being included at an appropriate place within the preexisting organized network of our memory.

Organization as a Generative Scheme

One characteristic of efficiently organized knowledge sets and behavior is that they can be produced with great speed and ease. In fact, the speed with which an overlearned sequence such as the alphabet can be produced indicates that interitem associations could not be the generative mechanism. The response must be planned and organized ahead of overt production. That also is suggested by the fact that if the speaker is distracted or interrupted, he will continue the response for a short time, as if the short segment he is producing had already been programmed and was not disrupted by the distraction. Finally, if subjects are probed with a question such as "What letter comes after H?" they usually find it necessary to get a running head start and say something like "F, G, H, I" to themselves before they can come up with the answer.

These considerations suggest that subjects may plan responses in terms of chunk-size units with all of the decisions made at chunk boundaries. Once the subject has made the response decisions for a chunk, he can begin producing it and at the same time start making the response decisions for the next chunk. This view suggests that subjects plan their responses ahead of their overt production. If they encounter difficulty, it should be at the point where they make their decisions. These points are the chunk boundaries. The fact that TEPs are higher there than anywhere else is consistent with that view. In addition, as chunk size (and presumably difficulty) increases, there seems to be a linear increase in the TEP on the transition to the beginning of that chunk. Furthermore, if a difficult item is introduced at the end of a chunk, there is a marked increase in the TEP at the beginning of the chunk. These findings are consistent with the supposition that even the decision about the last item is made at the beginning of the chunk.

A simple demonstration of this function of organization is to ask someone to say the alphabet employing a rhythm other than that provided by the familiar alphabet song. Most people find the task almost impossible. In addition, if they are asked to say their phone number as fast as usual, but with pauses after the first, fourth, and seventh digits, most subjects will be unable to do it. Those that can produce the proper speed often have a marked tendency to make mistakes and give the wrong number. All of the above results seem to suggest that chunks represent planning units during the production of a response. It may be quite reasonable to view the overall organization for a sequence as a generative plan that allows the subject to work ahead of his overt production, and thereby facilitate performance (Johnson in Melton and Martin, 1972).

Semantic Memory as an Organized Network of Knowledge

A fascinating and perplexing issue for students of learning and memory has always been the speed and efficiency with which humans can recover knowledge from memory. When asked a question, even about a long past and seldom recollected experience, subjects often can retrieve the appropriate knowledge almost instantly, and recognition, if it occurs, is almost always instantaneous. The fact that recovery of stored knowledge is usually so swift and effortless requires some assumptions regarding the nature of the storage. The major problem is to explain why it is unnecessary to scan the entire contents of memory.

As one explanation, Mandler (Dixon and Horton, 1968) has suggested a hierarchical organization of the contents of memory with a semantic structure determining the organization. Such a view of memory assumes that: (1) the contents of our memory are organized in a hierarchical manner; (2) similar items are in some sense stored "near" one another; (3) our knowledge can be accessed at any level in the hierarchy; and (4) memory searches are efficient, because the organization provides pathways for us to get from one feature or concept to another without considering irrelevant information.

In order to understand the use and efficiency of such a system, it is necessary to realize that the system is usually probed with a question, and the content of the question specifies an entry point. For example, knowledge of objects may be divided into many classes, one of which is *living things. Living things* can be subdivided into many classes, one of them might be *animals,* and that in turn could be subdivided into classes, with one being *birds.* Now, if one is asked if a *bird* is a *living thing,* it is possible to take either *bird* or *living thing* as an entry point and move through the pathways defined by the hierarchical organization. If the pathways define *bird* as a subentry of *living thing,* the appropriate response is "yes." The organization allows much irrelevant search to be excluded, because each move down a level in the hierarchy obviates the need to search through the subentries of other higher-order nodes. Only more recently has there been much research on this type of conception of long-term memory.

Learning as Organization

One of the interesting and suggestive implications of the prior considerations is that organization is an all-pervasive phenomenon in learning. A tempting further conclusion is that learning is just another name for an organizational process. The research on the issue of learning as organization has focused on both organization as a generative scheme and as a system for the storage of knowledge in permanent memory. Regarding organization's function as a generative scheme, most of the work has involved requiring subjects to change the organization they use for a given sequence or set of information. In one type of free-recall situations, a subject might be asked to learn a list followed by the learning of a second list, where the second list consists of all of the first-list items plus an equal number of new items. Under these circumstances, there is strong evidence of negative transfer and interference if the organization for the first list is in some way inappropriate for the total organization of the second list. If the second list can be acquired by simply expanding the first list organization, there is usually positive transfer. Similarly, if subjects learn a sequence, such as SB JFQ LZ, and then they learn the same letter sequence but organized differently (e.g., SBJ FQLZ), there is marked negative transfer during second-list learning, and evidence of forgetting from retroactive interference when they are asked to recall the original list. Finally, if a particular sequence is repeated on many trials, but with a different rhythm each time so that the learner organizes it differently, there is no evidence of learning across trials. If, however, the same rhythm is used on every trial, there is a marked facilitation. In all of these experimental situations, subjects are presented with material that they have encountered in the past, but if they are induced to organize it in a new way, they treat it as if it were new material. It would appear that the critical item is the organization rather than the specific information to be learned.

The above research is complemented by the work on long-term memory as an organized network of knowledge. The basic paradigm has been to present a subject with a set of words and simply ask him to find a way to organize them into a set of classes, using any system that is meaningful to him. He is then asked to recall the items, although he did not know in advance that he would be given that test. Performance is then compared to that of subjects who had been instructed to memorize the list and to another group that had just sorted the words into random and arbitrary categories. The results of these studies have indicated that the instruction to organize results in the same amount of learning as does the instruction to memorize.

Taken as a set, these experiments suggest that learning may be an organizational process. If a learner is deprived of his ability to use a previously learned organization, or to use a consistent organization, he seems to operate as if the experience is totally new, even though the material is something that is already known. Furthermore, if he can be induced to organize the material in some way, the resulting memory trace is indistinguishable from that which is formed if he deliberately attempts to memorize the items.

Overview

Although the first explanations of organization effects were in terms of meaningfulness, positive transfer, and a reduction in the amount needed to be learned, it soon became apparent that the major factor was grouping or unitizing processes in memory. The basic organizational process seems to be one of grouping or recoding information sets into small units or chunks of about three items each. The codes for these chunks can themselves be recoded into higher-order units, and the organization for a sequence can be viewed as the recoding pattern. In that such a recoding process seems to occur in all situations, it may not be meaningful to ask whether organization facilitates learning, but rather one should ask whether learning can take place at all without organization.

Considerations such as these have led many to the conclusion that learning itself may be an organizational process. If learners change the organization for a known set of information, there seems to be no positive transfer. If they are prevented from developing a stable organization during learning, no learning takes place even though the material is presented over and over again. Finally, whatever processing mechanisms are engaged by the instruction "memorize," also seem to be equally engaged by the instruction "organize."

BIBLIOGRAPHY

DIXON, T., and HORTON, D. *Verbal behavior and general behavior theory.* Englewood Cliffs, N.J.: Prentice-Hall, 1968.
EBBINGHAUS, H. *Memory: A contribution to experimental psychology.* New York: Columbia University Press, 1913.
MELTON, A., and MARTIN, E. *Coding processes in human memory.* Washington, D.C.: Winston, 1972.
MILLER, G. The magical number seven plus or minus two: Some limits on our capacity for processing information. *Psychological Review,* 1956, *63,* 81–97.
TULVING, E., and DONALDSON, W. *Organization of memory.* New York: Academic Press, 1972.

See also SEMANTIC MEMORY

NEAL F. JOHNSON

MEMORY: THE ROLE OF REHEARSAL

If a subject is stopped during the course of studying a list of items in a memory experiment and asked what he has been doing, only rarely will he report that he has been passively attending to the items as they were presented. Instead, the subject nearly always describes himself as engaging in some active manipulation of the material being studied. These manipulations, which range from repeating items over and over to the formation of complex interitem groupings of images, are usually referred to as rehearsal.

Rehearsal has only recently become a topic of serious investigation. There seem to be at least two factors which have led to neglect of this area. First, rehearsal has often been viewed in a negative way as a source of error precluding precise experimental control over the subjects' processing of a list. Researchers attempted to gain control over study of a list of items by presenting the items one at a time for fixed presentation times, assuming that such a procedure would equate the study accorded each item. Unfortunately, it was noted that if the study time per item was fairly long (e.g., 2–5 seconds) subjects would often report thinking about, or rehearsing previously presented items during a subsequent item's presentation period. If the presentation rate was more rapid, subjects often reported virtually ignoring some items so that they could continue to rehearse other previously presented items. There were even indications that instructing subjects to attend only to the presented item during its presentation interval could not completely eliminate the tendency to rehearse some items of a list more than others.

A second problem which has hampered the

study of rehearsal has been the lack of agreement among researchers as to the function or functions of rehearsal. Examples of the roles proposed for rehearsal include the maintenance of information in short-term storage, the transfer of information from short-term to long-term storage, the production of elaborative codes of stimuli, and practice at retrieving information. The single term rehearsal has thus been applied to a wide variety of cognitive activities. Rehearsal, in this broad sense, might be defined as any cognitive manipulation of encoded information undertaken by a subject for the purpose of making that information available for future use. While such a definition is consistent with the way in which the term rehearsal has been used, the breadth of this definition has discouraged the investigation of rehearsal processes.

Methods of Studying Rehearsal

Four general approaches have been used in the study of rehearsal: (1) minimizing or precluding rehearsal, (2) using incidental learning procedures to control type of rehearsal, (3) structuring rehearsal by imposing particular rehearsal strategies, and (4) monitoring spontaneously produced rehearsal activity. Studies which have attempted to minimize or preclude rehearsal have been directed less toward understanding rehearsal than toward eliminating it so that other memory processes could be examined. The distractor technique, introduced to study short-term memory, is an example of this approach. The aim of this technique was to explore the loss in retention of a small amount of information, usually three letters, words, or trigrams, over a brief period of time, up to 30 seconds, after study. It was immediately apparent that unless subjects were engaged in some distracting task during the time between study and test they would rehearse the to-be-remembered material and perform perfectly on the test. In order to prevent rehearsal during the study-test delay, subjects were instructed to perform some attention engaging activity (e.g., counting backwards rapidly by threes) during the study-test interval. One important function of rehearsal is illustrated by this procedure. Rehearsal can serve to maintain a small amount of information in memory

for as long as rehearsal is continued. Those researchers favoring a dual-storage conception of memory have gone on to suggest that active rehearsal is necessary to prevent the loss of information from short-term storage and recent evidence supports this hypothesis. It should be pointed out that distractor tasks do not completely preclude rehearsal. Studies of the effects of various distractor tasks on rehearsal have shown that even complex distractor tasks cannot prevent surreptitious rehearsal; therefore, procedures of the type just described would be best interpreted as ways of minimizing rehearsal.

Incidental learning paradigms have recently been employed in the study of rehearsal processes. In the incidental learning procedure, items are presented to subjects, but the subject is not told that he will be tested on his memory for the items. As a rationale for presenting the items, subjects are asked to perform some operations on the items, for example, crossing out all vowels or rating the pronounceableness of the words. Since the subject does not expect a subsequent memory test it is assumed that he will only study the items to the extent required by the experimental cover task; thus, the incidental learning procedure attempts to gain control over rehearsal by eliminating its apparent value to the subject. In addition, the nature of the cover task determines the type of processing in which the subject engages. For example, asking the subject to simply repeat each item as it is shown should result in different processing than would asking the subject to produce a synonym for each word shown. At least one important result has already emerged from the study of rehearsal using incidental learning. If the subject rehearses items by simply repeating them over and over, (i.e., maintaining the items in short-term storage), then the length of time for which an item is thus rehearsed is not related to the recall probability of the item on a later test. Rehearsal, at least rehearsal whose purpose is simple maintenance, does not result in an automatic increase in long-term recallability. Some forms of rehearsal do, however, result in such an increase, thus providing evidence for at least two types of rehearsal.

A third approach to the study of rehearsal has involved attempting to structure the pattern of rehearsal employed by a subject (Atkinson and Shiffrin, 1971). The most common rehearsal pattern used has been repeated rehearsal of each item of a list during its presentation interval; however, other, more complicated patterns have also been tried. Attempts to structure rehearsal have met with the same difficulty as attempts to preclude rehearsal. Subjects often rehearse items other than those desired by the experimenter. The most consistent result emerging from structured rehearsal studies has been the observation that imposing any particular rehearsal pattern results in a reduction in recall when contrasted with recall performance of subjects whose rehearsal is unconstrained.

In the past few years techniques have been developed which allow the direct observation of rehearsal (Rundus, 1971). The most straightforward technique involves requiring a subject to rehearse aloud while studying a list of items, tape recording this overt rehearsal, and tabulating and analyzing (usually with the aid of a computer) the recorded rehearsal protocols. Subjects are not constrained to any particular pattern of rehearsal; rather, they are told to study in a "normal" way and to try to make their overt rehearsal correspond to whatever they arc "thinking about." To facilitate analysis, subjects are told to rehearse aloud only words from the list being studied (i.e., whenever they are thinking about a list item in any context they are to say that item aloud but not other extralist words which may be part of their rehearsal context). The overt rehearsal procedure appears to be minimally disruptive since neither level of recall nor the subject's ability to organize items shows significant impairment when compared with performance in silent study. The overt procedure does not allow the investigator to tell exactly what the subject was doing during study. That is, if the subject rehearses the word "fish" aloud it is not possible to tell if he was forming an image, attending to the word's auditory characteristics, imbedding the word in a sentence or story with other list items, or processing the item in some other way. However, it is assumed that the overt rehearsals produced by the subject provide an indication of how much rehearsal was accorded an item, how that rehearsal was distributed during the study, and what items were temporally contiguous in the subject's rehearsal. Thus far, the major thrust of experiments using this procedure has been the examination of particular memory phenomena to ascertain whether they are explicable as resulting from particular study strategies. It would seem that the overt procedure should also serve as a useful tool in the theoretical examination of rehearsal processes themselves. For example, examination of actual rehearsal protocols might provide insight into the decision rules employed by a subject in choosing how to study a particular item and how or when to integrate several items. The principal drawbacks to the observed rehearsal procedure are that (1) as already mentioned, it is not possible to determine exactly what cognitive operations are represented by a particular overt rehearsal of an item, and (2) it is not possible to manipulate the amount of rehearsal given a particular item. Any comparisons between observed rehearsal of an item and recall of the item must, therefore, be correlational.

Two Types of Rehearsal

As mentioned earlier, one of the barriers to the systematic study of rehearsal has been the breadth of phenomena and processes subsumed under that single term. One resolution of this problem is to identify and label particular types or classes of rehearsal. Data appear to allow the identification of two distinct types of rehearsal, maintenance rehearsal and coding rehearsal. There is not enough information available to clearly specify the cognitive operations unique to each of these two classes; instead, they are perhaps best delimited by the purpose of each type of rehearsal.

Maintenance rehearsal refers to those rehearsal activities which serve to hold a limited amount of information in a highly available state. An example of this type of rehearsal would be finding a telephone number in a directory and rehearsing that number until dialing is completed. Unless there is some distraction, the number will usually be maintained perfectly until the rehearsal is terminated following dialing. While this form of rehearsal may appear to be used in only a limited number of situations, it is quite possible that its use is more pervasive. Except for those cases where incoming information is rapidly encoded to the desired level, maintenance rehearsal might be used to hold presented information in a highly available state while decisions are made as to how the material is to be coded and while coding is occurring.

One important characteristic of maintenance rehearsal is its apparent ineffectiveness in forming memory traces which will be usable at some time after rehearsal ceases (Craik and Watkins, 1973). Several incidental learning studies which required only that the subject hold items in memory for varying amounts of time but provided no reason for other processing, have shown that the amount of time which the subject spent maintaining an item was not related to the later recallability of the item. Thus a widely held assumption that long-term recallability increases as a function of amount of rehearsal must be modified by considering the type of rehearsal being employed.

Of the four types of experimental procedures used to examine rehearsal, the *incidental learning* procedures appear to hold the most promise as means of elucidating maintenance rehearsal. Since the purpose of the rehearsal and not its frequency seems to be of major importance, both structuring and monitoring procedures would appear to be of limited use. While the restricting or precluding procedures are primarily aimed at eliminating maintenance rehearsal (i.e., preventing the subject from holding information in short-term storage via rehearsal) these procedures will probably not be useful in determining the characteristics of the cognitive operations of maintenance rehearsal. In contrast, manipulating the type of processing required in an incidental task should help identify those types of codes involved in maintenance rehearsal. Current evidence suggests that maintenance rehearsal entails manipulations of sensory (e.g., acoustic, visual) features of items but not more complex semantic or imaginal attributes. To confirm the sensory nature of maintenance rehearsal, it would be necessary to show that the incidental learning cover tasks which direct subject processing toward sensory features, give rise to the good immediate recall and lack of increment in long-term recall which characterizes maintenance rehearsal. Cover tasks involving other attributes must

then be shown not to yield such data. By testing a variety of processing tasks in this way it should be possible to establish the set of cognitive operations utilized in maintenance rehearsal.

The other proposed class of rehearsal processes, *coding rehearsal,* is also characterized mainly by its purpose—to make information available for recall at some time after rehearsal has ceased. Examples of the types of rehearsal activities subsumed under this label include rehearsing together items which the subject perceives as being related in an attempt to emphasize their interrelationships and create retrievable item groups, rehearsing items together in an attempt to integrate them into phrases, sentences, stories, or images which would serve to make the items more recallable, and rehearsing items in conjunction with some extra-list retrieval aids (e.g., peg-word or method-of-loci mnemonic strategies). Unfortunately, little is known about the actual operation of coding rehearsal. Studies have shown that coding rehearsal usually requires more time during study, either for the discovery of appropriate codes or for the adequate storage of such codes, than does maintenance rehearsal. Also, there appears to be a maintenance-coding tradeoff. Subjects who are aware that they will be given both a short-term and a long-term test on studied material can alter their rehearsal to produce better recall on one of the tests, but only at the expense of recall ability on the other test. Among the things which are as yet unknown are how a subject decides upon a particular coding rehearsal strategy; how potentially usable interitem relationships are detected; whether retrieval strategies or cues are also rehearsed with the to-be-remembered items and, if they are, how they are rehearsed; and how maintenance rehearsal, which may be required to hold items in immediate memory until coding can occur, shares attention with coding rehearsal processes.

The preceding description should not leave the impression that all memory research concerned with the ways in which information is stored and retrieved is really the study of rehearsal. The term *rehearsal* has as its domain active strategy decision processes and their implementation rather than the resulting codes and their utilization. At least this much restriction is necessary if the term is to be theoretically useful.

The Contribution of Rehearsal Investigation

From the variety of experimental aims of researchers investigating rehearsal emerge three types of contributions which the study of rehearsal processes may make to a general understanding of memory. First, the observation of rehearsal processes has already proven valuable in aiding in the interpretation of phenomena often seen in memory research. The following two examples illustrate this contribution. First, when a list of words is presented one-at-a-time to a subject and the subject is then asked to recall the words in any order (free recall) words which are related, for example, instances of a particular category, usually appear together in the subject's recall even if the words were not presented contiguously. One explanation of this finding assumes that the subject stores information about each item separately during study but then at recall employs a strategy which gives rise to the observed organization. An alternate explanation suggests that rehearsal allows organization of the items during study and this organization is then manifest in recall. Observing rehearsal during the study of a list has shown that as each list item is presented subjects tend to rehearse that item along with other previously presented items which are related to the new item. Thus organization does appear to be occurring during study contrary to the independent storage hypothesis. As a second example, in a free recall task in which a series of study-test trials are given using the same list of words, a priority effect for newly recalled items is observed. This priority effect refers to the fact that when words are recalled which had not been recalled on earlier trials these words tend to be recalled early in the recall protocol. One explanation of this effect proposes that the subject recognizes that the previously unrecalled items are only tenuously stored in memory and will recall them first so that they will not be lost due to interference caused by recall of previously recalled items. An alternate hypothesis suggests that the subject recognizes previously unrecalled items when they are re-presented for study and concentrates rehearsal on these items thus making

them highly available and likely to appear early in recall. When rehearsal is examined the latter hypothesis is clearly supported.

Rehearsal data may also serve as a source of theoretical insight. Inspection of rehearsal protocols illuminates the multiplicity of possible encoding schemes available to a subject and analysis of the recall resulting from particular encoding strategies may assist in discovering commonalities among various coding processes. The decision to cease rehearsal of some particular information may reflect the operation of some internal "recallability" monitoring system and examination of rehearsal data may suggest how such a system operates. When a subject chooses to rehearse two or more items together this may indicate that he has perceived a similarity among them. By analyzing such observable rehearsal decisions it may be possible to arrive at hypotheses concerning the dimensions of item similarity existing in memory. Rehearsal is an empirically analyzable manifestation of cognitive processes and as such surely has much to offer theoreticians and model builders.

Finally, rehearsal is an important part of our repertoire of mental skills and as such is worthy of examination in its own right. Rehearsal abilities, like the ability to read, develop with practice. Studies of rehearsal in children and adults suggest that children begin with minimal rehearsal strategies usually relying on simple repetition of each item as it is presented and only slowly acquire the rich variety of adult rehearsal skills. Studies of the development of rehearsal processes may isolate deficiencies (and perhaps their remedies) and suggest ways of optimizing the acquisition of efficient study techniques.

In summary, several useful procedures currently exist for the study of rehearsal and others are likely to be developed. Since its emergence as a topic of investigation, the study of rehearsal processes has proven useful in resolving empirical questions and giving direction to theory and model formulation.

BIBLIOGRAPHY

ATKINSON, R. C., and SHIFFRIN, R. M.   The control of short-term memory. *Scientific American*, 1971, *224,* 82–90.
CRAIK, F. I. M., and WATKINS, M. J.   The role of rehearsal

in short-term memory. *Journal of Verbal Learning and Verbal Behavior,* 1973, *12,* 599–607.

RUNDUS, D. Analysis of rehearsal processes in free recall. *Journal of Experimental Psychology,* 1971, *89,* 63–77.

DEWEY RUNDUS

MEMORY: STAGE MODELS AND ALTERNATIVES

It is currently fashionable in experimental psychology to regard man as a processor of information. Various psychological functions such as perception, memory, learning and thinking can be described in terms of hypothesized structures and processes whose function is to interpret the pattern of incoming stimulation, to store relevant new information and to organize appropriate responses. One valuable feature of this approach is that memory functions can be seen as part of a larger system and described in the same terms—"the flow of information through the organism," as Broadbent puts it. Although earlier hopes of information theory providing a rigorous system of measurement for human performance have not been fulfilled, the concepts of information processing still provide an extremely useful framework which researchers and practitioners can use to guide their experiments, to help formulate reasonable questions and to suggest reasons for memory failure.

Broadbent's Model

In applied studies of human performance, it is important to know the extent to which an operator can attend to two information sources at the same time. It was established in several laboratories during the 1950s that the operator could report rather little about a second source of information provided the first was sufficiently demanding. The person behaved as though the information-processing system had a central "bottleneck" which could only pass a limited amount of information in a given time. The English psychologist Donald Broadbent (1958) suggested that when there were several sources of information, one was selected by a filter mechanism prior to the central limited-capacity channel (or bottleneck). If the filter is efficient, then the person should be able to report very little about rejected sources of information and, in general, this was found to be true. However, in the case of two simultaneous auditory messages, it was found that when the messages ended, the subject was able to switch from the accepted message and also report the last few items from the rejected, or unattended, source. This result could only be obtained if the rejected message remained in a storage system prior to the filter, and this is what Broadbent suggested (see Fig. 1). In Broadbent's model, conscious perception corresponds to the item's entry into the limited-capacity channel; from there, a response could be initiated, or the item could be rehearsed by looping it back into the prefilter store. Thus, so far, Broadbent's model has two memory systems: a store for items which have not yet been fully processed or perceived, and a system whereby perceived items can be maintained in conscious perception by recycling them through the preperceptual store, the filter and the central channel. Further experimental work established that the first storage system held sensory material rather briefly (about 2 seconds in the case of auditory items) and that the second system imposed a limit on the number of items that could be recycled (about 7 or 8 digits, the "memory span"). The second system was named "short-term memory" since the material being rehearsed is rapidly lost when the limited-capacity channel is occupied by some different activity. However, both of these two systems hold material briefly, whereas plainly we can retain some items over lengthy periods regardless of whether or not we continue to keep them in conscious attention. Thus a third, "long-term" system was required, and Broadbent suggested that this long-term store was closely connected to the central channel, in that learned material was transferred from short-term to long-term storage and also, of course, items could be retrieved from long-term memory and reenter conscious awareness.

Figure 1 shows the main features of Broadbent's model as it was published in 1958. Information from the sense organs is first held briefly in a sensory storage area, if the information is selected by the filter, that is, attended to, it is passed on to conscious awareness where it may help to form a response, be recycled, or transferred to long-term memory for more permanent retention. A link is also shown between long-term memory and the filter, since presum-

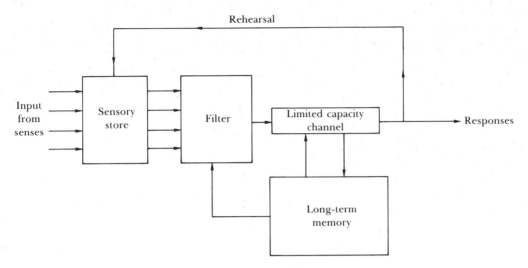

Fig. 1.   Model based on Broadbent's (1958) ideas. (Adapted from Broadbent, D. E., *Perception and Communication*, p. 299. © 1958, Pergamon Press Ltd. Reprinted with permission.)

ably the most important source of information is selected by the filter on the basis of previous experience.

Three-Store Models

The notion that the memory system could usefully be divided into three major compartments, gained wide acceptance in the 1960s. Broadbent's model was elaborated and modified by several theorists on the basis of further experimental work. In a series of experiments Sperling demonstrated a visual sensory store which held material very briefly, only 200–300 milliseconds under some circumstances. It seemed likely that each sense modality was associated with a specific storage area which held relatively "raw" unprocessed information. Thus, for verbal material, the relevant sensory store would hold the word's visual or acoustic features—the *meaning* would not be perceived until the stimulus pattern reached the limited-capacity channel and made contact with the semantic features stored in long-term memory. It was generally assumed that material was forgotten from the sensory store by a passive decay process, although presentation of additional, similar items also led to decrements. As an example of the latter point, Crowder and Morton found that the last digit in an auditorily presented string of numbers was particularly well remembered; they attributed this good performance to the fact that the last digit was still well represented in the auditory sensory store

("echoic memory"). These researchers also found that if a further auditory word was inserted after the end of the list, even the instruction "recall," performance on the last digit was markedly reduced. Thus, items in sensory memory are easily lost from the system by one means or another, unless they are "selected" by the processes of attention and thus passed on to short-term memory.

The principal features of the short-term store are its limited capacity, the suggestion that verbal items are stored in terms of their "acoustic" features and the finding that items in this store are forgotten largely by a process of active displacement. The limitation on capacity is demonstrated most simply by the fact that memory "span," the longest string of items that can be reproduced in the correct order, is quite short—only about 9 digits, 7 letters, or 5 words. Further, it has been found that short-term memory for visually presented items, though not for auditory items, is reduced if the subject is asked to carry out a second task at the same time. With regard to the "coding" of items in short-term storage, both Sperling in the United States and Conrad in Britain showed that verbal materials were apparently held in acoustic terms. If subjects were given a string of letters to recall, the errors they made typically *sounded* like the correct letter—*C* for *V, S* for *X,* and so on. This result was found even when the letters were presented visually. It was originally argued that the visual material was "recoded" into acoustic terms, but a later and more plausible suggestion was that both auditory and visual material is translated into a speech code and it is this code which is rehearsed—since the articulatory patterns of verbal items are necessarily similar to the acoustic patterns, confusions of the speech code might well appear to be acoustic in origin.

A further focus of research in short-term memory was the mechanism of forgetting. It was universally agreed that if the subject carried out a task which prevents him from rehearsing the memory items, retention drops to a very low level within 10–30 seconds. It was then of interest to determine whether the items simply decayed in the absence of rehearsal, or whether they were actively interfered with in some way by further items. The balance of the evidence is in favor of an "interference" theory although decay may play some part. As an example, Glanzer and his associates showed that the last few words of a memory list were forgotten more readily when 6, as opposed to 2, further words were interpolated between the end of the list and recall; it did not matter whether the interpolated words were presented in 2 or 6 seconds—the number of items, not the length of the interval, determined the amount of forgetting.

According to a generalized version of the three-store model, when an item is rehearsed, information about it is gradually copied or transferred into long-term storage. In this third memory system, there is no problem of capacity; despite some parents' fears that their children are "cramming their heads with nonsense" while reading comic books and thereby leaving less room for more important material, there is no evidence for a limit to human learning. If anything, the reverse is true—the more we learn about some topic, the *easier* it is to learn and retain further relevant facts. A second difference between long-term and short-term memory is that while verbal items are held in the latter system in terms of relatively superficial features (e.g., articulatory features or the *name* of the item), in long-term storage, meanings and relationships are the dominant characteristics. This does not mean that visual and auditory features cannot be held in long-term memory—our recognition of pictures, faces and voices attests to the fact that they can. By and large, however, long-term storage appears to deal with abstract semantic properties

of events rather than with their literal "surface" features. A third distinguishing characteristic of long-term memory is the forgetting function. Here we are on very speculative ground; some theorists have suggested that there is *no* forgetting from long-term memory, we fail to remember because some pieces of information become temporarily or permanently inaccessible. The problem of retrieval is particularly acute in this part of the system. At the very least, we can say that while items remain in the sensory store and short-term memory for seconds or minutes, we can retain information in long-term memory for months and years.

The general features of three-stage models were summed up in a sketch by Murdock (Figure 2), although Murdock did not himself advocate such models. While the boxes in the flow chart do represent discrete stages, they need not necessarily refer to different *structures* —they could just as well be interpreted as distinct psychological *functions*. In fact, however, three-stage models have usually been interpreted in terms of separate structural mechanisms. The model shown in Figure 2 leads to a research program whose aims are to specify the capacity, coding characteristics and forgetting functions of each store more precisely, also to work out how information is transferred from store to store. Many memory researchers were concerned with these problems during the 1960s.

Clinical studies provided a further source of evidence in favor of discrete stages in human memory. The notion of separate short-term and long-term stores would obviously be strongly supported if brain-damaged patients could be found with one store intact and the other destroyed. One such case has been described in detail by the Montreal psychologist, Brenda Milner. This patient has a normal short-term memory—he can repeat back strings of digits and carry on a conversation—but seems unable to transfer new material to long-term memory, thus can learn nothing new. More recently, a patient with the converse syndrome has been described by Warrington and Shallice; this person shows long-term memory function within the normal range, but has a specific deficit of auditory short-term memory. The finding of a deficient short-term store, yet normal learning, requires the modification to Figures 1 and 2

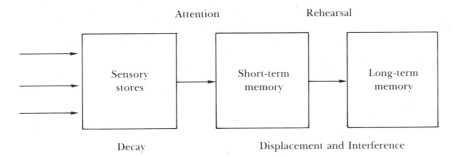

Fig. 2. A generalized three-stage model. (From Recent Developments in Short-Term Memory by B. B. Murdock, Jr. In *British Journal of Psychology*, 1967, *58*, 421–433. Printed by permission of Cambridge University Press.)

that material can sometimes be passed *directly* to the long-term store; apparently the short-term stage is not an inevitable link between perception and learning. A further piece of evidence supporting separate stages comes from experiments on amnesic patients and normal elderly subjects; both groups show impaired learning and long-term retention, but their short-term performance, measured by "span" techniques or short-term interference tasks, is unimpaired. Thus findings from various "abnormal" groups can corroborate theoretical models or force a revision of them.

Revisions of the Stage Model

One early opponent of the dichotomy between short-term and long-term stores was the American, Arthur Melton. In an influential paper published in 1963, Melton argued in favor of a "continuum" view of memory and against a series of discrete stages. He took several established phenomena from the classic verbal learning literature and demonstrated that essentially the same results were found in short-term memory experiments. For example, items in short-term memory were gradually learned; also, their retention was impaired by interfering items presented either before or after them in the experimental series. Since the same pattern of results obtained in "short-term" and "long-term" situations, why distinguish between them?

Waugh and Norman provided an answer in 1965. They suggested that Melton and most other theorists at the time had confused the notions of short-term *retention* with a postulated short-term *mechanism*. While it had been as-

sumed that items held for a few seconds or minutes were necessarily retrieved from the short-term store, Waugh and Norman suggested that information could be copied into the permanent memory system rather rapidly, while it was also maintained in the short-term stage. This means that information about an item can reside in both systems and that, even a short time after presentation, recall performance will reflect the characteristics of both stores. In this way, Waugh and Norman argued that while Melton's examples dealt with "short-term memory," in terms of the task or the retention interval, the information was being drawn in part from the long-term store and thus classic learning and interference effects were reflected in performance. Waugh and Norman's version of the stage model is shown in Figure 3. To avoid confusions with previous concepts, they termed the initial stage "primary memory" and the subsequent stage "secondary memory." Items in primary memory are consciously perceived; they may be maintained in primary memory by a process of rehearsal and this process also serves to transfer information about the items to the more commodious and permanent secondary memory system.

Probably the most sophisticated version of the discrete stage model was presented in the late 1960's by Atkinson and Shiffrin. They distinguished between the relatively "built-in," *structural* aspects of the memory system and the more flexible, optional strategies or *control processes* at the subject's command. As Figure 4 shows, information is first held in the relevant sensory register, read out into the short-term store, and finally transferred to the long-

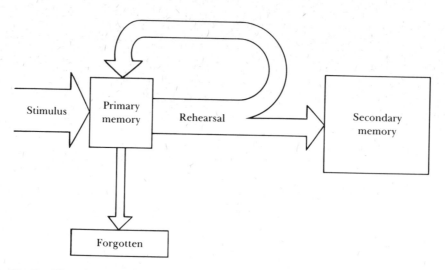

Fig. 3.   Waugh and Norman's model. (From Primary Memory by N. C. Waugh and D. A. Norman. In *Psychology Review,* 1965 (March), *72,* 89–104; © 1965 by the American Psychological Association. Reprinted by permission.)

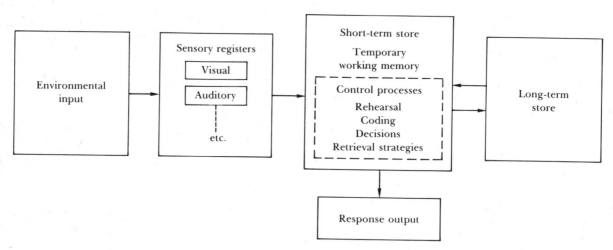

Fig. 4.   Atkinson and Shiffrin's model (1971). (From Atkinson, R. C., and Shiffrin, R. M., The Control of Short-Term Memory. Copyright © 1971 by Scientific American, Inc. All rights reserved. Reprinted by permission.)

term store. Within the short-term store the subject could set up a "rehearsal buffer," and by this means maintain three or four items. Rehearsal, as in the Waugh and Norman model, had the dual function of maintaining information in the short-term store and transferring it to long-term storage. Characteristics of the buffer and transfer functions were worked out in considerable detail. The model gives a good account of many experimental findings. For example, if a list of unrelated words is presented to the subject for recall in any order, the first few words are recalled relatively well, the mid-

dle terms poorly and the last few words are recalled best of all. According to the buffer model, the last few words are still being rehearsed and thus are well recalled. Also, the first few received relatively more rehearsals, since there were no competing words and were thus well transferred to the long-term store. In general, the short-term store with its control processes, occupies an important, pivotal position in the model, since it is here that information is transferred to long-term store, retrieved from long-term store, combined with other information and translated into responses.

Alternatives to Stage Models

Despite the success of such multistore models, the usefulness of splitting up the information flow into stages or compartments has been questioned. If the stages are distinguished on the basis of their different capacities and forgetting functions, a minimal requirement would seem to be that these distinguishing features are invariant across a variety of experimental situations. This does not appear to be the case: the estimated capacity of the short-term store varies from 2 to 20 words; also, forgetting functions for the representational aspects of visual material range from less than 1 second to well over 2 minutes (Craik and Lockhart, 1972). In the light of these empirical observations, it is extremely difficult to draw hard and fast lines between the postulated stages. An alternative viewpoint is to focus on the encoding operations themselves and to suggest that rates of forgetting are a function of the amount and qualitative nature of the processing carried out on the stimulus.

Craik and Lockhart suggested that when a stimulus enters the information-processing system it is subjected to a series of analyses, from those concerned with superficial physical features to analyses of "deeper" semantic features. Thus a continuum was envisaged, with deeper levels of analysis being concerned with the extraction of meaning. A slightly different way of expressing these ideas is to say that the encoded stimulus is progressively enriched as it is interpreted in the light of past experience. The rate of forgetting is then seen as inversely related to depth or richness—the greater the depth of analysis, the slower the forgetting. This approach implies that the memory trace is formed automatically, as a by-product of operations which are primarily concerned with perception and thought. In this model there is still a role for a separate "primary memory," but it is now seen as a functional process (as opposed to a different structure) whose role is to rehearse or maintain information about the stimulus at an intermediate level of analysis. By this view, the contents of primary memory will depend upon which features of the stimulus have been selected for rehearsal. Also, "maintenance rehearsal" of this type keeps the information at a high level of accessibility but does not lead to a stronger trace unless deeper analyses are involved. Thus, rather than partition memory into discrete sensory, short-term and long-term stores, the "levels-of-processing" model suggests that the memory trace results from the nature and depth of the initial encoding; performance reflects an interaction between the characteristics of the trace and the demands of the test.

To summarize, there has been a growing trend throughout the 1960s and 1970s to describe memory in terms of processes and operations rather than in structural terms. To return to the information-processing analogy—the present emphasis is on the programming capabilities of the mind, rather than on its "hardware" structure.

BIBLIOGRAPHY

ATKINSON, R. C., and SHIFFRIN, R. M.   The control of short-term memory. *Scientific American,* August 1971, pp. 82–90.

BROADBENT, D. E.   *Perception and communication.* New York: Pergamon, 1958.

CERMAK, L. S.   *Human memory: Research and theory.* New York: Ronald, 1972.

CRAIK, F. I. M., and LOCKHART, R. S.   Levels of processing: A framework for memory research. *Journal of Verbal Learning and Verbal Behavior,* 1972, *11,* 671–684.

MURDOCK, B. B., JR.   *Human memory: Theory and data.* New York: Halsted Press, 1974.

NORMAN, D. A.   *Memory and attention.* New York: Wiley, 1969.

FERGUS I. M. CRAIK

MEMORY AND IMAGERY

The history of imagery as an explanatory concept in memory and thought has a long and turbulent history. The main issue concerning the role of imagery in thought is whether thinking can be based on a series of mental images, which in turn hinges on the question of whether abstract concepts and relationships can be expressed as visual images. The basic question on the role of imagery in memory is whether our remembrance of things past includes mental images which bear more resemblance to raw perceptual experience than to either verbal descriptions or abstract networks of propositions.

A mental image is often defined as the experiencing of a sensation in the absence of the original stimulus; such an image could thus be visual, auditory, tactual, gustatory, or olfactory, as in remembering the visual appearance of an apple, how it sounds when bitten into, how it feels to the hand, how it tastes, or how it smells. Here we confine ourselves to visual images and visual imagery.

Imagery is used in common discourse and in psychological research to cover two kinds of activity—*remembering* the appearance of an experienced event, which results in an image of memory, and *imagining* the appearance of an unexperienced event, which results in an image of imagination. We remember the appearance of a collie that we saw jumping over a fence yesterday, and we can imagine the appearance of a dog jumping over the moon, even though we have never experienced the latter event. Images of imagination are based on objects and actions which we have seen, but which we appear to be able to manipulate into novel combinations. Both kinds of visual images are used in memory research. Images of memory are based on actual spatial-pictorial information presented by the experimenter to the subject, as when a subject is tested for recognition of a previously exposed picture, and images of imagination are generated by the subject in response to verbal materials, as when a subject is instructed to imagine a pair of words in an interacting relationship in a paired-associate learning task.

Few psychologists today believe that all ideas are concretized as mental images or that all information that we store about the world is represented as mental images. The alternative to the strict imagist position has traditionally been the verbal-linguistic view: that thought and memory are based on the verbal-linguistic system, so that thought is formed in language, and memory is based on verbal descriptions. Neither the strict imagist nor the strict verbal position seems tenable either on the basis of introspection or on the basis of current experimental evidence. The two most prevalent views of how knowledge is represented in memory are the *dual-coding* position and the *conceptual-propositional* position.

The dual-coding hypothesis, most vigorously espoused by Paivio (1971), holds that there are two memory systems, the visual-spatial system and the verbal-symbolic system. These two systems are differentiated by neural locus and by differential specialization for different tasks.

However, the two systems are richly interconnected, and many types of material may be encoded into both systems. For example, a subject attempting to remember a concrete word may store both the word itself and its visual image. Conversely, a subject shown a simple picture of a namable object may store both the memory image of the picture and its name. On the other hand, there may be some verbal material which is so abstract that it is only encoded into the verbal system, and there may be some visual material, such as faces of strangers and abstract paintings, which is so indescribable that it is only encoded into the visual system.

The conceptual-propositional view questions the assumption that the visual and verbal memory systems are qualitatively different (Anderson and Bower, 1973; Pylyshyn, 1973). The major instigation for this position has been the development of computer simulation programs to mimic various human performances, including those which are usually thought to require mental imagery and imagined spatial movement for their solution. Such programs do not store information about the world in either visual or verbal terms, but rather in terms of abstract propositions and relationships. Since such programs are often adequate simulations of human performance, the conceptualists argue that human knowledge about the world, including memories about things seen and heard, might also be stored in such an abstract form. Thus, in their view, knowledge obtained from a visual representation and that obtained from a linguistic representation are stored in the same way in memory, as a system of abstract propositions and relationships. The conceptualists do not deny the introspective reality of mental imagery, or of verbal thinking, but simply regard them as epiphenomena which do not in themselves constitute evidence for two types of memory storage.

Ever since the behavioristic revolution, psychologists have been wary of using the results of introspection as evidence for psychological processes, although they have not hesitated to use them as a guide to research. In that tradition, we turn to experimental evidence on imagery variables in memory. These constitute two areas of research: (1) empirical evidence for the superiority of imagery over nonimagery in memory, and (2) evidence on the degree to which the visual image is similar to a perceptual event.

Superiority of Imagery in Memory

Two types of imagery-related variables have been manipulated experimentally: variables related to stimulus materials, and variables designed to manipulate subjects' encoding strategies.

Stimulus variables have been manipulated by using pictorial representations of objects, names of those objects (concrete words), and names of abstract concepts (abstract words). When pictures are used as stimuli, the experimenter provides the subject with a prefabricated memory image, and when concrete words are used, the subject generates his own visual image. For a wide variety of paradigms, including item recognition, item recall (in which the name of the picture is the recall response), and paired associate recall, memory performance progressively increases as the concreteness of the stimulus increases; from abstract words, concrete words, line drawings of objects, photographs of objects, to the objects themselves.

The dual coding hypothesis accounts for these results by assuming that pictorial materials are most efficient in arousing a pictorial code, concrete words are less efficient, and abstract words least efficient. Because pictures and concrete words are more likely to be dually coded, and perhaps because the visual code is stronger or less subject to interference than the verbal code, pictures and concrete words are remembered better than abstract words. The conceptual hypothesis accounts for these results by assuming that a picture generates more spatial predicates than its word referent.

The dual-coding hypothesis has received rather direct support from a study of types of confusions in recognition memory (Snodgrass, Wasser, Finkelstein, and Goldberg, 1974). Subjects learning a set of concrete words and simple pictures found it more difficult to distinguish an old picture from its new corresponding word than vice versa. That is, they made more errors in choosing between the previously seen picture "hand" and its verbal label which had not previously been exposed, than in choosing between the previously seen verbal label and the new picture, despite the fact that

picture memory was generally superior. These results were interpreted as indicating that dual codes were generated to both types of stimuli. However, verbal codes of old pictures were more likely to match the picture's name than visual codes of old words were to match the name's picture, since there are more ways to image a word than to name a picture.

Encoding strategies have been manipulated by explicit instructions to subjects to form visual images of words or word pairs, either in single-item situations or in serial-list learning situations. Instructions to image have been used more often, and more successfully, in the paired-associate paradigm than in the single-item recall or recognition paradigm. Instructions to form interacting images of the referents of pairs of words in the paired-associate learning task improves memory performance. Initially it was thought that the use of bizarre as well as interacting images was crucial, but evidence indicates that bizarreness of images is not an important variable. Evidence that imagery instructions improve performance in single-item recall or recognition has been equivocal, perhaps because subjects often form images of concrete words spontaneously (Paivio, 1971).

The most striking improvement in memory by imagery training occurs in the serial recall situation. The Greek orators introduced the "method of loci" as a memory aid, in which prominent locations in the oratory hall were picked as "pegs" on which to hang key points in the speech. Luria's study of the mnemonist "S" revealed that "S" employed the method of loci, pegging his to-be-remembered stimuli on locations along a familiar street. Another well-known technique is the "one-bun" method, in which subjects learn rhyming concrete words to the first few digits, and then associate, by imagery, items on a to-be-learned list to each of the peg words associated with each of the digits.

These empirical data show that visual memory images, whether provided by the experimenter in the form of pictures or generated by the subject to words or word-pairs provide a powerful alternative to the verbal-associative-semantic system of verbal encoding. The question remains, however, whether the imaginal encoding system is qualitatively different from the verbal encoding system. Clearly, the visual system is different from the auditory system, so that the question is whether, and to what extent, the visual image partakes of the spatial-parallel properties of visual pictures, and whether, and to what extent, visual imaging is like visual perception.

Is the Picture in the Mind's Eye Like the Picture in the Brain's Eye?

If a visual memory image is like a perceptual image, then we might expect the visual image to have some, if not all, of the following properties: (1) it can be scanned; (2) it cannot be distinguished from a weak perception; (3) the process of imaging will disrupt the process of perceiving; (4) similarity of visual images will act in the same way as similarity of visual perceptions; and (5) visual images will function differently from verbal symbolic codes.

Scanning Visual Images

Whether memory images can be scanned is one of the oldest questions in the history of experimental psychology. It has long been known that subjects find it difficult to spell an imagined word backwards, although this poses no problem when the word is present. One of the oldest tests of visual memory is the letter square; subjects learn a square of letters, and then are asked to read them off in columns or diagonally. This posed a problem for all subjects, even those who claimed good visual imagery. Thus scanning a visual image is much more difficult than scanning a visual stimulus.

Distinguishing Visual Images from Weak Perceptions

If images are somehow like perceptions, then subjects should have difficulty distinguishing the two. In a classic study, Perky (1910) instructed subjects to image specific objects and then surreptitiously showed them weak projections of the same objects while they were imaging. No subject reported being aware of any external stimulus, even though their reported images were obviously influenced by the weak stimuli in that they resembled them in color, orientation, and so on. This result, which has been replicated, suggests that images and weak stimuli share many of the same characteristics,

and under some conditions cannot be distinguished.

Shared Neural Pathways

If imaging is somehow like perceiving, then imaging in a particular modality should affect the ability to perceive in that modality, and conversely, perceiving in one modality should interfere with imaging in that modality.

Segal and her students (1971) have found that imaging in one modality affects signal detection in that modality more than detection in another. Thus, imaging a visual stimulus interferes more with visual signal detection than with auditory signal detection, and vice versa.

Interference in the opposite direction has been studied by several investigators. Brooks (1968) has shown that performing a task which presumably involves visual memory, for instance, categorizing the corners of block letters according to whether they are extremes or not, is slowed significantly by requiring a visual pointing response rather than a vocal response, whereas categorizing each word of a sentence according to whether it is a noun or nonnoun, a linguistic-verbal task, is slowed more by requiring a vocal response than a pointing response. Thus, the type of memory task—visual versus verbal—and the type of output response—pointing versus vocal—interacted in such a way as to suggest competition between memory and response modalities.

Similarly, Atwood (1971) has shown that having to process visually-presented stimuli interferes with memory for high imagery associates, whereas processing the same stimuli delivered in an auditory mode interferes less. Conversely, memory for abstract paired-associate pairs, which are presumably handled by the verbal-auditory system, are interfered with more by the auditorially than by the visually presented stimuli.

These results taken together suggest that imaginal processes share some of the same neural pathways as perceptual process, thereby supporting the notion that imaging and perceiving are similar sorts of activities.

Similarity of Visual Images

A fourth area of research which studies parallels between visual imagery and visual perception compares similarity as measured by ratings or reaction time between pairs of visual images and pairs of visual stimuli.

Similarity ratings of shapes of the various states of the United States show the same pattern regardless of whether subjects are making judgments on pairs of physically present state shapes, or whether they are making judgments based on the names of such states (Bower, 1972). Presumably, when names of states are presented, the subject transforms the names into visual memory images of their shapes, and compares the imagined shapes, much as he might the physically present shapes.

Similar results have been obtained with judgments of object size, using reaction time as the dependent variable. When subjects must choose which of two physically present stimuli has more of some characteristic, such as length, brightness, or size, time to choose the greater stimulus decreases as the difference between the pair of stimuli increases. Thus, reaction time to discriminate two stimuli can be used as a barometer to determine the modality of comparison. In several experiments, subjects were presented with pairs of animal names and the time to choose the name of the larger animal was measured. Reaction times decreased as size differences between the physical sizes of the animals increased; thus, the reaction time to choose elephant was smaller for the pair "elephant–mouse" than for the pair "elephant–lion." Paivio (1974) has argued on the basis of these data that subjects were converting words to images, and basing their decisions on object size as somehow represented in the visual image. Further support for this inference is provided by experiments using pictures of animals rather than names; a similar function between rated size difference and reaction time was obtained, and the picture pairs produced faster reaction times than the word pairs, presumably because the extra step required to convert words to images had been eliminated.

Functional Differences Between Visual and Verbal Codes

If there are at least two codes in memory, one might expect them to show functional differences. Several differences between the two systems have been proposed. One is that visual codes are specialized for parallel-spatial processing, whereas verbal codes, depending as they do on the linguistic system, are specialized for sequential-temporal processing. Some evidence for the superiority of verbal codes over visual codes in maintaining serial order has been found for recall experiments, although the results for recognition of temporal and spatial order have been equivocal. A second difference, at least for complex visual material, has been the lack of serial position effects in recognition, and the lack of an interstimulus interval effect, suggesting that complex pictures, unlike words, cannot be rehearsed. Finally, there is the large literature on hemispheric effects in storage and manipulation of language and spatial relations. Evidence from both brain-damaged patients and from normal subjects suggest that one hemisphere, the left in right-handed subjects, is specialized for verbal-linguistic functions, whereas the other hemisphere is specialized for visual-spatial relationships.

A final source of experimental evidence for the perceptual-spatial character of visual memory images is the mental rotation paradigm first introduced by Shepard and Metzler (1971). In their paradigm, subjects were presented successive pairs of visual displays of three-dimensional figures, and asked to indicate whether the second figure was the same as or different from the first. Reaction times to same figures rotated by various numbers of degrees showed a linear increase with degree of rotation, suggesting that subjects performed mental rotation on the mental image of the first figure to determine if it was identical to the second.

The mental rotation results pose perhaps the most difficult problem for the conceptualist position. However, final resolution of the question whether there are two or more distinct memory systems awaits future theory and research.

BIBLIOGRAPHY

Anderson, J. R., and Bower, G. H. *Human associative memory.* Washington, D.C.: Winston, 1973.

Atwood, G. An experimental study of visual imagination and memory. *Cognitive Psychology,* 1971, *2,* 290–299.

Bower, G. H. Mental imagery and associative learning. In L. W. Gregg (Ed.), *Cognition in learning and memory.* New York: Wiley, 1972.

Brooks, L. R. Spatial and verbal components of the act of recall. *Canadian Journal of Psychology,* 1968, *22,* 349–368.

PAIVIO, A. *Imagery and verbal processes.* New York: Holt, Rinehart and Winston, 1971.

PAIVIO, A. Images, propositions, and knowledge. Paper presented at the Interdisciplinary Workshop on Images, Perception, and Knowledge, University of Western Ontario, May 9–12, 1974.

PERKY, C. W. An experimental study of imagination. *American Journal of Psychology,* 1910, *21,* 422–452.

PYLYSHYN, Z. W. What the mind's eye tells the mind's brain: A critique of mental imagery. *Psychological Bulletin,* 1973, *80,* 1–24.

SEGAL, S. J. Processing of the stimulus in imagery and perception. (Chap. 5). In S. J. Segal (Ed.), *Imagery: Current cognitive approaches.* New York: Academic Press, 1971.

SHEPARD, R. N., and METZLER, J. Mental rotation of three-dimensional objects. *Science,* 1971, *171,* 701–703.

SNODGRASS, J. G.; WASSER, B.; FINKELSTEIN, M.; and GOLDBERG, L. B. On the fate of visual and verbal memory codes for pictures and words: Evidence for a dual coding mechanism in recognition memory. *Journal of Verbal Learning and Verbal Behavior,* 1974, *13,* 27–37.

JOAN GAY SNODGRASS

MENNINGER, KARL AUGUSTUS (b. 1893)

Karl Augustus Menninger completed medical school cum laude at Harvard University in 1917. While an intern at Kansas City General Hospital, he became interested in neurology and psychiatry. He went to Boston Psychopathic Hospital, where Elmer Ernest Southard was superintendent, to continue his work. Menninger credits Southard, who urged him to return to his native Midwest to pursue his career, as the inspiration that led him to become a researcher, author, and teacher in his chosen field.

Returning to Kansas in 1919, he set up practice with his father, Charles F., already established as a physician in Topeka. In 1925, they were joined by his youngest brother, William C. The Menninger Clinic, a group of practicing physicians, and the Menninger Psychiatric Hospital, based entirely on psychoanalytic principles, were organized. In 1944, the Menninger family reorganized their enterprises into the nonprofit Menninger Foundation in order to expand its programs of education, research and prevention.

Although psychiatry was little known Menninger realized that people had an innate longing and need for its benefits. *The Human Mind,* published in 1930, was his first effort to explain psychiatry to the laity, and it promptly became a best seller. This book leaned on Freud's concepts, as did his next one, *Man Against Himself* (1938), focusing on destructiveness. He then turned to the constructive drive in *Love Against Hate* (1942).

Menninger was one of the first physicians in the United States to complete psychoanalytic training, holding certificate number 1 from the Chicago Institute for Psychoanalysis. He cofounded and was the first director of the Topeka Institute for Psychoanalysis in 1942, then the only institute west of the Mississippi River. He has served as president of the American Psychoanalytic Association. He, with others, founded the American Orthopsychiatric Association and the Central Neuropsychiatric Association. He has served the American Psychiatric Association as counselor, chairman of the Committee on Legal Aspects of Psychiatry, and as a member of its Reorganization Committee.

Karl Menninger, aware that the need for psychiatrically trained personnel was critical, conceived the idea for the Menninger School of Psychiatry in 1945. In 1946 the Veterans Administration asked the Menninger Foundation for assistance in training psychiatrists and Menninger became the manager of the Winter Veterans Administration Hospital in Topeka, establishing it as a pilot teaching hospital. In 1948 he became the chief consultant to the Kansas state hospital system. In both posts he became a reformer and teacher, noted for his dedication to the interdisciplinary team concept in psychiatry. In his role as educator of psychiatric professionals, he wrote *A Guide to Psychiatric Books* and *A Manual for Psychiatric Case Study.*

Menninger's theoretical views are at once philosophical and clinically detailed. They reflect the influence of Freud and Adolf Meyer, as well as Southard. His *Theory of Psychoanalytic Technique* (1958) examined the psychodynamic processes in psychoanalytic practice. In *The Vital Balance* (1963), he offered a new diagnostic understanding in the perspective of a unitary concept of mental health and illness, after a gigantic review of historical nosologies and classification systems.

Menninger's *The Crime of Punishment* (1960) describes the "sins" of the public against criminals, exuding a reformer's zeal for overhauling the penal system. In the ensuing years, his work has focused increasingly on the broader social problems of mistreatment among human beings. *Whatever Became of Sin?* (1973) deals with individual and collective sin, expressing his belief that mental health and moral health are identical, and that there is hope of preventing destruction.

The establishment of The Villages, Inc. in 1966 to provide a permanent home for homeless, neglected, and abandoned children, sums up much of Karl Menninger's life work. Like his lifetime efforts at conservation, his work as a naturalist, and his advocacy of oppressed and neglected groups such as American Indians, this project is attuned to hope and love and compassion, prevention of waste and destruction, and conservation of resources.

Karl Menninger is the Chairman of the Board of Trustees of the Menninger Foundation, spending much of his time in consulting and educative work with government agencies, a variety of schools and other organizations across the country. He continues to live in Topeka, Kansas.

VERNE B. HORNE

MENNINGER, WILLIAM C. (1899–1966)

William Claire Menninger was born in Topeka, Kansas, October 15, 1899. He received an A.B. degree from Washburn University in 1919, an M.A. in zoology from Columbia University, New York, in 1922, and an M.D. from Cornell University Medical College, New York, in 1924. He subsequently received honorary degrees from six other institutions.

With a strong interest in general medicine, he returned to Topeka in 1925 to join the Menninger Clinic, established with his father, Dr. C. F., and his elder brother, Dr. Karl Menninger. He gained psychiatric experience in 1927 at St. Elizabeths Hospital, Washington, D.C.; and in the early 1930s, he received training at the Chicago Institute for Psychoanalysis.

As director of the Menninger Hospital, he applied his psychoanalytic understanding to psychiatric hospital treatment and developed a concept of milieu treatment that was unique at the time. The C. F. Menninger Memorial Hospital has retained the psychoanalytic emphasis that he and Karl Menninger initiated.

During World War II, Colonel and later Brigadier General Menninger was named chief neuropsychiatric consultant to the Surgeon General of the Army. In this capacity, he increased the numbers and quality of psychiatrists in the Army, substantially improving psychiatric treatment in all phases of Army operations. He undertook a revision of the psychiatric nomenclature, which was adopted by the Navy and Veterans' Administration as well as the Army, and which also served as the basis for further revision by the American Psychiatric Association. He was instrumental in achieving parity for psychiatry as a distinct medical specialty with medicine and surgery in the Army. Menninger summarized his military experience in *Psychiatry in a Troubled World* (1948), to document the lessons psychiatry learned during the war. For his contributions to military psychiatry, he was awarded the Distinguished Service Medal (1946) and the French Legion of Honor (1948).

Aware of the need for more progressive views in American psychiatry, he spearheaded a group of fellow psychiatrists who organized the Group for the Advancement of Psychiatry (1946), and he became its first chairman (1946–1951). In recognition of his leadership in psychiatry, he was elected president of the American Psychoanalytic Association, American Psychiatric Association and Central Neuropsychiatric Association in the same year (1948). Maintaining his liaison with general medicine, he was long active in the American College of Physicians serving as governor for Kansas (1949–1958), chairman of the Board of Governors (1957–1958), member of the Board of Regents (1958–1963), and first vice-president (1964).

He became increasingly convinced that psychiatric knowledge could and should contribute substantially to the general welfare. At the Menninger Foundation, he initiated seminars on human motivation and behavior for industrial and governmental executives. He championed the cause of the institutionalized mentally ill; in response to invitations in the 1950s, he challenged federal and state governmental agencies to improve the treatment of the mentally ill. Addressing legislators in 27 states, he stressed the priority of providing trained personnel before building new hospital structures, "Brain before Bricks."

In 1957, Menninger was elected president of the Menninger Foundation, a nonprofit institution dedicated to treatment, education, research and prevention of mental illness. In 1962, he received the Gold Medal of the National Institute of Social Sciences for "distinguished service to humanity."

He died September 6, 1966, of pulmonary carcinoma.

ROY W. MENNINGER

MENNINGER FOUNDATION

The Menninger Foundation is known primarily as a psychiatric, diagnostic, and treatment center with highly diversified inpatient and outpatient facilities, but to many segments of society it is known as a center where efforts are made to apply what has been learned about human behavior to other settings.

Educators in the mental health profession know the Menninger Foundation as a training center of some renown for its emphasis on the joint education of psychiatrists, psychoanalysts, psychologists, social workers, clergy, nurses, and others. Lawyers and judges know its staff not only as expert witnesses in clinical cases but as advisors to courts, penal institutions, and police departments. Its staff and students practice in and consult with public schools (from nursery school to college levels), juvenile homes, churches, welfare agencies, retirement homes, and rehabilitation centers. The scientific community knows the Menninger Foundation for its extensive involvement with research and for research done elsewhere by people who have received a substantial part of their training there, or began their research careers in projects sponsored by the Foundation (including such outstanding scientists as David Rapaport, George Klein, Gardner Murphy, Lois Murphy, Sibylle Escalona, Roy Schafer, Riley Gardner, and Robert Wallerstein).

Over 50 years the Menninger Foundation has developed from a group practice by physician members of the Menninger family, specializing early in psychiatry, pioneering in the application of psychoanalytic principles beyond the reaches of the private office and couch, to become a nonprofit organization. In the 1940s

the Menninger Foundation formed a psychiatric training program. Today the professional staff numbers 72 psychiatrists, 6 neurologists and neurosurgeons, 3 internists, 39 psychologists, 27 psychoanalysts, 45 social workers and one social scientist. The staff includes scientists with specializations in child and adult psychiatry, psychoanalysis, psychophysiology, developmental psychology, perceptual psychology, social psychology, psychopharmacology, ethology, cultural anthropology, behavior measurement theory, and statistics. Nearly all investigators and scholars at the Menninger Foundation are involved in multidisciplinary team work with another or a group of colleagues practicing in the field of mental health service. The result is a unique atmosphere particularly hospitable for multidisciplinary work.

The Menninger Foundation traces its beginnings to 1889 when Dr. Charles F. Menninger began a general medical practice in Topeka, Kansas. As his practice developed, he sought to overcome the isolation of the general medical practitioner by establishing a working relationship with colleagues so there could be an environment of mutual encouragement and learning by sharing experiences. His answer was to establish a group practice with his sons, patterned after the Mayo practice in Minnesota.

In the summer of 1919, C. F. Menninger's oldest son, Karl, returned from Harvard Medical School and he and his father attempted to interest other doctors in joining a cooperative medical effort in Topeka. Although the plan was rejected, the following spring the Menningers took two young Topeka physicians into the family practice and complete diagnostic laboratories were set up in the office of the group. The practice was known as the Menninger Diagnostic Clinic.

At the time, the clinic was envisioned as one of general medicine, but Karl Menninger's interest was in psychiatry. His psychiatric patients were first treated in a local hospital but when alarmed citizens obtained a court injunction barring the creation of a "maniac ward," Menninger smuggled his psychiatric patients into the hospital through disguised diagnoses.

In 1925, the year C. F. Menninger's youngest son, Will, joined the family practice, a subscription drive was launched to establish a small mental hospital. Topeka businessmen and physicians were encouraged to buy stock in the project and the Menninger Sanitarium and Psychopathic Hospital was established in a farm house on 40 acres of land on the western edge of Topeka. The 13-bed facility was half-filled the first day with psychiatric patients transferred from their sub-rosa quarters in a local hospital.

The initial contribution of the Menninger family to the psychiatric profession was simply the idea of gathering a group of medical colleagues to practice together. The opening of a psychiatric clinic in the 1920s occurred at a time when the public attitude toward mental illness was indifferent at best and negative at worst. Mentally ill people were looked upon as pariahs, relegated to isolated buildings and forgotten. From the outset the Menninger hospital was a radical statement to the contrary: that psychiatric patients are treatable and can get better.

The Menningers joined two concepts: the *psychoanalytic* understanding of behavior and the concept of using the *milieu,* the environment, as part of the treatment process. Psychoanalytic theory had not previously been applied to the treatment of hospital patients. The Menningers applied psychoanalytic understanding to the more seriously disturbed people who sought help and needed hospitalization. To this was added the intentional use of the environment, enlisting the attention and help of not only the nurses but also the aides, the recreational, art, and music therapists, even the housekeeping staff, as well as the mental health professionals. From this experience comprehensive concepts about the social environment of the patient emerged.

There have been other notable achievements as well, such as the development of one of the first day hospitals in the late 1930s. An unusual aspect of this setting has been the central clinical role played by psychologists almost from the beginning. Under the tutelage of David Rapaport and later Gardner Murphy the psychologists on the staff made significant contributions to the diagnostic testing process.

In 1926 the Southard school for mentally retarded children (which later became a facility for children with all types of psychiatric conditions) was opened. In 1931 the Menninger Sanitarium was the first institution to be approved for training psychiatric nurses. In 1933 the sanitarium initiated a residency program in neuropsychiatry for physicians specializing in psychiatry. The Topeka Psychoanalytic Society was established in 1938 and the Topeka Institute of Psychoanalysis was formed in 1942. In 1941 a nonprofit Menninger Foundation for psychiatric education and research through which funds could be raised for educational research programs was established, and by 1945 the Menninger Foundation was expanded to become the umbrella organization for the clinic, the sanitarium and the school for children.

Public Involvement

Outside the clinical setting, Karl and Will Menninger worked to gain public acceptance of psychiatry.

In 1930, Karl Menninger's first book, *The Human Mind,* was published; it helped establish public acceptance of psychiatry as a legitimate science. His book argued that the forces which motivate ill people are not so different from those which motivate all human beings, that the difference is one of degree, not kind.

During World War II, Will Menninger was brigadier general in charge of the Army's neuropsychiatric program. He demonstrated that psychiatry could add to the understanding of groups, maintenance of morale, and the nature of leadership. Psychiatry soon achieved status equal to surgery in the Army.

When the war ended, Will Menninger emerged as a leading public spokesman for long overdue reforms in civilian hospitals. Concurrently, Karl Menninger was crusading for reforms in psychiatric hospitals. Part of the Menninger solution to mental health care was to train additional psychiatrists.

In 1945, the Menninger Foundation's School of Psychiatry was formed. In 1946, Karl was hired by the Veterans Administration to manage the Winter General Hospital in Topeka and to establish a psychiatric residency training program. Using the Menninger School of Psychiatry as a base, Karl, in his 30 months as manager, assembled a teaching faculty, many of whom were Foundation staff members, and developed a broad curriculum.

In 1948, Karl Menninger was appointed by Kansas Governor Frank Carlson to the Committee for the State Mental Hospitals. The committee recommended that the Menninger Foundation assume responsibility for reforming the state mental hospital systems. A state system of psychiatric training was established. Today, residents in the Menninger School of Psychiatry are assigned to the Topeka State Hospital, the Veterans Administration Hospital, the C. F. Menninger Memorial Hospital, and numerous other community agencies and institutions. Alumni of the Menninger School of Psychiatry are practicing in 43 states, the District of Columbia, and 22 other countries.

In the last two decades the Menninger Foundation has emphasized its programs to prevent mental illness by sharing psychiatric information with people outside the foundation. Initial work began in 1949 in four primary areas: mental health in industry, law and psychiatry, marriage counseling, and religion and psychiatry. These programs continue today within the Department of Preventive Psychiatry and the Department of Education.

In 1974, the foundation's work with industry expanded with creation of a new division, the Center for Applied Behavioral Sciences. The center conducts approximately 50 seminars a year for businessmen, physicians, management personnel, government executives, and others; the seminar alumni number approximately 4,000. The seminar, entitled "Toward Understanding Human Behavior and Motivation," is basic to the nature of human psychology and therefore applicable to persons from widely varying occupations. Seminar issues such as personal value systems, self-perceptions, objectives and goals, and managing a variety of human feelings are significant to everyone. The center also is involved in consulting with businesses and executives on a variety of industrial problems ranging from conflict management to alcoholism policies, to individual life assessment programs for executives.

In the history of the Menninger Foundation, the concern of the 1920s was diagnosis, followed by an emphasis in the 1930s and 1940s on treatment as new methods, especially psychoanalytic knowledge became available. Then in the subsequent two decades, the 1950s and 1960s, education was the major focus with the beginning of The Menninger School of Psychiatry. As each preceding focus consolidated

its initial growth, it became a platform on which the next phase was launched.

ROY W. MENNINGER

MENTAL HEALTH: ISSUES AND PROGRAMS

AGING: MENTAL HEALTH PROGRAMS

ASIA: MENTAL HEALTH AND PSYCHIATRY

HEALTH SERVICE PROVIDERS IN PSYCHOLOGY: THE NATIONAL REGISTER

INDUSTRIAL MENTAL HEALTH

INTEGRATION OF MENTAL HEALTH IN PUBLIC HEALTH PROGRAMS

MENTAL HEALTH: PSYCHOLOGISTS AS MENTAL HEALTH SERVICE PROVIDERS

MENTAL HEALTH ADMINISTRATION: PSYCHOLOGISTS AS ADMINISTRATORS

MENTAL HEALTH IN THE SCHOOLS

MENTAL HEALTH AND SOCIAL PSYCHOLOGY

NATIONAL INSTITUTE OF MENTAL HEALTH

NORMALITY: THE CONCEPT OF MENTAL HEALTH

SOCIAL SYSTEMS AND HEALTH

SOCIOECONOMIC STATUS AND MENTAL DISORDERS

MENTAL HEALTH: PSYCHOLOGISTS AS MENTAL HEALTH SERVICE PROVIDERS

Psychologists provide direct health services in many settings: state hospitals, Veterans Administration hospitals, private psychiatric hospitals, general hospitals, comprehensive mental health centers, mental hygiene clinics, rehabilitation facilities, schools, facilities for the mentally retarded, long-term care facilities, counseling centers, industrial programs, alcohol and drug abuse treatment centers, developmental disabilities facilities, head start programs, private practice, health maintenance organizations and other prepaid plans (federations), correctional facilities, medical schools, and a variety of other facilities.

In those settings in which the psychologist is reimbursed by a salary or on a fee for service basis, qualified psychologists are now recognized as independent and autonomous health service providers. It is only when third parties pay for health services that full recognition is not yet complete.

The major breakthrough in third party reimbursement for services of licensed or certified psychologists occurred in 1970 when the Department of Defense authorized CHAMPUS (Civilian Health and Medical Program of the Uniformed Services) to pay for professional health care provided to dependents of military personnel and retired armed services personnel and their dependents by qualified psychologists without referral or supervision by physicians. In 1973 CHAMPVA (Civilian Health and Medical Program of the Veterans Administration) followed with similar recognition for services provided to dependents of totally disabled veterans.

The Rehabilitation Act of 1973 (PL 93–112) recognized the qualified psychologist as one who could diagnose and treat mental disorders as an independent practitioner. This was the first instance of federal legislation recognizing professional psychologists for third party reimbursement.

Clinical psychologists were recognized as independent and autonomous practitioners in all insurance policies in the Federal Employees Health Benefits Program in PL 93–363. Although Aetna Insurance had reimbursed qualified psychologists before this legislation was passed, Blue Cross and Blue Shield had required referral and supervision by a physician. The law removed this requirement, so that beginning in January, 1975 federal employees and their dependents in the Federal Employees Health Benefits program carrying a policy with Blue Cross and Blue Shield have had the freedom to choose a practitioner.

At the state level, 18 states covering well over 50% of the population of the United States have enacted freedom-of-choice legislation which prohibits insurance carriers from restricting the provision of mental health services to physicians; insurance carriers must reimburse for services of that state's licensed or certified psychologists without requiring referral or supervision by a physician.

In the Medicaid program, which is a state operated health program for the medically and categorically needy, 12 states reimburse psychologists licensed or certified in their state for health services provided.

The Work Injuries Compensation Act (PL 93–

416) covering federal employees also recognized the clinical psychologist as an independent provider of health services.

In prepaid health plans, psychologists are participating as independent practitioners such as in the San Joaquin Foundation plan.

The federal regulations of the Health Maintenance Organization Act (PL 93–222) recognize clinical psychologists as health practitioners and therefore eligible to become participating members of the organization.

Disappearance of resistance to third party reimbursement for services of qualified psychologists seems to accompany these steps toward full recognition of the qualified psychologist as an independent and autonomous health service provider.

ARTHUR CENTOR

MENTAL HEALTH ADMINISTRATION: PSYCHOLOGISTS AS ADMINISTRATORS

The expansion of professional psychological functioning beyond its traditional roles of psychodiagnosis, psychotherapies, and research has taken a quantum leap in the past decade. The professional psychologist now finds himself being called upon to undertake tasks in the human services field for which very few universities or graduate schools have adequately prepared him through formal curricula or field experience. One such area includes the field of mental health administration.

Due to vast organizational changes in mental health delivery systems brought about through federal and state legislation in the 1960s, there became available to professional psychologists for the first time an opportunity to play key roles in the mental health administrative arena. The forerunner of this organizational change was the report of the Joint Commission on Mental Illness and Health, which was established in 1955 during the Eisenhower administration. In 1961, the commission's final report *(Action for Mental Health)* urged a movement away from custodial care in large impersonal institutions for the mentally ill and a strengthening of community mental health programs in geographic areas of 200,000 population or less. The report also recognized that manpower problems would preclude all the administrative roles in the community mental health movement being occupied by psychiatrists or physicians and suggested that nonmedical professional mental health experts be recruited to fill some of these administrative posts as they were established.

In 1963 the basic concepts of the Joint Commission's report were translated into Federal law in the Community Mental Health Centers Construction Act of 1963, followed in 1965 with the Community Mental Health Centers Staffing Act. Under these federal acts monies were allocated to each state to plan for its reorganization in the delivery of mental health services in order to be eligible for these funds. Many states passed laws making psychologists (among other nonmedical professionals) eligible to fill top level administrative posts in institutions, clinics, area, regional, and central offices of the Department of Mental Health. In Massachusetts, for example, psychologists may now compete for administrative posts ranging up to and including the commissioner's position. Salary differentials between nonmedical and medical administrators are gradually being abolished and the "quality principle" rather than the "discipline principle" is being applied.

One might well ask what there is in the background and training of a professional psychologist which would equip him to function successfully in the administrator's role (as opposed to, say, a hospital administrator or management analyst). A professional psychologist possesses at least three qualities which facilitate successful functioning in the administrator's role: (1) an ordered concept of normal as well as abnormal human behavior, (2) an understanding of dyadic relationships, (3) a proclivity toward objective assessment of mental health administrative issues and crises.

Since a primary portion of the mental health administrator's role is devoted to planning effective ways of promoting positive mental health and preventing or ameliorating mental illness an understanding of human behavior and of aberrations of that behavior is vital in the planning process. The traditional psychiatrist focuses upon abnormal aspects of behavior; the hospital administrator emphasizes organizational arrangement for effective service delivery; the management analyst promotes

cost effectiveness. While the psychologist-administrator has to take account of all these processes, he is helped by his background also to determine priorities and to try to find a place for programs emphasizing prevention of emotional illness as well as programs for ameliorating it.

The psychologist-administrator is required to interact with a wide variety of individuals in the performance of his duty ranging among citizen groups, politicians, other mental health professionals, and so on. It is frequently of inestimable value to be able to understand the dynamics, the motivations, the aspirations, and the goals of these individuals. While most of them genuinely wish to better the lot of the mentally handicapped, their personalities, life styles, personal experiences, and needs often influence their actions and effectiveness. The psychologist can react more effectively in his dealings with these persons if he applies his psychological understanding to what makes them tick. This is not to say that he "psychoanalyzes" them or "reads their mind" in the lay understanding of these terms; rather, he can respond more effectively to their needs by his understanding of the dynamics of their behavior.

With his background in research and objective methods the psychologist-administrator is in a position to view administrative issues and crises from many angles and to make objective assessments before embarking upon a course of action. Anyone with experience in the research method knows that "things are not always what they seem." In dealing with administrative crises, the same maxim frequently obtains. By garnering data from a variety of sources and checking their validity and reliability, the psychologist-administrator is in a position to make decisions which are not as likely to backfire on him.

The one pitfall which psychologist-administrators must learn to avoid, however, is what Hirshowitz (1971) calls the "clinician-executive" dilemma in which a clinical stance which serves the psychologist well in a medical or psychological setting becomes a crippling bind for planning and executive functions. A psychologist who practices an analytic or nondirective approach to clinical situations may find himself at a loss when placed in an administrative role which requires decisive political responses, direct actions, and negotiation with community agencies. The administrator, says Hirshowitz, is more than a reactor: he is a proactor, a transactor and an interactor and must accommodate his psychological background to this reality.

Rosenblum (1975) identified 17 distinguishable roles which had to be learned by him over a span of years in order to carry out his administrative responsibilities satisfactorily. While they are not all-inclusive they hopefully will convey to the reader the diverse range of activities which the psychologist-administrator role encompasses. The roles are as follows:

Planner. This involves assessment of unmet needs of a community and available resources, and planning for development of new resources, better utilization of existing resources, and establishment of meaningful priorities.

Educator. This includes education of citizen groups, mental health professionals, and local and state legislators.

Organizer and Grant Writer. This applies particularly to federal grants although it includes grants from private foundations, drug companies, and so on.

Mental Health Consultant. The mental health administrator frequently receives calls from local organizations who either wish help in resolving internal organizational struggles or who would like assistance in improving their effectiveness.

Communicator. The purpose of this function is to make readily available to all interested parties materials and information about current happenings and recent changes which may affect the decision-making process.

Lobbyist. The lobbying role is an important one for effective mental health administration. It is essential in convincing authorities to fund vitally needed programs.

Architectural Consultant. In order for an architect to formulate effective architectural plans for a mental health program he needs the assistance of a mental health administrator who can not only spell out a viable program in terms the architect can comprehend, but who also understands the language and drawings of architects and the construction industry.

Coordinator. To be effective in the coordinating role between mental health professionals and citizen groups the psychologist-administrator must be perceived as knowledgeable and cooperative and, at the same time, objective and fair minded in mediating differences which may arise between groups.

Expeditor. This role moves beyond the coordinating function in that it facilitates the forward progress of planning and implementation of new or modified programs.

Conceptualizer. The conceptualization of mental health goals is a role well suited to the psychologist who has been trained in conceptual analysis, in an understanding of human development and behavior, in a grasp of motivational determinants, and in experiences in dyadic relationships.

Fund Raising Advocate. The mental health administrator is frequently called upon to appear before mayors, selectmen, boards of health, and school committees at the behest of local mental health and mental retardation associations and area citizen boards to aid in their quest of obtaining local funds to support their programs.

Personnel Recruiter. An important administrative function is the search for and recruitment of qualified professionals to fill key positions in clinics and state hospitals.

Budget Analyst. Understanding the intricacies of the budget process is essential in the efficient operation of clinical programs.

Planned Change Agent. The mental health administrator is frequently asked to participate in task forces or boards of organizations which are concerned with changing health and/or mental health systems.

Inspector and Standard Setter. This role is to ensure that mental health institutions, both public and private, maintain professional standards of operation as defined by state regulations and national accrediting organizations.

Primary Prevention Facilitator. The mental health administrator can play an important role in educating his colleagues of the merits of primary prevention efforts and in facilitating the development of such programs through his influence over budgetary priorities.

Evaluator. Evaluation is an essential aspect of program development. It is not enough merely to conceptualize programs, to plan programs, or to implement programs; it is essential that the efficacy of those programs be assessed through the "scientific method." The psychologist-administrator has a responsibility to his profession, as well as to the public who pays the tax dollars, to see that programs are operated ethically, efficiently, and effectively.

Heraclitus, the Greek philosopher, once remarked that the only thing that is permanent is change. In this context one might speculate how psychologists might have to adapt to changing concepts of the mental health administrator's roles as they evolve during the next decade.

It appears probable that a major shift in responsibility for the psychologist-administrator in the late 1970s and early 1980s will be away from direct supervision of the delivery of mental health services and a move toward contractual arrangements with a variety of community private nonprofit agencies who will provide services under guidelines established by a coalition of mental health professionals and local citizen groups. The administrator will continue to assist in the process of program conceptualization, planning, development, implementation, evaluation, and standard setting while nongovernmental agencies will operate the programs and be accountable annually to him for their quality and effectiveness.

Another likely change in the administrator's role will be toward closer collaboration and involvement in a broad human services delivery system which will include mental health, public health, rehabilitation, welfare, the youth and elderly in a network of services which will integrate the total needs of an individual from economic and physical to psychological and social. Within this context there is an exciting future for psychologists as human services coordinators and facilitators as well as mental health administrators.

BIBLIOGRAPHY

HIRSCHOWITZ, R. Dilemmas of leadership in community mental health. *Psychiatric Quarterly,* 1971, *45,* 102–116.
JOINT COMMISSION ON MENTAL ILLNESS AND HEALTH. *Action for mental health.* New York: Basic Books, 1961.
ROSENBLUM, G. Community psychology and mental health administration: From the frying pan into the fire. In S. Golann and J. Baker (Eds.), *Present and future trends in community psychology.* New York: Behavioral Publications, 1975.

GERSHEN ROSENBLUM

MENTAL HEALTH CONSULTATION: THE ROLE OF PSYCHOLOGISTS

With the advent of an increased public interest in the area of prevention of mental and emotional disorders, many psychologists are shifting the major focus of their professional activities from diagnosis and treatment to mental health consultation in the community. The term *consultation* has been diversely interpreted and practiced and this has often resulted in a diffuse and ambiguous role definition. Riesman (1963) defined consultation as "a helping process, an educational process, and a growth process achieved through interpersonal relationships."

When functioning as a mental health consultant, the psychologist attempts to assist key caregivers in a community in improving their role functions through discussions of case studies or administrative problems or through discussions of mental health principles. This effort involves three aspects. First, it implies that the consultant is knowledgeable about the mental health needs of the community. Second, it stresses the goal of improved functioning of the consultee in his professional role. Third, it focuses on the work problems of the consultee rather than upon personality problems or on dissemination of mental health concepts. Central to these endeavors is the nature of the colleague relationship which minimizes the transference and stresses the ego strengths of the consultee.

Consultation Models

One may distinguish seven consultation models (Rosenblum, 1970). These varied from the *traditional medical consultant* model (in which an "expert" is requested to interview or evaluate a colleague's client in order to make recommendations for program resolution) to the *intramural administrative consultant model* (in which a top administrator in an organization provides consultation to other personnel within the same organization). Of the seven models, three appear to be particularly well suited to be applied by the professional psychologist who wishes to provide a consultation function. These include:

The Consultant-Trainer Model. A consultant meets regularly with a group of consultees to discuss problems that the consultees face in their professional functioning. The method employed is a case seminar approach in which a group member presents case material for discussion by the group. The consultant acts variously as a group leader, teacher, clinician and facilitator of communication among the members of the group.

The Change-Agent Model. A consultant meets with key caregivers in the community or key professionals in agencies and institutions in order to bring about changes in the organizational or social system. The intervention may be active and politically oriented or may be catalytic and neutral.

The Mental Health Consultant Model. A consultant meets regularly with a consultee with the specific goal of enabling the consultee himself to solve mental health problems which he encounters in his professional capacity, in order that he might be able to handle similar problems in the future more competently.

Qualifications

Although there is a divergence of opinion regarding the optimum qualifications for a mental health consultant, what follows are considered to be basic requirements. Even though these are not the exclusive purview of the professional psychologist, they are consonant with the psychologist's background and training in understanding human behavior and his ability to relate meaningfully to others dynamically:

1. The mental health consultant must possess a solid grounding in the "helping relationship" (i.e., transactional analysis).

2. The mental health consultant requires special training and understanding of the mental health consultation process (e.g., Caplan's theory of mental health consultation).

3. The mental health consultant must have the ability to perceive the consultee as a qualified practitioner of his profession (i.e., education, religion, law enforcement, etc.).

4. The mental health consultant must be able to assume a collegial, rather than a professional-patient, relationship with the consultee.

5. The mental health consultant must be able to maintain awareness of his own feelings and reactions to the consultee as a person.

6. The mental health consultant must be flexible in his approach in differing consultee settings.

7. The mental health consultant must recognize that his expertness is in the realm of mental health and that the consultee is the legitimate authority in his chosen profession.

8. The mental health consultant must use his clinical insights to enhance the consultee's awareness and understanding of mental health issues in a manner that will improve the consultee's functioning within his profession.

In mental health consultation a peer relationship is developed between a mental health specialist and a member of another profession who may have a need to talk about the mental health problems of a client. The consultee may be a teacher with problems about children in her class, a principal, a school administrator, a supervisor, a psychologist, or nurse. The client whose problems are the center of the consultation process is the person or persons for whom the consultee is responsible.

Consultation Phases

The consultation process involves eight phases. Gibb (1959) described them as follows: entry (into consultation), diagnosis (definition of the problem), data collection (kinds of data and method of data gathering), relationship (mutual acceptance of consultant and consultee), boundary definition (limits of the relationship), resource development (nature of the relationship), decision making (the process), and termination (with minimal disruption to the social system).

As the psychologist moves into the mental health consultant role he must learn to collaborate successfully with many caregivers in the community and to be prepared, if he is successful in his consultation efforts, to be replaced by those consultees who have acquired insight and enhanced skills as a result of the consultation process.

BIBLIOGRAPHY

GIBB, J. R. Sequences in the consultation process. *Journal of Social Issues,* 1959, *15,* 1–4.

RIESMAN, D. W. Group mental health consultation with public health nurses. In L. Rapoport (Ed.), *Consulta-*

tion in social work practice. New York: National Association of Social Workers, 1963. Pp. 85–98.

ROSENBLUM, G.   Social intervention-consultation to organizations. *Mental Hygiene,* 1970, *54,* 393–396.

GERSHEN ROSENBLUM

MENTAL HEALTH AND POLITICS

Unlike other branches of medicine, psychiatry has depended more on the sociopolitical climate of the times than on the accumulation of technical knowledge. Between 1832 and 1855, moral treatment in America represented a high spot of humane psychiatric practice, but soon fell upon hard times as a result of the industrial revolution, the influx of foreign born, the expansion of mental hospitals, and the deterioration of close personal relationship to a low point of custodialism and neglect.

We have now seen a slow return to humanism as the plight of our emotional casualties has been moving more and more into the central focus of the body politic. Two world wars have demonstrated beyond denial that emotional disorders are rampant in the nation and take a heavy toll of conscriptable manpower; also, that casualties from psychiatric disorders during combat are often as high as from physical trauma. The great economic depression of the 1930s alerted the nation to the vast human expense of uncontrolled laissez-faire economics. Thus, the national government has moved progressively into the field of human salvage, welfare, and care and treatment of the mentally ill, retarded, alcoholic, and drug-dependent. Establishment of the National Institute of Mental Health (NIMH) was followed in the 1960s by enlightened legislation to assist hard-pressed mental hospitals, train personnel, encourage innovative clinical programs, build comprehensive mental health centers, and staff them. Programs attacking poverty and efforts to rehabilitate the handicapped have greatly assisted the mentally ill. Citizen organizations fighting on behalf of the mentally ill have helped enormously, supported as they have been by federal mandate requiring maximum consumer participation in programs receiving federal aid.

A few of the specific areas of sociopolitical change affecting mental illness practice and theory are considered below.

The New Accountability.   This flows from Professional Standards Review Organization (PSRO) and Health Services Review Organization (HSRO) regulations that hold physicians accountable for standards and review of patient care, physician practice, and institutional profiles of treatment. The first level of accountability is for institutional practice, but outpatient, extended care, and office practice surveillance is expected to follow. This legislation heralds a new day of collaboration between the medical profession and the political arm of government.

Coordination of Services.   The high cost of medical care, which to a large extent has motivated PSRO, plus claims of duplication and waste in overlapping services, and the inefficiency of multiple bureaucracies has led many states to establish human service superagencies—embracing usually mental health, retardation, welfare, public health, and often corrections. This change results in a relative loss of autonomy and identity for mental health agencies, and may in the long run put psychiatry into the hands of management specialists with their emphasis on fiscal economy, accountability, efficiency, and computerized criteria for performance.

Racism and "Minority" Psychiatry.   The black riots, the civil rights legislation, and the growing awareness by the nation of the social injustices suffered by minority groups have significantly affected the psychiatric scene. Among others, blacks and Spanish-speaking subgroups have received increasing attention with respect to the unique life situations and stresses that relate to the causes and treatment of their emotional disabilities. Much thought is being given by the psychiatric establishment to better representation for minority groups, and specialized training for professionals who serve them.

Mental Health and Sexual Politics.   Accompanying the socioeconomic and political upheavals of the last decades has been a great change in the sexual, marital, family, economic and professional roles of women. Women are demanding equality in every sphere—sex, child rearing, jobs, professional status, and political power. Many shibboleths regarding the biological inferiority of women, and the inevitability of male dominance are being overthrown. Major changes in concepts of psychosexual development of women and in definitions of normality and maturity, together with active and open experimentation with new types of pairing arrangements that might replace conventional marriage require a reorientation of psychiatric goals and practices in dealing with the modern liberated female.

Urbanization and Poverty. The culture of poverty and its ravages on the human spirit and the inadequacies of present mental health techniques and systems in dealing with human casualties of poverty have become challenges to psychiatry in the last few decades. This problem is intermixed with that of race, minority disfranchisement, civil rights; it is also related to questions of superurbanization in the twentieth century, and the inability of large bureaucracies to attend to the needs of the common man. Thus, another great challenge to psychiatry for treatment techniques and treatment systems to meet critical needs of the larger population has arisen.

Legislative Therapy. In many states, legislators have shown a desire to regulate the practice of mental health care and treatment, to the consternation of highly individualistic professionals, and the disruption of the status quo. In some instances, legislation has intruded unduly upon the subtleties of the physician-patient relationship, and upon their freedom to carry out studies and investigation that might advance the body of knowledge and contribute to theory and practice of benefit to future generations of patients. A new balance between professional and political forces is slowly emerging in which the autonomy of the profession is gradually being subordinated to overall health planning by the political bodies of government.

Psychiatric Impairment of Political Leaders. In a highly unstable world threatened with nuclear disaster, the public has great anxiety about the maturity and mental stability of its leaders. Accordingly, it has been recommended that services of psychiatric professionals be sought in evaluating the personality and mental competence of candidates for high office. These professionals would presumably look after the mental health of these leaders in much the same sense as nonpsychiatric physicians look after their physical health.

Three questions exist with respect to this hope: (1) whether psychiatry has enough knowledge to predict the performance of potential leaders; (2) whether psychiatry has enough technology to buffer the strains of high office; and (3) whether at this time in history, considering the reputation of psychiatry in political circles and in the public mind, such recommendations would be acceptable to political man.

BIBLIOGRAPHY

American Psychiatric Association official actions: Position statement on Public Law 92–603 (PSRO). *American Journal of Psychiatry,* 1974, *131*(9), 1072.

GREENBLATT, M. Psychopolitics. *American Journal of Psychiatry,* 1974, *131,* 1197–1203.

GREENBLATT, M. Psychopolitics and the search for power. *Psychiatric Annals,* 1975, *5,* 71–83.

GREENBLATT, M. Towards a definition of psychopolitics. *Psychiatric Annals,* 1975, *5,* 6–11.

GREENBLATT, M.; YORK, R. H.; and BROWN, E. L. *From custodial to therapeutic patient care in mental hospitals.* New York: Russell Sage Foundation, 1955.

GREENBLATT, M.; EMERY, P. E.; and GLUECK, B. G., JR. (Eds.). *Poverty and mental health.* Washington, D.C.: American Psychiatric Association, 1967.

JACO, E. G. *The social epidemiology of mental disorders.* New York: Russell Sage Foundation, 1960.

JOINT COMMISSION ON MENTAL ILLNESS AND HEALTH. *Action for mental health.* New York: Basic Books, 1961.

SULLIVAN, F. W. Professional standards review organization: The current scene. *American Journal of Psychiatry,* 1974, *113,* 1354–1358.

MILTON GREENBLATT

MENTAL HEALTH IN THE SCHOOLS

Adaptive Problems

In school, the young child must meet two critical sets of adaptive demands. He must master increasingly complex bodies of knowledge, and he must do this within a sometimes stringent set of behavioral and interpersonal limits. These requirements often have reciprocal consequences. Adaptive problems can restrict the child's ability to learn just as failures in educational mastery can produce psychological problems. School mental health services originated at, and still find their prime justification in, the intercept of these two sets of demands.

School social work services began early in the twentieth century when the first compulsory school attendance laws were passed

(Wrenn, 1968). In that era, children's education often suffered or ended because of nonattendance due to economic hardship or family disinterest. The first school social workers or "visiting teachers" (a term still widely used) sought to develop family contacts to improve children's attendance and hopefully to forestall such adverse social consequences as ignorance and delinquency. School psychology, by contrast, grew out of an evolving psychometric tradition. Its first, all-encompassing emphasis was on the slow-learning or problem child. The psychologist's job was to assess children's skills, potentials, and deficits in an attempt to find for them more appropriate school experiences (e.g., specific instruction, special class placement).

A common feature of these early school mental health roles was their emphasis on the casualties of the system. The numbers and types of casualties for whom services, however defined, could be provided depended on a system's resources. Since the latter were characteristically thin, most services went to a small fraction of visibly maladapting children.

Many factors have contributed to school mental health's later growth and development. For one thing, some school people found such services useful and relevant to their everyday concerns. Evolving social philosophies, especially the conviction that *all* children have the right to a meaningful, contributory educational experience, also supported the field's growth, as did technological advances in testing and treatment. In practice, however, the development of school mental health services has principally meant (1) more resources and (2) role expansion and liberalization that allows professionals to do more varied things than before. Even so, today's roles still reflect the clear imprint of their original definition; they remain directed primarily to the serious problems of a small minority of the most maladapted children.

School mental health's most important current challenges stem from the fact that its resources cannot meet evident needs. Glidewell and Swallow's (1969) survey of school maladjustment incidence studies, done for the Joint Commission on Mental Health of Children (1969), indicates that 30% of American children are experiencing school adjustment problems. And for 10% those problems are suffi-

ciently serious to require immediate professional help. Given the original Joint Commission's (1961) contention that education, like coal and iron, is a major natural resource, Glidewell and Swallow's findings suggest a tragic national waste. The challenges posed by these data are: how to extend the reach of effective school mental health services and how to redefine such services, and attendant professional roles, to optimize the school experience for the many (Fein, 1974).

Preventive Action

Such questions have fueled recent explorations of new school mental health conceptualizations and roles. Although primary prevention seems to be an attractive *ideal,* it is abstract and futuristic. Hence, concrete efforts to increase school mental health's scope and effectiveness have had more immediate, achievable goals, such as developing techniques for prompt, accurate identification of school maladjustment. *Early detection* is a critical gateway to effective early intervention. Recent years have witnessed many constructive attempts to develop early identification methodologies. These efforts have been based on one or a combination of the following approaches: direct behavioral observation, interview methods, psychodiagnostic evaluation, and the use of symptom surveys. They have often included teacher inputs, since the teacher's daily contacts with children enable her to provide unique information about how children meet the school environment's adaptive demands.

In addition to early identification, promising new professional roles such as the *elementary counselor* (Faust, 1968) and the *school mental health consultant* (Newman, 1967) have been identified, as have a variety of new approaches (e.g., "schools without failure," encounter groups, and behavior modification) to helping youngsters cope effectively with the school experience. More systematically, some (Cowen, Trost, Lorion, Dorr, Izzo, and Isaacson, 1975) have called for school mental health delivery systems with a combined emphasis on (1) the very young child; (2) widespread screening and early detection of school adjustment problems; (3) use of nonprofessional help-agents to expand the reach of effective services geometrically; and (4) changing professional roles toward such "quarterbacking" functions as education, training, supervision, and consultation in order to bring meaning and substance to expanded delivery systems.

School mental health's resource limits dictate that difficult but realistic choices be made among alternatives. Decisions must be made about apportioning finite time between (1) younger versus older children; (2) actively promoting the health and well-being of the many versus dealing reactively with the dysfunctions of the few; (3) engineering school environments that maximize learning and development (Sarason, 1971) versus focusing on individual children. Although all the preceding objectives are laudable, society cannot generate the resources needed to achieve them. School mental health may be more rewarding and socially contributory if it develops approaches that (1) reach out effectively to many more, and younger, children; (2) reach the heretofore unreached; and (3) build effectiveness and competence in all children from the start rather than focusing exclusively on repairing dysfunction.

BIBLIOGRAPHY

BARDON, J. I. School psychology and school psychologists. *American Psychologist,* 1968, *23,* 187–194.

COWEN, E. L.; TROST, M. A.; LORION, R. P.; DORR, D.; IZZO, L. D.; and ISAACSON, R. V. *New ways in school mental health: Early detection and prevention of school maladjustment.* New York: Human Sciences, 1975.

FAUST, V. *The counselor-consultant in the elementary school.* Boston: Houghton Mifflin, 1968.

FEIN, L. G. *The changing school scene: Challenge to psychology.* New York: Wiley, 1974.

GLIDEWELL, J. C., and SWALLOW, C. S. *The prevalence of maladjustment in elementary schools: A report prepared for the Joint Commission on the Mental Health of Children.* Chicago: University of Chicago Press, 1969.

JOINT COMMISSION ON MENTAL HEALTH OF CHILDREN. *Crisis in child mental health: Challenge for the 1970s.* New York: Harper & Row, 1969.

JOINT COMMISSION ON MENTAL ILLNESS AND HEALTH. *Action for mental health.* New York: Basic Books, 1961.

NEWMAN, R. G. *Psychological consultation in the schools.* New York: Basic Books, 1967.

SARASON, S. B. *The culture of the schools and the problem of change.* Boston: Allyn-Bacon, 1971.

WRENN, C. G. The movement into counseling in the elementary school. In V. Faust (Ed.), *The counselor-consultant in the elementary school.* Boston: Houghton Mifflin, 1968.

EMORY L. COWEN

MENTAL HEALTH AND SOCIAL PSYCHOLOGY

Social psychology has contributed to the field of mental health in the following ways:

1. Social psychology emphasizes the social context of behavior, and attempts to measure and understand the relational and interactive qualities of interpersonal behavior. It examines social interactions in relation both to intrapsychic constructs and to extrinsic social concepts. Thus, destructive patterns of family relationships are studied in conjunction with the disturbed behavior of the individual; such patterns may actually be perpetuated by their role in preserving the microsocial system of the total family. The interview or testing situation may be viewed as a two-person social system. In this microsystem, the tester's role, his values, and his power over the subject will all be reflected in the type of identity, values, and attitude toward authority that the subject displays.

2. Social psychology stresses the importance of values in definitions of mental health and illness. It distinguishes among "personal maladjustment," "social deviance," and "productive nonconformity." Therapeutic goals such as adaptation, self-realization, and maturity are seen in the context of the values held by the society in which the individual lives.

3. Social psychology not only examines maladaptive behavior, but also studies the executive and adaptive functioning of the healthy individual under different social conditions.

4. Social psychology examines the influence of the social system on the progress of the mental patient, in terms of etiology, maintenance, and therapeutic procedure. Additionally, the psychological correlates of basic variables such as social class and sibling order, have been investigated. Social class itself can be viewed as a complex function of such factors as value system, social deprivation, standard of living, and methods of child rearing.

5. The analysis of interpersonal interaction on the individual level offers help in transcending the limitations imposed on therapeutic theory and practice by traditional medical models. The study and classification of various types of

family interaction have been especially helpful in this regard.

6. The social psychologist utilizes research in such areas as addiction and juvenile delinquency in his approach to the problem of mental health. Furthermore, the cross-cultural comparison of symptom patterns can be useful in understanding the relationship between social environment and mental illness.

7. In "action research" (K. Lewin) the investigator becomes directly involved with the system he is studying in order to understand it and change it.

Mental Illness as a Social Issue

The basic reasons for considering mental health as a social issue are the following:

1. Mental health problems involve a huge number of people; some estimates place the proportion of people presently suffering from some form of mental disorder as high as one in three.

2. The cost of mental illness is very high, not only in human terms, but in social and economic terms as well. Loss of productivity and waste of human resources must be considered in addition to the direct outlay of capital and operational funds in assessing the total cost.

3. Present resources cannot deal with the mental health problem adequately; sufficient facilities and personnel are simply not available.

4. The prevalence of mental illness varies among different sectors of society, and is inversely related to the availability of treatment within those sectors.

5. A wide variety of social forces, including automation, overpopulation, poverty, racism, and international conflicts, are likely to influence the formation of mental symptoms.

6. The widespread occurrence of mental disorders, and the comparative scarcity of resources for relieving those disorders, may themselves be symptomatic of the pathology of a social system. The social psychologist may ask how the society itself can be changed to fulfill fundamental human social needs. Thus, one task of the social psychologist is the determination of psychological "tolerance limits" in the areas of population density, social depriva-

tion (especially in childhood), and interpersonal conflict.

Social psychologists attempt to analyze the progress of the mental patient, from the prepatient to the expatient phase, in terms of his interaction with a variety of "micro" social systems with which he comes into contact. The patient's social class, his family, his role in the community, his response to the culture and values of the psychiatric institution, and the small face-to-face treatment group in which he may find himself—all are examined in an effort to understand their psychological meaning to the patient, and the influence they may have upon him.

The Definition of Mental Health and Illness

Mental illness can be seen in purely sociological terms, as a deviation from socially approved standards of interpersonal behavior, or as an inability to perform one's sanctioned social roles. Conversely, mental health can be defined as behavior that meets the demands of social roles and norms. But when social norms cease to be well-defined, when anomie and family instability come to characterize an entire society, then the criteria for mental illness also become vague and uncertain. Under these circumstances, interpersonal behavior that would be classified as "pathological" at other times may actually serve an important, if temporary, adaptive function. Medical and psychophysiological observations alone cannot give an adequate picture of the individual experience of mental illness; that picture must be seen in the context of the interpersonal relationships that surround the individual. Mental health or illness is determined by the person's interaction with his social matrix; any personal decisions, any plans he makes must be formulated with regard to the social expectancies of which he is constantly aware. Interpersonal behavior is always organized by social setting and context.

In social science literature it is generally agreed that the term *mental illness* refers to dysfunctional interpersonal behavior, judged to be "dysfunctional" in terms of the norms and values held by the observer. The fact that this judgment is frequently made in the absence of any evidence of somatic or physiological disorder has led a large number of social scientists to argue that the "medical model" is totally inapplicable to the study of problems in interpersonal behavior. Many others challenge the medical model on purely practical grounds, arguing that methods of therapy based on this model have not been found to be effective.

The Mental Hospital: Effects of Institutionalization

Goffman (1958) has investigated and systematically described what it feels like to be cast in the role of a "mental patient." He accomplished this task by becoming a "participant observer," working as an assistant athletic director in a large mental hospital with psychotic patients. He described the process of self-transformation that begins with the decision to commit the person and ends when he has become a stabilized mental patient. This process is accompanied by experiences of family betrayal, loss of social identity, self-humiliation, and diverse forms of mortification; all are experiences that, taken together, would be bound to have a devastating effect even upon a "normal" person. Goffman's essential point is that the "total institution" of the mental hospital degrades the patient and denies his personal dignity. Since all power in the institution is concentrated in the hands of the staff, the patient exerts virtually no influence over institutional decisions that may drastically affect his life. To justify the patients' powerlessness, the institution must become increasingly committed to defining all patients as "mentally ill," and thus presumably incapable of rational decision making. The institution structures the daily activity of its inmates so that they are constantly in the company of a large number of other patients; they are all treated alike, and are all required to do the same thing at the same time. Schedules are highly routinized, and are maintained through a rigid system of regulations. Contact with the world outside the institution is minimized. By narrowing the scope of the patients' lives in all of these ways, the institution makes it possible for a small group of untrained supervisory personnel to control a much larger population of inmates with a minimum of effort.

The constraints of the institutional environment have been shown to have definite adverse effects on patient behavior. Wing (1968) has demonstrated that the degree of institutional restrictiveness and patient understimulation correlate with the extent to which the inmates become socially withdrawn, underactive, silent, and emotionally dulled. Improving the social environment leads to definite changes in these behavior patterns; the "time spent doing nothing" decreases considerably in the patient population. Similar results have been reported in the studies of Hunter et al. (1962); Klein and Spohn (1962; 1964); and Wolman (1964).

While Goffman has accurately characterized the environment provided by the custodial hospital, he has not dealt with the question of how different types of patients may interact with that environment. The "aggressive psychopath," the "withdrawn paranoid schizophrenic," and the "severe psychoneurotic" all respond very differently to common institutional pressures, while at the same time their behavior probably elicits different responses from the staff.

The Therapeutic Milieu

The concept of a total treatment environment, or "therapeutic milieu" originally proposed by Maxwell Jones, has led to the development of several innovative treatment programs (Raush and Raush, 1968; Spohn, 1958; Ellsworth, 1968). All of these approaches stress social interaction of patients and staff (with a minimum of status differentiation), a democratic political structure (patient government or participation in making the rules), and the blurring of patient-staff distinctions so that they are likely to stand together on certain issues. Programs to change patient behavior rely primarily on informal group pressure, and on systems of positive rewards that are individualized for each patient.

Wax (1963) has described the salient features of the therapeutic community:

1. Attention is focused on the current social behavior of the patient.

2. Responsibility for the progression of treatment is shared by the patients and staff; the patient is expected to take an active role in his own treatment, as well as in other patients.

3. Social stratification among patients and staff is minimized to allow for freer exchange

of information and emotional communication.

4. The patient's psychopathology, and the goal of attaining psychodynamic insight into its causes and manifestations, are deemphasized.

An important question must be asked as to whether the patient who improves in a hospital setting might not necessarily be able to function better when he rejoins his family and community outside the hospital walls. Ellsworth (1968) has posed the specific question of how symptom reduction in the hospital can be expected to correlate with improvements in family relationships and job performance when the patient is released. A complete understanding of the *patient's* community is necessary before the patient can be prepared to leave the total treatment environment; the expectations of the expatient's family, employer, and co-workers are of primary importance.

This consideration of community dynamic raises another question: Is it possible to design a social environment to maximize the opportunity for informal "treatment relationships" to develop? Such a social environment would be of value not only to the expatient who has just left the hospital, but to "normal" individuals subjected to the unavoidable pressures of daily social life. In the final analysis, the problem of designing social environments for the prevention and treatment of mental disorder cannot be separated from the attempt to design social environments that promote positive mental health among "normals" as well.

BIBLIOGRAPHY

ELLSWORTH, R. B. *Nonprofessionals in psychiatric rehabilitation.* New York: Appleton, 1968.

GOFFMAN, E. Characteristics of total institutions. In *Symposium on preventive and social psychiatry, 15–17 April 1957.* Walter Reed Army Institute of Research. Washington, D.C.: U.S. Government Printing Office, 1958.

HUNTER, M.; SCHOOLER, C.; and SPOHN, H. E. The measurement of characteristic patterns of ward behavior in chronic schizophrenics. *Journal of Consulting Psychology,* 1962, *26,* 69–73.

JAHODA, M. *Current concepts of positive mental health.* New York: Basic Books, 1958.

JONES, M. *The therapeutic community.* New York: Basic Books, 1953.

KLEIN, E. B., and SPOHN H. E. Behavioral dimensions of chronic schizophrenia. *Psychological Reports,* 1962, *11,* 777–783.

RAUSH, H. L., and C. L. RAUSH. *The halfway house movement: A search for sanity.* New York: Appleton, 1968.

WECHSLER, H.; SOLOMON, L.; and KRAMER B. M. (Eds.). *Social psychology and mental health.* New York: Holt, Rinehart and Winston, 1970.

WING, J. K. Social treatments of mental illness. In M. Shepherd, and D. L. Davies (Eds.), *Studies in psychiatry.* London: Oxford University Press, 1968.

WOLMAN, B. B. Nonparticipant observation on a closed ward. *Acta Psychotherapeutica,* 1964, *12,* 61–71.

LEONARD SOLOMON
HENRY WECHSLER
BERNARD M. KRAMER

MENTALLY RETARDED CHILDREN AND THE SCHOOL PSYCHOLOGIST

Teamwork

The current concept of the role of the school psychologist working with the retarded is much changed from the traditional function. Under this new formulation the psychologist becomes the member of a team which provides a full range of diagnostic, remedial, and developmental services. The team which is ad hoc and changes as needs dictate, consists of psychologists, speech therapists, special education teachers, social workers, medical personnel, and any other consultative personnel required by the situation. The team is designed to serve the immense needs of the retarded. It provides academic and vocational testing; remediation; guidance for faculty, child, and parents; social services; speech and hearing testing and therapy; language development; instructional services, both formal and informal; and medical referrals. It also provides any other neurological, psychological or psychiatric services that might be required. The team concept stresses the close relationship between the educational and psychological knowledges available to serve the retarded child.

The Role of the School Psychologist

The range of the school psychologist's responsibilities include the following areas:

1. Help to students through assessment of the educational and psychological patterns of performance and the child's needs on a short/

long-term basis; the making of recommendations as to programs and services based upon that assessment.

2. Consulting with other team members, other community facilities and agencies for implementing the recommendations.

3. Providing counseling to parents and child to assist in optimizing functioning through a problem-solving procedure.

4. Help to parents through interpretation of the assessment, and giving them a realistic picture of the educational and psychological needs of their child.

5. Providing suggestions as to ways parents can assist the child to develop better cognitive, affective, and social skills.

6. Making appropriate referrals to agencies and specialists.

7. Educating parents individually and through parent-group programs on the nature of retardation and its social, emotional, and educational effects.

8. Help to teachers through interpreting the diagnostic protocol so that planning to meet the needs of the child can take place.

9. Working directly with acting-out children and assisting the teacher in planning and managing these children.

10. Attendance at conferences; keeping up with new concepts and knowledge.

In the utilization of the educational team concept the psychologist functions as the coordinator. His responsibility is the integration and interpretation of educational and psychological information which the team has developed so that the formal protocol becomes useful to faculty, administration and parents. Thus, it can be utilized as a tool to help the retarded child maximize his potential.

ROBERT HOLZBERG

MENTAL RETARDATION

MENTAL RETARDATION: DEFINITION, INCIDENCE, AND CLASSIFICATION

Definition of Mental Retardation

One definition of mental retardation calls it a condition which "refers to significantly subaverage general intellectual functioning existing concurrently with deficits in adaptive behavior, and manifested during the developmental period" (Grossman, 1972, p. 11). This definition, which is widely accepted among clinicians and academicians working with mentally retarded persons, is in itself a complex combination of terms filled with potential semantic pitfalls. Nevertheless, the definition represents the distillation of the best thinking of authorities in the field and serves as the basis for the remainder of this article. The following dissection of this definition also simultaneously reveals or implies many of the salient considerations and features of *incidence* and *classifica-*

tion. Consequently, less attention will be given to these latter two considerations.

In order to provide additional definitional perspective, it is important to understand that mental retardation is a condition that falls within the larger category of *developmental disabilities.* The Developmental Disabilities Act (Public Law 91–517) defines the term developmental disability as:

a disability attributable to mental retardation, cerebral palsy, epilepsy, or another neurological condition of an individual found by the Secretary (U.S. Department of Health, Education, and Welfare) to be closely related to mental retardation or to require treatment similar to that required for mentally retarded individuals, which disability originates before such individual attains age eighteen, which has continued or can be expected to continue indefinitely, and which constitutes a substantial handicap to such individual (P. L. 91–517, 1970, p. 10; parenthetic item added for clarification).

A more recently proposed revision of P.L. 91–517 adds *autism* and suggests *specific learning disabilities* as additional legitimate developmental disabilities. Although the definition of developmental disabilities does shed some light on where mental retardation is thought to fit in the continuum of handicapping conditions, it implies that mental retardation is exclusively a neurological condition.

This underscores another feature of definition, namely that a complete definition should have both inclusive and exclusive stipulations. It should state both what something is and, when it is likely to be confused with something else, what it is not. A person who is mentally retarded due to neurological causes would generally fall under the classification of developmental disability, whereas a person whose mental retardation is a function of inadequate environmental enrichment would not legitimately be included in the definition of developmental disability even though his intellectual functioning might be equally defective.

A good example of a more complete definition of a related condition is that proposed for *specific learning disability,* which has been defined as:

a disorder in one or more of the basic psychological processes involved in understanding or in using language, spoken or written, which disorder may manifest itself in imperfect ability to listen, think, speak,

read, write, spell, or do mathematical calculations. Such disorders include such conditions as perceptual handicaps, brain injury, minimal brain dysfunction, dyslexia, and developmental aphasia, but such a term does not include children who have learning problems which are primarily the result of visual, hearing, or motor handicaps, or mental retardation, or emotional disturbance, or environmental disadvantage (Meier, 1971, pp. 9–10).

The difficulties and misunderstandings surrounding definitions of various disorders of child growth and development and the resultant tragedy of misclassification and mistreatment are readily acknowledged. Ample testimony to the controversy surrounding the labeling of children is found in Hobbs (1975a,b), which is discussed in a later section dealing with classification.

The preceding definition of mental retardation should be construed as a relative definition which is explicitly inclusive and only implicitly exclusive. It states what mental retardation is relative to normal intellectual functioning and adaptive behavior, but it does not state which similar conditions are to be excluded. The following three sections address the logical divisions of the definition of mental retardation and include observations germane to incidence and classification.

Significantly Subaverage General Intellectual Functioning

The word *significantly* here typically refers to a statistical concept which in turn refers to measured performances that are one standard deviation below the average measured performance of the referent population, in this case groups of normally developing humans in the United States. It has been statistically determined that approximately two-thirds of all persons taking the Stanford-Binet Test of Intelligence or the Wechsler Intelligence Scales, two commonly used measuring instruments, fall within a range of about 30 intelligence points around the preadjusted average of approximately 100. With reference to the normal distribution curve, this means that nearly 70% of the entire population on which these tests were standardized have intelligence scores between about 85 and 115. It also means that approximately 15% of the population have intelligence scores below 85, which in the past was used as the sole criterion for establishing that a person was mentally retarded, that is, his test performance indicated that he was significantly less mentally able than the majority of the population. This is usually borne out by the fact that such individuals have significant difficulty in benefiting from the standard school program in comparison with their age peers of normal and above-normal measured intelligence. In this fashion, such tests of intelligence are said to have predictive validity within the limitations to be discussed later.

It is critical to specify the characteristics of the population on which the given test is normed or standardized, since what is normal or standard intellectual performance, as presently measured, among college graduates versus impoverished and/or brain-damaged children would be poles apart. In a pluralistic society, with multiple diverse cultural values, it is extremely important to measure intellectual functioning with procedures or instruments that are appropriate to the subject's background and that have been normed on a comparable reference group. The same intelligence scores, which correctly predicted the ability of a person to get along in a less complex society, may no longer be sufficient in a society that requires increased levels of sophistication and ability to deal satisfactorily with the many abstract and symbol-laden daily problems. It can be argued that the incidence of mental retardation is increasing, not only as a result of more persons of significantly subaverage potential being kept alive due to recent medical advances long enough to enter the schools and in some cases the adult world, but also as a result of there being relatively fewer occupations or life situations in which those with subaverage general intelligence can perform satisfactorily.

The word *general* is intended to include only those whose intellectual functioning is impaired across a broad spectrum of cognitive categories and to exclude those who have cognitive deficits in one or two specific domains but are generally intellectually competent. For example, there are many cases reported in the literature of persons with exceptionally high measured intelligence who may have specific intellectual deficits in a verbal domain such as spelling, or a mathematical domain such as solid geometry, or a performance domain such

as assembling puzzles. Such persons may have specific learning disabilities and even be legitimately defined as developmentally disabled yet their overall intellectual functioning would not permit them to be called mentally retarded. On the other hand, there are cases reported of persons (sometimes called idiot-savants) who exhibit general mental retardation but have one or two specific intelligence-related functions developed to a very high degree of excellence, such as reading or spelling very long and tricky words, but not being able to define or properly use most words in the language, or who are able to deal with spatial relations problems, such as assembling puzzles at the concrete level of operation, but are not able to abstract or verbalize these operations for more general problem-solving applications.

If a definition of mental retardation relative to each individual's native or inborn learning capacity is accepted, it is quite probable that the majority of persons in the society at large do not realize their fullest capacity for learning and are thus retarded below what they could be if they had the opportunity to fully realize their intellectual capacities. Although intelligence tests purport to measure intellectual capacity, they in fact measure achieved levels of information and skills in the verbal and nonverbal areas. It is then inferred that, based on previous achievements, there is a reasonably high probability that the individual will continue to derive in the future a similar amount from his environment, which includes all of the people, places, and things he experiences in his daily living. Since most individuals do not radically alter their life circumstances, the constancy of their environment tends to ensure that their measured intelligence will not fluctuate appreciably, provided that they continue to function at the same rate of learning and with the same degree of exposure to their environment.

The actual assessment of an individual's ability to learn new skills and apply this new learning to either old or new problems is rarely done and yet this is what intelligence is allegedly thought to be. Clearly, the person in a deprived environment, regardless of his native intelligence, will be severely limited in the acquisition of new knowledge and the development of new skills. He will probably test as significantly subaverage in general intelligence, remain in or be placed in settings for mentally subaverage individuals, and in prophecy-fulfilling fashion continue to perform at a subaverage level on tests of intelligence.

Directly related is the word *functioning,* which is inextricably woven into the fabric of intelligence as measured. In fact, the phrase *as measured* relates to this important consideration of function, which is to be differentiated from absolute status. Functional intelligence refers to the contextual aspects of a person's performance and is frequently qualified by such phrases as *under the circumstances, all other things being equal,* and *conditions being what they are.* The diagnosis of functional mental retardation refers to the fact that on the basis of a person's intelligence test performance he receives a score that falls in the range of mental retardation, that is, significantly subaverage; however, the word *functional* indicates that there is some doubt as to whether this is an immutable status or relative to one or more extenuating circumstances.

This designation further underscores the relativity feature in the currently accepted definition of mental retardation. A person, for example, whose mother tongue is different from that of both the examiner and the test materials will likely function much as a retarded person in attempting to solve verbal problems or to understand verbal directions. In a pluralistic society, the environments in which people are born and reared vary greatly along a continuum from poverty to affluence, and typically vary in degree of deprivation to enrichment insofar as the availability of the content of the intelligence tests is concerned. It is, therefore, necessary to take the relativity feature into consideration before attributing absolute mental retardation to a given individual. The assumption "all other things being equal" is seldom if ever met; if an intelligence test is fundamentally a reflection of the learning on the part of the individual, and the environment in which he grows up is not equal in many of the sources of skill and information enjoyed by the majority, he may also function as relatively mentally retarded, although his basic intellectual capacity and learning ability is equal to his peers.

Many subcultures in a pluralistic society have not only different languages but different cultural expectations which may unduly influence a person's general experience for better or for worse, insofar as his functioning on intelligence testing is concerned. Such realizations have given rise to euphemisms, such as "six-hour retarded children," who find it difficult to function normally in school settings, which represent a generally foreign culture to them. Similarly, children of average or above intelligence in mainstream America would have considerable difficulty functioning at the same level of competence in a country where a completely foreign language is used exclusively. Contrariwise, the child who develops language relatively very late or very poorly, given all of the same opportunities sufficient for his peers to master the language, should be considered to have at least a communication disorder. If such a child were tested in a different language from his vernacular, his delay may be even more pronounced but should not be attributed entirely to the unfamiliarity of the new language. A child who has difficulty learning English and displays a significantly subaverage acquisition of speaking and listening vocabulary will likely manifest similar delays in learning Spanglish, Creole Black dialect, smoke signaling, or other languages because of a fundamental deficit in language ability. Since expressive and receptive language are critical to intellectual functioning as measured by most current intelligence tests, a child with such a specific language disorder may be assessed as mentally retarded in spite of normal or above-normal capacities to learn in other nonverbal areas.

Many environmentally deprived or culturally different individuals have intelligence scores that are just below the average level and have in the past been designated as "borderline" mentally retarded. They have been called "slow learners" or "educables" by the mainstream public school system and were grouped with others having similar deficits, thereby further depriving them of learning from their more enlightened and able peers. This particular classification has been deleted from the more recent classification language, since so many of these individuals have demonstrated at least average inherent capacities for learning when given sufficient opportunity to compensate for previous deprivations or differences in experience.

Existing Concurrently with Deficits in Adaptive Behavior

This phrase represents a formal acknowledgement of the fact that a person can demonstrate significantly subaverage general intellectual functioning and at the same time get along in his social surroundings. The individual who has mastered those behaviors necessary to adapt to his given environment, regardless of how simple or complex it may be, cannot be legitimately labeled mentally retarded. He has, in fact, learned what is necessary to cope with and survive in his own peculiar life situation, which has its own limitations on the extent of information and skills available to be learned. The Eskimo or Tlingit Indian in Alaska, the Amish in the northeast United States, the coal-miner in Appalachia, or the native Hawaiian on the Island of Molokai may all test as mentally retarded on the Wechsler or Stanford-Binet Intelligence Tests, even if the test is translated into their vernacular. Nevertheless, they are behaving satisfactorily and normally in their peculiar native environs. And just as the immigrating Puerto Rican may psychometrically test in the mentally retarded range, his ability to behaviorally adapt to and satisfactorily function in the Miami or New York City environs speaks well of his mental capacity to learn new information and skills. If an individual cannot satisfactorily behave in his own native environment without extraordinary support from others, he is regarded to have deficits in adaptive behavior not only in his native environment but most probably in any other "normal" situations as well.

The description of deficits in adaptive behavior is more complex than for measured intelligence because of the former's lack of objective measures. The level of deficiency in adaptive behavior is expressed in four levels, which roughly correspond to standard deviation units. Level I, which is about two standard deviations below the population mean, represents some noteworthy adaptive difficulties, whereas Level IV represents almost total lack of adaptive behavior.

The Vineland Social Maturity Scale—supplemented where possible by portions of the Gesell Developmental Schedules, the Bayley Infant Scales, the Cattell Infant Intelligence Scale, and the Kuhlmann Tests of Mental Development—is recommended for use at the preschool level as a measure of adaptive behavior. During the school-age period, standardized achievement tests serve as the initial measure of adaptive behavior in the academic world. The Vineland Scales may have to be used to differentiate among the lower levels of mental retardation. At the adolescent and adult level, adaptive behavior is best seen in social adjustment, but there are few instruments available that adequately assess this. Therefore, the level of social adjustment is frequently determined by the clinician's assessment of the individual's social and vocational adjustment, often in combination with ratings on the AAMD Adaptive Behavior Scale.

The AAMD Adaptive Behavior Scale provides scores that measure a number of separate aspects of adaptive, as well as maladaptive, behavior. A forthcoming edition of the Scale's Manual offers the procedure by which some of the scores can be combined to derive an individual's overall level of adaptive behavior. For younger children, the adaptive behavior level is determined by a composite of measures that include the degree of self-sufficiency, sensory-motor development, language development, and socialization. For older children and adults, the adaptive behavior level is determined by the same composite of measures augmented by measures of domestic skill, vocational potential, and responsibility.

At the present time, the value of a *single score* for adaptive behavior level classification is limited largely to certain administrative purposes and has little diagnostic or program planning import for the individual. Assessment of performance in *specific domains* of behavior, however, can be very useful in identifying deficits and training needs. As with I.Q. scores, individuals who are classified at the same overall level of adaptive behavior may not be "clinically equivalent" in that they may vary significantly in the various domains of behavior that comprise the overall rating (Grossman, 1973, pp. 19–20).

The final clinical judgment as to a person's adaptive behavior level is arrived at only after considering the multiple factors that contribute to the development of adaptive behavior. These must include repeated observation of the individual in his natural setting, reports from others who have observed his behavior in other regular settings, recognition of the limitations and opportunities imposed by a given setting, including others in the environment, and consideration of general intellectual functioning from a more structured test situation. When this deficit in adaptive behavior exists concurrently with inadequate intellectual functioning, a second important criterion of mental retardation is fulfilled.

Manifested During the Developmental Period

Since even the term *developmental* is subject to various and sundry interpretations, these ambiguities have been essentially eliminated, though not illuminated, by simply designating the chronological age of 18 years as the upper limit of the developmental period. For persons who are over 18 years of age and meet the preceding two main criteria of mental retardation, it is necessary to derive thorough histories in order to determine whether the condition of mental retardation was manifest in the individual's intellectual functioning and adaptive behavior before 18 years of age. This history should include pertinent data about (1) family background (and pedigree charts if readily available); (2) living conditions plus estimate of socioeconomic status; (3) physical characteristics; (4) medical conditions; (5) education and training experiences; (6) academic achievement and skills; (7) several breakdowns of measured intellectual functioning; and (8) several estimates of adaptive behavior. In light of this stipulation, if whatever condition that is responsible for a person's functioning in a mentally retarded fashion occurred after he was 18, he is not technically mentally retarded and would have to be classified under some alternative nomenclature.

Current Measures for Defining Mental Retardation

Table 1 summarizes the measures for defining mental retardation which are widely used in the current state of the art and knowledge. The preceding discussion has underscored the complexities and controversies involved in the use of these pragmatic definitional criteria.

Incidence of Mental Retardation

Incidence and prevalence studies which have attempted to document the extent and degree of mental retardation have yielded highly variable results. The wide range of such findings are a function of several inconsistencies from study to study: (1) variations in the definitions of mental retardation; (2) variations in tests and procedures used to assess mental retardation; (3) variations in the characteristics of the population used as a referent group; and (4) all of the above variations in combination, plus other uncontrolled contaminants. A marked difference in incidence of mental retardation would be expected between two studies, one of which employed a rather loose relative definition, and another based on a rigid and absolute definition. For example, mental retardation could be defined as any deficiency in mental functioning relative to what reasonably would be expected of an individual given full physical integrity and environmental enrichment. This might legitimately include all persons who have failed to fully realize their presumed potential, or whose scores are lower than the highest possible scores in any of several dimensions of mental functioning; by this criterion, 99% of the population would appear retarded in mathematical reasoning relative to Albert Einstein.

If individually and competently measured intelligence scores alone were used, approximately 16% of the population would fall at least one standard deviation below the average. Using the United States population of over 200,000,000 persons, this would calculate to over 32,000,000 mentally retarded persons. With the elimination of the "borderline" segment, the estimate drops to about 3%, or 6,000,000 persons with intelligence scores below 70. It is estimated that at least 0.35% of the population, that is, about 7,000,000 persons, are moderately to profoundly retarded and would be recognizable in any society as incapable of independent existence, since their adaptive behavior would also be so highly limited. In the milder forms of intellectual deficit and where the environment demands are relatively simple, a person's adaptive behavior may be adequate to disqualify him from the designation of mental retardation. On the contrary, as suggested in preceding sections, when the environment or culture demands more abstract reasoning skills for successful adaptation, a higher incidence is likely. This largely explains why there is a considerably higher estimated prevalence of mentally retarded individuals during

Table 1. Mental Retardation Criteria

Adaptive Behavior Levels	Intellectual Functioning Deficiency	Approximate Percentage		Standard Deviation (SD)	Measured Intelligence Score	
		Mentally Retarded	Total Population		Stanford-Binet SD = 16	Wechsler SD = 15
	(borderline)	67	13	−1.01 to −2.00	68–83	70–84
I	mild	22	2.7	−2.01 to −3.00	52–67	55–69
II	moderate	6	.2	−3.01 to −4.00	36–51	40–54
III	severe	3	.1	−4.01 to −5.00	20–35	25–39
IV	profound	2	.05	−5.00	20	25

school age than for preschool or postschool ages.

Classification of Mental Retardation

Several systems of classification of mental retardation have been used during the past several decades. Each successive system has usually reflected the advancing state of the art and knowledge with respect to defining mentally retarded individuals. As more is learned about the many complexities of mental retardation, the classification systems have become increasingly detailed and correspondingly more complex. The inadequacy of earlier classification and labeling systems have been periodically challenged when enough data accumulate to demonstrate that persons have been previously misclassified and as a result have endured many inappropriate and inequitable placements in institutions, special classes, sheltered workshops, and the like. The United States Department of Health, Education, and Welfare commissioned a Task Force (Hobbs, 1975) to address the various issues involved in the classification of exceptional children, many of whom are labeled mentally retarded. This comprehensive and thoroughgoing investigation finds that many of the past practices of pigeon-holing individuals and labeling them with indelible ink has in the long run done more harm than good for the individuals and probably for the society.

Children who are categorized and labeled as different may be permanently stigmatized, rejected by adults and other children, and excluded from opportunities essential for their full and healthy development. *Yet* categorization is necessary to open doors to opportunity: to get help for a child, to write legislation, to appropriate funds, to design service pro-grams, to evaluate outcomes, to conduct research, even to communicate about the problems of the exceptional child.

Children may be assigned to inferior educational programs for years, deprived of their liberty through commitment to an institution, or even sterilized, on the basis of inadequate diagnostic procedures, with little or no consideration of due process. *Yet* we have the knowledge needed to evaluate children with reasonable accuracy, to provide suitable programs for them, and to guarantee them recognized due-process requirements.

Large numbers of minority-group children—Chicanos, Puerto Ricans, blacks, Appalachian whites—have been inaccurately classified as mentally retarded on the basis of inappropriate intelligence tests, placed in special classes or programs where stimulation and learning opportunities are inadequate, and stigmatized. *Yet* these children often do need special assistance to manifest and sharpen their unappreciated competences. Improved classification procedures could increase their chances of getting needed services.

Classification of a child can lead to his commitment to an institution that defines and confirms him as delinquent, blind, retarded, or emotionally disturbed. The institution may evoke behavior appropriate to his label, thus making him more inclined to crime, less reliant than he could be on residual vision, less bright than his talents promise, more disturbed than he would be in a normal setting. *Yet* families and communities are not equipped to sustain or contain some children; families require relief, and the child himself may need the protection and specialized services of an institution and the opportunity it presents for instruction and treatment on a twenty-four-hour basis.

We have a multiplicity of categorical legislative programs for all kinds of exceptional children. *Yet* the child who is multiply handicapped, who does not fit into a neat category, may have the most difficulty in getting special assistance.

The juvenile court system was designed to guide and protect the delinquent child, as well as to protect society, with the judge serving a near-parental function. *Yet,* because of inadequate procedural safeguards, children classified as delinquent or in need of supervision may receive harsher treatment than would an adult who had committed the same offense.

Voluntary and professional associations, organized around categories of exceptionality, have effectively pressed for financial appropriations for exceptional children. Funds and services have increased substantially in the past decade. Federal, state, and local bureaus, also organized by categories of exceptionality, are well staffed and busy. *Yet* associations, bureaus, and service agencies compete for scarce resources; there is much duplication of effort; services for children are poorly coordinated; continuity of care is seldom achieved; and children get lost in the system over and over again (Hobbs, 1975, pp. 3–4).

In addition to the above rather generic concerns about classification, there has been considerable criticism of the use of the traditional medical model for classifying mental retardation, since it relies upon the diagnosis of the etiology or cause of mental retardation. In more than half of the cases which meet the aforementioned definitional criteria, a clear-cut medical or physical etiology cannot be detected or described. This has given rise to the acronym somewhat euphemistically applied to children for whom no clear diagnosis is forthcoming, namely, GORK, which stands for God only really knows. It is of course useful to know the etiology of the mental retardation in any given individual, especially if there are known treatments which will either cure the condition or prevent further deterioration in mental functioning. Some 10% of mental retardation cases do have a clear-cut organic cause which is amenable to physical, biochemical, or perhaps surgical intervention and arrest. These are quite infrequent but sufficiently dramatic to hold out encouragement to the other 90% who would desire similar relatively simple cures. Although research for these cures continues and occasionally yields new and exciting findings, the vast majority of mental retardation is due to far more complex interactions between a person's native endowment and his environmental experiences. Therefore, any classification scheme which is based solely upon the etiology determined by a medical diagnosis is now considered to be simplistic and usually grossly inadequate for treatment planning. An etiological classification is only useful if it demonstrates the causes of a condition for which there are known cures or, at best, enables one

to make accurate predictions about the outcome of the condition.

In spite of the above reservations with respect to the medical model, the clinician is nevertheless encouraged to identify a primary cause and specific disorder whenever possible. These classification schemata follow essentially those advanced by the World Health Organization's International Classification of Diseases (1968) and the American Psychiatric Association Diagnostic and Statistical Manual of Mental Disorders (1968), both of which ascribe numerical categories to each condition. It is not within the scope of this discussion to elaborate further on the nomenclature used in the classification of mental retardation according to its many possible causes. Suffice it to say that the causes of mental retardation, regardless of its severity, are grouped under the following main headings: following infection and intoxication; following trauma or physical agent; with disorders of metabolism or nutrition; associated with gross brain disease (postnatal); associated with diseases and conditions due to unknown prenatal influence; with chromosomal abnormality; gestational disorders; following psychiatric disorder; environmental influences; other conditions.

Under each of the aforementioned headings are numerous highly specific subheadings, each having additional qualifiers. For example, in the case of mental retardation due primarily to an organic cause, an individual may have a congenital brain injury with a secondary cranial anomaly such as hydrocephalus caused by a chromosomal aberration resulting in some impairment of vision, a convulsive disorder of petit mal seizures, and a motor dysfunction of spasticity with mild diplegia. Such a classification of a condition, its cause(s), and results may be arrived at through careful physical, developmental, and neurological examinations and assigned an impressive multidigit number for the above condition. However, if the mental retardation is due to "environmental influences" or "other conditions," as is true in a majority of the less serious forms of the condition, the classification is not helpful except, perhaps, by ruling out any suspected organic causes.

One of the surest ways of preventing an individual's getting an unwarranted and perhaps permanent label is to employ an ongoing evaluation-remediation process of merely tentatively identifying the strengths and weaknesses of the client and then further refining the assessment of these as the client's ability to profit from trial remediation procedures is observed and evaluated. This approach does not commit a client to a hard and fast label. Using the scientific method, it proposes a series of hypotheses about the causes and care for an individual's apparent mental retardation. These hypotheses are confirmed or abandoned as new data are discovered while the individual grows and develops, thereby revealing new aspects of his potential. Any mental retardation classification system, which is appropriately linked to remediation, postulates only tentative categories of mental deficit with a common understanding that such a deficit may be temporary and functional or at least amenable to amelioration. Thus, with the increasing efficacy of intervention/prevention efforts, such as those by Heber et al. (1974), who authored the first major reference for classification of mental retardation (Heber, 1961), the acceptance of multidetermination and the rejection of predetermination characterize the current state of the art and knowledge. The definition of mental retardation is understood to be complex, relative, and multidimensional, requiring a vast array of interdisciplinary personnel to describe and deal adequately with its many facets. Estimates of incidence and prevalence, having abandoned the simplistic genotype-phenotype definition of mental retardation, fluctuate as functions of varied definitions.

BIBLIOGRAPHY

Developmental Disabilities Act (Public Law 91–517), 1970. P. 10.

Diagnostic and statistical manual of mental disorders (2nd ed.). Washington, D.C.: American Psychiatric Association, 1968.

Grossman, H. J. (Ed.). *Manual on terminology and classification in mental retardation* (Rev. ed.). Baltimore, Md.: Garamond/Pridemark, 1973.

Heber, R. *A manual on terminology and classification in mental retardation* (Monograph Supplement, 2nd ed.). Washington, D.C.: American Association on Mental Deficiency, 1961.

Heber, R. et al. *Rehabilitation of families at risk for mental retardation: A progress report.* Madison: University of Wisconsin, 1972.

Hobbs, N. *The futures of children, categories, labels, and their consequences.* San Francisco, Calif.: Jossey-Bass, 1975a.

Hobbs, N. (Ed.). *The classification of exceptional children.* San Francisco, Calif.: Jossey-Bass, 1975b.

Hunt, J. *Intelligence and experience.* New York: Ronald Press, 1961.

International classification of diseases (8th rev. ed.). World Health Organization, 1968.

Meier, J. H. Prevalence and characteristics of learning disabilities in second grade children. *Journal of Learning Disabilities,* 1971, *4* (1), 1–16.

John H. Meier

MENTAL RETARDATION: ETIOLOGY

It is basic in understanding the complex issues of mental retardation to recognize that it is not a single disease entity. Mental retardation is merely a symptom, a signpost that signifies all is not well, that developmentally some things have gone wrong. The what, when, and how may arise prenatally, perinatally, and/or postnatally and may consist of numerous and varied separate afflictions.

The time from conception to labor (the prenatal period) may give rise to problems that are genetic, to defects produced by the genes—such as a dominant gene (e.g., epiloia), a single recessive gene (e.g., gargoylism), or chromosomal defects (e.g., Down's syndrome). Other defects may stem from an abnormal intrauterine environment due to such factors as the mother's poor physical condition, heart ailment, or hypertension, which prevent proper growth and development of the fetus.

The perinatal period (the time immediately surrounding labor and delivery) is a crucial time for susceptibility to trauma. The birth process may be held up by slowed-down muscular contractions, possibly due to anesthesia given to the mother or analgesics given for pain relief. Outside assistance may then be necessary, and the nurse may pull and tug and thus inadvertently harm the infant. Likewise, if the size of the baby's head is disproportionate to the maternal pelvis, forceps may be used, possibly resulting in head injury and subsequent mental retardation. The change in temperature from the intrauterine environment immediately after delivery may also adversely affect the neonate and induce brain injury with mental retardation.

After birth, infectious diseases of bacterial or viral etiology may afflict the brain. Although infants frequently have accidents such as falling out of cribs and high chairs without any serious damage, sometimes a fall or a blow to the head causes brain injury with serious neurological complication. Lead poisoning often leads to tragic irreparable damage of brain tissue and consequent limited intellectual functioning.

The growing infant is an incipient social creature and an imitator. He needs to see, hear, babble, and play, even if his social responses are simply smiling or kicking hands and feet. If his environment lacks sights, sound, communication, and friendly human faces, the infant has no experiences in social response, physical response, or the joy of bodily movement. He will then fail to imitate, kick, follow lights and sounds, or squeal in delight. Lying in silence without stimulation, the infant missing the activities necessary to healthy growth will remain inert and underdeveloped.

Critical and frequent illnesses, lack of proper food, and parental indifference and/or neglect may in combination with the absence of stimulation eventually produce a child with little interest, no curiosity, poor attention, and lack of wholesome functioning and adjustment. Such children are frequently found in lower socioeconomic groups living in deteriorated homes, overburdened with other poorly nourished and unstimulated family members.

The term *mentally retarded* embraces the entire gamut of patients from the one totally helpless in the crib with complete lack of self-help skills to the child whose handicap is apparent only in school. *Mental retardation* is not synonymous with *mental illness,* which however, may occur as a concomitant of retardation because of associated stresses and problems. Basically the retardate's problems are his limited capacity to absorb, process, maintain, and utilize his own experiences relevantly and to acquire new experiences and learning.

It has not been easy to establish a viable definition or set of definitions of mental retardation which are clear-cut and useful. An interdisciplinary organization of professionals, the American Association on Mental Deficiency (AAMD), concerned with the complex problems of retardation, set up its own definition. According to the AAMD, *mental retardation* refers to subaverage general functioning

which originates during the developmental periods and is associated with impairment in adaptive behavior. This definition reflects a specifically developmental approach, which stresses comparisons based on standards appropriate for the child's chronological age and with emphasis on different aspects of functioning at different ages. This definition is stated in terms of general intelligence, which is evaluated together with evaluation in other areas, as motor skills, academic achievement, self-help skills, vocational skills, social skills, and community adjustment.

Causes of mental retardation may be classified temporally (prenatal, perinatal, postnatal) or in accordance with anatomopathologic and biochemical factors.

Temporal Classification

A. Prenatal Factors
   1. Hereditary—e.g., familial, metachromatic, leucoencephalopathy, cerebral sclerosis, craniostenosis
   2. Acquired in utero—e.g., infection (rubella), anoxia, hemorrhage, isoimmunization, endocrine, roentgen-ray irradiation

The prenatal influences on the fetus which relate to mental retardation arise from the effect on the dividing and differentiating embryonal cells. By the end of the first trimester of pregnancy, the fetal systems, except for the genitourinary system, are completely differentiated from the ectoderm, mesoderm, and endoderm. For this reason, it is all-important to protect from and prevent any assault on the embryonal cell via the placenta which would prevent its proper differentiation and its normal maturation. Such first-trimester assaults frequently create abortions, or worse still, viable monsters such as the anencephalic.

Assaults upon the differentiated cell in the second and third trimesters do not occur with impunity, however. In these situations, the intactness of the cell may be destroyed or its molecular function abrogated.

Prenatal assaults include untreated infection in the mother, such as syphilis, toxoplasmosis, and cytomegalic inclusion bodies, and viral disease, which can create a fetal meningoencephalitis in addition to infection of all fetal organs. Rubella can be transplacentally transmitted to the fetus. Maternal rubella has in the past been considered a cause of mental retardation in offspring. Although a typical rubella syndrome exists consisting of opthalmological and cardiac defects with microcephaly and low birth weight, the British showed that rubella infants have the same IQ curves as their controls. Other prenatal assaults include the allergic phenomena of isoimmunization (RH, ABO, etc.) leading to hyperbilirubinemia and staining of the basal ganglia. The trauma of pelvic radiation in the first trimester can kill the neural cell. Abnormal endocrine assaults from the mother which can block the fetal thyroid development or function, or render the fetus athyrotic, will cause a hypoplasia of the neural axons and dendrites and reduce neural cell mass. Fortunately, the retardation associated with athyrosis and cretinism may be happily influenced when substitution therapy is commenced prior to the infant's age of six months. Uterine abnormalities, abortive assaults, and placental deviations in the prenatal area, because of their tendency to diminish placental circulation to the fetus, create fetal anoxemia and injure neural cells in part or in toto.

B. Perinatal Factors
   1. Anoxia, hemorrhage
   2. Birth trauma

The perinatal assaults which lead to retarded mental development are those which create infantile cerebral anoxia of long degree. The trauma of the delivery, infant hemorrhage due to cord abnormalities or of clotting disorders, prematurity, postmaturity, infant respiratory distress of all variations give in common the production of cerebral anoxia by deficient cerebral blood supply or by oxygen desaturation of the circulatory system.

C. Postnatal Factors
   1. Trauma—e.g., accidental skull fracture
   2. Infections—e.g., meningitis, encephalitis
   3. Toxic—e.g., lead, arsenic, coal tar derivatives
   4. Vascular accidents—e.g., congenital aneurysms, cerebrovascular thrombosis
   5. Anoxia—e.g., carbon monoxide poisoning
   6. Neoplasm

In the postnatal period, the assault on the brain derived from infection, skull trauma, uncontrolled seizures, toxins and poisons such as carbon monoxide and lead can lead to mental retardation either by deprivation of cerebral oxygen supply or by interference with cellular structure and function.

Anatomopathologic and Biochemical Factors

A. Primary Cerebrocranial Developmental Defects
   1. Cerebral malformations—e.g., cerebral agenesis, cerebral hypoplasia, cerebral hyperplasia (macrocephaly)
   2. Cranial defects—e.g., craniostenosis, hypertelorism
   3. Congenital ectodermosis—e.g., tuberous sclerosis, cerebral angiomatosis (Sturge-Weber syndrome), neurofibromatosis
   4. Mongolism
   5. Familial defect (defective or inferior intelligence in one or both parents and in other siblings)
   6. Undifferentiated cerebrocranial defect (primary amentia) (As our knowledge of cerebral physiology and pathology increases, the number of cases placed in this last category will decline.)
B. Secondary Cerebral Malformations
   1. Porencephaly—e.g., from trauma
   2. Hydrocephalus—e.g., from congenital anomalies of the central nervous system, intracranial hemorrhage associated with birth trauma or anoxia, infection of neoplasm
C. Central Nervous System Abnormalities Associated with Metabolic Defects
   1. Phenylpyruvic oligophrenia
   2. Galactosemia
   3. Cretinism (congenital hypothyroidism)

4. Gargoylism (Hurler's syndrome, dysostosis multiplex)
5. Hepatolenticular degeneration (Wilson's disease)
6. Reticuloendotheliosis—e.g., Gaucher's disease, Niemann-Pick disease
7. Maple syrup syndrome

D. Acquired Focal or Disseminated Central Nervous System Lesions
   1. Posttoxic and infection—e.g., lead encephalopathy, viral encephalitis, kernicterus
   2. Posttraumatic lesions
   3. Posthypoxic lesions

E. Degenerative Disorders of the Central Nervous System
   1. Cerebroocular degeneration (Tay-Sachs disease, amaurotic familial idiocy)
   2. Demyelinating encephalopathies

F. Functional Mental Retardation (Pseudoretardation) (These conditions may sometimes be confused with psychosis because of the severity of the secondary, overlying emotional problems. They have been discussed above as comprising visual, auditory, and speech handicaps, which by leading to problems in communication may cause a spuriously low IQ to be recorded by the psychologists. A similar situation may pertain in the case of the hyperkinetic dyslexia with reading problems and inability to concentrate.)

BIBLIOGRAPHY

CARTER, C. H. (Ed.). *Medical aspects of mental retardation.* Springfield, Ill.: Thomas, 1965.
FORD, F. R. Intoxications, metabolic and endocrine disorders, dietary deficiencies and allergies involving the nervous system. In *Diseases of the nervous system in infancy, childhood and adolescence* (Rev. ed.). Springfield, Ill.: Thomas, 1966. Pp. 549–800.
NYHAN, W. L. (Ed.). *Amino acid metabolism and genetic variation.* New York: McGraw-Hill, 1967.
PENROSE, L. S. *The biology of mental defect* (Rev. ed.). London: Sidgwick and Jackson, 1966.
PURPURA, D. P., and REASER, G. P. (Eds.). *Methodological approaches to the study of brain maturation and its abnormalities.* Baltimore: University Park Press, 1974.

See also MENTAL RETARDATION: ORGANIC ASPECTS

MARGARET J. GIANNINI

MENTAL RETARDATION: GOVERNMENTAL POLICIES

The President's Committee on Mental Retardation (PCMR) has an executive mandate to advise the President of the United States on the effectiveness of the national effort to combat mental retardation, and on the potential of federal programs for achieving the president's goals in this field. The committee also provides liaison between government and private organizations, and develops and disseminates information about mental retardation.

The committee has seen much progress in the field since PCMR was established in 1966 in terms of prevention, humane services, full citizenship, and public attitudes—the four major areas of committee concern.

One must be aware of unmet needs and great gaps in our knowledge of biomedical and environmental causes, and of insufficient application of existing knowledge about ways to minimize the occurrence of retardation. Many communities lack the spectrum of quality services that would enable retarded people to live full lives and they continue to fail in upholding the legal rights of retarded citizens. The residue of unfavorable attitudes stemming from earlier misconceptions about retardation remains in our society.

Etiological Factors

In the field of prevention, medical science has learned, for example, how to deal with the Rh factor in a relatively simple way; there is now a vaccine against rubella, and there are improved tests and treatments for phenylketonuria (PKU). However, current medical research knowledge is not yet being applied to all affected mothers and infants and the rate of immunization against rubella has declined. Forty-three states require testing of newborns for phenylketonuria, with the result that, since 1966 when PKU screening was first performed, there have been no new admissions to institutions of children retarded because of PKU.

There is the need to alert both the health professions and the general population, especially those at greatest risk. For example, although women over 35 account for only 13% of all pregnancies, 50% of babies with Down's syndrome are born to women over 35. If all women in this age group were informed of this risk, more of them might ascertain through amniocentesis whether their fetus has this defect, and if so, decide whether to continue to term.

Family planning can be used in order to have children when their chances of being well-born are best, that is, when the mother is between the ages of 18 and 34. Between amniocentesis and family planning, it should be possible to reduce the incidence of Down's syndrome by more than 50%.

There are many gaps in the understanding of the causes and treatment of mental retardation. Although more than 1,800 genetic disorders have been described in scientific literature no specific biomedical cause has been found for more than 20% of all cases of mental retardation. Even though one can assume that a significant portion of the remainder are attributable to socioenvironmental causes, it seems reasonable to expect that intensified research will find more biomedical causes—poor nutrition, for example.

The National Institute for Child Health and Human Development funds research and research training in both the biomedical and behavioral aspects of mental retardation, which in fiscal 1975 amounted to more than $18 million.

Conley (1973) cited a study in a Maryland county showing that children born into the lowest socioeconomic class were almost 13 times as likely to be retarded as those born into one of the upper three social classes. Although the disadvantages associated with poverty will not be eliminated in the near future, it does seem possible to focus preventive activity on some of the factors most relevant to mental retardation.

Governmental Preventive Action

The federally funded Milwaukee project of Heber (President's Committee on Mental Retardation, 1972) strongly suggested that the cycle of retardation that exists in perhaps 10% of disadvantaged families can be broken by a program of developmental stimulation beginning in infancy, combined with assistance to the parents. Making the parent a partner helps assure continuing stimulation once the child leaves the program and enters an elementary school. This may counter the regressive trend

observed in some children after they leave the beneficial environment of an early childhood program like Head Start projects for young children.

Two other important aspects of the environment influencing retardation which are the subjects of government programs are maternal and child health care from the prenatal stage onward, and nutrition for mothers and children. They bear particularly on the matter of prematurity and low birth weight, both associated with a higher risk of mental retardation.

Under the Social Security Act, the federal government assists the states in providing a variety of maternal and child health services. These include prenatal and postnatal care, family planning services, genetic counseling, clinical services for mentally retarded children from diagnosis through treatment, and training personnel to work with mentally retarded children.

For example, 335,200 mothers received care in maternity clinics during the year 1973, and 75,618 children were served by mental retardation clinics. The latter not only provide treatment plans that minimize disability, but in many cases "unlabel" children—10,786 of those classified were found not to be retarded.

Appropriations for maternal and child health services in fiscal year 1975 totaled $294,868,000, including both formula grants to the states, and research and training grants for projects such as cytogenetic laboratories. These figures of course cover all mothers and children who are served, not just those where retardation is involved.

It is estimated that all expenditures by the United States Department of Health, Education, and Welfare (HEW) on behalf of the retarded (including income maintenance and the prevention of retardation) totaled $1.75 billion in fiscal 1975, an increase of 16.7% over 1974. State and local governments' expenditures are far greater. Conley (1973) estimated that in 1970 these jurisdictions spent $2.5 billion just for residential and community care services.

The federal money can have a significant catalytic effect, however, in funding demonstration projects that break new ground. And new ground is being broken, in all sectors of the mental retardation field.

There is a definite trend to minimize placement of retarded persons in institutions, and to provide residential and service alternatives in normal community settings. HEW's developmental disabilities program assists through formula grants to the states, grants to projects of national significance, and support of research and training programs at university-affiliated facilities. Public institution populations were reduced almost 9% between fiscal years 1970 and 1974 (Scheerenberger, 1975). PCMR seeks an acceleration of this trend.

The public school systems are opening to hundreds of thousands of mentally retarded children previously barred. In some cases, this is the result of landmark court decisions, such as *Mills* v. *Board of Education of the District of Columbia*. In others, state legislatures have set firm dates for providing public education to all children regardless of handicap. HEW's Bureau of Education for the Handicapped has several programs that contribute to this process.

The legal rights of retarded persons are recognized on many fronts. For those in institutions, this means a right to habilitative treatment, to pay for work done, and to periodic review of the need to remain as residents. For those in the community, it means a right to protection against compulsory sterilization, the right to marry, the right to vote, the rights of citizens generally. In this process, PCMR has played a leadership role, convening the first national conference on The Mentally Retarded Citizen and the Law, and cooperating with the United States Department of Justice as it participated in suits, first as *amicus curiae* and then as plaintiff.

Public Opinion

Public attitudes toward retarded persons also appear to be improving. A Gallup poll commissioned by PCMR in 1974 showed that 85% of those polled would not object to mildly or moderately retarded persons occupying a home on their block, and 91% would not object to having a trained worker who is mildly or moderately retarded employed where they work. These are considerably better responses than those given to questions in a 1970 survey (Gottwald, 1970) that were similar though not identical. The gains may be attributable to the public information efforts of PCMR and other organizations, via radio, television, and print channels.

PCMR is preparing a report to the President on the needs in the field until the year 2000. The volumes in this report are called the *Century of Decision* series.

BIBLIOGRAPHY

Conley, R. W. *The economics of mental retardation.* Baltimore, Md.: Johns Hopkins University Press, 1973.

Gottwald, H. *Public awareness about mental retardation.* Reston, Va.: The Council for Exceptional Children, 1970.

President's Committee on Mental Retardation. *MR 71: Entering the era of human ecology.* Washington, D.C.: PCMR, 1972.

Scheerenberger, R. C. *Current trends and status of public residential services for the mentally retarded, 1974.* Madison, Wisc.: National Association of Superintendents of Public Residential Facilities, 1975.

Fred J. Krause

MENTAL RETARDATION: MOTOR LEARNING AND PERFORMANCE

Mental retardation is almost invariably accompanied by impairment in both fine and gross motor skills. The greater the intellectual deficit, the more pronounced is the motor inadequacy. Impairment in motor behavior is usually seen early in life, for the retarded infant is slow in the development of such postural and locomotor functions as sitting, creeping, crawling, standing and walking. Similarly, he is late in acquiring control of the muscles of the fingers and hand. Historically, the mentally retarded child's movements have been perceived as being clumsy and awkward, a characteristic believed to hold little promise for improvement.

The exact causes of the general motor impairment of retardates are not yet fully understood. It is clearly a central nervous system deficit, for the receptor mechanisms of these children seem to function within the normal range. Reflex responses of the mentally retarded have been shown to be normal, but both simple and choice reaction times are slower than in intellectually normal children.

Motor Performance

The assessment of the motor abilities of the mentally retarded have traditionally used one of two general procedures: (1) the age of acquisition of particular motor functions, such as standing and walking; (2) tests of fine and gross motor performance that have been used with normal children. The former are employed primarily with infants and preschool-age retardates, the latter with those of school-age and adults.

Tests of fine motor skill designed to assess such capabilities as tracking, speed and precision of placing, positioning and turning small objects have been successfully used with retardates. These include such tests as the Minnesota Rate of Manipulation, the Purdue Pegboard, and the pursuit rotor. Physical fitness and gross motor performance has traditionally been tested by measures of strength, power, agility, coordination, balance, flexibility, and physical work capacity. The use of track and field tests is often employed under the assumption that these measures draw upon the above components of motor performance in addition to assessing types of movement that are used in recreational pursuits.

The Lincoln-Oseretsky Motor Development Scale (Sloan, 1955) standardized on 749 children (ages 6 to 14 years) separately normed, for boys and girls, has been rather widely used in research with retarded children. This Binet-like test, a reduction from the original 85-item Oseretsky Scale to 36 items, has acceptable reliability and purported validity based on test content and the age discriminatory power of the test items.

Gross Motor Performance. The muscular strength, power, and gross motor coordination of educable mentally retarded (EMR) children has been shown to be well below that of intellectually normal children (Francis and Rarick, 1959). While the age and sex trends are similar to those in normal children, the performance lag of educable retardates is two to four years. The magnitude of the lag increases with age and with the complexity of the motor task.

Exceptions to the above noted lag are not uncommon for Rarick, Dobbins, and Broadhead (1976) have shown that on both fine and gross motor tests many EMR children perform above the seventy-fifth percentile of their intellectually normal counterparts. However, the overall magnitude of motor deficiency of some 261 EMR children (ages 6–13 years) based on 39 gross and fine motor tasks was substantial, that of the retarded boys and girls being .91 and 1.56

standard deviations below their respective normal counterparts. The reason for the relatively greater deficit in motor performance of retarded girls is not clear. It may be that more boys than girls are mistakenly assigned to special classes because of behavioral or learning problems rather than for clear-cut evidence of mental retardation.

Few large scale investigations have been done on the gross motor performance of trainable mentally retarded (TMR) children. Clinical observations of TMRs indicate substantial retardation in the acquisition of postural, locomotor and self-sufficiency skills—the age of first sitting unsupported, 10 to 24 months; walking alone, 14 to 36 months; toilet trained, 24 to 72 months; and dressing unassisted, 5 years and over. Findings by Londeree and Johnson (1974) on the gross motor performance of a large sample of institutional TMRs, ages 6–19 years, shows that the extent of motoric impairment in measures of strength, power, coordination, and endurance is indeed great, much greater than might be predicted from the performance of EMR and normal children. The data suggest that the relationship between intelligence and gross motor performance becomes exponential when the population includes both EMR and TMR children.

Fine Motor Control. The performance of retardates on tasks requiring fine motor control is generally substandard. Rarick, Dobbins, and Broadhead (1976) report that on five fine visual-motor tasks EMR girls were on the average 2.1 standard deviations below the mean of normal girls, whereas the deficit in the retarded males was 1.38 standard deviations. On none of the five tasks were the girls as a group better than the boys. The magnitude of impairment in the fine visual-motor tasks was relatively greater than the previously cited impairment in the gross motor tasks.

Clinical observations of the fine visual-motor performance of TMR children indicate that they respond at a level consistent with what has previously been noted on their gross motor proficiency. However, with proper training many adult retardates can and do perform rather intricate visual-motor tasks as skillfully as most normals.

Physical Work Capacity. The physical work capacity of retarded children, as assessed by either maximum aerobic capacity or by the physical work performed at a given heart rate, is generally less than of intellectually normal children. While the difference in aerobic capacity between marginally retarded girls and normal girls is not great, the difference between similarly classified boys is substantial (Bar-Or et al., 1971). Likewise, the physical work capacity of retarded boys and girls at a heart rate of 170 beats per minute is less for retardates than for normals, the difference being greater for boys than girls. The lower work capacity of retardates is in all probability a reflection of the more sedentary mode of life of these children.

Variability of Motor Performance. Wide individual differences in motor performance are as characteristic of mentally retarded children as is their relatively low level of motor skill. The coefficient of variation on most fine and gross motor tests is from 25–50% greater in retardates than in normals (Rarick, Dobbins, and Broadhead, 1976).

Motor Performance and Intelligence. Within a limited IQ range the correlation between measures of intelligence and measures of gross motor skill is positive, but low. In a national survey of the gross motor performance of 4200 EMR children, 152 of 154 correlations were positive, but the majority were in the .20s and .30s (Rarick, Widdop, and Broadhead, 1970). Correlations between intelligence and measures of fine visual-motor coordination are also low and of approximately the same magnitude as the correlations with gross motor tasks. Those activities that are relatively complex have higher correlations with measured intelligence than do less complex tasks.

The fact that many high functioning retardates perform effectively in sheltered workshops suggests that their motor impairment may be as much a function of limited opportunity as of mental deficiency. Furthermore, the limited opportunities for these children to engage in the usual physical education and perceptual-motor training programs may well be a contributing factor in their motor inadequacy.

Interrelationships Among Motor Abilities. The interrelationship among motor abilities in retardates is moderate to low. This is true for both fine and gross motor skills (Rarick, Dobbins, and Broadhead, 1975). Tests that require similar capabilities show moderate intercorre-

lations. Measures of dynomometric strength have intercorrelations for both sexes (age span of three years) in the range of .30 to .80. Tasks requiring elements of speed, power, and coordination generally show intercorrelations in the range .40 to .70. Intercorrelations among measures of fine visual-motor abilities are in the range .35 to .75. Intercorrelations among measures requiring different capabilities are generally low. The magnitude of the intercorrelations among motor tests in retardates is similar to that in normals.

Factor Structure of Motor Abilities

Factor analysis has been effectively used in identifying the basic components of motor performance in normal children and adults, and has in recent years been used successfully with mentally retarded children. The factor structure of motor abilities of normal and educable mentally retarded children is indeed quite similar as evidenced by a factor analysis study (Rarick, Dobbins, and Broadhead, 1976) in which a battery of 47 measures of body size, gross motor, and fine visual-motor performance was administered to a sample of 406 normal and EMR boys and girls (two groups of normal and four groups of EMRs). The comparable common and comparable specific factors extracted from each of the six intercorrelation matrices were indeed similar as evidenced by the similarity of variables with high loadings on each. The comparable common factors were tentatively identified as strength-size power, gross limb-eye coordination, fine visual-motor coordination, fat or dead weight, balance, and leg power and coordination. A quantified comparison of the factor structures of the six groups of subjects was made employing the procedure of Kaiser, Hunka, and Bianchini (1971). Using as the base the orthogonally rotated incomplete principal components solution, the consistently high cosines among comparable factors verified the previously noted similarity in the factor structures of the six groups.

Similar results using the technique described above were obtained by Rarick and McQuillan (1976) in a factor analytic study of seven sex-age groups of TMR children. Comparable common factors identified as fine visual-motor coordination, balance, fat (dead weight), upper limb-eye coordination, hand-arm strength, leg power-coordination, and spinal flexibility were extracted in each group from the intercorrelation matrices of 45 variables. Thus the factor structures of normal, EMR, and TMR children regardless of disability, age, and sex are indeed quite similar. While a factor structure is a reflection of the variables used (almost identical in these investigations), the fact remains that the several factor structures were so much alike that one must conclude that given a common set of variables the motor abilities of children are structured in much the same way regardless of age, sex, and intelligence.

Motor Learning

The difficulty that retarded children have in acquiring both fine and gross motor skills is widely recognized. The exact reasons for this difficulty are not well understood. Clearly, some motor tasks have many intellectually dependent factors, others have few. It is generally agreed that the retarded's learning problems relate to such factors as task complexity, past experience with similar tasks, the steps involved in task execution, and the attention given to the task. However, most retardates can acquire simple motor skills and many can with extensive practice learn to master reasonably complex coordinations.

Research on the impact of mental retardation on motor learning has used both short-term (within day) controlled experiments and experiments conducted over weeks and months under conditions less well controlled, but designed to simulate conditions in the real world. The former have been patterned after traditional learning experiments, using primarily fine visual-motor tests such as the pursuit rotor, maze learning, and tasks of manual dexterity.

More recently learning experiments with retardates have used the stabilometer, a device designed to assess an individual's ability to maintain equilibrium while standing upright on a delicately balanced platform supported at its midline by a knife edge. This is an unfamiliar but reliable gross motor task, one in which good learning curves can be established in ten to twelve 30-second trials.

Fine Visual-Motor Learning. Early research has shown that in maze learning moderately retarded children learn somewhat more slowly than normal children of the same age, the young retardates using trial-and-error learning, whereas the older retardates tend to employ a strategy of *general orientation,* an approach characteristically used by older normals. Thus, the learning characteristics of older moderately retarded would seem to be more like that of older normals than like that of younger normals.

Studies with the pursuit rotor, comparing the learning curves of mildly retarded and normal subjects of equal chronological age (CA) have clearly demonstrated the superiority of normals in terms of both massed and distributed practice with no differential effect of practice schedules. Larger reminiscence gains regardless of practice schedule favor the normals.

The relative effects of CA, IQ, and MA (mental age), on the learning of fine motor tasks are still not clear. With moderately retarded groups, the correlations between MA and learning scores are generally low. Learning experiments using normals and mildly retarded children (equal CA groups) give positive correlations between IQ and initial trials although retardates tend to show the greater performance gains. The research generally supports an equal MA advantage for retardates on such fine motor tasks as object assembly, card sorting, and letter coding. Findings on pursuit rotor or mirror drawing tasks are still not sufficient to postulate an equal MA deficit. It is apparent that both task difficulty and amount of practice are both factors of major importance in perceptual motor learning of retardates. It is the general concensus that MA determines the upper limit of task complexity that the retarded can master. However, the initial performance disadvantage of the retarded can with practice be overcome if the task is within the range of his ability.

Gross Motor Learning. The gross motor learning of EMRs (stabilometer) compares favorably with the learning of normals (equal CA), although the retardates' initial scores tend to be significantly poorer. Variability in learning is substantially greater in EMRs than in normals. The older children learn significantly more than the younger, and the boys learn more than the girls. Poor initial performance is often associated with no measurable improvement or with a performance decrement. Overlearning on the stabilometer has been shown to be almost as effective in skill retention in EMRs as in normals. Stabilometer learning of TMRs is negligible under the experimental conditions used with EMRs and normals.

Little systematic attention has been given to the relationship of gross motor performance and learning to mental age. The limited data available suggest that with equal MA retardates perform and learn the less complex gross motor skills as well or better than normals. The physical maturity and greater body size of the older retardate would seem to be critical factors for their success in these tasks.

The evidence is reasonably clear that well designed and carefully administered programs of physical education result in substantial improvements in the gross motor performance of EMR children. Improvements in gross motor performance of EMR children occur more readily from individualized than group oriented instruction and performance gains are greater in older than younger children (Rarick, Dobbins, and Broadhead, 1976).

It is reasonably well established that most moderately retarded boys can achieve performance levels in many sports skills on par with average normals, if properly motivated and if given instruction by a patient and knowledgeable teacher. No well-controlled investigations of the impact of organized physical education programs on the development of gross motor skills in TMR children have been conducted. Investigations of this kind are long overdue.

Several theories have been proposed to explain the general performance and learning inadequacies of the mentally retarded. Those in support of the *big deficit* theory postulate that the deficiency is based on a single factor, such as long-term retention deficit, incidental learning deficit, attention deficit, or a faulty association of verbal and motor signaling systems. Others support the *little deficits* theory which holds that learning deficiencies stem from an interaction of many conditions which together adversely affect performance and learning. In view of what is known today about the specificity of motor behavior and the many variables which affect motor learning, it is difficult to accept a single general factor as the cause. Furthermore the *little deficits* theory recognizes the probability that certain deficits are more critical than are others at different levels of retardation and have different etiological classifications.

Motor performance and motor learning tasks have in the past been useful in testing learning theories and will undoubtedly be used for this purpose in the future. However, much of the motor learning research in the future will be used not only as a tool for studying how retardates learn, but as a means of determining how the lives of such persons can be enriched.

BIBLIOGRAPHY

BAR-OR, O.; SKINNER, J. S.; BERGSTEINOVA, V.; SHEARBURN, C.; ROYER, D.; BELL, W.; HAAS, J.; and BUSKIRK, E. R. Maximal aerobic capacity of 6–15 year-old girls and boys with subnormal intelligence quotients. *Acta Paediatrica Scandinavica Supplement,* 1971, *217,* 108–113.

FRANCIS, R. J., and RARICK, G. L. Motor characteristics of the mentally retarded. *American Journal of Mental Deficiency,* 1959, *63,* 292–311.

KAISER, H. F.; HUNKA, S.; and BIANCHINI, J. D. Relating factors between studies based on different individuals. *Multivariate Behavioral Research,* 1971, *6,* 409–422.

LONDEREE, B. R., and JOHNSON, L. E. Motor fitness of TMR vs EMR and normal children. *Medicine and Science in Sports,* 1974, *6,* 247–252.

RARICK, G. L.; WIDDOP, J. H.; and BROADHEAD, G. D. The physical fitness and motor performance of educable mentally retarded children. *Exceptional Children,* 1970, *36,* 509–519.

RARICK, G. L.; DOBBINS, D. A.; and BROADHEAD, G. D. *The motor domain and its correlates in educationally handicapped children.* Englewood Cliffs, N.J.: Prentice-Hall, 1976.

RARICK, G. L., and MCQUILLAN, J. P. *The factor structure of motor abilities of trainable mentally retarded children: Implications for curriculum development.* Final Report for HEW, Office of Education funded project no. H0006SN. Berkeley: University of California, 1976.

SLOAN, W. The Lincoln-Oseretsky motor development scale. *Genetic Psychology Monographs,* 1955, *51,* 183–252.

G. LAWRENCE RARICK

MENTAL RETARDATION: ORGANIC ASPECTS

Historical Review

Mental retardation may be viewed as medical, psychological, or educational, but in its final analysis it is primarily a social problem. This explains the fact that throughout history the attitude toward the mentally retarded often reflected the general social attitudes of a people or culture.

In more recent times there were three distinct junctures characterized by great public interest and professional creative thinking in the field of mental retardation. Characteristically, they all followed periods of great social upheaval, resulting in a popular adoption of more liberal attitudes toward society's less fortunate members, including the mentally retarded.

The first germinal period in the field of mental retardation coincided with the time of the French and American Revolutions and their ideas of equality and rights for all men. These upset the feudal, vertical social structure. The times of Itard and his pioneering labors were also the times of Pinel, who unchained the insane, and facilitated the beginning of a popular vote and social legislation.

The second period followed the revolutions that swept Europe in 1848. In the wake of this period a further liberalization of public opinion and gradually increasing legislative justice took place.

The third, our present period, followed World War II. The great resurgence of professional and public interest in mental retardation and its sudden respectability are the result of several, not necessarily related, factors. Again, probably the most important was the radical change in the social climate felt everywhere on the local, national, and international level. As if to atone for the ravages of World War II, the postwar trend has been toward securing equal rights and opportunities for all human beings. These include the colonial nations of Asia and Africa, racial and religious minorities everywhere, the old, the very young, the poor, the sick, as well as the retarded.

Thus, the social climate has been favorable for overcoming the traditional public inertia regarding mental illness and mental retardation. Suddenly, in the early 1960s the retarded were viewed as individuals with inherent needs and rights. Various civic groups became champions of those rights in the forum of the federal, state, and local governments. In the United States, in the best American tradition of self-help, the National Association for Retarded Children, founded in the 1950s by groups of parents of retarded children, has been the *spiritus movens* of the radical change in public opinion in favor of the retarded. This had its greatest momentum from John Kennedy's President's Panel on Mental Retardation.

Definition

The biomedical and sociocultural adaptational models represent the two major approaches to the conceptual definition of mental retardation. The adherents of the former insist on the presence of basic changes in the brain as a sine qua non in the diagnosis of mental retardation. The proponents of the latter, on the other hand, emphasize the social functioning and general adaptation to accepted norms. Each of these approaches has many ramifications that complicate the issue even further.

The sociopsychological approach focuses on the developmental impairment in infancy and preschool years, on learning difficulties in school age, and on poor social-vocational adjustment in adulthood.

Most people agree that mental retardation has to be considered as a multidimensional phenomenon that involves overlapping physiological, psychological, medical, educational, and social aspects of human functioning and behavior.

Nomenclature

Mental deficiency, which is one of the terms used in the American Psychiatric Association's manual on terminology and classification to designate subaverage intellectual functioning, is often used interchangeably with *mental retardation.* Recently, however, the World Health Organization recommended the use of the term *mental subnormality,* which in turn is divided into two separate and distinct categories: mental retardation and mental deficiency. According to this nosology, mental retardation is reserved for subnormal functioning due to pathological causes, while mental deficiency results from environmental deprivation.

Classification

The pluridimensional character of mental retardation is also reflected in the various approaches to classification of this condition. Essentially, they all deal with the developmental characteristics, potential for education and training, and social and vocational adequacy.

The degrees of levels of retardation are expressed in various terms. The following terms are recommended by the World Health Organization: *mild subnormality* (IQ 50 to 69); *moderate subnormality* (IQ 20 to 49); and *severe subnormality* (IQ 0 to 19). The American Association on Mental Deficiency and the American Psychiatric Association adopted the terms *borderline* (IQ 70 to 89); *mild* (IQ 55 to 69); *moderate* (IQ 40 to 54); *severe* (IQ 25 to 39); and *profound* (IQ 0 to 24). The terms *idiot, imbecile,* and *moron* still enjoy some popularity in Europe but are seldom used in the United States. In addition, the mentally retarded are often divided into educable, trainable, and custodial to reflect their level of competence, which has become the principal guideline for establishment of suitable programs, particularly educational and vocational.

Epidemiology

It is estimated that 3% (6,000,000) of the United States population are mentally retarded. This often quoted estimate is only approximate, since there are no precise data available, except in a few areas of the country.

The overwhelming majority (87%) of the mentally retarded fall into the mild category, and the remainder (13%) belong to the moderate, severe, and profound groups. Many mildly retarded and those of borderline intelligence are not innately retarded, but rather victims of environmental deprivation. Mild remediable handicapping conditions which could lead to learning disorders often are unrecognized and dealt with when they could be corrected.

Etiological Considerations in Organically Based Mental Retardation

Since Garrod's original description of alkaptonuria in 1908, the inborn errors of metabolism have commanded the attention of researchers and clinicians, exceeding by far their relative frequency. The total of all the known hereditary metabolic defects probably accounts for only a minority of mental defectives, but the lessons already learned from the study of these disorders point to exciting diagnostic, therapeutic, and preventive possibilities. Further biochemical research may bring the number of metabolic disorders to at least 10% of the mentally retarded group.

The success of dietary measures in phenylketonuria (PKU), maple syrup disease, and galactosemia represent a major triumph in the medical treatment of mental retardation which heretofore had operated on a hit-or-miss basis. Although the mechanism or injury to the central nervous system in these disorders is not known, it is believed to be a result of abnormal accumulation of metabolites. The therapy is based on the principle of dietary omission to circumvent a specific enzymatic block. This in turn helps to eliminate potential injury to the central nervous system. Another therapeutic approach consists of dietary *addition* of essential metabolites, such as the addition of cystine in homocystinuria. Following are some representative examples of the various etiological groupings.

Disorders of Amino Acid Metabolism

Phenylketonuria (PKU). First discovered by Folling in 1934, phenylketonuria has become known as the inborn error of metabolism associated with mental retardation, par excellence.

PKU is transmitted as a simple recessive autosomal Mendelian trait. Its frequency in the United States and various parts of Europe ranges between 1 in 10,000 to 1 in 20,000. The basic metabolic defect in PKU is an inability to convert phenylalanine, an essential amino acid, to para-tyrosine because of the absence or inactivity of the liver enzyme phenylalanine hydroxylase, which catalyzes this conversion. This in turn gives rise to several abnormal biochemical findings, such as (1) elevated phenylalanine in the blood (10 to 25 times normal) and cerebrospinal fluid, excretion of an abnormal metabolite, phenylpyruvic acid, in the urine as well as phenylalanine (30 to 50 times normal) and several derivatives; (2) a related disturbance of tryptophan and tyrosine metabolism, leading to a marked decrease in serum serotonin and lower than normal blood levels of epinephrine and norepinephrine.

The majority of patients with PKU are severely retarded, but some patients are reported to have borderline or normal intelligence. Eczema and convulsions are present in about a third of all cases. Electroencephalogram (EEG) is abnormal in about 80%, even in patients without convulsions, showing irregular spike and wave discharges. The majority of patients are undersized, have light complexion, coarse features and the head tends to be small. Although the clinical picture varies, typical PKU children are hyperactive and exhibit erratic, unpredictable behavior, which makes them difficult to manage. Verbal and nonverbal communication is usually severely impaired or nonexistent. Coordination is poor, and perceptual difficulties are many. The original description of PKU patients as blond and blue-eyed (due to a relative deficiency of melanin, a by-product of tyrosine) applies to some, especially in the younger age group.

Early diagnosis is of extreme importance, since a low phenylalanine diet, in use since 1955, results in significant improvement in both behavior and developmental progress. The best results seemed to be obtained with early diagnosis and the start of the dietary treatment prior to 6 months of age.

Disorders of Fat Metabolism

Cerebromacular degenerations. The cerebromacular degenerations represent a group of disturbances in which there is progressive mental deterioration and loss of visual function. They are all transmitted by an autosomal recessive gene. The four types of cerebromacular degeneration differ as to the age of onset. The earliest one, Tay-Sachs disease, occurs chiefly among Jewish infants, particularly those from Eastern Europe; the others are found in members of all races.

Disorders of Carbohydrate Metabolism

Galactosemia. Galactosemia is transmitted by an autosomal recessive gene. Its metabolic defect, detected in 1956 by Kalckar et al., consists of the inability to convert galactose to glucose, because of the enzymatic defect of galactose 1-phosphate uridyltransferase.

The clinical manifestations begin after a few days of milk feeding and include jaundice, vomiting, diarrhea, failure to thrive, and hepatomegaly. If milk is not eliminated from the diet, the disease may be fatal within a short time, or it may lead to progressive mental deterioration, associated with cataracts, he-

patic insufficiency, and occasional hypoglycemic convulsions.

Hormonal Disturbances

Goitrous cretinism. Cretinism as a condition associated with mental retardation has been known since antiquity. Throughout modern history up to the middle of the nineteenth century, all forms of mental retardation were considered as variants of this condition.

The classical endemic variety occurs in certain regions as a result of iodine deficiency in the diet. Sporadic athyreosis, congenital absence of the thyroid gland, is the common variety in this country and may be caused by transplacental transmission of immune bodies against thyroid from the mother.

The clinical signs in all varieties include hypothyroidism, goiter (except in athyreosis), dwarfism, coarse skin, disturbances in ossification, hypertelorism, and a large tongue. Mental retardation becomes a part of the clinical picture if the disease is unrecognized and untreated in infancy.

The children are sluggish, their voices hoarse, and speech does not develop. Among the laboratory findings are a low basal metabolism rate, depressed protein-bound iodine, and a high cholesterol level. The radioactive iodine uptake is low, except in the variety reported by Stanbury, which is recessively inherited.

Treatment with thyroid extract may avert most of the symptoms if instituted early in life. It is not effective in adult cretins. Endemic goitrous cretinism is treated and prevented by the ingestion of small amounts of iodine.

Chromosomal Aberrations

Down's syndrome (mongolism). Since the classical description of mongolism by the English physician Langdon Down in 1866, this syndrome has remained the most discussed, most investigated, and most controversial in the field of mental retardation.

1. Patients with trisomy 21 (3 on chromosome 21 instead of the usual 2), who represent the overwhelming majority of mongoloid patients, have 47 chromosomes, with an extra chromosome 21. The karyotypes of the mothers are normal.

2. Nondisjunction occurring after fertilization in any cell division will result in mosaicism, a condition in which both normal trisomic cells are found in various tissues.

3. In translocation, there is a fusion of two chromosomes, mostly 21 and 15, resulting in a total of 44 chromosome material. This disorder, unlike trisomy 21, is usually inherited, and the translocation chromosome may be found in unaffected parents and siblings. These asymptomatic carriers have only 45 chromosomes.

Mental retardation is the overriding feature of Down's syndrome. The majority of patients belong to the moderately and severely retarded groups, with only a minority having an I.Q. above 50.

There are over 100 signs or stigmata described in Down's syndrome, but they are rarely all found in one individual. Among the most frequently encountered are a high cephalic index, epicanthal folds, fissured tongue, dwarfed stature, small rounded ears, strabismus, white speckling of the iris (Brushfield spots), and lax ligaments. The dermal ridges on the palms and soles have a characteristic configuration, which is often diagnostic.

Infections During Pregnancy

Syphilis. Syphilis in pregnant women used to be a major cause of a variety of neuropathological changes in their offspring, including mental retardation. Today the incidence of syphilitic complications of pregnancy fluctuates with the incidence of syphilis in the general population. Some recent alarming statistics from several major cities in the United States indicate that there is still no room for complacency.

Rubella (German measles). This disease has replaced syphilis as the major cause of congenital malformation and mental retardation due to maternal infection. The children of affected mothers may present a number of abnormalities, including congenital heart disease, mental retardation, cataracts, deafness, microcephaly, and microphthalmia. Timing is crucial, since the extent and frequency of complications are in inverse proportion to the duration of pregnancy at the time of maternal infec-

tion. When mothers are infected in the first trimester of pregnancy, 10 to 15% of the children will be affected, and the incidence rises to almost 50% when the infection occurs in the 1st month of pregnancy. The situation is often complicated by subclinical forms of maternal infection, which often go undetected.

Erythroblastosis fetalis. This is the most common cause of nonphysiological jaundice and is due to mother-child incompatibility regarding the Rh factor, A or B, or (rarely) Kell, Kidd, and Duffy factors in the blood. The resulting breakdown of the infant's red cells causes bilirubinemia and anemia. Stillbirth due to a generalized edema, hydrops fetalis, occurs in some. In others kernicterus will develop. This name refers to yellow staining of the basal ganglia, cerebellum, and brain stem, resulting frequently in cerebral palsy, mental retardation, and hearing deficit.

Sociocultural Factors. It was mentioned previously that the overwhelming majority of the mentally retarded in the United States come from the lowest socioeconomic group. The frequency of the battered-child syndrome, burns, serious accidents, and ingestion of toxic substances, with inherent risks to the central nervous system, is disproportionately high in this group.

In addition, as a result of living in a world that seems hostile, without encouragement and praise, the child's self-concept, including his body image, may be faulty. The fatalistic, hopeless attitudes of the slum environment can stifle initiative and motivation.

Personality Development in Mentally Retarded Children. Differences in the degree of intellectual functioning in the mentally retarded are compounded by the divergence of etiological factors, ranging from clearly demonstrable brain damage to emotional and cultural deprivation. The resulting extreme heterogeneity of the mentally retarded group is probably responsible for the often conflicting and confusing views about the personality development and frequency of psychopathology of its members, which range widely from the assumption of little or no difference from the normal population in the frequency of emotional disturbance, to the contrasting opinions that assign to the mentally retarded a very high risk of psychotic illness—up to 40% in some studies.

Given an accepting and adequately stimulating family environment and appropriate educational and vocational training facilities, the majority of retarded children can develop good social and vocational adjustment and capacity for appropriate interpersonal interactions and attachments. However, in the process, they face hazards along the way that exceed the ones facing the normal population. Such hazards seem to increase in direct proportion to the degree of retardation.

Emotional Vulnerability

Constitutional Factors. Many mentally retarded children are unable to process and adapt to levels of sensory stimuli of more than low intensity. A rising intensity of such stimuli is perceived by the child as disturbing or even painful and may lead to behavioral disorganization. Such hypersensitivity may involve one or more sensory pathways. In cases of auditory hypersensitivity, the child may perceive noises and loud voices as painful. Infants with this handicap will become upset when exposed to the sounds of a vacuum cleaner, electric shaver, radio or television. Others cannot tolerate strong visual stimuli such as very bright and strong colors. Finally, there are infants who don't like to be touched as most infants do and show discomfort when picked up or cuddled and are at hazard for the normal type of relationship experience for which they are otherwise available.

Low Self-Esteem. The growing mentally retarded child can become progressively aware of being different from other normal people. Such an awareness may result from a self-evaluation and comparison of his performance to that of other members of his family or social group. On the other hand, it may be a reflection of the negative evaluation of the mentally retarded child by people in his environment.

Role of the Family. The child's mental retardation often induces parental inner turmoil, grief, a sense of disappointment, shattered hopes, and sometimes feelings of guilt and failure. These feelings, if unresolved, make it difficult for many parents to accept the child, to be proud of him, and to give him affection and recognition.

Psychopathology of the Mentally Retarded. While few people dispute the high frequency of psychopathology in the mentally retarded, there is less unanimity as to the nature of psychiatric disorders in this group. The most frequently seen disorders are: adjustment reactions (which frequently mask an underlying depression); chronic brain syndrome with behavior disturbance; and psychotic reactions (both process and reactive).

Prevention and Treatment

A preventive approach to mental retardation can only succeed in an educated, enlightened community. Without wholehearted support of the people for whom it is intended, the best conceived plan is doomed to failure. Basic to any real improvement in this area is the raising of the standards of living and education among disadvantaged, forgotten citizens. Improvement of prenatal care is a recognized cornerstone in all efforts to prevent mental retardation. Genetic counseling helps to clarify the question of the desirability of future offspring by the parents, siblings, and sometimes more distant relatives.

Despite considerable progress there are still only a few conditions in which early detection and treatment of hereditary disorders may prevent mental retardation. For example, prompt diagnosis and treatment of bacterial meningitis with antibiotics and occasionally with steroids may prevent neurological sequelae, including mental retardation. Prenatal diagnostic techniques have much promise in defining preventable conditions.

Acceptance by his parents despite his handicap is the best assurance of an adequate self-image of the mentally retarded individual. An opportunity for learning and developing social, academic, vocational and motor skills in a good school setting is also essential. Of special importance is the early identification and treatment of the culturally deprived child by providing a stimulating environment.

The emotional problems of the mentally retarded differ in many ways from similar ones of children with normal intelligence. Consequently, they often require methods of treatment not commonly employed with the latter group. Parent counseling is of paramount importance to ensure an optimal mileu for the retarded child and reduce the impact on the family.

The pioneers of residential care for the mentally retarded stressed education and training. The failure to realize early hopes caused a shift of emphasis. Institutions took on a custodial character, protecting the retarded individual and isolating him from the community. Today the thinking in this field has come full circle. Training, education, treatment, and rehabilitation are once again the primary goals. The area of vocational training and rehabilitation must be stressed in the overall educational program for the mentally retarded. The education of the mentally retarded shares, with the education of normal children, the goal of preparing the student for future satisfactory life adjustment and helping him develop his full potential.

Conclusion

The change in psychiatric thinking, which now stresses the interplay among biological, psychological, and cultural factors in the shaping of human personality, permits the integration of mental retardation into psychiatry, the latter seen broadly as a science concerned with human behavior.

The many hazards in the process of personality development faced by the mentally retarded point to the pivotal role of the psychiatrist in the prevention of retardation, as a consultant to other physicians, educators, and rehabilitation programs and as a direct participant, when indicated, in the treatment, care, and rehabilitation of the retarded. His training helps him recognize the innate developmental forces and environmental influences. By timely intervention, he may direct the handling of distorted personality patterns so as to identify and help interrupt patterns of pathological interaction between the retarded patient and his family or his caretakers. His training in identifying sources of anxiety and the nature of defensive maneuvers helps him in bringing about a reduction of tension, thus promoting emotional maturation and motivation for learning.

The psychiatrist's role as an interdisciplinary coordinator, currently emphasized in psychiatric training, seems especially applicable to the field of mental retardation. The complexity of the problem calls for cooperation of many medical and nonmedical specialties. His

knowledge of group dynamics and training in recognition of and dealing with the interaction of social, biological, and psychological factors places the interested psychiatrist on at least a par with the other candidates for leadership. Furthermore, as an expert in human personality development, he should play an important role in the training and education of physicians, psychologists, social workers, and educators in the field of mental retardation. His clarification of the sometimes bizarre behavior of the mentally retarded and the intrafamily tensions provoked by a retarded family member will greatly increase the effectiveness of all disciplines.

The reasons behind the institutionalization of the majority of the retarded are the behavior and attitudes that make it difficult or impossible for the individual to function in the community. The retarded child has as much right to have help with such personality disturbances as his brighter brothers and sisters. Thus, the psychiatrist has an obligation to be equally available to the retarded child and adult.

BIBLIOGRAPHY

CYTRYN, L., and LOURIE, R. S. Mental retardation. In A. M. Friedman and H. I. Kaplan (Eds.), *Comprehensive textbook of psychiatry.* Baltimore: Williams and Wilkins, 1967. Pp. 817–856.

CYTRYN, L., and LOURIE, R. S. Prevention of mental illness in the mentally retarded. In E. Katz (Ed.), *Mental health services for the mentally retarded.* Springfield, Ill.: Thomas, 1972.

HAYWOOD, H. C. (Ed.). *Socio-cultural aspects of mental retardation.* New York: Appleton-Century Crofts, 1970.

KATZ, E. (Ed.). *Mental health services for the mentally retarded.* Springfield, Ill: Thomas, 1972.

KOCH, R., and DOBSON, J. C. (Eds.). *The mentally retarded child and his family.* New York: Brunner/Mazel, 1970.

LOURIE, R. S., and RIEGER, R. Psychiatric and psychological examination of children. In S. Arieti (Ed.), *American handbook of psychiatry* (2nd ed.). New York: Basic Books, 1974.

MENOLASCINO, F. J. (Ed.). *Psychiatric aspects of the diagnosis and treatment of mental retardation.* New York: Basic Books, 1972.

PHILIPS, I. (Ed.). *Prevention and treatment of mental retardation.* New York: Basic Books, 1966.

ROBINSON, H. B., and ROBINSON, N. M. *The mentally retarded child.* New York: McGraw-Hill, 1964.

STANBURRY, J. B.; WYNGAARDEN, J. B.; and DRIEDRICKSON, D. S. (Eds.). *The metabolic basis of inherited disease.* New York: McGraw-Hill, 1972.

LEON CYTRYN
REGINALD S. LOURIE

MENTAL RETARDATION: SOCIAL ASPECTS

Capacity for social adjustment is, in most instances, the primary determining factor in designating mental retardation. Of the 3% usually referred to statistically for all categories of mental retardation, epidemiological studies of severe mental handicap adhere almost universally to a figure of only .4%. The great majority of the handicapped are therefore capable of some measure of adaptation to societal demands. Sociocultural, social class, and individual family factors determine the level of adaptability that is acceptable and the point at which the unachieving individual is perceived as socially handicapped and subject to societal concern and special planning, or disparaged as deviant and undesirable, to be ignored, scorned, or put out of sight.

Social Attitudes

Attitudes toward the retarded have not been fixed historically and have undergone major shifts consistent with social and ideological change, as well as fluctuations in popular fads and fashion. Presently, in the United States there is a strong forward movement to improve the condition of the retarded and to modify social pressures. Yet perspectives from the past remain rooted in the national consciousness and may even have been reeinforced by the increased complexity of contemporary living. The prejudices of the past are still reflected in segments of our thinking, and the heritage of unconscionable victimization of the retarded has not yet been undone.

A society committed to the Calvinist ethic of present and future reward for diligence and purposeful work, the worship of individual achievement, the inordinate valuation of physical appearance, and fear and suspicion of difference, has created a singularly hostile environment for the mentally handicapped.

In colonial America the feebleminded, like the mentally ill, were usually treated with cruelty and contempt. The suffering of the handicapped was looked upon as a judgment of providence responding to sin and wickedness. The limited institutions for the insane also admitted those termed feebleminded, and little distinction was made until well into the nineteenth century. The great majority of the institutionalized retarded were placed in poorhouses or jailed. Progress toward humanizing the condition of the retarded was well underway in Europe, particularly under the guidance of Seguin in France, when the first state institution and school for the feebleminded was established at Waverly, Massachusetts. The first institutions were conceived in an atmosphere of enthusiasm. Treatment was based on Seguin's methods, which were sound and progressive. Expectations of cure were high, but failure to reach unrealistic objectives led to disappointment and reaction. An experiment that held great promise deteriorated into pessimism and gloom. A period of hysteria and alarm was soon to follow, with beginnings approximating the appearance in 1859 of Darwin's "Origin of the Species" and the evolving concept of natural selection and the survival of the fittest. In 1877, Dugdale's study of family degeneracy, "The Jukes," was published. Its readers were quick to generalize that many social problems resulted from biologically determined "bad stock." Social Darwinism, the application and misapplication of Darwin's thinking to social processes, became a dominant intellectual theme.

In 1905, the Stanford-Binet test was developed as a way of grading and categorizing intelligence. There was growing interest in Mendelian theory, with its implication that feeblemindedness is inherited and transmitted in accordance with natural laws. The most widely read and influential of the heredity studies arrived in 1912, Goddard's "The Kallikak Family." Feeblemindedness was isolated as the primary source of social ills. The "moron" had been discovered as a major menace to society.

Professional and scientific circles accepted the new findings and almost universally regarded feeblemindedness as hereditary. There was much concern over the alleged prolific birthrate of the retarded who could eventually outnumber the normal population. Demands arose for segregation, sterilization, even euthanasia. The peak of this period was to last through the first two decades of the century. Social Darwinism posed a biological explanation for maintaining inequality and justifying lack of commitment to programs of betterment. It gave rise to the eugenics movements and its widespread abuses leading to laws requiring sterilization of the retarded in 23 states and restrictive marriage laws in others. It strengthened the worship of individual ability and competitive skill, encouraging even further devaluing of the limited. The retarded suffered in the past and are still residually affected from the uncritical and inappropriate application of the idea of natural selection in relationship to social change. The individual in society is not reducible to biology and can only be explained in terms of cultural analysis. Social improvement results from advances in technology and social organization, not from breeding and selective elimination.

The retarded have posed special dilemmas for social reformers and helping professionals. It is only more recently that either has assumed a sustained advocacy role for the rights and quality of care of the retarded and their families. The retarded have been a testament to the gap between the stated values and behavior of the community as a whole and in particular for those who should have been concerned. When the retarded were seen as a threat to civilization and somehow responsible for a multitude of social afflictions, society mobilized itself to place them under restraining observation and social control. The reformers and the professional elite of the early part of the century did not pick up their cause. Some agreed with the attacks, others were silent. From the mid-1920s through the early 1950s, the retarded were no longer denounced, but were largely disregarded in planning services and evaluating health and social needs. The substantial social adjustment problems they presented and what appeared to be their limited capacity to participate in helping processes seemed overwhelming and beyond the interest of the helping professions.

Until this time there was emphasis on social deviance. The mildly retarded, with their need for control and social planning, received most of the public attention. The severely retarded were herded off to isolated institutions or ignored in the homes of their overburdened families. It was the parents of this latter group who caused a major social shift as a result of their sustained and highly successful actions in bringing the needs of the retarded to public awareness. The parents' movement, which was middle-class-dominated, moved the concentration of concern from the mildly retarded, so-

cially deviant, mainly from the lower socioeconomic groups to the severely retarded, who are equally distributed among social and economic groups. The multiple health and special care needs of ths group encouraged the ascendancy of the medical model in understanding and servicing of the retarded. The mildly retarded were initially little differentiated, even though their needs required other kinds of intervention.

Labeling

Jane Mercer (1973) has called attention to the destructive social effects of "labeling" the mildly retarded with its built-in self-fulfilling prophecy of failure and damage to the self-concept and ego structure of the labeled individual. A social system perspective rather than a clinical one reflecting the medical model is seen as the more valid approach for the mildly retarded. Mercer differentiates the two approaches. Within the *social system perspective,* mental retardation becomes an achieved status in a social system and the role played by persons holding that status. A person is deviant if he does not meet the norms of the social system. Socialization factors determine the impact of the labeling process. Intelligence tests and clinical instruments are judged to be codifications of the middle-class norms of the American core culture. Except for gross disability, it is not possible to conceptualize intelligence as existing apart from the sociocultural matrix which creates that intelligence. The *clinical* or *medical* model, on the other hand, highlights pathology, the search for biological symptoms, and the use of statistical averages and norms. The clinical perspective views mental retardation as an individual attribute rather than a social phenomenon.

In our complex industrial society, the response to the label of mental retardation is severe and carries a host of negative cues and responses. Inability or limited capacity to contribute to the good of society is viewed as a major social disability with painful consequences for the retarded person and his family. Within this generalization there are class, economic, ethnic, and psychic factors that point up the multiplicity of social factors interacting when we attempt to understand and deal with retardation in individual human terms.

The Family

The consequences for the family of the destructive definition of retardation requires further exploration. The family is, of course, the primary social unit for the continuity and transmission of the values of the culture. Mental retardation complicates severely the family's ability to carry through this goal and prepare the child for an acceptable and contributing role in society. If labeling the individual as retarded suggests that he will not be qualified to function adequately within society, the family may also be perceived, by implication, as deviant because it has failed one of its major functions.

The retarded child can mean a crucially changed life cycle for the whole family. The presence of a family member so negatively defined in social terms can result in a family preoccupied with disability and its consequences. Society's attitudes intensify reality problems of adjustment and can present countless barriers to the natural flow of family life. The support of parents in normalizing the social functioning of the retarded is burdened by society's unwillingness to allow the normalization of the family itself. The degree to which the family accepts or rejects this vision of itself as deviant varies with its relationship to social institutional factors in the community and the family's intrapsychic strength and weaknesses.

Farber (1968) found that the level of interaction between the family and the community was influenced by the presence of retardation. Families tended to disengage from community activity and to focus their energy on intrafamily matters. The social mobility of the family is affected, particularly when a severely or moderately retarded child is born early in the marriage. Siblings are influenced in personality and life orientation, and this is more pronounced the closer they are in age to the retarded child.

Sociological findings are highly significant to the perspective of the intricate totality that is mental retardation. In immediate professional contact with families, however, it is necessary to move from an academic framework to the reality of what is being confronted. When the problem is individualized, social factors are translated into unique person-to-person terms, with the intrapsychic taking equal priority with the social forces that are engaged.

Environmental Factors

The most damaging impact of adverse social factors is encountered when we attempt to investigate the nature and extent of environmentally determined retardation. There is little agreement about terminology, and such terms as *environmental retardation, cultural disadvantage, cultural deprivation* and other so-called poverty-inspired labels are considered to have judgmental and disparaging connotations. There is little question, however, that many children are born into an impoverished and disinherited milieu with a potential for normal intellectual functioning and adequate social adaptation but fail to thrive and develop adequately. Others are the victim of the fixed kinds of assault that are a corollary of poverty—poor prenatal care, a high incidence of premature birth, nutritional deficiencies, a higher incidence of infectious illness in infancy, more frequent accidents, the danger of lead poisoning, and the infinity of other hazards in a hostile and callous environment.

The early months of life, and what the infant experiences and is exposed to is crucial. The quality of mother-child interaction, the nature of stimulation offered the child, and the extent of exposure to language, symbolic representations, and social exchange, are interrelated elements affecting the intellectual, social, and emotional adjustment of the child. Many parents in the most adverse circumstances can offer a nurturing and supportive atmosphere for the child's development. Other parents from the same impoverished world who have severely retarded children are often able to provide extraordinary acceptance and creativity in relating to their child and helping him reach his optimal level of functioning.

Those mothers of children categorized as retarded who appear unable to provide minimal stimulation to their young children are those who are most psychically traumatized by their own life experiences and the brutality of poverty life. There is often a sense of hopelessness, inertia, and indifference, which inhibit them from relating affectively to their growing children. Their anomie is characterized by an overwhelming sense of powerlessness, pessimism, and immobility. While those mothers may not be representative of mothers in poverty, they are often encountered in clinical programs for the retarded. Conventional methods of helping are usually inappropriate; flexible, innovative, outreach styles of working with clients must be introduced.

The whole question of mild retardation among low socioeconomic groups requires much further investigation. Most knowledge is speculative and presumptive. There is a strong possiblity that we are dealing with a selective or focal kind of retardation, related to distinctive presumptions and perceptions of social reality. These differ from the standard norms, particularly in relationship to the valuation of and investment in the achievement of academic goals. Often these school failures show little measurable deficits in other areas of functioning.

Social factors assume a major part in understanding the totality of mental retardation. We are often measuring deficits in societal awareness, attitudes, and commitment to human needs rather than irreversible deficits in the assumed retarded individual.

BIBLIOGRAPHY

ADAMS, M. *Mental retardation and its social dimensions.* New York: Columbia University Press, 1971.

DAVIES, S. *The mentally retarded in society.* New York: Columbia University Press, 1958.

DEUTSCH, A. *The mentally ill in America.* New York: Columbia University Press, 1949.

FARBER, B. *Mental retardation: Its social contexts and social consequences.* Boston: Houghton Mifflin, 1968.

HAYWOOD, H. C. (Ed.). *Social-cultural aspects of mental retardation.* New York: Appleton-Century-Crofts, 1970.

HOBBS, N. (Ed.). *Issues in the classification of children* (Vols. 1, 2). San Francisco: Jossey-Bass, 1975.

MERCER, J. *Labeling the mentally retarded.* Berkeley: University of California Press, 1973.

LAWRENCE GOODMAN

MENTAL RETARDATION AND ENVIRONMENT

"Mental retardation refers to significantly subaverage general intellectual functioning existing concurrently with deficits in adaptive behavior, and manifested during the developmental period." This definition of the American Association on Mental Deficiency in the 1973 edition of its *Manual on Terminology and*

Classification is probably the most used definition today. It has been adopted, sometimes with slight modifications, by other professional organizations and appears in many state regulations or laws. The significance of widespread use of this definition in a discussion of mental retardation and the environment is evident when explanation of the terms within the definition are examined.

General intellectual functioning is defined in terms of the results obtained by psychological assessment with one or more of the individually administered general intelligence tests. Since many of the tasks on such tests are related to the individual's understanding of the environment and ability to solve problems requiring such understanding, measured intelligence is not independent of the individual's history of interactions with the environment. *Significantly subaverage* refers to a score that is two or more standard deviations below the mean, or population average, of the normative sample of individuals on whom the test was standardized.

Adaptive behavior is defined as the effectiveness or degree with which an individual meets the standards of personal independence and social responsibility expected for age and cultural group. Thus, an individual in one environment may demonstrate adaptive behavior deficits whereas the same individual may not have deficits in a less demanding environment. Since both measured intelligence and adaptive behavior must be impaired in order for the designation of mental retardation to apply, it becomes clear that an individual with limited intellectual functioning may be considered retarded or not, depending in part on environmental demands.

The *developmental period* is defined as the period of time between birth and eighteenth birthday even though it has been clearly demonstrated that environmental variables which impinge on the fetus prior to birth may be associated with later mental retardation. For example, certain viral diseases in the mother or blood incompatibilities between mother and child may affect the fetus adversely. However, this definition denotes a level of behavioral performance, which cannot be reliably measured prior to birth, or even in the neonatal period. For those children who have medically diagnosed disorders discovered during the neonatal period, mental retardation as defined by behavioral deficits can be predicted for later years, but the behaviors indicating retardation cannot be demonstrated readily.

The definition refers to functioning, and thus it is predicated on assessment of current behaviors without necessarily implying prognosis. By emphasizing this aspect of the concept of mental retardation, it is recognized that an individual may be retarded at some time in his life and not at other times. Both intellectual status and adaptive behavior levels may change across time. Such changes have been well documented in longitudinal studies and appear to relate to such factors as associated physiological conditions, motivation, treatments, training opportunities, or to other factors. Further, changes may relate to the measurement of the two relevant variables, especially adaptive behavior, which is closely associated with the environment and its demands. Deficits in adaptive behavior during infancy and early childhood are often reflected most strongly in development of sensory-motor skills, communication skills, and self-help skills, as well as simple socialization skills. During the school years, retarded persons may show the same deficits as in early childhood, or they may be deficits only in the use of basic academic skills, reasoning and judgment in mastery of the home and community environment, and in social skills. During late adolescence and adult life, the deficits may include any of the above or be demonstrated only in vocational and social responsibilites. Thus, to an extent, the environment itself determines the identification of individuals as "retarded." In practice, the minimal requirements of the general culture rather than subculture may be used in decision making because an individual who shows retardation in measured intelligence but who is able to function in a highly protective environment which makes minimal demands (such as a very overprotective home or a residential facility requiring only very minimal self-dependence) might well be retarded if additional demands were made.

Environment and Heredity

Defining retardation in terms of current functioning recognizes the role of environment in the identification of an individual as re-

tarded, but does not provide evidence about the effects of environmental factors in determining the current retarded status of the individual. The followers of Binet and the users of his test (and its descendents) developed a body of literature which was believed by many to support the notion that most of what is measured by the intelligence tests is due to heredity. Evidence was also accumulated to indicate that intelligence, at least as measured by tests, was generally constant in a given individual. Numerous correlational studies were done with twins, siblings, cousins, and other relatives. In general, results indicated a very high correlation in IQ scores between monozygotic twins; for such twins reared together, correlations in the various studies using individually administered intelligence tests ranged around .90 and for those reared apart around .85. For dizygotic twins and for siblings, the correlations generally were found to be about .50; some studies reported somewhat higher correlations for dizygotic twins than for siblings not born at the same time, suggesting that perhaps the environments were less alike for siblings born at intervals than for those born at the same time. Parent-child IQ correlations usually were reported to be about .50. Correlations for children not related to each other, but reared together were around .25, and correlations for nonrelated children reared apart were of zero order. Such results were interpreted to indicate that the greater the gene pool in common, the greater the relationship and therefore, heredity was a predominant factor in determining intelligence.

However, other studies, many appearing in the late 1930s and the 1940s, challenged that interpretation with results which showed correlations between intelligence test scores of adopted children with those of the biological mother were much lower than those of biological mother-child living together. In one study, a group of children whose biological mothers had a mean IQ of 49 were separated (not for purposes of the experiment) into two groups and it was found that those who remained at home with their retarded mothers obtained IQ scores quite similar to the mother's, but that for the group separated from the mother before age two, the mean IQ was at the average for the general population. As longitudinal studies were done, it was found that the idea of immutable IQ was erroneous, for children tested at differing times in their lives obtained different scores. Further, a number of studies reported that psychoeducational interventions were responsible for changes in IQ. Methodological problems with the human studies led investigators to the study of animals in efforts to determine factors which might interfere with learning. The animal studies were done with rats, dogs, fowl, monkey, and other primates. Investigations were made of such effects as extreme sensory deprivation in visual, auditory, or tactile modalities, social isolation, single sense deprivation and environmental enrichment. Taken together, results of the animal studies indicated that restrictions or deprivations in the environment did impair learning as measured by the "animal IQ tests" such as Hebb-Williams maze, Dashiell maze, T-maze, and shock avoidance apparatus. Early interventions, positive or negative, seemed to have a greater effect than later ones. On the basis of these experiments, it is possible to form some hypotheses to be tested about humans even though the precision of control possible with animals is prohibited in human research.

Some human experiments were conducted in populations where "accidental" circumstances made possible comparisons between children reared under differing conditions. Among the best known are the infant studies of children in "sterile" nursery environments as compared with those in enriched environments. In most studies, infants cared for under conditions of minimal stimulation tended to fare worse, especially in language and perceptual development, than those in environments providing a variety of visual, auditory, and tactile stimulation. The study of Skeels and Dye reported in 1938, with a follow-up in 1965, provided striking evidence of the effects of environmental enrichment on retarded children. In that study, the experimental group of retarded young children was removed from an orphanage which was basically a custodial care facility to an institution for retarded persons and was given a variety of environmental stimulations by a group of mildly retarded women, and was later adopted; the striking improvement in the enriched group, initially and on follow-up, contrasted markedly with the tendency toward further retardation of the contrast group.

Whether animal studies can be generalized to man, whether factors such as illness in control or comparison groups of humans made a difference, or whether chance may have accounted for some results kept alive the debate on the relative importance of environment versus heredity.

In part, some of the disagreement may have been related to a failure to differentiate between factors which were responsible for transmission of across generations through genes and factors which were constitutional and present at birth, but were related to prenatal environmental factors rather than genetic ones. Environmental stimuli which impinge on the organism and may be reflected in mental retardation include not only family and community and other social institution variables, but diseases, trauma, and various deprivations both prenatally and postnatally. Some confusion may have been due to the relatively immature state of the sciences (as they relate to this issue) during the first half of twentieth century. Although Gregor Johann Mendel began his studies of hybrid sweet peas about 1856 and ten years later published results which indicated that there must be unitary elements within cells which exert control over inherited characteristics, it was not until about a century later that efficient techniques were developed for study of chromosomes and some insight was gained into the structure and functioning of genetic material. Emphasis on chromosomal abnormalities stems from Lejeune's report that individuals with the retardation-associated condition known as mongolism (Down's syndrome) carried extra chromosomal materials.

More recently numerous abnormalities in structure or number of chromosomes have been found in syndromes which are associated with mental retardation. In some of these abnormalities the defect is associated with either dominant or recessive autosome transmission; others, usually with lower incidence of retardation in the group, are associated with abnormal numbers of sex chromosomes. Although there have been reports of a wide variety of chromosomal abnormalities reported in mentally retarded populations, it is often unclear whether the abnormality is a mutation and it is even less clear what is the specific mechanism relating chromosomal abnormality to mental retardation.

In some other disorders, heritability is clear. Most of these are rare disorders, but they are usually associated with rather severe retardation if no biomedical treatment is available. Disorders in which parents are known to be carriers are, for example, phenylketonuria, with an incidence of about 1 in 10,000 births in the general population; Tay-Sachs disease, with the carrier population among Ashkenaze Jews being about 1 in 30; and other rare disorders such as Hurler's syndrome and Sanfilippo's syndrome, Krabbe's disease, maple syrup urine disease, some forms of hydrocephalus and cretinism, and Gaucher's disease. These disorders are used as examples here despite their rareness because for some of the clearly genetic disorders treatments have been developed which make it possible to use "environmental manipulation" in the form of medication or dietary control to mitigate the effects of the physiological abnormality which is associated with the disorder. That such interventions may determine whether a child becomes retarded or not is another illustration that intelligence is determined by the interaction between heredity and environment.

Environmental Interventions

Sophisticated techniques have been developed to study the physiological concomitants of mental retardation. Effective techniques for remedying gene defects in the human are not yet available and the current state of our ignorance makes genetic engineering taboo. At this time, interventions are limited in variety. For known genetic defects, which make up a minute proportion of the total population of the retarded, in some disorders genetic counseling can be provided for known carriers who may then make decisions on parenthood, or may seek laboratory tests such as amniocentesis or determination of sex of the fetus in cases carrying risk of a sex-linked disorder and, where appropriate, have pregnancy terminated, thus preventing birth of a child destined for retardation.

For several of the rare metabolic disorders, simple neonatal screening procedures are available to aid in early diagnosis of the disorders. For some of these, medication or diet may aid in preventing the severe mental retardation usually associated with the disorder.

For disorders such as Kwashiorkor, which appears to be due to severe deficiency of protein in the diet during the early developmental stage, the solution of adequate diet is obvious even when it may not be available in the areas of starvation where the disorder occurs.

Treatments of diet or medication in disorders with substances missing (e.g., for hypothyroid children) follow the medical model of determining a cause and seeking a remedy. For the majority of retarded persons, estimated from 75 to 90% of the retarded population, neither the specific syndrome or specific medical intervention is possible. Most retarded individuals fall into the mildly retarded (educable mentally retarded) group and usually do not show any specific syndrome or disease. For a small number of these individuals, and some moderately retarded (trainable mentally retarded) with behavior problems tranquilizers may be used effectively, but only to affect such behavioral problems as hyperactivity, aggressiveness, or withdrawal; tranquilizers appear to do nothing to enhance intelligence and may even interfere with learning. Control studies using stimulants such as methylphenidate (Ritalin) and dextroamphetamine (Dexedrine) have not shown any appreciable changes in intelligence, although they are sometimes prescribed in efforts to reduce hyperactivity. Nor do the anticonvulsants such as diphenylhydantoin (Dilantin) appear to improve intelligence, although they are useful in control of seizures which are not an uncommon finding in the more seriously retarded population.

The most obvious remaining environmental manipulation falls in the psychosocial or psychoeducational realm. Included in this class are environmental stimuli such as parents, teachers, therapists, other adults, and a wide variety of objects and actions of others. Most retarded individuals are in the group which has been attributed to environmental influences, a category of the medical classification system of the American Association on Mental Deficiency which includes those cases in which there are indications of adverse environmental conditions and in which there is no evidence of other significant organic disease or pathology; the category is subdivided into two groups. One group is labeled "psychosocial disadvantage" and described as a group in which at least one of the parents and at least one sibling (if any) also show subnormal functioning, and is further delineated as usually coming from impoverished environments with poor housing, inadequate diets, inadequate medical care. The other, much smaller group in this category is called "sensory deprivation" and refers to evidence of atypical parent-child interactions such as severe maternal deprivation or severe sensory deprivation during the developmental years. The children in the psychosocial disadvantage group have been designated by some writers as probably having retardation at least in part because of polygenic inheritance factors, but direct evidence on this point is difficult to establish. These children often come from urban slums or from rural, isolated areas. The prevalence of mild mental retardation in ghetto areas has been reported in different surveys as being between 5% and 15%, although the prevalence in the general population is usually estimated at no more than 1 or 2%. Incidence is estimated at about 3% who will at some time in their lives be regarded as retarded, but at any given time the prevalence is lower because some individuals, especially the mildly retarded, are not identified until the school years and often function adequately in society as adults, and can thus no longer be legitimately classified as retarded.

Identification has yet to be made of specific cultural environmental variables which are associated with mental retardation in a sizable minority of children in economically deprived areas. However, the research on animals, some of the studies made of comparisons of groups living under differing conditions of environmental stimulation, the early childhood studies, and increased sophistication in theory suggested approaches for intervention. The massive Head Start programs for children deemed to be "high risk" for mental retardation were an effort in providing psychoeducational and medical intervention. The Head Start programs differed in different communities and results of efforts to evaluate their impact resulted in mixed findings. A smaller, carefully controlled study, initiated prior to Head Start, is the Peabody College work under the direction of Susan Gray. Gray and her colleagues developed a program in which evaluation of effects were carefully planned and has followed the children of her experimental group, her local control group, and another control group located in a nearby town. The deprived Negro children in Gray's study were given direct preschool experiences which emphasized language, perceptual-cognitive development and development of motivation; parents of the children were given specific training in techniques of stimulation and reinforcement of children in the home. Like children in culturally deprived areas elsewhere, the control groups in Gray's study tended to decline in intelligence, but the environmentally enriched children gained in intelligence as measured by standardized tests. Superiority of the specially trained group over the control groups was maintained on school entrance, although the groups were somewhat more similar in test scores after a few years in school; an important point in this work is the finding that younger siblings of the enriched group were superior to siblings of the other groups.

Another environmental intervention program in Milwaukee under the direction of Rick Heber chose infants whose mothers were retarded, who lived in poor homes, and who came from the area of the city which produced the majority of educable retarded children in the schools. Beginning at ages below one year, children in the enriched group were provided with intensive training, with heavy emphasis on language development. Mothers also were aided occupationally and in caring for their children. Early results indicated that children in the environmentally enriched program did not suffer the progressive decline in intelligence typical for the ghetto and found in the control children, but were actually well above average in intelligence when they entered school. Later results indicated some decline in test scores for both groups, but the children with environmental stimulation remained above average as they went through the early school grades whereas the mean IQ for the control group of children declined to a dull normal level and was still low at last report.

Educational Intervention

These studies, as well as a number of others on preschool and early intervention, strongly suggest that the adverse effects of an environment which is associated with a high prevalence of retardation can be mitigated by carefully planned strategies of the environmental intervention generally known as "education." Extensive use has been made of a psychoeducational type of environmental intervention which is known under a variety of names such as behavior therapy, behavior modification, contingency management, token economy, environmental design. This approach is derived from the operant conditioning work of B. F. Skinner and his colleagues and is essentially the systematic application of established principles of learning (primarily from reinforcement theory) to the acquisition and maintenance of "desirable" behaviors and the weakening of "undesirable" behaviors. This approach emphasizes observable behaviors and their relationships with environmental stimuli. Skinner's early work was with animals and the first reported use of operant conditioning with a child was the training of a profoundly retarded boy. These procedures have been used on a great variety of behaviors with retarded children and adults: improvement of self-help skills, sign language training, language development, reading, arithmetic, occupational and work behaviors, personal independence skills, social skills, attention span, and posture, as well as decrease in tantrums, stereotyped movements, aggressive and assaultive acts, and self-mutilations. Behavior management which emphasizes programming objects and persons in the child's environment in a manner designed to facilitate development of adaptive behaviors in the child is currently the single most used psychological treatment modality with retarded children today. When used by well-trained perceptive personnel, it is highly effective in increasing those skills needed for coping with the environment.

Other environmental change approaches currently in vogue include foster home placements for retarded children, community group living for retarded adults, reintegration into regular classes of many of the educable children from special classes (mainstreaming), and efforts to provide an environment which is as near normal as possible (normalization) for retarded individuals. There is not yet sufficient evaluation of most of these programs to warrant statements about their effects on mental retardation or mentally retarded individuals. It suffices to say that a very large number of environmental changes have been attempted in efforts to reduce the incidence and prevalence or severity of mental retardation and to improve the intellectual and adaptive functioning of retarded persons. Recognition of the interaction of constitutional and environmental factors has somewhat reduced debates on relative importance of these factors and research has turned toward developing strategies for intervention and to basic research in understanding how neurophysiological and environmental factors facilitate or impede development of cognitive skills.

BIBLIOGRAPHY

BALTHAZAR, E. E., and STEVENS, H. A.   *The emotionally disturbed, mentally retarded: A historical and contemporary perspective.* Englewood Cliffs, N.J.: Prentice-Hall, 1975.

DINGMAN, H.   Social performance of the mentally retarded. In R. K. Eyman, C. E. Meyers, and G. Tarjan (Eds.), *Sociobehavioral studies in mental retardation.* Washington, D.C.: American Association on Mental Deficiency, 1973.

GRAY, S.   An experimental preschool program for culturally deprived children. *Child Development,* 1965, *36,* 887–898.

GROSSMAN, H. J.; BEGAB, M. J.; EYMAN, R.; NIHIRA, K.; O'CONNOR, G.; and WARREN, S. A. (Eds.).   *Manual on classification and terminology.* Washington, D.C.: American Association on Mental Deficiency, 1973.

HAYWOOD, H. C.   Some perspective on socio-cultural aspects of mental retardation. In H. C. Haywood (Ed.), *Social-cultural aspects of mental retardation.* New York: Appleton-Century-Crofts, 1970.

HEBER, R., and GARBER, H.   *An experiment in the prevention of cultural-familial retardation.* Madison: University of Wisconsin Press, 1971.

HUNT, J. McV.   *Intelligence and experience.* New York: Ronald Press, 1961.

JENSEN, A. R.   A theory of primary and secondary familial mental retardation. In N. R. Ellis (Ed.), *International review of research in mental retardation* (Vol. 4). New York: Academic Press, 1970.

KANNER, L.   *A history of the care and study of the mentally retarded.* Springfield, Ill.: Thomas, 1964.

McCANDLESS, B. R.   Relation of environmental factors to intellectual functioning. In H. A. Stevens and R. Heber (Eds.), *Mental retardation: A review of research.* Chicago: University of Chicago Press, 1964.

SKEELS, H. M.   Effects of adoption on children from institutions. *Children,* 1965, *12,* 33–34.

SKODAK, M.   Adult status of individuals who experienced early intervention. In B. W. Richards (Ed.), *Proceedings of the first congress of the International Association for the Scientific Study of Mental Deficiency.* Reigate, Surrey: Michael Jackson, 1968.

SUE ALLEN WARREN

MENTAL RETARDATION AND FAMILY LIFE

In most societies, the nuclear family serves as the primary socializing agent for today's children and tomorrow's adults. It is in this setting that children learn right from wrong, how to share, respect for the rights of others, and the values of their culture. Here, too, personality development is formed, language and communication abilities are acquired, and the child learns the beginning skills for mastery of his environment.

Most families discharge this responsibility well, despite the complexities of the child-rearing task and the periodic crises that arise in the normal course of child development. When the child, because of biological damage or deficiencies, falls far below parental and societal expectations, the task is immeasurably more complicated, and the coping strategies of the family to maintain its stability, integrity, and life-style are sorely taxed. No problem is more vexing or potentially more disruptive to family life than that posed by the retarded child.

Although the *initial* impact of mental retardation on the average family is universally devastating, its long-range consequences are as varied and complex as the symptom itself. Some families never get over the intense feeling of disappointment, disillusion, and despair occasioned by the birth of a retarded child. For them, it is a human tragedy of the utmost magnitude, a pervasive source of chronic stress, a threat to family unity. To other families, it is a crisis, more serious than most, perhaps, but within their capacity to handle in time and without harmful self-sacrifice. To still others—intellectually limited families in particular—the child's difference is neither acknowledged nor recognized, but is one element among many that chains them even more securely to their disadvantaged life circumstance.

Parents of the mentally retarded come from every walk of life. All are vulnerable more or less to the damaging effects of genetic disease, complications of pregnancy, prematurity, infectious processes, physical trauma, and the myriad of other factors that impede brain development before or after birth. Children born under these conditions are generally moderately or severely retarded and often have as-

sociated physical handicaps or stigmata as well. The overwhelming majority of the mentally retarded population, however, are mildly retarded and neurologically intact. They are heavily concentrated in our rural and urban slums and ghettos.

While parents of the retarded clearly share many common problems, sweeping generalizations regarding the impact of retardation on family life are hazardous. Much depends on their own childhood experiences; on their income, education, and culture; on their religious beliefs and value system; on the stability of the marital relationship; and perhaps most important, on the psychological and material resources available to them for handling stress. The physical appearance of the child, too, his degree of disability, and the pattern of his behavior will influence family adjustment. Nor can the attitudes of relatives, neighbors, and the larger community be overlooked. And finally, since few families can cope with the burdens of care, training, and management unaided, the availability of community services and programs must also be considered.

Thus, families perceive and react to their retarded members according to a wide range of differentiating characteristics. Nevertheless, certain problems occur with sufficient frequency to merit some common observations. They can be roughly classified into two areas: (1) psychological and emotional reactions of parents and normal siblings and their affect on intrafamily relationships and adaptation; and (2) practical problems of care, training, and management of the retarded person. The problems that predominate in a specific family depend on the factors mentioned earlier. For many, both areas intrude on family integrity with equally disruptive force.

Emotional Reactions of Parents

Parents of mentally retarded children represent the total spectrum of human personality variation and capacity for parenthood. Where the intellectual disparity between parent and child is marked, as in the case of the average family and severely damaged child, the psychological impact is great. Parenthood has special meaning in our culture, and it is enhanced in large measure by the expectations we have for our children. In a society that values physical and intellectual prowess, the retarded child is a threat to parental self-esteem. Parents think of children as extensions of themselves, and they are assailed with feelings of self-doubt and guilt when their offspring is glaringly imperfect. While guilt is not the universal reaction it is sometimes reported to be, few persons reach the stage of parenthood completely free of guilt-producing experiences. Taboos regarding sex in childhood and adolescence and its obvious association with the reproductive process is an important source of this guilt.

Shame and embarrassment are common corollaries of guilt. They are reflected in the withdrawal of parents and child from ordinary social contacts, in attitudes of overprotection toward and overindulgence of the retarded child, in feelings of lethargy, chronic sorrow, hopelessness, and immobility. These reactions are most intense when the retarded infant is the product of an unplanned and unwanted conception. In this situation, defenses tend to crumble and hostility may be generated between the parents, especially if either one was an unwilling partner to the pregnancy.

Some parents, despite overwhelming evidence to the contrary, deny their child's limitations. For them, denial is a basic form of self-protection against the intolerable pain of reality. They become preoccupied with the few things the child does well and ignore the major functions he performs poorly. They attribute his limited skills to laziness, lack of motivation, and "not trying hard enough." Fathers in particular who see the child for only a small part of the day "see nothing wrong with him." These parents reject professional diagnosis and shop around from clinic to clinic seeking magical cures which do not materialize and further frustrate them.

In the face of severe and prolonged handicap, denial becomes increasingly difficult and self-blame too painful to endure. The tendency is to place the blame elsewhere. The obstetrician is blamed for improper prenatal care or induced labor, the pediatrician for inadequate treatment of infection or injury, the teacher for deficiencies in education or training. Often the parents themselves are the scapegoats for one another's attacks, especially if marital tensions existed before the child's birth. Even more disconcerting are the parents who place the full burden of the child's deficiencies on the child

himself. Pressures are imposed to improve language skills and school grades, and the child's body also may be subjected to frantic and ill-founded attempts at surgical correction or chemical treatment. The anger underlying projection of this kind, if unresolved, can absorb parental energies in counterproductive activities and alienate the professionals who would help them.

Not all of the feelings and defenses noted are experienced by all parents, nor characterized by the same intensity or duration. For the most part, these are not pathologic reactions and can be so regarded only when they persist over an unduly long period of time and seriously interfere with the family's adaptation and normal problem-solving behavior. In time, many parents—more than would be presumed from a reading of the clinically oriented literature—maturely acknowledge their child's condition and adjust satisfactorily. These parents compromise their original aspirations for the child and accept him as he is. They maintain their normal social contacts and share responsibility for the retarded child's care and rearing. He is protected from danger and exploitation but assigned responsibilities he can handle and given opportunity for emotional growth and development. Equally important, the needs of other children in the home are not neglected, and parental love and attention are properly distributed.

Many of the emotional reactions described heretofore do not apply to the large number of retarded children whose intellectual defects do not set them apart from other family members. In these families, the child is not viewed as deviant or different. Here, guilt feelings are uncommon and there is little anxiety, ego threat, or despair about the future, at least for the reasons encountered in the intellectually average parent. Problems are more likely to be precipitated by the child's failure in school, conflicts with neighbors and law-enforcement agencies, child neglect and abuse, and limited work skills and earning capacity.

These families represent the marginal segment of our society. Almost invariably, they have limited education and income, are of low occupational status, and live under generally unfavorable health and housing conditions. Some are welfare recipients and are chronically unemployed or underemployed. Psychological aberrations and other personality defects in the parents are not unusual, and broken homes are fairly commonplace. For these parents, child achievement is not a fundamental value, and mental retardation is only one—and sometimes the least important—of the multiple problems disrupting family life.

The daily survival problems of disadvantaged families are even more difficult to solve because of the suspicion and distrust with which they regard agency intervention. They are confronted by society on many occasions with evidence of their shortcomings as wage earners, parents, and citizens and have little confidence or self-esteem. As a consequence, many become "social isolates," divorcing themselves from community activities and gradually caring less and less what their neighbors think of them. Lacking motivation to improve their living conditions and knowledge of sound child-rearing practices, these parents have little to offer their mildly retarded children.

Limited intelligence in parents does not by itself disqualify parents to care for their children properly. Despite highly inadequate resources, some of these parents are very devoted to their children and, given supplementary help in home management and community programs to stimulate the child's mental development, discharge their responsibilities reasonably well.

Although the problems experienced by socially disadvantaged families with retarded children are not readily distinguished from those of their social-class counterparts with normal children, the factor of retardation is nevertheless further incapacitating in its impact on family life. If the child is severely handicapped, the practical burdens of care and management to be discussed below become almost insurmountable. Whereas the average family can obtain diagnostic and medical services and find surcease through private facilities and community-based resources of various kinds, the limited family has few alternatives to public institutional care. The mildly retarded child poses different but no less consequential problems. As a school failure, he focuses negative attention on himself and his family, which is aggravated even more should he respond to his frustrations by antisocial or delinquent behavior. This background is a guarantee of social immobility, a fate other families sometimes escape through achievements of their children.

Impact on Normal Siblings

The impact of retardation on the family is not confined to parental stress but includes normal brothers and sisters as well. Here, too, reactions vary considerably from one family to the next. Generally, disturbances in the parents coincide with disturbances in the normal siblings. The well-adjusted parent can relieve many of these conflicts, but some disturbances stem from sources outside the home and are beyond parental control. The normal sibling of a retarded child, for example, cannot always escape the unkind words or unwanted pity of peers or adults. They cannot easily disregard a sense of disappointment when friends boast about the achievements of brothers and sisters, or their feeling of embarrassment at large family affairs. Nor, in cases involving genetic transmission, can they rid themselves of the pervasive anxiety that they, too, may carry deleterious genes.

Some of the adjustment difficulties faced by normal siblings derive from a lack of intrafamily communication and parental inattention to their individual needs and feelings about retardation. Although professional perspectives have shifted somewhat in recent years, parents are still sometimes advised to place their severely retarded infants outside the home very early in life. If the child's deficiency and the reasons for this action are not openly discussed with the normal children in the family, it may arouse deep-seated anxieties and fears that they, too, may be unwanted. There is also the fear that destructive sibling rivalry fantasies may have caused the condition and forced the separation. Open communication and the judicious enlistment of support of all family members in caring for the retarded child can avoid these emotional conflicts and resultant insecurity. Knowledge about retardation and the cause of it in their own family, even where genetics may be involved, is far less damaging than the fantasies of uncertainty.

Adverse effects on normal children are most likely to occur when parents become fully absorbed in their retarded child and overindulge him to the neglect of other children. Under these conditions, the retarded child becomes a tyrant in his own household, generating in his brother or sister a feeling of deep resentment and sense of parental unfairness. Similar reactions may be aroused in older sisters who are pressed into service as "mother surrogates" prematurely and denied the opportunity for normal childhood play experiences. Attention-seeking behavior, overcompensation in school work, and social withdrawal are possible responses.

The effect of retardation on normal siblings assumes different dimensions at various stages of development. During preschool years, the child may protest parental inattention by extreme negativistic behavior or by excessive co-operation to curry maternal favor. The former pattern may foster hostility, whereas the latter may reflect an unhealthy inhibition of normal childhood demands. Entry into school exposes the child to the social implications of his sibling's deviancy at a time when he is already unsure of himself. And as he grows older, pressure for scholastic achievement can create doubts that he is loved for himself rather than his accomplishments. Adolescence in turn arouses feelings about future parenthood and embarrassment in dating and courtship relationships. Finally, as adults there is the prospect of caring for a dependent sibling when the parents can no longer do so and other alternatives are psychologically unacceptable.

The adverse consequences outlined above are neither universal nor inevitable. In fact, many normal children can handle the problem of retardation without undue stress or harmful outcomes. Much depends on the adaptation of the parents and the stability of the family unit prior to the birth of the retarded child. The crises of retardation imposed on a precarious marriage or general family disharmony can prove devastating. However, where intra-family relationships are strong and the status and roles of each member well defined, crises may bring the family even closer together. Normal children can be invaluable assets to parents. They can compensate for disappointment in the retarded child and help in his social and emotional development through empathy, acceptance, stimulation, and modeling behavior. This experience has promoted in many normal siblings a high level of patience, tolerance of individual difference, greater emotional maturity, and a keen sense of social responsibility.

Practical Problems in Care and Management

Problems in care and management, sometimes distinct from yet often interrelated with feelings and attitudes, also impact on family life. As families move from acute crises to chronic stress, these problems are often the most crucial.

The nature of problems presented are directly related to the degree of dependency in the child. Among the severely handicapped, many—in the absence of special training in self-care skills—require complete nursing care around the clock. The health of the mothers, who bear the brunt of care, can be affected drastically. They often suffer from chronic fatigue and occasionally verge on mental breakdown. The emotional strain is further heightened by the frequent medical attention the child requires and the severe financial drain this represents. Extra costs are involved in securing diagnosis and treatment for some and training and recreational opportunities for others. Even the cost of board and lodging, from which parents of normal children usually obtain relief when the children are grown, may continue indefinitely. Not uncommonly, the depletion of the family's resources may have far-reaching consequences on its mobility, earning power, and educational level.

Management problems frequently stem from retarded psychological, social, and sexual development. Some of the more handicapped are hyperactive, aggressive, and destructive and are commonly preoccupied with bodily needs and masturbatory behavior and have little impulse control or awareness of common dangers. The constant supervision these children require is a physical impossibility for most parents. Such children, however, are not generally a threat to the safety of others, have little sex drive or interest, and usually lack the capacity for reproduction. Their management problems derive from their prolonged and total dependency and need for constant protection and supervision.

While intellectual criteria alone cannot precisely differentiate among subgroups of retarded persons, behavioral dimensions do expand as intelligence increases, bringing into management considerations factors of personality, interests, motivations, and likes and dislikes. Delinquent behavior or sexual misconduct is more likely to occur among the mildly retarded. In these instances, the behavior is heavily influenced by the same social-environmental and family forces found in antisocial and asocial persons of average mentality, but low intelligence may nevertheless play a contributing role, at least indirectly.

The current emphasis on normalization and caring for the retarded in the community compels an increasing proportion of parents to care for their retarded children in their own homes. In most instances, the child's presence has a significant and lasting impact on family life. For some, it signals a distortion of roles, intolerable tensions, and a drastic change in life-style. For others, adaptations are made to maintain and possibly even strengthen family stability without undue sacrifice. To a considerable extent, these differential outcomes depend on the psychological, material, and spiritual resources the family can bring to bear on the problem. But even the most capable need the support of accepting public attitudes and extensive community-based services to supplement parental efforts.

BIBLIOGRAPHY

ADAMS, M. *Mental retardation and its social dimensions.* New York: Columbia University Press, 1971.

BEGAB, M. J. *The mentally retarded child: A guide to services of social agencies.* Children's Bureau Publication no. 404. Washington, D.C.: U.S. Government Printing Office, 1963.

BEGAB, M. J., and RICHARDSON, S. A. (Eds.). *The mentally retarded and society: A social science perspective.* Baltimore, Md.: University Park Press, 1975.

FARBER, B. *Effects of a severely mentally retarded child on family integration.* Monograph of the Society for Research and Child Development no. 71, 1959.

FARBER, B., and JENNE, W. C. Interaction with retarded siblings and life goals of children. *Marriage and Family Living,* 1963, *25,* 96–98.

GOFFMAN, E. *Stigma: Notes on the management of spoiled identity.* Englewood Cliffs, N.J.: Prentice-Hall, 1963.

GROSSMAN, F. K. *Brothers and sisters of retarded children: An exploratory study.* New York: Syracuse University Press, 1972.

KESSLER, J. *Psychopathology of childhood.* Englewood Cliffs, N.J.: Prentice-Hall, 1966.

MATTINSON, J. *Marriage and mental handicap.* Pittsburgh: University of Pittsburgh Press, 1970.

PHILLIPS, I. (Ed.). *Prevention and treatment of mental retardation.* New York: Basic Books, 1966.

SCHREIBER, M. *Social work and mental retardation.* New York: John Day, 1970.

WOLFENSBERGER, W., and KURTZ, R. *Management of the family of the mentally retarded.* Chicago: Follett, 1969.

MICHAEL J. BEGAB

MERCIER, DESIRÉ JOSEPH (1851–1926)

A Belgian cardinal, philosopher, and psychologist, Mercier founded the Institut Supérieur de Philosophie at Louvain (1889) whereupon, commissioned by Pope Leo XIII to take note of the "new psychology," he undertook the study of psychology under Charcot. Consequently, he procured A. Thiéry, Wundt's student, to organize the first Catholic experimental laboratory (1891). Mercier fought via the *Revue Néo-Scolastique* the "exaggerated spiritualism" and mechanism that he believed flowed from Cartesian dualism. He appealed to biology, physiology, and neurology to show the substantial unity of man, explaining this unity through hylomorphism. He founded with Michotte (1923) the School of Pedagogy and Applied Psychology in Belgium.

S. M. FLORIANNE ZACHAREWICZ

MERLEAU-PONTY, MAURICE (1907–1961)

Merleau-Ponty was a French existential philosopher who tried to integrate phenomenology and psychology. He made perception the foundation of his philosophy because he considered it as man's primordial contact with the world. Merleau-Ponty's *The Structure of Behavior* (1942) and *Phenomenology of Perception* (1945) are his main works.

VIRGINIA STAUDT SEXTON

MESMER, FRANZ ANTON (1734–1815)

Mesmer was the discoverer of hypnosis and the originator of a line of thinking in medicine that went directly through the nineteenth century to hypnosis, psychotherapy, and dynamic psychiatry. He was the son of a forester at Iznang, in Swabia, Germany. In 1766, he received his doctorate in medicine from the University of Vienna, and then joined the faculty of that illustrious school. Two years later he married a wealthy widow, and they established in their home one of the cultural centers of Vienna. Mesmer took from Richard Mead the idea of gravitational influences on fluids in the human body, and built it into the idea that his patients might be benefited by "animal gravitation."

Later, the work of Maximilian Hell, an astronomer and priest, came to his attention. Hell was using magnets to effect cures. Mesmer saw at once that the power of healing lay not in the magnets but in the effects of the magnets on the body fluids, and he called the new power animal magnetism. He was particularly successful in the case of a hysterical girl in 1773–1774, and he announced his new discovery in 1775.

For ten years after his marriage he practiced successfully, and then in 1778, he removed to Paris, where he created a sensation with his claims and demonstrations. Mesmer himself had abandoned magnets, but continued to think in terms of magnetic fluids as he treated his patients. A difficult and egotistic person, he was said once to have claimed to have magnetized the sun. After a report of a joint commission of the French Academies of Medicine and Science, which denied the existence of mesmeric fluid and attributed his influence to the imagination, Mesmer in 1785 left Paris. After some years he settled in Switzerland, where he remained in obscurity until his death.

His followers split into various groups. They persisted throughout the nineteenth century all over the Western world but usually outside of the medical tradition. One line, going from Faria, who came to believe the imagination was the principle involved, to Bernheim, led to the suggestion theory of hypnosis and psychotherapy. Other lines contributed likewise to new explorations of the physician-patient relationship, and ultimately, dynamic psychopathologies.

JOHN C. BURNHAM

METABOLISM

See BIOCHEMISTRY

METACHROMATIC MATERIALS IN NEURAL TISSUES

Metachromatic materials are those that take on a color different from that of the dye which is used. Toluidine blue is commonly employed for their demonstration. This stains metachromatic materials pink or violet in contrast to the blue orthochromatic staining of most other substances. The mucopolysaccharides of mesenchymal tissues are among the most strongly metachromatic substances; their metachromasia is attributed to the presence of acid sulfate groups. The metachromasia exhibited by these materials often persists as the stained sections are dehydrated and mounted permanently in a nonaqueous medium.

In the brain, metachromatic materials of the type just described are not infrequent in mesenchymal tissues, notably in the walls of blood vessels. A variety of other metachromatic materials may also be found in the neural parenchyma. Their chemical significance is less clearly understood. They may be sulfate esters, such as sulfatides. However, sulfate-free substances that contain many acidic groups may also exhibit metachromasia. These materials stain pink or violet with toluidine blue; in addition, they are stained brown by cresyl violet in an acid medium, while the orthochromatic materials are violet. This brown metachromasia is not exhibited by the mucopolysaccharides in mesenchymal tissues. The metachromasia of these neural substances is less intense than that of the mesenchymal substances, is more readily demonstrated in frozen than in paraffin sections, and is lost if the stained sections are dehydrated in alcohol and mounted in a nonaqueous medium. The loss of staining is not due to the extraction of the metachromatic substances since these materials can be restained when again placed in an aqueous medium.

In the brain substance, metachromasia is exhibited by normal myelin in frozen sections, but not in paraffin sections. Not unexpectedly, it may be demonstrated in some of the irregular clumps and masses of materials present in neural tissues undergoing degeneration, some of which may originate from myelin. Some of these materials are metachromatic in paraffin sections as well, as is also true for materials which may have arisen in degenerated axons. Corporea amylacea are regularly meta-chromatic even in paraffin sections. Some of the lipids associated with calcific deposits in the brain, such as those in oligodendrogliomas, are metachromatic.

The greatest quantities of metachromatic materials are observed in the degenerated white matter in some cases of diffuse sclerosis. In one group of these, termed metachromatic leucodystrophy, the material has been identi-fied as sulfatides; in other cases the meta-chromatic materials are heterogenous in na-ture, the other staining characteristics being quite diverse. In some such cases, two classes of metachromatic materials may be separately identified. In some of these latter cases, the metachromatic materials may not represent the end-product of a specific metabolic disorder of the lipidosis type, as is thought to be true of the metachromatic leucodystrophy group, but may reflect a less specific abnormality in mye-lin catabolism. Abnormalities in myelin forma-tion may also be associated with the deposition of metachromatic materials.

BIBLIOGRAPHY

AUSTIN, J. Metachromatic form of diffuse cerebral sclero-sis. III: Significance of sulfatide and other lipid abnor-malities in white matter and kidney. *Neurology,* 1960, *10,* 470–483.

BRAIN, W. R., and GREENFIELD, J. G. Late infantile meta-chromatic leucoencephalopathy with primary degen-eration of the interfascicular oligodendroglia. *Brain,* 1950, *73,* 291–317.

FEIGIN, I., Diffuse cerebral sclerosis (metachromatic leucoencephalopathy). *American Journal of Pathol-ogy,* 1954, *30,* 715–737.

FEIGIN, I., and BUBELIS, I. Lipids deposits in the brain in non-specific conditions histochemically like those in the lipidoses. In *Cerebral sphingolipidoses—A sym-posium on Tay-Sachs disease and allied disorders.* New York: Academic Press, 1962. Pp. 125–128.

VON HIRSCH, T., and PFEIFFER, J. Über histologische Me-thoden in der Differentialdiagnose von Leukodystro-phien und Lipoidosen. *Archiven der Psychiatrie und Neurologie,* 1955, *194,* 88–104.

IRWIN FEIGIN
ABNER WOLF

METAPSYCHIATRY: THE CONFLUENCE OF PSYCHIATRY AND MYSTICISM

Metapsychiatry is a term born of necessity to designate the hitherto unclassified interface between psychiatry and mysticism. Metapsy-chiatry encompasses not only parapsychology, but also all other "supernatural" manifesta-tions of consciousness that are in any way rele-vant to the theory and practice of psychiatry. Thus, metapsychiatry may be conceptualized as the base of a pyramid whose other sides are psychiatry, parapsychology, technology and mysticism. First proposed by Dean in 1971, *metapsychiatry* is found in the newest edition of the official psychiatric glossary of the Ameri-can Psychiatric Association.

Psychic research is a legitimate concern of psychiatry, the specialty best qualified to inves-tigate phenomena, assess validity, and expose fallacy in matters of the mind. As yet there is no general agreement, even among parapsy-chologists, as to what is or is not *psychic.* The term encompasses a heterogeneous assortment of superstitions, beliefs, and procedures rang-ing, for example, from witchcraft at one ex-treme to biofeedback monitoring at the other. In between are a large number of diverse ele-ments related to each other only by an underly-ing current of mysticism. Some are little more than fanciful superstitions; others hover on the brink of natural law, seemingly within reach of scientific validation. An updated system of *psi* classification is needed.

Richard Maurice Bucke, the 1890 President of the American Medico-Psychological As-sociation, read a paper titled "Cosmic Con-sciousness" at the annual meeting of the as-sociation in 1894 and four years later published a book under the same title (Bucke, 1964). He developed the theory that a seemingly miraculous higher consciousness, appearing sporadically throughout the ages, was a natu-ral rather than an occult phenomenon, that it was latent in all of us, and was, in fact, an evolutionary process that would even-tually raise all mankind to a higher level of existence. He predicted that psychic re-search would eventually become a major con-cern of psychiatry.

Cosmic consciousness refers to a suprasen-sory, suprarational level of mentation that transcends all other human experience, and creates a sense of oneness with the universe. Its existence has been known since antiquity un-der a variety of regional and ritual terms—*nir-vana, satori, samedhi, unio mystica, Kairos,* to name but a few. For purposes of standardiza-tion, Dean has proposed the term, *ultracon-*

sciousness, because it has closer semantic ties to current psychiatric nomenclature.

Miraculous powers have been attributed to the ultraconscious, and from it have sprung the highest creativity and loftiest ideals of man. Yet it still remains the greatest enigma of the mind. All but neglected by science in the past, it has in recent years attracted ever increasing interest for a number of reasons:

1. Accelerated communication and travel have forged closer transcultural links between Western empiricism and Eastern mysticism, thereby creating a cross-fertilizing continuum wherein ancient truths can be reexamined in the light of modern technology.

2. Transcultural psychiatry has become increasingly interested in shamanism and psychic healing (Dean, 1972; Kiev, 1964).

3. Psychedelic drugs, their uses and abuses, have dramatically focused attention upon extraordinary levels of consciousness.

4. Computer technology has made available vast reservoirs of integrated data that have broken down many of the barriers which previously isolated the behavioral from the physical sciences. As a result, it will become feasible for many sciences to coordinate the findings of various centers.

5. Space exploration has ushered in an enormous and imminent awareness of the universe, and with it a corresponding desire to expand the horizons of consciousness.

6. Today's technology makes possible more sophisticated scientifically "respectable" research on consciousness, for example, REM (rapid eye movement) dream monitoring, modern meditation techniques, and physiological self regulation through biofeedback training. These developments have added an important new dimension to psychiatry and psychosomatic medicine (Ornstein, 1972).

A special high-frequency photographic technique, known as the *Kirlian effect,* after its Russian proponents, has allegedly revealed halo-like, pulsating, bioenergetic emanations that are emitted into the atmosphere by all forms of life; they presumably intermingle and interact with other emanations, past, present, and future, and can theoretically be detected by properly developed human and mechanical sensors. Cults and commercial enterprises have sprung up exploiting meditation, biofeedback, mind control, and higher states of consciousness. It is important to differentiate true ultraconsciousness from the pseudoprofundity of the charlatan.

The concept of metapsychiatry was developed at a series of symposia on psychiatry and mysticism presented at four consecutive annual meetings of the American Psychiatric Association (1972–1975). The results of this development in professional orientation are presented in *Psychiatry and Mysticism* (Dean, 1976).

BIBLIOGRAPHY

BUCKE, R. M. *Cosmic consciousness.* New York: Dutton, 1969.

DEAN, S. R. Shamanism vs. psychiatry in Bali, "island of the gods." *American Journal of Psychiatry,* 1972, *129,* 91–94.

DEAN, S. R. Metapsychiatry: The interface between psychiatry and mysticism. *American Journal of Psychiatry,* 1973, *130,* 1036–1038.

DEAN, S. R. *Psychiatry and mysticism.* Chicago: Nelson Hall, 1976.

KIEV, A. *Studies in primitive psychiatry today: Magic, faith, and healing.* New York: Free Press, 1964.

ORNSTEIN, R. E. *The psychology of consciousness.* San Francisco: Freeman, 1972.

SHAPIRO, D. Recommendations of ethics committee regarding biofeedback techniques and instrumentation: Issues of public and professional concern. *Psychophysiology,* 1973, *10,* 533–535.

STANLEY R. DEAN

METAPSYCHOLOGY
See PSYCHOANALYTIC METAPSYCHOLOGY

MEYER, ADOLF (1869–1950)

Meyer was the most influential American in giving psychiatry its modern form. Meyer was originally Swiss, born in Niederweningen near Zürich. Heir to liberal religious and political traditions as well as a special theological strain that celebrated the unity of mind and body, Meyer studied medicine at the University of Zürich, particularly psychiatry with Forel and neuropathology with von Monakow. He chose neuropathology for a career, and failing to receive an appointment at the university, he emigrated to the United States in 1892. After some difficult times, which required his entering the practice of neurology in Chicago, he began to teach at the University of Chicago. Already at that time he advocated a biological approach to neurology. From 1893 to 1895 he was pathologist at the new state mental hospital at Kankakee, Illinois. There he worked in the laboratory, as well as with both patients and staff, trying to integrate the scientific approach with clinical practice.

American psychiatrists at that time were anxious about their scientific status, and Meyer's demonstrations on pathology promised to help redeem that status. He was invited to the state hospital at Worcester, Massachusetts, where he was influential in establishing systematic records and patient descriptions. This aspect of Meyer's contributions made a fundamental and lasting impression on clinical practice in the United States. He insisted that case records be of a caliber that they could be used in clinical investigations. Meyer himself carried this new standard to New York when he was made director of the Pathological Institute of the state hospitals system in 1902, and he continued this influence in his prestigious post, beginning in 1910, as professor of psychiatry and head of the Phipps Psychiatric Clinic at Johns Hopkins Hospital and Medical School.

Inseparable from Meyer's passion for completeness in case histories was his conception of *psychobiology*. His approach to the patient was holistic, and he insisted that all facts—organic, psychological, and social—that went into the development of a case should be searched out and noted. This broad and inclusive approach involved eclecticism, and such undogmatic but still scientific thinking fitted in very well with the existing inclinations and tastes of American physicians. Both Meyer and his followers were deeply influenced by Darwinian thinking and perceived the patient as an organism adapting to an environment.

In the course of upgrading hospital procedures, Meyer effectively introduced Kraepelinian classification into American psychiatric practice. He had visited Kraepelin's clinic in 1896, just after the latter's nosological innovations were first published. From Worcester and the New York state systems, Kraepelin's diagnostic-prognostic system came into general use in the United States.

Meyer very early encouraged physicians on the staff of both the New York state hospital system and Phipps Clinic to investigate psychoanalysis. Meyer himself absorbed from Freud the importance of both early childhood and sexuality in the patient's life history, and emphasized these aspects in interviews with patients. This practice, in turn, affected practice in many places across the country.

Meyer emphasized the importance of social factors. Already in Chicago, Meyer had become acquainted with Jane Addams and other reformers, and he subsequently was one of the first to introduce psychiatric social work. He was a sponsor of Clifford Beers when he began the *mental hygiene movement*. Meyer often lent his name and counsel to other social reform efforts, as Forel did in Switzerland.

Meyer's long career falls into two general periods. In the first, before about 1920, he was an inspiring innovator. In his later years, perhaps beginning with a period of serious depression, he viewed himself a competitor with Freud and others and did not keep his most able students with him. His shrewd denunciation of the mere labeling of patients by Freudians and Kraepelinians came to have a peevish quality. He attempted to introduce a new nosology, but it failed to gain adoption despite Meyer's power and influence. In spite of many opportunities, he was not a successful lecturer or explicator of his ideas. He retired from the Phipps Clinic in 1941 and spent much of his retirement working on his favorite subject, neuroanatomy.

Meyer's work is described in John C. Burnham's *Psychoanalysis and American Medicine, 1894–1917: Medicine, Science, and Culture* (New York: International Universities Press, 1967), and Alfred Lief's *The Commonsense Psychiatry of Dr. Adolf Meyer* (New York: McGraw-Hill, 1948).

JOHN C. BURNHAM

MEYNERT, THEODORE (1833–1892)

Theodore Meynert, a leading Viennese neurologist, neuroanatomist, and histopathologist, is noted for his fundamental descriptions of the central structures of the brain. Although some of his discoveries could not be verified, he did demonstrate many association tracts. He considered a number of mental illnesses to be the result of inadequate blood supply of the brain. Depression, he believed, was due to excessive flow of blood in the cerebral vessels. He introduced the term *defense,* one of two ways the organism can respond; the other being attack.

His famous pupils included Carl Wernicke and Sigmund Freud. It was Meynert who recommended Freud for the office of Privatdocent in neuropathology in 1885. He also assisted in getting Freud a traveling scholarship which brought him to study with Charcot. Following this, Meynert broke with Freud, one cause being his inability to conceive that a male could suffer from hysteria. Meynert also opposed hypnosis because of the strong sexual feelings that were aroused.

Meynert was described as having a striking appearance, short body, large head, and wavy hair. Despite being a poor lecturer and uncordial in behavior, Meynert attracted a large following. In his textbook he cautioned against the word *psychiatry,* saying, "The historical term psychiatry, i.e., 'treatment of the soul' implies more than we can accomplish and transcends the bounds of accurate scientific investigation." His main work is *Psychiatry* (New York: Putnam, 1885).

LEO H. BERMAN

MICHOTTE VAN DEN BERCK, ALBERT E. (1881–1965)

A Belgian psychologist who investigated human action through use of the experimental phenomenological approach, Michotte was concerned with the relationships between experience and behavior. He is renowned for his investigations of perception, particularly of phenomenal causal impressions, and for his search for the precise spatiotemporal conditions that prompted them. Michotte investigated self-determination, logical memory, motor activity, rhythm, and movement, and expressed a dynamic (both functionalistic and structuralistic) orientation to psychological investigation that viewed all experimental problems of psychology from the standpoint of action. He shared his techniques and ideas with scholars worldwide who visited the University of Louvain laboratory he directed.

EILEEN A. GAVIN

MILITARY PSYCHIATRY

Historical Review

Experiences of warfare, both ancient and modern, have demonstrated a marked attrition of military manpower from infectious disease, climatic extremes, and other environmentally induced nonbattle injury and disease which was of greater magnitude than battle casualties. However, it was not until the latter half of the nineteenth century that advances in medicine gave military services an increasing technical capability of safeguarding personnel from environmental disease and injury.

Military medicine has pioneered in the development of prevention and treatment techniques for disease and injury of undoubted environmental causation, including combat casualties. These contributions have been readily applicable to the civil setting in such areas as infectious disease, trauma, and transportation of the sick and injured. Military medicine continues to make major contributions to civil medicine, as wartime conditions serve as a vast arena of environmental stress and strain which demands efforts to conserve military strength and provides a prompt feedback upon the efficacy of such endeavors.

Military Psychiatry Before World War I

Only since World War I has military psychiatry become established as a regular component of military medicine of the Armed Forces of the United States and many other nations. Prior to World War I, mental illness in military personnel was narrowly defined to include mainly severe abnormalities of psychotic proportions. For example, only 2410 cases of "insanity" were recorded from the Union Forces during the Civil War. Later, rates of 2 to 3 per 1000 troops per annum were reported from the Franco-Prussian, Spanish American, Boer, and Russo-Japanese wars, which although higher than peacetime rates, clearly indicated that mainly psychotic type mental disorders were recorded (Glass and Bernucci, 1966).

It was not until 1912 that mental disorders in the United States Army were broadened from a single diagnostic entity of *insanity* to the category of *mental alienation* which included subcategories of organic and functional psychoses, defective mental development, constitutional psychopathic states, hypochondriasis, and nostalgia. Promptly thereafter, the incidence of mental illness in the United States Army rose from 1 to 2 per 1000 troops per annum to 3 to 4 per 1000 troops per annum.

The concept of *neurosis* or *psychoneurosis* was still in various stages of formulation by Freud and others and apparently not widely known or accepted. Little consideration was given to situational causation of mental disorders in military personnel in the decades prior to World War I. Then, as in civilian life, causation of mental illness continued to be regarded as due to pathology within the individual either from hereditary influences, constitutional "weakness," intrapsychic conflict or disease or injury of the nervous system.

Thus it was, because of the relatively small incidence of mental illness in military personnel, as then defined, which was not ascribed to environmental causes, that there was little interest or concern for these problems by the expanding activities of military medicine. Personnel of the United States Army and Navy with mental disorders were either discharged from the service or transferred to the Government Hospital for the Insane in Washington, D.C. (now St. Elizabeths Hospital).

World War I

From early reports of the fighting on the Western Front in 1914, there appeared accounts of a new psychiatric disorder in Allied troops termed *shell shock* which was of such frequency as to constitute a major military medical problem. Similar but less frequent failures of adaptation in previous wars were regarded as cowardice, poor motivation, weakness, or other expressions of moral condemnation to be dealt with punitively. However, changes of attitude made possible the acceptance of combat psychiatric breakdown as legitimate casualties of war.

In World War I, warfare had reached new heights of destruction and terror. In its early phases, optimum conditions were present for the emergence of psychiatric casualties, in that troops new to battle were locked in intense prolonged combat with heavy concentrations of artillery fire and a high incidence of battle losses.

Advances in psychiatry and the social sciences in the decades prior to World War I facilitated awareness that mental disorders could be situationally induced. But it was necessary that failure in the battle role be manifested by symptoms or behavior which are accepted by the combat reference group as constituting an inability rather than an unwillingness to function. For this reason, manifestations of psychiatric casualties beginning in World War I, and usually their terminology, have indicated a direct causal relationship with traumatic conditions of the battle environment rather than poor motivation, personality weakness, or other innate vulnerability to situational stress. Thus, initially, psychiatric casualties in World War I seemed to occur as a direct result of enemy shelling. Individuals, so involved, appeared dazed and tremulous with or without dissociative behavior or major conversion reactions which were apparently an immediate consequence of nearby shell explosion; hence the terminology *shell shock*. Thus, in the beginning of World War I, psychiatric disorders of combat were accepted on the basis of organic injury much like brain concussion. However, by 1915–1916, Allied medical services clearly recognized that shell shock was entirely a psychological disorder, and the terminology of *war neuroses* came into usage. But by this time, shell shock had achieved fixation and legitimacy as a disease and thus an inability to function in combat (Medical Department of the U.S. Army, 1929).

Treatment

Location. In 1914, shell shock casualties from British troops were evacuated to the distant rear where they quickly overtaxed existing civil and military psychiatric facilities. Later, special military neuropsychiatric hospitals and psychiatric units of military general hospitals were established for the treatment of shell shock and other functional nervous disorders. In all of these facilities which were located in Great Britain, shell shock was refractory to treatment.

Similar unsatisfactory results with shell shock evacuees to rear bases were experienced by the French medical services. For this reason, advanced neuropsychiatric hospitals for the war neuroses were established in the rear zone of active military operations. Treatment in these more forward locations gave significantly improved results.

Because increased German submarine warfare imperiled shipping in the English Channel, many elements of the British medical services, including special treatment units for the war neuroses, were relocated to France. Again, it became evident that treatment of shell shock was more effective in forward locations.

The better results obtained by forward facilities prompted a further extension of treatment to locations nearer to the battle front in British casualty clearing stations and similar advanced posts of the French medical services. In 1916, Allied medical services reported that from 66% (British) to 91% (French) of the war neuroses were returned to combat duty by forward treatment.

Network of Services. Upon entry of the United States into World War I, Major Thomas Salmon, Chief Psychiatrist of the American Expeditionary Forces (AEF) and his associates, fully aware of the British and French experiences with the war neuroses, gradually established an integrated network of services for mental disorders of United States troops as follows:

1. Divisional psychiatric facilities which held cases of shell shock and similar mental disorders for 3 to 10 days of respite from combat which included sleep, reassurance, and suggestion, under the supervision of the division psychiatrist.

2. Neurological hospitals, which received refractory cases from divisional facilities for 2 to 3 weeks of treatment.

3. A psychiatric base hospital in the advanced communication zone which provided prolonged treatment for the most severe mental disorders to prevent chronicity and evacuation to the United States.

The three-echeloned system became fully operational during the final United States offensive in the last several months of the war.

Environment of Treatment. Major Salmon and his associates noted an important aspect of treatment at all levels to be "an intangible and mysterious therapeutic influence termed *atmosphere.*" By this was meant the feelings and attitudes of all personnel of the treatment

facility relative to providing an urge or incentive for return to duty.

Contributions of Military Psychiatry in World War I. In retrospect, World War I provided much of the basis on which the current conceptual and operational framework of military psychiatry has been developed. Major contributions in this regard include:

1. Repeated demonstrations that environmental stress and strain caused mental disorder in so-called normal personnel as well as in those of neurotic or vulnerable predisposition. Previously, mental illness had been considered as originating almost exclusively from individuals with physical or psychological abnormalities.

2. Treatment of mental illness, particularly the war neuroses, early and near the site of origin, although developed by trial and error was a logical consequence of the recognition that mental disorder could be caused or precipitated by environmental circumstances. It made practical sense to promptly aid psychiatric casualties to cope with the combat situation rather than their evacuation to remote hospitalization with its implication of failure and the consequent development of chronic disability.

3. A network of mutually linked and supportive treatment facilities for mental disorders from front to rear was first established by the AEF medical services. Only recently has civil psychiatry recognized the value of a system which provides for a comprehensive continuity of services.

4. Perhaps for the first time, military psychiatry noted and utilized attitudes and feelings of treatment personnel as an important therapeutic instrument for inpatient services. Much later, this important finding became the principle of providing *expectancy* for return to duty which, together with *proximity* and *immediacy* derived from location constitute the three cardinal principles of treatment in military psychiatry (Artiss, 1963).

Between World War I and World War II

After World War I, military psychiatry became a recognized branch of military medicine. Clinical psychiatric units, consisting of open and closed wards and outpatient services, were provided as a section under the medical services at all major United States military hospitals. The practice of psychiatry at these larger military hospitals was similar to the diagnostic and treatment procedures in comparable civil mental hospitals. However, neither locally based treatment or other concepts of military psychiatry as practiced by the AEF seemed to have survived after World War I.

Civil psychiatry, also, was not prepared to grasp the significance of either the situational causation of mental disorder or the importance of location in treatment. Perhaps due to the relatively brief experiences of AEF psychiatry (1917–1918), war neuroses became regarded in the United States as a special type of *traumatic neurosis* which occurred only under the extraordinary circumstances of combat and had little relevance for mental illness of civil life. But the persistent residual syndromes of World War I psychiatric casualties comprised a high proportion of veterans receiving hospitalization or disability compensation. Although these chronic refractory mental disorders were considered to have been precipitated by battle conditions, extensive clinical experience engendered a widespread belief that the war neuroses originated mainly from individuals who were vulnerable to battle stress by reason of neurotic predisposition. This limited ability to cope with combat was deemed the result of faulty personality development which conformed to increasing acceptance of the psychoanalytic model during the decades prior to World War II.

Curiously, or because of the above trends, during this era it was generally believed by military and civil psychiatrists that the major lesson learned in World War I was the importance of psychiatric screening at induction to exclude vulnerable individuals from entering military service and thus prevent the mental breakdown of troops during peace or war. Yet none of the experiences of World War I indicated that studies were conducted or observations made upon the validity of psychiatric screening. Indeed, psychiatric screening was not performed in any extensive or uniform manner in World War I.

World War II

Before and during the early phases of World War II, the contributions of military psychiatry in World War I were completely ignored. Instead, reliance was placed upon psychiatric screening. The subsequent failure of psychiatric screening in World War II has been well documented. Despite rejection of approximately 1,600,000 at Army induction stations, a rate of 7.6 times as high as in World War I, the incidence of hospitalization for mental disorders was three times that of World War I or approximately 1,000,000 admissions to medical facilities.

In retrospect, it is evident that medical screening in World War I rejected only obvious neuropsychiatric disorders, including mental deficiency and epilepsy. In contrast, psychiatrists in World War II endeavored as instructed to identify and reject the potential as well as the relatively fewer overt neuropsychiatric disorders. It was this effort to eliminate potential mental disorders which was responsible for the much higher rate of psychiatric rejections in World War II over that of World War I.

The major lesson learned from the psychiatric screening experiences of World War II lies in appreciating the almost insurmountable limitations inherent in any single psychiatric or psychological examination which, prior to induction, attempts to predict future effectiveness or mental breakdown during military service. Clearly, psychiatric prediction or any medical effort to forecast future disability is much more accurate when symptoms of abnormality or disease already exist (as apparently was the case in most psychiatric rejections in World War I) than are attempts to predetermine the behavior of individuals, particularly when the later circumstances of assignment, associates, leadership, hardships, hazards, and other environmental variables are unknown.

Emphasis upon psychiatric screening served to deny the magnitude of wartime mental disorders, since psychiatric screening was expected to eliminate the problem. Thus, there was little preparation for the management of mental disorders, combat or otherwise. For example, for reasons of economy, the organization of psychiatric services in combat divisions which had been established in World War I was discarded just prior to World War II.

The inevitable occurred. With expanding mobilization and the onset of war, a high incidence of mental disorder soon overwhelmed existing meager psychiatric facilities. The major diagnostic category for these mainly situationally induced mental disorders was *psychoneurosis,* with its implication of unresolved internal conflict from which symptoms were unconsciously derived.

The newly built cantonment hospitals of World War II became half-filled with patients having refractory psychiatric syndromes, often including somatic symptoms to which "gain in illness" had been added. The only solution to the problem seemed to be medical discharge from the Army. Thus, mental illness became the major medical cause of manpower loss from troops within the United States.

Mental disorders also occurred with high frequency during the Tunisia campaign, the first large scale combat experience of the United States Army in World War II. As in the early phases of World War I, psychiatric casualties were evacuated hundreds of miles to distant medical facilities in Algiers, Oran, and Casablanca where symptoms became fixed and few could be returned to overseas duty. Again, terminology for these cases was mainly *psychoneurosis.* Such labeling with its connotation of personality defect or weakness was not acceptable to the combat reference group as being the result of battle conditions; rather they were considered a consequence of failure in induction screening.

Efforts were made initially by individual psychiatrists and later by coordinated programs to move the site of treatment out of hospitals and establish locally based services for most psychiatric disorders. However, over two years elapsed after Pearl Harbor before the development of psychiatric services in the field achieved sufficient operational capability to deal adequately with wartime mental disorder, both at home and overseas. These changes occurred in 1942 and 1943, initially in training camps in the United States and later in overseas combat theatres.

Consultation Services. Beginning in early 1942, independently and almost contemporaneously, psychiatric outpatient units termed *Consultation Services* were established in various training centers in the United States.

Psychiatric personnel of Consultation Services worked closely with trainers in aiding the newly inducted soldier to adapt to separation from home, lack of privacy, regimentation, and other changes incident to the transition from civilian to military life. Consultation Services not only provided outpatient treatment for referred symptom disorders, but participated in the orientation of trainees and in planning the activities of the training program. Consultation Services also became involved in the continued education of trainer personnel in upgrading their understanding of adjustment problems. It became evident that if psychiatric illness were to be prevented, control or modification of one or more of the pertinent situational determinants of mental disorder would be necessary. Since this was the responsibility of command, psychiatrists in World War II endeavored to function as staff advisors to commanders at various levels. Experiences revealed that the effectiveness of the psychiatrist in prevention was equated with the quality of relationships that were established with commanders and other supervisory personnel based on the practical management of referred psychiatric problems.

Combat Psychiatry. In March 1943, during the latter phase of the Tunisia campaign, successful attempts were made to reestablish the World War I forward type treatment for psychiatric casualties. Cases were held for 2 to 5 days of treatment in a field medical facility near the fighting. Treatment included sedation to insure sleep and rest, ample food, reassurance, and suggestion, along with opportunity to discuss battle experiences. As in World War I, it was found that "forward" treatment could return a majority of psychiatric casualties to combat duty.

Soon after this demonstration, a new terminology for psychiatric casualties or the war neuroses was officially established. By directive from the Senior United States Army Commander (Major General Omar Bradley), all psychiatric disorders occurring in the combat zone (divisional level) were designated as *exhaustion.* Other and more definitive diagnoses were permitted in rear medical facilities (Glass, 1973). Exhaustion was selected because it best described the appearance of most psychiatric casualties and indeed most combat participants at this time. The following description by the well-known battlefield reporter, Ernie Pyle, is pertinent:

For four days and nights they have fought hard, eaten little, washed none and slept hardly at all. Their nights have been violent with attack, fright, butchery, and their days sleepless and miserable with the crash of artillery. The men are walking. . . . Their walk is slow, for they are dead weary, as you can tell, even when looking from behind. Every line and sag of their bodies speaks their inhuman exhaustion. On their shoulders and backs they carry heavy steel tripods, machine gun barrels, leaden boxes and ammunition. Their feet seem to sink into the ground from the overload they are bearing. They don't slouch. It is the terrible deliberation of each step that spells out their appalling tiredness. (Pyle, 1943)

World War I was characterized by trench warfare with limited movement during which receiving shell fire was the most common traumatic experience. Thus shell shock was an apt description. In contrast, World War II was a war of movement with objectives to be achieved in successive phases by troops, mainly on foot, who fought up and down hills and valleys, carrying on their persons much of the needed weapons, ammunition and other supplies. In this type of warfare, which included physical fatigue and the strain of continued battle, *exhaustion* served as an appropriate terminology for psychiatric casualties.

Exhaustion was readily accepted by both psychiatric casualties and the combat reference group. Almost all participants in battle could understand that anyone could become temporarily unable to cope with the stress and strain of continued combat conditions. Again, as in World War I, psychiatric breakdown in battle became legitimized as a rational consequence of unavoidable battle conditions.

With acceptance of *exhaustion,* manifestations of combat psychiatric breakdown became less dramatic. Psychiatric casualties did not need to portray *psycho* to communicate inability to function in combat. During the Sicily campaign of July 1943, most psychiatric casualties seen early in rear hospitals mainly exhibited tension, tremors, irritability, noise sensitivity, and verbalized that they "couldn't take it anymore," or "stand the shelling" with or without evidence of physical fatigue, which depended upon prior duration of participation in continued combat. There were relatively few instances of dissociative or regressed behavior or major hysteria.

As the war proceeded, psychiatric services were expanded to include combat units with the assignment of division psychiatrists. In the early months of 1944, a three-echeloned network of services, similar to that of World War I, was established in most overseas combat theatres.

Contributions of Military Psychiatry in World War II

The prolonged and diversified experiences of psychiatry in World War II, not only fully confirmed the validity and usefulness of the concepts and practices of psychiatry in World War I, but further refined and elaborated upon these contributions as follows.

Causation and Frequency. It was evident that the continued threat of external danger was an essential element in the causation of combat psychiatric casualties. However, the frequency of psychiatric casualties was related to situational circumstances which either reduced or enhanced the capacity of combat participants to cope with battle conditions. Most important in this regard was the influence of the small combat group (squad, platoon, or company) or particular members thereof, termed group identification, group cohesiveness, the buddy system, morale, or leadership which served to sustain the individual in battle. Repeated observations demonstrated that the absence or inadequacy of such sustaining relationships or their disruption during combat was mainly responsible for psychiatric breakdown. Also it became evident that the existence of varying degrees of this supportive group relationship, corresponded to marked differences in the psychiatric casualty rates of combat units which were exposed to a similar intensity of battle stress. This recognition of mutually supportive influences from within the group in combat or other stress situations was perhaps the most significant contribution of World War II psychiatry. In effect, experiences of World War II clearly showed that circumstances external to the self were at least as important as personality configuration in the effectiveness of coping behavior. Indeed, the frequency of psychiatric casualties seemed to be more related to the characteristics of the group than the character traits of individuals. From this insight came increasing awareness of the social and situational determinants of behavior which facilitated the development of prevention, intervention, and treatment techniques in military psychiatry.

Other circumstances of lesser but pertinent significance to combat adjustment included: lowered physiological capacity because of fatigue, intercurrent illness or inadequate physical conditioning, and insufficient training in battlefield tactics and the use of weapons.

Treatment. It was readily apparent that forward treatment provided prompt relief for fatigue and other physical deficits of psychiatric casualties. However, it was not until recognition of the sustaining group relationships in combat that the significance of treatment near or at the site of origin became fully appreciated. Proximity of treatment to the combat unit tended to maintain relationships and investment in the core group and motivation to rejoin the combat group was further heightened by improvement in physical well-being because of a respite from combat and recuperative measures of sleep, food, bathing, and the like.

In addition, brief, simplified treatment in the battle zone clearly communicated to both patients and treatment personnel that psychiatric breakdown in combat represented only a temporary inability to function and it provided the atmosphere of expectancy for return to duty. In contrast, evacuation of psychiatric casualties to distant medical facilities weakened emotional ties with the combat group making continuation of the sick role the only honorable explanation for "failure in battle."

Diagnosis. Even in World War I, Salmon and his associates were aware of the potential adverse effects of a definitive diagnosis for the early and field manifestations of psychiatric casualties. For example, shell shock conveyed the impression of brain damage. The war neuroses also implied a continued or chronic mental illness. For this reason field medical personnel were encouraged to utilize the vague and tentative category *NYD*—not yet diagnosed—*(Nervous)*, but shell shock was too firmly established for such change.

As previously indicated during the initial combat experiences of World War II, the widely used diagnosis of psychoneurosis for U.S. psychiatric casualties produced such deleterious effects that a new terminology, *exhaustion* was created.

Similarly, *psychoneurosis* was utilized for most nonpsychotic situational disorders of noncombat origin. As in combat, psychoneurosis conveyed the impression of serious psychopathology from which symptoms were unconsciously derived. For this reason, at the termination of World War II, new categories were established for noncombat situationally induced emotional disorders. One of these categories, the *immaturity reactions* with various subcategories of *passive-dependent, passive-aggressive,* and *aggressive reactions* largely replaced the ubiquitous psychoneurosis which had become the single most common cause of medical discharge in World War II. As a result, during the Korean War, the diagnosis of psychoneurosis for combat or noncombat situational disorders was infrequently used.

Post-World War II Psychiatry and the Korean War

Following World War II, United States military psychiatry, medicine, and surgery maintained the coequal status which had been achieved in the later stages of the war, so that specialty training was instituted at large military general hospitals, creating in the course of several years a cadre of career military psychiatrists.

As following World War I, little attention was paid to the contributions of World War II psychiatry. Instead, military psychiatry endeavored to emulate the prevailing concepts and practices of civilian psychiatry. Psychiatric services of the larger military hospitals provided somatic therapy (electroshock and insulin coma) for the psychoses and psychoanalytically oriented psychotherapy for the personality and neurotic disorders. Wartime consultation services of the major training bases were steadily diminished in number and importance along with the termination of the draft (1948) and the decreasing strength of the Armed Forces. During these years one heard little of forward treatment and the principles of *proximity, immediacy,* and *expectancy.*

With the abrupt onset of the Korean conflict in late June, 1950, United States Army psychiatry moved promptly to reestablish the World War II system of mental health care, both at home and overseas. A three-echeloned network of psychiatric services was established in Korea and Japan within several months after the onset of fighting. The ineffective psychiatric screening program of World War II was discarded. A rotation policy of 9 to 12 months in combat which had been unsuccessfully urged in World War II was established after the first year of the Korean War. Within the United States, Mental Hygiene Consultation Services were reestablished at all major army bases. These locally based services provided an expanded and flexible utilization of psychiatrists, psychologists, social workers, and enlisted technicians. Brief inpatient services and outpatient evaluation and treatment were furnished along with indirect consultation and education services for unit commanders and other post military agencies much like that of the current community mental health approach.

As a result of the rapid implementation of the psychiatric lessons learned in World War II, even during the initial year of intense combat of the Korean conflict, psychiatric rates were less than one-half of the high incidence in World War II. Thereafter, a steady decline occurred and in the last year of the Korean War reached to almost peacetime levels.

The Post-Korean War Era (1954–1964)

Following the Korean War, military psychiatry continued to elaborate and implement the concepts of social psychiatry. This direction was most likely the result of the momentum developed during wartime. Also, in part, it reflected a nationwide movement toward a community mental health approach. At this time, military psychiatry was preeminent in the establishment and utilization of locally based psychiatric services which provided intervention rather than distant hospitalization.

During this era, Mental Hygiene Consultation Services (MHCS) and divisional psychiatry were expanded particularly in the sphere of disciplinary problems and the utilization of consultation. A *field approach* was instituted in which enlisted specialists dealt directly with referred mental disorders near or at their work location rather than in the outpatient clinic setting. This more informal approach diminished the "sick" role and permitted more realistic information to be obtained relative to situational problems.

Also in this decade a collaborative program was initiated involving the Offices of the Army Provost Marshal General and the Army Surgeon General aimed at the reduction of major disciplinary offenders (Glass et al., 1962).

In this intervention endeavor, all personnel placed in post stockades for less serious offenses were interviewed by members of the Mental Hygiene Consultation Service who would then consult with the appropriate unit commanders and other post agencies involved to resolve individual problems to prevent recidivism with subsequent confinement in an army prison and dishonorable discharge. Over several years, this screening and problem solving program was largely instrumental in eliminating four of the five existing army prisons.

Child psychiatry training and service programs were also introduced during this era. This effort was in response to awareness that mental disorders of children in the increasing number of military families contributed significantly toward the maladjustment or noneffectiveness of military personnel.

It became more and more evident during this decade that military psychiatry must broaden its objectives and scope to include noneffective behavior from various psychological and sociological reasons rather than limiting its programs to traditional overt mental disorders.

Vietnam Era

1965–1968. In the early years of the Vietnam conflict, according to published reports, army psychiatry achieved its most impressive record in conserving the effective strength. Psychiatric casualties were treated at secure forward combat bases, often as outpatients by enlisted specialists supported by unit general medical officers, with supervision by the roving division psychiatrist and/or division social worker (Tiffany, 1967; Office of the Surgeon General, 1968).

So few psychiatric casualties required evacuation to rear medical facilities as to create the impression that "classical" or "genuine" *combat fatigue* was infrequently produced by the decentralized and relatively brief episodic nature of the Vietnam fighting.

1969–1973. Reports of the later years are

fragmentary and scant. Following the enemy Tet offensive in 1969 which produced high casualties on both sides and the growing unpopularity of United States involvement in the Vietnam War, psychiatric casualties and behavioral problems from American forces were significantly increased. Most important was the emergence of increasing drug abuse by United States troops in Vietnam paralleling the rise of drug abuse among the youthful population of the United States. Drug abuse by American troops in Vietnam became a significant problem because of the cheap and ready availability of almost pure heroin in Vietnam.

For the above reasons, United States military authorities moved toward the establishment of screening (detection from urine specimens) and treatment programs, initially in Vietnam and soon thereafter at most military bases in the United States. These programs represented a marked change in military policy since previously the small incidence of drug abuse in the Armed Forces was dealt with mainly on a punitive basis.

Current Trends in Military Psychiatry

During the post-Vietnam period, the draft was discontinued and a volunteer armed forces is being established. Military psychiatry continues to expand its scope to include additional categories of noneffective duty performance due to social or situational causation.

In addition to drug abuse programs, alcoholism treatment units have been established at all major military bases. Efforts are also being made by mental health personnel to institute programs that would identify and deal with problems of racism among United States troops.

Community services on each military post have been created under command auspices to provide needed social and welfare services for military families. These programs operated by social service personnel, with volunteers, deal with housing, financial, legal, school, and other family problems which may adversely affect the morale of the military member. Inevitably, community services, although not under medical-psychiatric auspices, uncover problems of neglected children, including child abuse, family disharmony, and other situations that require treatment by MHCS personnel.

Summary

As part of military medicine, military psychiatry was born of a need to conserve military manpower from losses due to situationally induced mental disorders.

From the experiences of military psychiatry has come:

1. recognition of the social and environmental determinants of mental disorder;
2. repeated demonstrations that locally based psychiatric facilities furnish optimum conditions for the intervention and treatment of mental illness;
3. awareness and utilization of therapeutic benefits that can be derived from the attitudes and actions of personnel, administrative structure, and other aspects of the treatment environment.

These contributions of military psychiatry have become gradually incorporated into current changes within the delivery of civilian mental health services from prolonged care in remote institutions to intervention and treatment by local psychiatric facilities.

BIBLIOGRAPHY

ARTISS, K. L. Human behavior under stress—From combat to social psychiatry. *Military Medicine,* 1963, *126,* 1011–1015.

GLASS, A. J.; ARTISS, K. L.; GIBBS, J. J.; and SWEENEY, V. C. The current status of army psychiatry. *American Journal of Psychiatry,* 1962, *117,* 673–683.

MEDICAL DEPARTMENT, UNITED STATES ARMY. *Neuropsychiatry in World War II,* vol. 1: *Zone of the interior* (A. J. Glass and R. J. Bernucci, Eds.). Washington, D.C.: United States Government Printing Office, 1966. Pp. 3, 5, 347–376, 737–740.

MEDICAL DEPARTMENT, UNITED STATES ARMY. *Neuropsychiatry in World War II,* vol. 2: *Overseas theatres* (A. J. Glass, Ed.). Washington, D.C.: United States Government Printing Office, 1973. Pp. 9–10, 15, 756, 990.

The Medical Department of the United States Army in the World War, vol. 10: *Neuropsychiatry.* Washington, D.C.: United States Government Printing Office, 1929. Pp. 271–523.

OFFICE OF THE SURGEON GENERAL, DEPARTMENT OF THE ARMY. *The mental health of U.S. troops in Vietnam remains outstanding.* Washington, D.C.: United States Government Printing Office, 1968.

PYLE, E. T. *Here is your war.* New York: Holt, 1943.

TIFFANY, W. J., JR. Mental health of army troops in Vietnam. *American Journal of Psychiatry,* 1967, *123,* 1585–1686.

ALBERT J. GLASS

MILITARY PSYCHOLOGY

April 6, 1917 marked the beginning of American military psychology. At the annual meeting of the American Psychological Association (APA) in Emerson Hall at Harvard University, a messenger brought the announcement that the United States had entered World War I. Robert Yerkes, president of the APA, immediately started what was the beginning of the first United States military psychological effort—to help mobilize great numbers of men through scientific screening and classification, so that training could be rapid and effective.

Today, military psychology makes its impact in the Defense Department, in the Congress, and in all the military services as a science and as an applied field. In the broadest terms the purpose of the military psychology program is (to quote an official directive):

to develop techniques, methods, and procedures to achieve maximum effective use of military manpower at minimum cost by (a) accession, classification, training, utilization, sustainment, and career management of an adequate manpower base to accomplish the DOD mission of national security; (b) maintaining and improving the performance of military personnel; (c) reduction of life-cycle cost of weapon system ownership; (d) improving the quality of life in military service; (e) developing data and investigating the decision-making process to enable DOD executives to make sound, factual, and cost-effective decisions about personnel, training, and manpower matters.

The Early Period—World Wars I and II

The early period of military psychology (WW I) drew heavily on the existing knowledge and research base to develop and introduce methods of classifying enlisted men —by constructing the Army Alpha Test (for literates) and the Army Beta Test (for illiterates), both group paper-and-pencil learning ability aptitude predictors. These tests drew on the existing knowledge of A. S. Otis's research at Stanford, aided by such early leaders of American psychology as Cattell, Thorndike, Whipple, Bingham, and Yerkes. Their participation was facilitated through many committees, including the Committee for Psychology under the sponsorship of the National Research Council and the Committee on Classification of Person-

nel of the Army. This was the big effort in World War I. It probably advanced industrial psychology in that period more than any other event, encouraging many to become preoccupied with psychometrics, selection, and aptitude testing as its most important aspect.

The beginnings of other activities on a small scale also took place. Some psychologists working for the Navy not only analyzed selection and assignment of gunners, but also began to concern themselves with training and to study training methods. Some psychologists working for the Division of Military Aeronautics explored the effects of a new military environment—the environment of aviators. And in what were the bare beginnings of human engineering, some psychologists became interested in the design of the gas mask.

However, the end of World War I resulted in virtually the complete loss of interest in military psychology, and it was not until 1939 with a new crisis facing the United States that Walter Van Dyke Bingham, as did Yerkes in 1917, urged the rekindling of these efforts. That year a *Personnel Testing Section* was established in the office of the War Plans Office, the Adjutant General's Office, War Department. Reserve officers and enlisted personnel and civilians with psychological training were assigned to the section. Other groups were established within the year, including the Applied Psychology Panel of the National Defense Research Committee, the Emergency Committee in Psychology in the Division of Anthropology and Psychology of the National Research Council (NRC), and the Committees on Selection and Training of Aircraft Pilots and on Classification of Military Personnel, also in NRC. Possibly the most widely used group test that came from these activities was the United States Army General Classification Test *(AGCT)*, which was administered to more than 12 million men in World War II. In addition, nonlanguage tests for illiterates, mechanical and clerical aptitude tests, and trade tests were developed and validated. At the same time research was conducted to develop selection techniques for officer candidate school selection. As one would expect, the early leadership research programs found ways to predict success in school more readily than success on the battlefield—or combat leadership. By 1942, 130 Army Specialists Corps psychologists had been commissioned and hundreds of enlisted men and women psychologists (called "rare birds") were working to develop aptitude tests for the Army Air Corps.

The Air-Crew Classification Battery was a major product of this effort, consisting of more than 20 tests used for classification of pilots, navigators, and bombardiers in the World War II heavy air-warfare type of conflict. Aptitude was measured and validated in specific training programs, with John C. Flanagan making a major contribution.

As recorded by C. W. Bray, its chief, the Applied Psychology Panel sponsored such projects as a study of Army antiaircraft artillery which developed a synthetic tracking trainer, a study to improve the training of Navy rangefinder personnel, and research on the selection and training of Army heightfinder personnel, on errors in Army field artillery, and in the design of gunsights in the flexible gunnery equipment of B-29 aircraft. Still other Applied Psychology Panel projects were studies of voice and Morse code communications and shipboard and laboratory investigations of Navy combat information centers. Thus, World War II saw the origins of system as well as training and human engineering research.

The Post-World War II Period

But since the early period put so much emphasis on selection, psychometrics, and aptitude measurement, and on the application of *existing knowledge,* it was not until after World War II that it became apparent that the military had to establish its own research facilities if the field of military psychology were to be responsive to a broader spectrum of problems, free of the current fashions of industrial psychology or civilian applied psychology.

This decision to develop a broader base has been facilitated in several major steps, first when the Army, requiring a substantial expansion of *training* research beyond that done in the late 1940s and early 1950s in the Personnel Research Section of TAGO—the oldest organizational entity in military psychology—established a Federal Contract Research Center in 1951 called HumRRO (Human Resources Research Office). Also in 1951 the Army founded the *Human Engineering Laboratory* at Aberdeen Proving Ground, which continues to conduct research in support of military equipment developers.

In 1954, J. R. Killian, chairman of the Army Scientific Advisory Panel, set up a working group headed by Harry Harlow to evaluate the Army's research and development (R&D) efforts. This group's report recommended the acceptance and integration of military psychological research as part of the Army's R&D activity. Behavioral and social science research activities were shifted to Research and Development, where nearly all the programs for *all* services dealing with these research problems are today, though operational placement of laboratories and technical supervision of contracts vary greatly.

In 1957 Arthur Melton, a leader in military psychology in the Air Force, reviewed military psychology in the United States. He estimated 729 psychologists were then working for the military departments and grouped their programs under three headings: (1) improvement of the military personnel management system, (2) contribution to the development and effective operational use of new weapons and weapons systems, and (3) the interactions of the personnel management system and the weapon system.

In 1960, J. E. Uhlaner called upon the military psychologists of the Army, Navy, and Air Force to "concern themselves with systems research" and presented a framework for systems research as applied to military psychology. These concepts have been extended and elaborated by Uhlaner and others in subsequent periods. Present-day military psychology treats personnel selection, training, and engineering psychology as independent areas of research, but most military psychologists realize that the variables in each of the human resources areas *interact,* and to give more meaningful products to the military user those interactions must be studied, measured, evaluated, and translated into operational terms for effective policy decisions.

In 1970–1971 a Defense Department panel recommended macroprojects rather than microprojects in behavioral and social science and urged establishment of "social processes," efforts dealing with values in American society, maintenance of an effective all-volunteer military force, and better understanding of social phenomena as they impinge on military operations. Programs were initiated in all services, especially in the Army (through the Army Research Institute for the Behavioral and Social Sciences—ARI) and in the Navy (through the Office of Naval Research), which sought to increase the individual soldier's ability to resolve problems associated with morale and discipline—racial tension, social change, career planning, socialization and adjustment to military life, drug abuse, or soldier-family-community relationships. Thus, improving the quality of life in the military services is an additional purpose of military psychology in the 1970s.

Military Psychology Products Relevant to Military Needs

The events in the post-World War II era (indicated above) led to many results and products relevant to the military user, of which only a few can be listed:

1. The Armed Forces Qualification Test (AFQT), introduced in 1950, was developed jointly by all services with the Personnel Research Section of the Army (now ARI) having primary responsibility. The AFQT was the first psychological test designated by Congress for a specific purpose—to determine mental acceptability for military service—with a mandatory qualifying score. It was also the first screening test used by all the services. The AFQT is a good predictor of performance in training for military jobs.

2. Aptitude area systems of classification were introduced. The desired object of differential classification is to train enlisted personnel according to the test scores which should indicate how well a man will perform, so that the available talent will yield the highest total of effective performance in Army jobs. By 1955 the combat aptitude areas were included in Army classification testing after a long period of unique development that included use of criteria based on actual combat performance. In 1958 the Air Force instituted preenlistment aptitude testing and centralized classification testing. The Navy classification tests are used in various combinations to assign recruits to training in about 60 naval ratings, or occupational fields. The test combinations also form aptitude composites.

3. A series of training products produced by HumRRO for ARI include TRAINFIRE, a new method of teaching combat rifle firing where the targets pop up simulating real combat environments; training courses of instruction in infantry and squad training; programmed instruction booklets for training in aerial observation; training programs and miniature devices for armor; techniques for training low aptitude level individuals; and techniques for teaching land navigation. Perhaps most significant was the development of the seven-step technology for "Effective Military Training": (a) an analysis of the military system from the human factors point of view, which is used in part of (b) the analysis of a particular job, from which grow (c) the specification of knowledge and skills and (d) the determination of training objectives—all of which becomes the base for a two-pronged, follow-on effort, (e) the construction of the training program (comprising programming of instruction, practice materials, and achievement testing) while at the same time (f) measures of job proficiency are being developed; finally there is (g) an evaluation of the training program.

4. Man/machine relationships in military weapon systems that *enhance,* not *degrade,* the performance of those systems were a contribution of human engineering research in the 1960s and early 1970s. Laser range-finder techniques developed by the Army Human Engineering Laboratory reduced forward observer error substantially, for instance; these findings and methods improved accuracy of artillery. The body of knowledge and development of data bases for use by human factors engineers have resulted in various guides. The *Human Engineering Guide to Equipment Design* sponsored by the Army/Navy/Air Force and NASA has data contributed by many engineering psychologists but is mainly applied by human factors engineers.

5. Simulation and systems research have also seen progress. Typically, the systems approach puts the research problem into an operations-like, though experimental, setting. Simulation is both useful and welcome because the actual system may not be available for experimental purposes and a systems measurement bed has to be built. Simulation of this type may even be preferred to the real thing because greater experimental control is generally possi-

ble. Research data thus gathered provided human factors answers needed by systems designers and users for future surveillance systems, future command and control systems, air defense systems, logistics organizations, and battlefield operations. Through systems research the team efforts of the military can be made more effective, as summarized by Parsons in 1972.

Manned systems research resulted in a major advance in *unit training* methods. In 1974 in a combined arms demonstration in Germany, the U.S. Army successfully used ARI's REAL-TRAIN I and II. The soldiers realized that they were learning tactical skills and that the built-in elements of competition and credibility —one side wins and the other side loses—were based not on luck or the subjective judgment of an umpire, but on the skill of the participating teams. Telescopes mounted on rifles, tank weapons, and antitank weapons make it possible to achieve and verify "hits" by identifying numbers on vehicles and on infantrymen's helmets. Many of the principles of learning and training were engineered into the REAL-TRAIN development.

Characteristic of military psychology today is the development of a technological base of knowledge—which often is documented in reports, books, guides, and handbooks—and the development of products for introduction and implementation by a military user or groups of users.

Practically every form of research method and design is used in testing of hypotheses or for gaining a better understanding of the variables and parameters relating to men, women, or teams. In this applied area, frequently a general criterion, or measure of performance effectiveness, is the underpinning of the research. The methods of research themselves run the gamut, including correlational designs, experimental designs, field test evaluations, complex systems measurement beds and application of cost-effectiveness techniques.

Much of the scientific development depends on the capability and willingness of the military user community to develop an appropriate delivery system for the potential military psychology products. If it is too costly to administer individual tests, even though they may be more predictive, group tests will be needed. Skill performance tests for evaluating demonstrated capability may or may not be developed depending on a variety of military policies, including sufficient funds for test administration and management. Elaborate test beds may be built to find out whether special training or new work methods (tactics and doctrine) can compensate for new equipment more costly than that already available. These products thus are of great variety and type. Another way to grasp the purposes of military psychology is to list some of these numerous products.

Enumeration of Other Military Psychology Products

The products of military psychology are: psychological tests of all kinds—personnel tests, both paper-and-pencil varieties or situational tests requiring performances of the examinee; interview techniques and methods; evaluation forms and procedures for associate supervisory or subordinate ratings; tests developed for groups to play out in a field setting; personal self-description forms with a variety of autobiographical materials; attitude scales and questionnaires; schedules of analyses of job requirements; specifications of knowledge and skills required for a particular job; development of training programs based on the determination of training objectives; measures of job performance and proficiency; reports on the evaluation of specific training program effectiveness, the development of training technology, and the need for training devices; reports evaluating the cost-effectiveness of training technologies; the development of technological research findings for cost-effective individual institutional and team and unit training; techniques and devices which tend to enhance motivation; reports on the evaluation of special training programs for drug abuse control and better race relations; techniques for socialization of men and women joining the military services; development of adjustment techniques; development of manned systems test beds for conducting research on interactions of selected variables and for testing and measuring weapon efficiency with specified personnel in the test bed and with varying training and work methods.

Much of what is described above is conducted as R&D activity by the U.S. Army Research Institute for the Behavioral and Social Sciences, Arlington, Virginia; the U.S. Navy Personnel and Training Research Development Center of San Diego, California; and the U.S. Air Force Human Resources Laboratory, San Antonio, Texas.

Additional products of military psychology are the development of information for human-factors requirements for classes of various weapons systems or for a specific weapon system; the development of principles to be used by the design engineer of a weapon system which would assure designing the machine or weapon system to fulfill its operational objective with available or specified (level of ability and training) manpower; research-based reports on effective design of dials, instrument panels, knobs, controls, and control devices to minimize error and enhance speed of perception; research-based reports on the evaluation of various displays and computer-related systems; information on the design of equipment so it is compatible with the characteristics of human operators, taking into account anthropometrics, visual and other sensory factors and environmental constraints.

Much of what is described above is conducted as R&D activity by the U.S. Army Human Engineering Laboratory, Aberdeen, Maryland, and the U.S. Army Research Institute for the Behavioral and Social Sciences, Arlington, Virginia; the U.S. Navy Laboratories at Pensacola, Florida, and at Groton, Connecticut; Aerospace Medical Research Laboratories, Wright-Patterson Air Force Base, Dayton, Ohio.

In 1975 these products were mainly produced through research and development by approximately 1,000 psychologists and related professionals, about half of them working in U.S. government laboratories and half in a variety of contract groups—nonprofit companies, profit-based companies or units, as part of aerospace companies, and in selected university centers. Many of the teams are indeed interdisciplinary and include industrial and organizational psychologists, engineering psychologists, psychometricians, statisticians, sociologists, computer scientists, engineers, experimental and physiological psychologists, training research specialists, and many other types of behavioral and social scientists.

Military Psychology and the Future

Although man will continue to condemn war, the threat of war is likely to continue; many psychologists will continue to study military psychology, most of them frankly to enhance the potential effectiveness of their country's defense; less effort will be devoted toward the scientific study of how to eliminate conflict. Limited-warfare problems will retain priority.

Secondly, research approaches of even greater variety will be utilized—fractionated and systemwide, laboratory and field, basic and applied, individual and team, in highly-controlled and loose demonstrations, action-oriented and science-oriented, not necessarily at the same time but as different policy makers, uniformed and politically appointed, occupy different decision-making posts. Should military psychology be dropped from defense RDT&E (and it could happen) the field would become relatively operational and nonscientific.

Military psychology will grow in size and influence, as new classes of users join the current groups in seeking advisory service and products. The field started with the assistance sought by the personnel and manpower manager. Next to seek products were the military training establishment and the equipment developers. More recently they were joined by the system developers, the operation test evaluators, and the tactical doctrine developers —and occasionally by the military policy makers. It is their job to concern themselves with the trade-off between quality of manpower and cost of training or the trade-off between the kind of weapon system and the ease or expense of staffing and training, while considering specific measured mission accomplishment. With man as the most costly and perhaps the least controllable part of the military system, as long as there is a need for a substantial military establishment, military psychology is likely to flourish in some form.

BIBLIOGRAPHY

BRAY, C. W. *Psychology and military proficiency. A history of the applied psychology panel of the national defense research committee.* Princeton, N.J.: Princeton University Press, 1948.

FLANAGAN, J. C. (Ed.). *The aviation psychology program*

in the Army Air Force. Washington, D.C.: U.S. Government Printing Office, 1948.

GRETHER, W. F. Engineering psychology in the United States. *American Psychologist*, 1968, *23*.

MELTON, A. A. Military psychology in the USA. In F. Geldard and M. Lee (Eds.), *Proceedings of the first international symposium on military psychology.* Washington, D.C.: National Academy of Sciences—National Research Council, 1961.

PARSONS, H. M. *Man-machine system experiments.* Baltimore: Johns Hopkins Press, 1972.

UHLANER, J. E. *Systems Research—Opportunity and challenge for the measurement research psychologist.* Personnel Research Branch Technical Research Note 108, 1960.

UHLANER, J. E. Human performance effectiveness and the systems measurement bed. *Journal of Applied Psychology*, 1972, *56*, 202–210.

UHLANER, J. E. Resolution of social problems aids Army productivity. *Defense Management Journal*, 1974, 35–38.

JULIUS E. UHLANER

MILL, JAMES (1773–1836)

James Mill was a British historian and politician who wrote a developed exposition of associationism, *Analysis of the Phenomena of the Human Mind* (1829) that viewed sensations and ideas as the elements of mental life. Mill considered contiguity to be the associative principle governing the perceived connection of elements and held that simple ideas unite to make up complex ideas. He believed that the principle of association testifies to the unlimited possibility of improving mankind through education and endorsed the utilitarianism of J. Bentham, which (while not explicit in Mill's associationistic doctrine) implied a theory of motivation based upon satisfaction of desire.

EILEEN A. GAVIN

MILL, JOHN STUART (1806–1873)

A British philosopher who laid the groundwork for scientific thought in his *Logic* (1843), Mill then stated that a science of human nature, although less exact than physics, can develop and achieve progressively greater exactness as it avails itself of methods successfully employed in the physical sciences. Mill influenced the thinking of Wundt and Helmholtz. He ad-

vocated a doctrine of associationism analogous to chemistry (hence "mental" chemistry) in which complex mental qualities are said to result from, or to be generated by, constituent elements no longer recognizable. He favored the cultivation of individuality, furthered by self-development, thereby becoming a forerunner of self-actualization theory.

His main work is *A System of Logic—Ratiocinative and Inductive—Being a Connected View of the Principles of Evidence and the Methods of Scientific Investigation* (2 vols.; London, 1875).

EILEEN A. GAVIN

MIMICRY IN ANIMALS

Most biologists define mimicry as a close resemblance between different species of organisms, implemented chiefly by features such as color and markings and brought about through natural selection, because the resemblance confers an advantage on one or both of the organisms. The concept is usually restricted —as it is here—to two classes of phenomena, aggressive mimicry, and defensive mimicry of two types, Batesian and Müllerian. Aggressive mimics resemble their prey and thus gain an advantage over them. Defensive mimics are protected from predators by their resemblance to an animal which is venomous or toxic and advertises its inedibility by its conspicuous appearance. Cryptic appearance or camouflage is usually excluded, although it could be viewed as mimicry of leaves, bark, or other background features of the habitat.

Wolfgang Wickler gave a broader definition, which includes not only aggressive and defensive mimicry, but also such diverse phenomena as camouflage, the resemblance of weed seeds to the seeds of cultivated plants, and intraspecific mimicry, such as the development in male hamadryas baboons of growths that mimic the genital swellings of the female and function as a greeting display. He believes that all of these phenomena are case studies in the evolution of inter- and intraspecific signals, and that all are fundamentally similar in that they involve the falsification of signals.

The outward appearance of animals is determined chiefly by superficial characteristics, such as color and markings. Nevertheless, appearance usually has an important effect on the individual's ability to function and survive. An understanding of this fact is prerequisite to a consideration of mimicry.

The colors and markings of most animals are aimed largely at escaping from predators, either as camouflage or as a warning of inedibility. Most edible species blend in with their backgrounds, thus obscuring characteristics that would betray their presence to predators. Other species flaunt themselves. Their markings—often combinations of black with white, yellow, or red—contrast with the colors of the habitat. Their movements or sounds often make them even more conspicuous. Most of these species are unsuitable as prey for one reason or another; some can inject a venom as do snakes, bees, and wasps; others can discharge a chemical defense as do skunks and bombardier beetles; and still others—for example many butterflies—contain a toxin which makes the predator ill if it eats one of them. Predators learn to avoid these species, associating their warning or aposematic appearance with the unpleasant consequences of attempting to eat them. A few predators, however, can utilize toxic or venomous prey. For example, some flycatchers and shrikes eat large numbers of stinging bees and wasps; the shrikes pull out the stinger before they swallow the prey.

M. Rothschild in England and L. Brower in the United States discovered that some aposematic insects do not synthesize the toxins that make them inedible, but rather sequester toxins that occur in their food plants. This is true of many species that feed on milkweeds (family Asclepiadaceae) and others that feed on birthworts (family Aristolochiaceae). The common North American monarch butterfly, for example, obtains cardiac glycosides from milkweed foliage, its only food during the larval stage. The glycosides are passed through the nonfeeding pupal stage to the aposematic orange and black adult, which otherwise could not obtain them, because it feeds only on nectar. Blue jays that ate monarchs in laboratory tests vomited profusely because of the emetic effect of the cardiac glycosides, learning to reject monarchs on sight after only one such experience. Most of the insects that feed on milkweeds or birthworts are aposematic.

Batesian Mimicry

Batesian mimicry—also known as pseudaposematic or false warning coloration, and probably the most widely known class of mimicry—is named for its discoverer, Henry W. Bates. In 1862, he reported that in the Amazon basin certain butterflies of the family Pieridae so closely resemble butterflies of the families Heliconiidae and Ithomiidae, that they are indistinguishable from them on the wing and difficult to distinguish even in the hand. The pierids in question differ markedly from other pierids in color, pattern, and manner of flight. He noted that the heliconiids and ithomiids were slow fliers, conspicuously colored, and surprisingly abundant in view of their apparent lack of defense against the insectivorous birds which were abundant in the area. Bates postulated that they are unpalatable, and that their conspicuous appearance advertises their unpalatability to predators, which learn to avoid them. He believed that the pierids are palatable, but are protected against predation by their mimicry of the heliconiids and ithomiids. Batesian mimics bluff by falsifying the warning signals of inedible species.

Batesian mimicry is a common and widespread phenomenon, both in the tropics and the temperate zones. It is most frequent among insects, but also occurs in other groups. Some spiders, for example, mimic ants. The black, red, and yellow bands of venomous coral snakes are closely mimicked by nonvenomous snakes. Among the insects, many kinds of conspicuous and unpalatable butterflies are models for Batesian mimics of various butterfly families, and even for an occasional moth. Various beetles are models for other beetles, crickets, moths, and even cockroaches. Stinging wasps and bees—often conspicuously marked with black and yellow—are mimicked by various flies, moths, beetles, and other insects. This list is by no means exhaustive.

The resemblance of Batesian mimics to their models usually includes behavior. Mimetic butterflies, for example, usually fly slowly and deliberately as do their models, although if actually threatened by a predator, the mimic may revert to the swift escape flight typical of its group. The sounds, jerky movements, or other showy behavior of the model are sometimes copied by mimics. For example, a wasp-

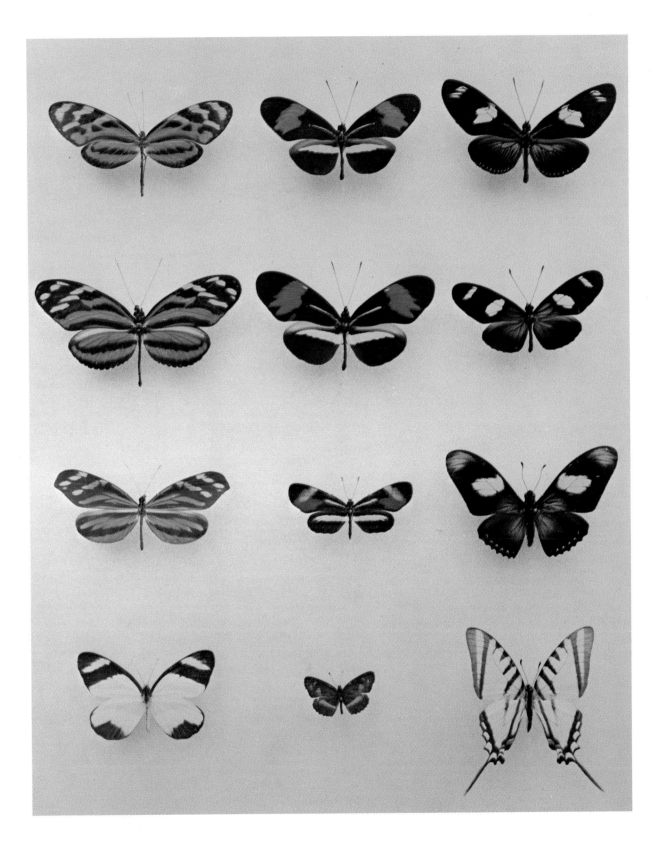

The top and second rows show three pairs of Müllerian mimics which are models for the Batesian mimics in the third row. In the bottom row are non-mimetic relatives of the Batesian mimics above them, showing the pattern more or less typical of the non-mimetic members of their group. Reading from left to right the species and families to which they belong are: top row: *Mechanitis polymnia* L. (Ithomiidae), *Heliconius erato* L. (Heliconiidae), *Heliconius doris* L. (Heliconiidae); second row: *Heliconius numatus* Cr. (Heliconiidae), *Heliconius melpomene* L. (Heliconiidae), *Heliconius sarae* Fab. (Heliconiidae); third row: *Dismorphia praxinoë* Dbl. (Pieridae), *Phyciodes lansdorfi* Godt. (Nymphalidae), *Eurytides pausanius* Hew. (Papilionidae); bottom row: *Perrhybris lorena* Hew. (Pieridae); *Phyciodes teletusa* Godt. (Nymphalidae), *Eurytides agesilaus* Guér. (Papilionidae). Specimens are from the collection of Dr. James G. Sternburg, University of Illinois.

mimicking flower fly (family Syrphidae) makes a high-pitched buzz almost identical in acoustical properties to the sound produced by its model. The same flower fly has short, inconspicuous antennae rather than long, black antennae like those which its model waves conspicuously in the air. The fly, however, mimics the antennae of the wasp by waving its anterior legs—which are black on the terminal half—in front of the head, a behavior seldom seen in other flower flies except for a few closely related wasp mimics.

It has been argued that Batesian mimics and their models must occur in the same geographic area and habitat, that both must occur at the same time of year, and that the model must always outnumber the mimic lest the predators recognize the deception. Lacking evidence to the contrary, it has also been assumed that predators do not respond innately to aposematic signals—that the aversion must always be learned. These views, however, have been tempered. It is at least theoretically possible that model and mimic could occur in different areas or even on different continents if they are both encountered by the same migratory predators. To what extent temporal separation of model and mimic can occur depends upon the memory of the relevant predators. In the laboratory, some birds have rejected aposematic insects as long as fourteen months after last seeing them. Obviously there must be an upper limit on the abundance of a Batesian mimic of any one model. However, the number of mimics which can be supported by a given population of models depends upon the availability of alternate prey and the severity of the discomfort caused to the predator. Evidence suggests that mimics may derive some protection even when they outnumber their models. There is abundant evidence that predators learn to avoid models and mimics on sight, but only more recently was evidence found which shows that the response to an aposematic pattern may be innate. One species of bird, a motmot, is known to respond innately to the coral snake's pattern.

In butterflies, Batesian mimicry is frequently sex-limited, with only the females being mimetic. Mimetic butterflies, whether their mimicry is sex-limited or not, some flower flies, and a few other insects may be polymorphic in another way. That is, they may produce two or more morphs (distinct types without intergrades) which mimic distinctly different models, or they may produce mimetic and nonmimetic morphs of the same sex. This polymorphism generally comes about because different model species occur in different parts of the geographic range of the mimic. The following examples in butterflies illustrate these points. Mimicry in the viceroy butterfly is not sex-limited. Over most of its range it mimics the abundant monarch, but in southern Florida and the southwestern United States it mimics the queen, an unmistakably different-looking toxic species which outnumbers the monarch in these two areas. Males of the North American tiger swallowtail are nonmimetic, but there are two female morphs, one which resembles its male and another which mimics the aristolochia-feeding pipe vine swallowtail. The range of the tiger swallowtail extends north and south of the range of the pipe vine swallowtail. Where the two ranges overlap, the mimetic morph is abundant, but to the north and south it is largely replaced by the morph that resembles the male. The African swallowtail *Papilio dardanus* has a bewildering variety of morphs. Mimicry is sex-limited in this species, and among females are found several nonmimetic morphs and several obviously mimetic morphs, each of which mimics a different model that is abundant in the morph's range.

In Batesian mimicry, both polymorphism and sex-limited mimicry should be favored by selection, since they reduce the number of individuals which resemble any one model, thus increasing the protection gained by the mimic. A plausible but as yet unsubstantiated explanation for the existence of sex-limited mimicry postulates opposing selective forces. Predators must exert selection pressure for mimetic resemblance on both sexes, but in the males this may be offset by the preference of the females for males that retain the ancestral pattern.

There was considerable debate as to whether or not mimetic resemblances actually evolve as a means of escaping predation. The dispute stemmed largely from two sources: the original dispute over Darwin's theory of natural selection, and a lack of evidence as to the genetic basis of mimicry. The Batesian mimicry concept was challenged, because it provided a most convincing example of natural selection in operation.

It was also challenged on biological grounds, the contention being that an incipient mimic could gain no advantage because it would lose the benefits of camouflage, but would not be deceptive enough to mislead a predator. Some researchers concluded that selection for mimetic resemblance is, therefore, impossible; others argued that mimicry could evolve only by macromutations, single mutations which affect many aspects of appearance and thus produce a near-perfect mimic in one step. The opposing view, in conformity with Darwin's ideas of natural selection, is that mimicry evolves through the selection of many small changes. These questions have been largely resolved by experimentation and observation.

There is now abundant experimental evidence demonstrating that Batesian mimicry does confer significant protection against predators, at least under laboratory conditions. Numerous tests with toads, lizards, and various birds have shown that these predators learn to reject inedible aposematic insects on sight, and that after this experience they usually also reject mimics of these insects. Laboratory work has also shown that predators tend to generalize, that is, once they learn to avoid a particular species of prey, they also tend to avoid species which are even vaguely similar. Thus, the evolution of mimicry in its early stages no longer presents a conceptual problem, since even an incipient mimic would probably gain some protection from even a vague resemblance to a model. Finally, it has been shown that mimetic resemblances are often under complex genetic control, a clear demonstration that mimicry must have evolved by gradual steps.

Müllerian Mimicry

In 1879, Fritz Müller described a completely different type of defensive mimicry. *Müllerian mimicry,* as it is now called, is not a bluff; two or more inedible species come to resemble each other, because it is economical to present predators with only one set of aposematic signals to learn. No matter how inedible they are, some individuals will always be killed in the process of educating and reeducating a population of predators. If several species look the same, then the loss will be shared by a larger number of individuals, an economy for each species. The gain for the members of each species will increase with the total number of individuals sharing that pattern and with the precision of their mimicry. Therefore, one would expect the evolution of Müllerian complexes consisting of many species, as has been the case. Müllerian mimicry is widespread, and there are many large complexes among butterflies, bees, wasps, beetles, and other insects.

Butterflies which are Müllerian mimics may be polymorphic, but their mimicry is not known to be sex-limited. There seem to be two major reasons for the absence of sex-limited mimicry. First, it has been suggested that, unlike the polymorphic Batesian mimics, the Müllerian mimics belong to groups that depend more upon chemical signals than visual signals in courtship and mating. Thus, it may be less advantageous for the males to retain the ancestral pattern. Second, while Batesian mimics benefit from a reduction in the number of mimics in their complex, this is obviously not the case with Müllerian mimics.

Two Central and South American species of *Heliconius* butterflies, *Heliconius erato* and *Heliconius melpomene,* are among the most complex of the polymorphic Müllerian species. Each occurs in over two dozen geographically limited morphs, most of which are mimetic. They are mostly black, and are variously marked with lines or patches of yellow, orange, red, green, or blue. In general, identical-looking morphs of the two species occur in pairs in the same area. In most of these areas, the pair mimics a third species of *Heliconius.* These facts have been difficult to reconcile with our understanding of Müllerian mimicry; normally there is strong selection against a Müllerian mimic changing its warning pattern unless the change results in greater conformity with the appearance of the other members of the complex. John Turner advanced an explanation of this seeming paradox. There is evidence that dry periods during the last Ice Age reduced the moist forest environment of *Heliconius* butterflies to relatively small "islands" surrounded by dry savanna. Turner believes that in these isolated environments populations of *Heliconius erato* and *Heliconius melpomene* coexisted with some other species of *Heliconius* which was more abundant and had a generally similar warning pattern. Different populations of *Heliconius erato* and *Heliconius melpomene* were selected to resemble the particular species of *Heliconius* with which they coexisted.

The colors and markings of animals do not function only as camouflage or warning signals. Some of them—as well as sounds and chemicals—may serve as intraspecific signals in the recognition of conspecifics, in courtship, or in territorial defense. One or more of the intraspecific signals of a prey species may be mimicked by predators, which thus gain an advantage over their prey. This form of mimicry, called *aggressive mimicry,* is probably less common than either of the previously described forms of defensive mimicry, but is known to occur among plants, insects, birds and fish. Even the plains Indians and other hunting groups practiced aggressive mimicry by covering their bodies with an animal skin during the hunt.

James Lloyd discovered an interesting example among the predaceous beetles of the family Lampyridae, commonly known as fireflies. Many fireflies locate mates by means of species-specific flash signals produced by a luminescent organ at the tip of the abdomen. At night, the males flash as they fly, and the females, resting in vegetation, flash replies to males of their own species. Females of *Photuris versicolor* mimic the replies of other firefly species in order to lure and eat the males. Individual females can mimic the replies of more than one species.

Most insect-pollinated flowers attract pollinators by means of color and odor and reward them with food—pollen and nectar. However, orchids of the genera *Ophrys* in Europe and *Cryptostylis* in Australia are aggressive mimics, achieving cross-pollination by exploiting the sexual urges of male wasps or bees. Their blossoms strongly resemble bees or wasps, and they produce odors similar or identical to the sex-attractant pheromone produced by the females whose males they exploit. The deception is sufficient to induce males to land on the blossom and to go through the movements of courtship and the beginning stages of copulation. Pollen sacs become attached to a specific part of the male's body, and cross-pollination occurs if the male is then deceived by another blossom of the same species.

BIBLIOGRAPHY

Cott, H. B. *Adaptive coloration in animals.* London: Methuen, 1957.
Ford, E. B. *Ecological genetics.* London: Methuen, 1964.
Rettenmeyer, C. W. Insect mimicry. *Annual Review of Entomology,* 1970, *15,* 43–74.
Wickler, W. *Mimicry in plants and animals.* New York: McGraw-Hill, 1968.

GILBERT P. WALDBAUER

MINERAL DEPOSITION IN NEURAL TISSUES

Chemical studies disclose many metallic elements in the brain. Metals of histochemical interest include copper, calcium, and iron. Rarely, silver or other components of a surgically applied silver clip may be deposited in the walls of adjacent blood vessels. Rarely, in generalized argyria, silver deposits are found in the choroid plexus.

Copper

Copper is normally present in brain tissue in a concentration too low for definitive demonstration by histochemical techniques. In Wilson's disease, copper is deposited in the brain in increasing concentration, a phenomenon that has been demonstrated histochemically. The most commonly employed technique utilizes rubeanic acid and depends on the formation of its copper salt, which is a dark green-black. Pretreatment of the tissues with hydrochloride acid vapors has been recommended as necessary to release bound, nonreactive copper. The presence of acetate in the rubeanic mixture will prevent the precipitation of cobalt and nickel salts of rubeanic acid. The technique is difficult to apply and may fail in instances in which chemical techniques have clearly demonstrated an appreciable amount of copper.

Calcium

Calcium is normally present in the brain in soluble form, but this is not generally of histochemical interest. Calcium salts are precipitated in many pathological conditions, and these often warrant histochemical demonstration. The most commonly employed histochemical technique is that of von Kossa, which actually discloses the carbonate and phosphate moieties precipitated with calcium. Citrates may also play a role. The section is treated with silver nitrate, the silver displacing the calcium to form silver carbonates and phosphates. The silver salt is reduced, either simultaneously by ultraviolet (UV) radiation or subsequently by chemical-reducing substances. The former method, with use made of a UV lamp rather than sunlight, is preferable. It is probable that in human and animal tissues calcium is always precipitated with these carbonates and phosphates, and the validity of the method is dependent on this assumption.

Calcium may be demonstrated directly by treating with alizarin, murexide, naphthochrome green, or other substances, the calcium lakes of which are colored in a characteristic fashion. While theoretically preferable to the von Kossa method in that they demonstrate the calcium itself, some difficulties have been encountered in their use, so that the advantage over the von Kossa method is not universally acknowledged. Some of the dyes commonly employed in neuropathological studies, such as hematoxylin and the Nissl dyes, also form lakes with calcium salts. These dyes reveal the sites of calcium salt deposition very accurately, even if further studies are required to establish the specific identity of the salt. Very similar deposits are formed as hematoxylin reacts with iron salts and at times with other substances in areas of degeneration. Some of the deep blue-black deposits in the stroma of the choroid plexus may be shown to contain calcium, or some iron, or neither calcium nor iron. In addition, many calcium deposits are also well stained by Luxol blue and by the para-aminosalicylic (PAS) techniques, probably reflecting the presence of other materials, such as glycolipids, deposited with the calcium salts. Such staining is not specific.

Deposits of calcium salts are frequently found in the pineal gland, where they may be of such quantity as to be visible by X ray. Areas of calcification and even bone formation may be noted in the cranial dura, and they, too, may be visible by X ray. Grossly visible calcific plaques, occasionally with bone formation, may be noted in the arachnoid membrane of the spinal cord, and rarely in that of the brain. Microscopically, calcium deposits may be found in the psammoma bodies of the leptomeninges and of the choroid plexus. Such calcific deposits are present in "normal" individuals free from disability related to the nervous system.

Calcium deposits may also be found as part of the atherosclerotic process affecting the larger cerebral arteries. They may occur in the tissues remaining in a subdural hematoma as the blood is resorbed. In some conditions associated with necrosis of the cerebral tissues, such as viral encephalitis, tuberculous infection, rare cases of coagulative infarction, and radiation injury, calcium salts may be deposited in the tissues. This is particularly frequent and particularly severe in the brains of children, and is noted in tuberous sclerosis, toxoplasmosis, and cytomegalic inclusion encephalitis. In these conditions, the quantity of calcium salts deposited may be sufficient to be visualized by X ray and may therefore be of diagnostic significance. The deposition of calcium salts in the subependymal tissues in cytomegalic inclusion disease may be so severe as to outline the ventricular system. In Sturge-Weber disease, large quantities of calcium salts are deposited in the cortical tissues adjacent to the angiomatous malformations characteristic of that disease. Calcium salts are also deposited in glial tumors, frequently in astrocytomas and in a higher proportion of oligodendrogliomas. They are less common in the more malignant gliomas. Calcification is very frequent in craniopharyngiomas, and is noted as well in many meningiomas. Extensive calcific deposits have been observed in some microcephalic infants.

In most instances of calcification, the mineral deposition is only part of a broader series of degenerative changes occurring at that site. Thus, materials which were metachromatic and stained with Sudan black and with the PAS techniques were demonstrated in calcified foci of the oligodendroglioma. The implication of specific metabolic abnormalities in this or in other types of calcification, because of the presence of such lipids, is probably not warranted.

Under each of these circumstances, small quantities of iron salts may be demonstrated at times at the same sites as the calcium deposits. It will be recalled that the calcium and iron lakes observed in hematoxylin-stained sections appear essentially the same, so that more specific techniques are required to identify the element or elements present in such mineral deposits. In the conditions already discussed, calcium deposits occur more frequently and in greater quantity than iron, though both may be demonstrated. Indeed, in one case of Sturge-Weber disease, iron salts were present to the exclusion of calcium.

A relationship to vitamin D or parathyroid metabolism is not clearly demonstrable in any of the conditions associated with calcification. It has, however, been suggested that hypoparathyroidism may be associated with calcific deposits in the walls of blood vessels in the globus pallidus and other portions of the brain. Calcification occurring with hyperparathyroidism is better documented. In any case, iron salts are almost always demonstrable in such calcific deposits and seem to occur with greater frequency than deposits of calcium. This is discussed further below.

Iron

Iron is normally present in the hemoglobin of red cells coursing in vessels of the central nervous system, and it is present also in the tissues. The precise nature of the iron deposits in normal tissues is not clear. Neither ferric nor ferrous ions are demonstrated in paraffin sections of normal neural tissues stained by the usual histochemical techniques. Iron may be stored as ferritin, a water-soluble iron-containing protein. It and its iron-free protein moiety, apoferritin, have been demonstrated by precipitation with cadmium sulfate, as a result of which characteristic octahedral yellow-brown crystals form. If ferritin were present in the brain, its iron component could be demonstrated by simple techniques. However, being water-soluble, it could readily be lost by processing in aqueous solutions.

Following hemorrhage, the iron present in hemosiderin, the major breakdown product of hemoglobin, is easily demonstrated. The same techniques which reveal the iron of hemosiderin will also bring out iron salts deposited in the course of pathological processes, excluding hemorrhage. The most useful technique is that which employs a ferrocyanide solution. This will precipitate as ferric ferrocyanide (Prussian blue) any ferric ions present in the tissue. In rare instances much smaller quantities of ferrous ions may be present in the tissues.

These can be demonstrated through precipitation as ferrous ferricyanide (Turnbull blue), utilizing ferricyanide solution for this purpose. In each instance, a slightly acid medium is used to free the weak bond which may exist between the iron and a protein or other substance.

Most of the iron deposits in the brain, other than those associated with hemorrhage, have no color. However, in hematoxylin-stained sections they form deep blueblack lakes, and they are also stained by the Nissl techniques. Iron in hematoxylin-stained lakes is indistinguishable from calcium. Thus, more definitive histochemical studies are required to determine if a given deposit contains calcium, iron, or both.

In the brain, iron salts are commonly found in the walls of small vessels within the globus pallidus, in the form of granules, irregular plaques, or linear deposits. At times the entire vessel wall is impregnated by such salts. When large quantities are present at this site, smaller amounts may be found free in the tissues. Very similar changes are often found in the cerebellum, particularly in the granular layer and about the dentate nucleus, and less often in the hippocampus; actually the salts may be deposited anywhere in the brain. Although such iron deposits are seen in approximately 40% of individuals past 40 years of age, a minor deposition of these salts in favored locations may be encountered in young individuals and even in infants. In most cases, no appreciable pathological change is noted in the cells and other tissue components of the affected area. Histochemically, iron is always demonstrable in these deposits. In cases in which iron salts are sparse, only iron can be identified, but when present in large quantity, calcium salts as well can be found (siderocalcification); although under the latter condition calcium salts may predominate, iron is almost never absent. Both iron and calcium salts are radioopaque, and large quantities of either of these salts or mixtures of both may be visible on X ray. Both iron and calcium in these siderocalcific deposits may be extracted by chelation with disodium ethylenediaminetetraacetate (EDTA). The iron of hemosiderin is not extracted by this procedure. In most instances, the iron deposits are only part of a broad series of local degenerative changes, as is true also for calcific deposits. Metachromatic glycolipids, possibly acid mucopolysaccharides, are regularly demonstrable at these sites.

Changes of this type are common past middle life and are seen with great frequency in the brains of older people who have had no neurological or psychiatric evidence of disease. Occasionally such changes are found in the brains of older individuals with clinical abnormalities; in some of these cases, the mineral deposits have been interpreted as a manifestation of a basic disease process, to which the term *Fahr's disease* has been applied. In these cases as well, very little pathological change is noted in other components of the mineralized tissues.

Iron salts are also present among the pigments deposited in tissues affected by Hallervorden-Spatz disease. They are also found in the cerebral cortex in general paresis, in degenerated areas in the choroid plexus, and, as already noted, following hemorrhage and in hemochromatosis.

BIBLIOGRAPHY

LIBER, A. F.   Chelatable iron in senile siderocalcification of the human brain. *Journal of Neuropathology and Experimental Neurology,* 1965, *24,* 675–681.
NEUMANN, M. A.   Iron and calcium dysmetabolism in the brain, with special predilection for globus pallidus and cerebellum. *Journal of Neuropathology and Experimental Neurology,* 1963, *22,* 148–163.
SLAGER, V. T., and WAGNER, J. A.   The incidence, composition, and pathological significance of intracerebral vascular deposits in the basal ganglia. *Journal of Neuropathology and Experimental Neurology,* 1956, *15,* 417–431.
UZMAN, L. L.   Histochemical localization of copper with rubeanic acid. *Laboratory Investigation,* 1956, *5,* 299–305.

IRWIN FEIGIN
ABNER WOLF

MINNESOTA MULTIPHASIC PERSONALITY INVENTORY (MMPI)

The Minnesota Multiphasic Personality Inventory is the best known and most widely researched psychological inventory in the area of psychodiagnosis and the assessment of psychopathology. Published in the early 1940s, the MMPI has remained essentially unchanged in format since that time, although considerable advances have been made in interpretive methods. The 1972 *Seventh Mental Measurements Yearbook* lists more than 3,000 publications on the MMPI.

The MMPI consists of 10 clinical scales and 3 validity scales (L, F, and K), based on 550 true/false items. Each clinical scale represents one of the major psychodiagnostic categories that were current in the late 1930s. The clinical scales, whose letter abbreviations are given below, are more appropriately known by their numbers (1 through 9 and 0), since a high score on a scale often does not automatically mean identification with that particular patient criterion group. The scales were developed primarily by the empirical method of test construction, a procedure that represented a significant advance for the time in the technology of psychodiagnostic test construction. In its many years of existence, the MMPI has served as a model for the construction of many other psychological assessment devices, and has also been the major vehicle for research on methodological topics, such as response bias and actuarial versus clinical prediction. The most authoritative reference work on the MMPI is the newly revised two-volume *MMPI Handbook* by Dahlstrom, Welsh, and Dahlstrom (1972–1975).

The MMPI is suitable for ages 16 and over, and is available in three main forms: (a) the card form, in which items are printed on individual cards and are sorted by the respondent; (b) the most common, the booklet form, in which responses are marked on an IBM-style answer sheet and are scored either by hand-scoring stencils or by machine, or can be mailed to a scoring service; and (c) Form R, a newer step-down booklet form with lap-board hard cover. The test takes 40–90 minutes to answer, and handscoring the booklet form takes about 10 minutes. Scores are transferred to a profile sheet, which converts them automatically to a normative standard score form (T-scores) with mean of 50 and standard deviation of 10, and permits the K-correction for defensiveness to be applied. The distributions of nearly all the scales are skewed in the positive direction. The MMPI is published by the Psychological Corporation.

Construction

Construction of the MMPI was begun in the late 1930s by Starke R. Hathaway and J. Charnley McKinley, who were motivated by their recognition of a need in both clinical psychiatric research and practice for an objective multidimensional instrument to assist in the identification of psychopathology. The instrument should provide for a comprehensive sampling of behavior of significance to psychiatrists, yet involve a simple presentation, so that it could be used with individuals of limited intelligence and education. They compiled more than 1,000 items from psychiatric examination forms, psychiatry textbooks, previously published attitude and personality scales, and from their own clinical experience, and prepared them in a self-report true/false format. The number of items was reduced to 550 through the course of revisions.

Generally speaking, each scale was empirically developed by contrasting the responses of nonpsychiatric control subjects with those of patients in a particular psychiatric diagnostic category, using the traditional system of diagnosis which stemmed from the work of Kraepelin in the late nineteenth century. More than 800 carefully studied psychiatric patients constituted the pool of clinical subjects, while approximately 1,500 control subjects were drawn from hospital visitors, normal clients at the University of Minnesota Testing Bureau, local WPA workers, and general medical patients. The individual diagnostic criterion groups generally numbered 50 or fewer, although in some cases, additional groups were utilized in efforts to improve the discriminating power of the scale. For example, more than a dozen scales were developed in an unsuccessful effort to obtain satisfactory discrimination among the subcategories of schizophrenia.

The usual method of item selection was to consider a basic pool of those items which showed a statistically significant percentage frequency difference between the responses of the criterion group and the control subjects. Items were excluded if the frequency of response for both groups was very high or very low, if they failed to differentiate among additional relevant groups, or if the group difference appeared to have an irrelevant basis, such as marital status. Further items were often eliminated from a scale if they showed an overlap in validity with some other diagnostic category. No item, however, was ever eliminated from a scale because its manifest content appeared unrelated to the category in question.

Individual Scales

The patient criterion groups are listed below, together with brief research-based notes on the meaning of high (and low) scores. It was the original hope of the test authors that a patient's appropriate psychodiagnostic category would be simply indicated by the highest scale score. Research has shown that the MMPI cannot be used in this manner, although considerable meaning can be derived from high scores on individual scales. More appropriate for psychodiagnostic purposes is the use of patterns or configurations of high scores, discussed in a later section.

Lie Scale (L). The L scale, intended to provide a basis for evaluating subjects' general frankness in responding to the test items, contains 15 items selected rationally to reflect behaviors that are socially desirable but obviously unlikely. High scorers have probably engaged in rather naive distortion in their responses to the remainder of the test, in an attempt to present themselves in a favorable light. They often come from the lower socioeconomic levels or have limited intelligence, a naive but genuine belief in their own virtues, and a lack of insight into their own motivation.

Infrequency Scale (F). The F scale contains 64 items which were endorsed by very few of the normal criterion subjects—usually less than 10%. Thus, a high F score indicates an atypical or deviant set of responses. Possible reasons are (1) technical difficulties, such as random responding, inadequate intelligence or education, lack of familiarity with English, inadequate vision, or a clerical error in scoring; (2) a deliberate effort by the subject to present himself in an unfavorable light, or to convey the impression that he is emotionally disturbed; and (3) actual deviance, or degree of psychopathology.

Correction Scale (K). The K scale was derived after the original development of the test as a correction scale for improving the discriminations of the clinical scales by correcting for test-taking defensiveness. Most of the items were selected by comparing the responses of normal subjects with those of 50 psychiatric patients who obtained high scores on the L scale but whose clinical scores were in the normal range. Various fractions of the K score are added to the raw scores of several clinical scales. Although

MMPI users have been encouraged to develop K weights that are optimal in their particular settings, use of the original weights as indicated on the profile sheet is almost universal. The K score reflects test-taking defensiveness of a more subtle nature than the L scale. The F minus K difference has been suggested as an index of exaggeration in a pathological direction.

Scale 1: Hypochondriasis (Hs). Hypochondriasis was defined as "abnormal psychoneurotic concern over bodily health." The criterion group contained 50 patients, and excluded any who showed indications of psychosis. High scores reflect undue concern about one's physical health; symptoms are often claimed for which no clear organic basis can be found, and the importance of any actual organic malfunctioning is exaggerated. When the two highest scores occur on the Hs and Hy scales, the likelihood of psychophysiological complaints is particularly high.

Scale 2: Depression (D). This scale was developed to measure symptomatic depression, referring to patients showing "a clinically recognizable, general frame of mind characterized by poor morale, lack of hope in the future, and dissatisfaction with the patient's own status generally." The main criterion group contained 50 patients, most of whom were in the depressed phase of a manic-depressive psychosis. This scale is the most frequent high point among psychiatric patients, and high scorers are readily aware of their proneness toward excessive worry and pessimism. It is sometimes suggested that patients who score high on the D scale but deny depressive feelings and in fact do not show depressive behavior should be watched carefully for possible suicidal intent.

Scale 3: Hysteria (Hy). The Hy scale was intended as an aid in the clinical diagnosis of hysteria. The criterion patients either had been diagnosed "psychoneurosis, hysteria," or had been observed to have hysterical components in their disturbance. High scores on the Hy scale are fairly common for women but rather infrequent for men, and suggest a tendency toward some particular somatic complaint or symptom, particularly when under psychological stress, with a simultaneous tendency to claim superior social adjustment. The "V" pattern of high Hs and Hy, and low D, has been interpreted as suggesting the clinical *belle indifference* of the hysteric.

Scale 4: Psychopathic Deviate (Pd). The main criterion group consisted of 100 persons who appeared to fit the asocial and amoral types of psychopathic personality. Those with psychotic or neurotic manifestations were eliminated. Most were in the age range 17–22, and all had long histories of minor delinquency, such as stealing, lying, truancy, sexual promiscuity, alcoholic overindulgence, and forgery. High scores on the Pd scale can be interpreted as nonconformity and rejection of normal social conventions. Prison and delinquent groups, as expected from the derivation of the scale, show marked elevations. Peaks on the D and Pd scales are not uncommon among alcoholics and drug addicts.

Scale 5: Masculinity-Femininity (Mf). The main criterion group consisted of 13 homosexual males, whose responses were contrasted with those of normal males. Use was also made of a group of feminine males identified by another inventory, and of differences in frequency of response to items by normal males and females. High scores on the Mf scale are designed to indicate feminine interests in men and masculine interests in women. Although homosexual men tend to show high scores, so do other groups, in particular those with artistic or literary interests.

Scale 6: Paranoia (Pa). The criterion patients were those judged to have paranoid symptoms including ideas of reference, feelings of persecution, and grandiose self-concepts; or, more mildly, suspiciousness, rigidity, and excessive personal sensitivity. The Pa scale is considered to be fairly weak. Although high scores suggest suspiciousness, fixed beliefs, and perhaps formal paranoid signs, the majority of paranoid patients do not achieve particularly high scores.

Scale 7: Psychasthenia (Pt). The term *psychasthenia,* now obsolete, was applied to individuals with compulsions, obsessions, unreasonable fears, and excessive doubts. The final criterion group contained 20 patients who had been studied intensively both medically and psychiatrically. The Pt scale is perhaps the best single MMPI indicator of general anxiety. High scorers tend to suffer from excessive doubts, to ruminate at length, and to have pervasive feelings of guilt and insecurity. Many such persons are compulsively introspective, and ruminate endlessly to no effect. This scale is highly correlated with the Sc scale.

Scale 8: Schizophrenia (Sc). Criterion patients for this scale were those diagnosed to have schizophrenia in one or another of its various subtypes. There were two partly overlapping criterion groups of 50 patients, of whom more were males than females. The final scale was one of a large number of preliminary scales, which included more than a dozen subscales derived from the four subclassifications of schizophrenia: catatonic, paranoid, simple, and hebephrenic. The Sc scale is also relatively weak; many schizophrenics do not score high on the scale, and the label "schizophrenic" should be used with great circumspection. Among known patients, peaks on the Pa and Sc scales sometimes suggest paranoid schizophrenia.

Scale 9: Hypomania (Ma). The term *hypomania* was employed to describe the milder degrees of manic excitement typically occurring in manic-depressive psychosis (elated but unstable mood, psychomotor excitement, and flight of ideas). The criterion group contained 24 patients, and excluded those with delirium, confusional states, signs of other psychoses, or agitated depressions. High scorers are hyperactive, impulsive, and unpredictable, elated but unstable in mood, restless, overoptimistic, and easily distractible. Moderate elevations on this scale suggest milder degrees of these characteristics. Peaks on scales Ma and Pd, or Ma, Pd, and Sc, are relatively common among prisoners and juvenile delinquents.

Scale 0: Social Introversion (Si). Although not one of the original clinical scales, the Si scale appears on the MMPI profile form and is widely used. Items were selected from among those which differentiated high scorers and low scorers on the social introversion-extraversion scale of the Minnesota T-S-E inventory. High scorers on the Si scale tend to be introverted, shy and socially inept, and prefer to avoid social activity. Low scorers are gregarious, outgoing, sociable, enthusiastic, assertive, talkative, and adept at interpersonal manipulation.

Interpretation

Basic interpretations of high scores on individual scales have been given above. It should be emphasized that these and the following interpretive statements apply to the MMPI profiles of patient populations only. For populations with greatly different frequencies (base rates) of psychological disorder, such as a college class, interpretive statements should be couched in nonpathological terms (Lanyon, 1968).

The most sophisticated interpretive procedures for the MMPI involve the use of profile patterns, usually defined mainly by the 2 or 3 highest scores (e.g., a "2–7" or a "4–8–9" profile), provided they exceed a certain minimum, usually a T-score of 70. Several such "code books," or collections of empirically derived MMPI patterns, are available, together with extensive interpretive information: the Marks and Seeman *Actuarial Description of Abnormal Personality,* and their *Actuarial Use of the MMPI with Adolescents and Adults;* the Gilbertstadt and Duker *Handbook of Clinical and Actuarial MMPI Interpretation;* and Lachar's *The MMPI: Clinical Assessment and Automated Interpretation.* Once again, these interpretations should be applied only if the population of which the patient is a member is similar to the one from which the interpretations were derived.

Also available are commercial MMPI interpretation services, which offer a computer printout of interpretive rules that are essentially a computerized code book. Despite the rapidly growing popularity of such services, readers should be warned that their use is hazardous because of the failure to allow for widely differing base rates of relevant patient characteristics. However, automated MMPI interpretation systems that are designed for a specific population or institution can be both valid and highly economical.

Variations in age, education, race, sex, and socioeconomic status affect certain of the scales in small but important ways. The interpretation of adolescent profiles tends to be substantially different from that of adults. It is extremely hazardous to utilize the MMPI in translation into languages other than English, though a number of translations have nonetheless been made.

Reliability and Validity

At the time that the MMPI was developed, test construction procedures lacked much of their current sophistication, so that the MMPI is much less than optimally efficient from a psychometric viewpoint. Two such problems are item redundancy and high interscale correlations. However, the volume of research on the MMPI is now so large that it is an extremely valuable tool despite these difficulties, and could not be changed without invalidating this extensive interpretive literature.

Reliability data are summarized in the two-volume *MMPI Handbook;* validity data are also reviewed there and in the code books listed above. Studies comparing the accuracy of MMPI interpretation with that of tests, such as the Rorschach and TAT, have shown the MMPI to be equal or superior on the average for general descriptive purposes; in addition, its much lower cost of use gives it high cost-efficiency. A common application in high-volume settings is the use of specifically trained clerical personnel for routine administration, scoring, and routine interpretations, using code books and objective rules that are specific to the particular setting, with the availability of an experienced consultant to design and monitor the system and to evaluate unusual cases.

Variations and Developments

Additional Scales and Indexes. The original (1960) *MMPI Handbook* lists, in addition to the 14 basic MMPI scales, approximately 200 additional scales and indexes that have subsequently been developed from MMPI items by other authors. Typical scales assess hostility, low back pain, underachievement, and ulcer personality. Many of these scales were, unfortunately, constructed with substantially less care than the original scales, and prospective users should study their derivation carefully. Several of the most popular scales are the following.

Factors A and R. It has been demonstrated through factor-analytic procedures that many of the MMPI items can be assigned to one of two general categories or factors. Scales A and R were constructed to assess these two main factors. Scale A appears to reflect anxiety or general emotional upset, and scale R has been considered related to the concepts of repression and introversion.

Ego-Strength (Es). This scale consists of items which discriminated 17 neurotic patients who were judged to have improved after six

months of individual psychotherapy from 16 patients who were judged unimproved. Although the criterion groups were small, subsequent evidence has shown the scale to be valid for predicting improvement in other psychotherapy settings.

Taylor Manifest Anxiety (At). The At scale was originally developed for use in basic research on Hullian drive theory. Items included were those that four out of five judges agreed upon as related to anxiety. There is research evidence for the validity of the scale, which correlates highly with the Pt and Sc scales.

Short Forms. A number of "short forms" of the MMPI have been developed, which attempt to predict scores on the basic scales from about 80–160 items. Studies have shown that while some of the short-form scales correlate highly with the full-length scales, the patterns of high 2-point and 3-point codes, on which interpretation tends to be based, show only limited correspondence, so that short forms are as yet not a feasible matter.

Other Variations. Taped forms of the MMPI are available for the hard-of-hearing; these appear to give essentially the same results as the booklet form. In regard to lifting individual scales out of context and administering them alone, this appears to have no ill effect on validity.

BIBLIOGRAPHY

DAHLSTROM, W. G. et al. *An MMPI handbook* (Rev. ed.). Minneapolis: University of Minnesota Press, 1972–1975.

LACHAR, D. *The MMPI: Clinical assessment and automated interpretation.* Los Angeles, Calif.: Western Psychological Services, 1974.

LANYON, R. I. *A handbook of MMPI group profiles.* Minneapolis: University of Minnesota Press, 1968.

RICHARD I. LANYON

MINORITIES IN PROFESSIONAL PSYCHOLOGY IN THE UNITED STATES

Minority representation in professional psychology in the past has been limited. There have been outstanding members of ethnic and racial minorities in professional psychology, but the numbers have been rather small.

Since the mid-1960s professional psychology

has attempted to meet the challenge to be more socially representative of the American population and has become more sensitive to the needs of society and to the social responsibility of psychology as a profession in meeting these needs. Psychologists have began taking on new tasks and attempting to solve new problems for new populations. These new sensitivities and attempts to serve different populations have spurred professional psychologists to examine more closely the racial/ethnic combinations within their own ranks.

No accurate assessment of the racial/ethnic distribution of psychologists has been made in the United States on a systematic basis. Bayton, Roberts, and Williams (1970) estimated that there were probably 200 black Ph.D.s in psychology in 1969 and even fewer who were members of other racial/ethnic minorities.

In 1972 the American Psychological Association (APA) conducted a survey (Boneau and Cuca, 1974) that included an optional question requesting respondents to identify themselves by racial/ethnic groups. As Table 1 indicates, minority representation in the APA is in general not proportionally representative of minority representation in the total population. Only the proportion of Orientals in the APA compares favorably with the total U.S. percentage.

The explanation for this low frequency of minority participation in professional psychology could be approached from a number of different levels. Psychology in general has been considered a "nontraditional" field for minority groups in the sense that they have not shared fully in the development of conceptual frameworks or training models in the field that would indicate sensitivity to minority concerns. Psychology has typically been responsible for exploitation and perpetuation of stereotypic views of minorities (Bayton, Roberts, and Williams, 1970; Boxley and Wagner, 1971; Sue and Sue, 1972). Hence, psychology in general has not been receptive to the needs of racial/ethnic minorities. This lack of sensitivity has often resulted in the field being unable to attract minority students who have the potential to alter the field's sensitivity.

Concerted efforts have been made to increase minority participation in psychology starting in the late 1960s. In 1969 the National Institute of Mental Health funded a conference with the expressed purpose of exploring the problems involved in increasing the numbers of minority group members in professional psychology (Bayton, Roberts, and Williams, 1970). One of the primary problems identified at that conference as limiting minority participation in psychology was the absence in numbers of successful minority psychologists, who could otherwise demonstrate the viability of psychology as a career for minorities.

From the late 1960s on minority psychologists have apparently felt the need to demonstrate psychology as a field viable for ethnic/racial minorities. A number of professional psychological associations were founded concerned specifically with the problems of certain ethnic groups and accelerating participation of specific ethnic groups in psychology.

Table 1. Minority Representation in the APA and U.S. Population

Racial/Ethnic Identity	Ph.D.s	% of Group in APA	% of Group in U.S. Population
White	14,864	93.6	87.7
Black	189	1.2	11.2
Oriental	128	.8	.8
American Indian	16	.1	.3
Middle Eastern	15	.1	NA
East Indian	27	.2	NA
Hawaiian-Polynesian	18	.1	NA
Other	628	4.0	NA
Total Responses	15,885	—	—

Note: NA = not available.
Source: Boneau and Cuca, 1974. © 1974 by the American Psychological Association; reprinted by permission.

Associations of Minority Psychologists

In 1968 the Association of Black Psychologists (ABPsi) was formed as a national organization addressing itself to the general problem of underrepresentation of black psychologists and the specific problem of critically conceptualizing the relationship between black people and the society in which they live (Williams, 1974).

The late 1960s also marked the beginning of the Association of Psychologists for La Raza and the Association of Asian-American Psychologists. These associations as well as ABPsi have been particularly responsive to the lack of reliable data and to misconceptions about mental health aspects of Mexican-Americans, Asian-Americans, and black Americans.

In 1968 the Black Students Psychological Association (BSPA) was founded. Among its goals was the establishment of a functional recruitment and training model that would be inclusive of many of the problems all psychology students face. The BSPA identified four areas of concern for program development and implementation: (1) recruitment of black students into psychology; (2) recruitment of black faculty members into psychology; (3) identifying programs offering meaningful community experience for black psychology students; and (4) developing programs at various degree levels to prepare black psychology students to return to the black community (1970). The BSPA identified ways in which the APA could aid in the implementation of these concerns.

CABPP

The APA responded to the stated concerns and objectives of the BSPA by expressing a commitment to work with the BSPA, including appropriating funds directly and indirectly to the BSPA, and by establishing the Commission for Accelerating Black Participation in Psychology (CABPP) (Simpkins and Raphael; 1970). One outcome of the commission's effort was the establishment of the Office of the Black Students Psychological Association in the APA building in Washington, D.C. The commission's final recommendations included a plea for members of APA to

accelerate the participation of black students and professionals in your own institution and try to understand the difference between involvement and tokenism. . . . As administrators, department heads, deans, therapists, trainers—stop trying to "fit" blacks into the white experience. Spend some time and effort to go beyond stereotypes to find what the black experience can offer the science of behavior and vice versa. (Blau, 1970)

Reported Progress

The *APA Monitor* reported that minority enrollment in graduate school departments of psychology was 10% in 1972 and 7% in both 1971 and 1970. The 3% increase in enrollment in 1972 was attributed to "a growing awareness on the part of psychologists that minorities have been underrepresented in the field" (Cuca, 1974). Recruitment of minority students was probably limited to a few schools. A study by Potter (1974) indicated that among 69 APA-approved programs in clinical psychology, 43 (66%) of the programs did not recruit minority group students. Padilla and Wagner (1973) reported that there was no significant increase in minority representation on the faculty level from 1970 (3.2%) to 1972 (3.3%). It was also reported in that same study that on faculties blacks were underrepresented by a factor of 5 and Chicanos by a factor of 50 and that Filipinos were not represented at all. El-Khanas and Kinzer (1974) indicate that in 1973 minority graduate student enrollment in psychology was 6.6% in public institutions and 6.1% in private institutions (based on data from 154 Ph.D.-granting institutions). This is not particularly encouraging if the 1972 enrollment was 10%, as reported by Cuca (1974).

Apparently, the increase has been slow on the student level and even slower on the faculty level, but there is some activity. The more important issues of minority life experiences being incorporated into the knowledge base of the field, the elimination of exploitative research in minority communities, and the elimination of stereotypical views of minorities have not yet begun to be evaluated. No systematic assessment has been made of what happens to minority Ph.D.s following graduation: what kinds of theoretical orientations are advocated, what kinds of jobs are accepted, and where the jobs are located. It can only be said that minority representation in professional psychology is increasing on all levels slowly.

BIBLIOGRAPHY

BAYTON, J. A.; ROBERTS, S. O.; and WILLIAMS, R. K. Minority groups and careers in psychology. *American Psychologist,* 1970, *25*(6), 504.

BLAU, T. APA Commission on accelerating black participation in psychology. *American Psychologist,* 1970, *25* (12), 1103.

BONEAU, C. A., and CUCA, J. M. An overview of psychology's human resources: Characteristics and salaries from the 1972 APA survey. *American Psychologist,* 1974, *29* (11), 821.

BOXLEY, R., and WAGNER, N. Clinical psychology training programs and minority groups: A survey. *Professional Psychology,* 1971, *2*(1), 75.

CUCA, J. Graduate enrollments level off, women and minority students increase. *APA Monitor,* 1974, *5*(11).

EL-KHANAS, E., and KINZER, J. *Enrollment of minority graduate students at Ph.D. granting institutions.* Higher Education Panel Reports no. 19. Washington, D.C.: American Council on Education, 1974.

PADILLA, E. R., and WAGNER, N. The representation of minority groups in clinical psychology. *APA Division 31 Newsletter,* March 1973, *4*(2), 2.

POTTER, N. D. Recruitment of minority group students and women. *American Psychologist,* 1974, *29*(2), 151–152.

SIMPKINS, G., and RAPHAEL, P. Goals of the Black Students Psychological Association. *American Psychologist,* 1970, *25*(5), xxii.

SUE, D. W., and SUE, S. Ethnic minorities: Resistance to being researched. *Professional Psychology,* 1972, *3*(1), 11.

WILLIAMS, R. A history of the Association of Black Psychologists: Early formation and development. *Journal of Black Psychology,* 1974, *1*(1), 9.

See also ETHNIC MINORITY GROUPS AND AMERICAN PSYCHIATRY

CAROLYN SUBER

MMPI
See MINNESOTA MULTIPHASIC PERSONALITY INVENTORY (MMPI)

MNEMONICS

Mnemonics (Gk. *mnēmonikos*) is defined as a "technique of improving the efficiency of memory." Presumably, such a technique would prove of immediate and persistent concern for psychologists interested in learning, and forgetting. However, psychologists had shown virtually no interest in mnemonics until about 1965 when a somewhat more than modest interest developed.

Psychologists' Disdain

The reasons for psychologists' disinterest in mnemonics is not difficult to appreciate.

1. The very definition is cast in *faculty* terms —one cannot improve something which does not exist.
2. A powerful negative opinion pronounced by William James after a heroic adventure in memorizing stated the basic position: one cannot improve the efficiency of memorizing by practice. This was interpreted to read: memorizing cannot be improved.
3. The art or skill of mnemonists, from what little was known about such stage performers appeared to be based in large part on imagery, and J. B. Watson's dismissal of imagery from the lexicon of psychology in 1913 closed the book on mnemonics for the next half-century.

The lack of interest in mnemonics does not mean that psychologists were not deeply involved in the study of learning and retention, if not memory, as some faculty of the mind. Methods of efficient learning were, of course, persistently studied. Such operations as active recitation rather than passive reading were found to be of high potency. In the decades following James, learning psychologists studied a whole variety of procedures and techniques for facilitating learning. Besides the active recitation procedure there was considerable investigation of such factors as whole-part learning, grouping and patterning, learning-how-to-learn, the influence of meaning, spacing versus massing, and so on. It was not then a lack of interest in retention that characterized psychologists but their reluctance to associate themselves with what they regarded as trickery or fraud. The "master mentalists" were put down as cheats or freaks, "idiot savants," and beyond the limits of the proper concern of psychologists with normal people. The notion that the study of the abnormal would help in the understanding of the normal did not seem to apply to memory.

The "Discovery" of Mnemonics

The first rumblings of a development of interest in mnemonics were heard when G. A. Miller, E. Galanter, and K. H. Pribram published their *Plans and the Structure of Behavior* in 1960. In this volume the authors argued that all learning is based on some sort of plan of how to learn, or of how to remember, and the structuring of the material to be learned. They argued further that with a plan much more is accomplished than without. They cited findings of increased retention with the use of some procedures (the plan) such as forming associations between words in some relationship with each other. Thus, they reported people remembering several hundred associated responses after one pairing when subjects were presented with the stimulus words they had formerly related to the response words. Miller, Pribram, and Galanter also described a mnemonic device which would facilitate learning ten items in a serial order. The device or, as they called it, the plan, consisted of first learning a 10-word nursery rhyme (1-bun, 2-shoe, 3-tree, 4-door, etc.) and then imagining any given object with its numerical listing; thus, if the fifth word mentioned is "knife", some kind of knife would be "imaged" with a hive (5-hive) and later the memorizer could report the fifth word by saying to himself "5-hive-knife", as the image of the hive would automatically arouse the image of a knife cutting through the hive or whatever the memorizer had previously imaged the knife to be doing. Similarly any of the other ten words could be reported in serial or any other desired order. The learning was not truly serial in nature; it was actually a set of ten paired-associates with the feature of a numerical value for one of the members of a pair which would thus permit a serial report.

The current and more active revival of interest in mnemonics can be attributed largely to the appearance of historian Frances Yates' *The Art of Memory* which traces the history of the mnemonic arts back to the early Greeks and Romans and the Ciceronian device, commonly attributed to him but actually not his invention of the associating through imagery of two items in terms of the location of the item of interest. The procedure called for being familiar with some structured *locus* (e.g., a house and its grounds). To remember an item or thing *(res)* one would imagine it at the front entrance. If there were more items to remember they would be imaginatively placed in a regular order around the several rooms and places in the home or garden. The procedure came to be identified as *loci et res* and works very effectively if one cares to remember a series of things or items in serial order. Thus Ross and Lawrence, in Australia (Richardson, 1969) familiarized subjects with the sequential location of some 50 buildings or structures on the campus and then asked them to "image" 50 items, one after another, on or in one of the 50 structures. Recall was virtually perfect for the 50 items in sequence. Such an astonishing performance of what would otherwise be regarded as mental wizardry led to a new concern with the formerly disregarded stage performers.

The publication of Luria's little book, *The Mind of a Mnemonist,* added to the growing interest in mnemonics. Here an internationally famous psychologist deigned to show interest in a professional mnemonist. Luria expressed his failure to understand the "unusual" capacities of his subject except for his use of the *loci et res* technique. What astounded Luria most was the capacity of Mr. S. to remember long lists of numbers for periods of years. Luria tested Mr. S. at various intervals over 30 years and was uniformly amazed at each test. The fact that Mr. S. is not unique, that many such mnemonists have been witnessed for centuries and are to be seen today, has led psychologists to a variety of conclusions:

1. the individuals possess a native talent, or
2. they are charlatans who have a bag of tricks by which they deceive audiences, or
3. they are not unusual, really, and any normal person could approximate their performances if he followed certain procedures he usually does not know about or does not care to practice.

The first conclusion might well be dismissed as might be the second in that there need be no deceptions involved. Performances like naming 200 people in an audience after having met them only briefly may be quite legitimate. Certainly naming all of the topics or sections of a magazine like *Time* by page numbers as they are called out at random is something well within the capacity of most literate people capable of reading the magazine. Remembering long lists of numbers is only slightly more troublesome and calls for an additional step. In the following paragraphs such "tricks" will be analyzed for those unfamiliar with what are now classical procedures.

The Tricks of the Trade

To learn the serial location of any item, take a critical review of a motion picture in a magazine, and to recall either the page number, given the item (or vice versa), it is first necessary to have a serial identifier, like 1-bun, 2-shoe, or the Ciceronian locus as, for example, the bathroom in one's home or some public place. If the series of items is extensive, say up to 100, then 100 serial identifiers are required and must be learned first. To facilitate learning and using 100 identifiers, mnemonists usually take advantage of a system first devised by Stanislaus Von Wenaussheim, otherwise known as Johann Wincklemann, in 1648. Leibnitz is said to have known or to have used or improved the system. The system consists of assigning a consonant to each numeral as: 1 = *t* or *d*; 2 = *n*; 3 = *m*; 4 = *r*; 5 = l; 6 = soft *g, j, ch,* or *sh*; 7 = hard *g* or *k*; 8 = *f* or *v*; 9 = *b* or *p*; and 0 = *s, z,* or soft *c*. Using such letters as substitute for numbers, one can then form simple, common words out of any numbers, for example any short word like "toe" could stand for 1. Vowels do not count. The number, 11, would be made up of a word with two ts or two ds and any number of vowels (e.g., dad, toot, teeth); 47 would call for a word beginning with r and having a k or g as the next consonant. Thus rug or rake would do. With 100 words prepared and memorized, the mnemonist is ready to undertake the magazine topic task. He sees on page 52 that the Queen of England is at a horse show. He "images" the Queen in some relationship

$$5 \quad 2 \quad \quad 5 \quad 2$$

with a word such as *loan* or *lion*—perhaps the Queen leading a lion around on a leash—and his task is done. Later when asked about page 52 he generates the word *lion* and automatically the image of the Queen is recalled. He could easily reverse the process if asked for the page with the story about the Queen. The same process is followed for each page and the mnemonist is then ready for the performance. What the mnemonist has done is to have used a set of preprepared distinctive "pegs" or "hooks" on which to hang a set of unassorted pictures. To remember a set of numbers is more troublesome and involves creating the second item of a pair. Having a list of 100 peg words manufactured out of numbers in the first place through translation the mnemonist must now translate a given number, say, 1485 into some word or phrase containing the consonants *t-r-v-l*, in serial order. The word "travel" is an obvious one and if 1485 is the first number group mentioned, the mnemonist images his word for 1 (e.g., "toy") in some relationship to travel. The second number group, say, 8397, calls for a word or words with the letters *v-m-b-k*, or *f-m-p-k*, or *f-m-p-g*, in that order. Here, if an obvious word does not spring up the mnemonist must fashion one for himself. He might try *f-m-p-g* and come up with *fame-pig* or *fame-book*. The generated phrase would then be associated to whatever he had previously prepared for 2, say *new* or *no*. If there were 10 such 4-place numbers, such as Luria's mnemonist could repeat after one hearing, he could then recite the numbers in any order upon request. He would have learned only 10 associations instead of 40 numerals. By a similar process he could remember a 40-place or 100-place number. It would be necessary only to group the original numbers into convenient words and associate them with their numerical pegs. Note that the number memorizer is not memorizing numbers at all—he is memorizing words or experiencing their substrates, namely images.

Mnemonists make use of another procedure called *linking*. Linking amounts to imaging and associating any pair of items, say *car* and *book,* and then associating *book* with a third item, say *spoon,* which is then associated with a fourth item, say *dog,* and so on. The imaging or association must be in the form of an interaction of the two items. Just "picturing" them side by side will not prove effective. To remember that spoon "goes with book," one could imagine the spoon being used as a bookmark. By this procedure an extended number of items can be recalled in serial order should one care to make the effort. Grammar school children do as well as college seniors with lists of 20 words, many earning perfect scores, with no prior training, if they are instructed to try to have interactive images.

Other mnemonic procedures make use of rhymes and rhythm (i before e, except after c; thirty days hath September). Apparently there is some inherent advantage to such linguistic features. For material with no inherent continuity, use is made of an additional device or procedure, that of substitution. The substitution can be applied to names which may have no meaning (e.g., Sokolov can become the *sock-i-love,* Talleyrand can be *tall-and-round* or whatever first occurs to the mnemonist). Abstract words can be "translated" into more concrete, imaginable items. "Justice" can be symbolized by the blind goddess, "freedom" becomes the Liberty Bell, and so on. Another form of substitution consists of making up words or acronyms from the first letters of the words to be remembered; thus Standard Oil Company becomes SOCONY in New York and in Ohio it becomes SOHIO. The National Organization of Women becomes NOW and so with hundreds of governmental agencies, clubs, and so on. Sometimes the "abbreviation" becomes somewhat involved as in the classical "On old Olympus tiny top a Finn and German viewed some hops" used by neurology students to remember the 12 cranial nerves.

The basic procedures employed by professional mnemonists have now been described. They consist of the use of pegs or hooks, linking, and substitution with a heavy reliance on imagery to function automatically in order to reactivate associations. One point commonly stressed by mnemonists is that the imagery has to be bizarre if it is to work. Commonplace associations are alleged to be forgotten quickly. In practice it becomes almost impossible not to use bizarre imagery with the kinds of randomly selected materials professional mnemonists are exposed to. If one is to remember an airplane or key in relation to a bun there is no ready-made prior association at hand. Any conceivable relationship will be bizarre. The point is that one need not look for bizarre relationships—they are already built into the systems employed. Experimental subjects instructed to use bizarre imagery show no advantage over uninstructed subjects.

Another point of importance is the need for practice. All mnemonists work at their systems until they become quite automatic, just as playing a musical instrument eventually becomes quite smooth and relatively effortless. Translating numbers into letters and grouping these becomes as easy as playing a new composition for the experienced pianist. Both the professional pianist and the professional mnemon-

ist follow the same road to success—practice.

The question is raised frequently as to whether the repeated use of some mnemonic system will not lead to interference. Both practical professional experience and laboratory studies indicate that there is no interference. The repeated use of a bun as a mnemonic in different contexts will result in the development of rather specific image combinations which apparently do not produce interference. The image of Olympic gods tossing buns at each other, for example, has little or nothing to do with the image of an alligator sandwich with the alligator reposing in a hot-dog bun.

Evaluation

The review of the achievements of mnemonists raises the question: are mnemonic systems of any value? Because their use is generally restricted to memorizing long lists of items having no sequence or relationship with each other it is obvious that they will have but little value for anyone but the professional mnemonist. The average citizen has little occasion to memorize lists of telephone numbers or even of names that accompany different faces in large groups. Children learn to pronounce the number system before they know what numbers are and they learn the alphabet in a sing-song (rhythmic grouping) fashion before they know much about letters or reading. Lists of states and state capitals might be required in some schools but they can probably be learned without the additional task of learning a mnemonic system. Shopping lists, by definition, need not be remembered if one actually has a list.

The chief value of mnemonics appears to reside in the entertainment world of stage and living room. If one chooses to learn a substitute pattern of pegs for playing cards, he can recite in order the name of the cards in a shuffled deck after seeing the order once. It calls for only a peg system and imagery association.

There have been some recent attempts to apply a peg operation to the learning of nouns in a foreign language. The method used involves pronouncing the foreign word (e.g., the French word *fenêtre*-window) and picking out some part of it that sounds like a familiar English word. In this case, it could be *net;* the learner then images some relationship between a net and a window. Subsequently when he hears "fenêtre" he automatically thinks of a net and window. The method has been shown to work with nouns. Other parts of speech have not been studied, and the method may be limited to those words that do have meaningful English-word sound components.

Mnemonics and the Psychology of Learning

Although the practice of mnemonics holds no great promise for making master memorizers of the citizenry it still has great value for the very people who avoided any contact with it for so long. Learning psychologists have finally ceased to expect that subjects would learn nonsense syllables by rote memory and repetition. Too many instances of one-trial learning finally brought them to realize that subjects were continually devising strategies and plans for achieving their goals. Many such subjects indicated that they were forming meaningful words out of the nonsense syllables and associating one with another through imagery or otherwise. The work of Miller, Pribram, and Galanter, and more recently of Paivio, among many others, has made the study of imagery respectable again. The renewed interest in imagery is reflected in a continuing stream of publications in experimental literature, with a lively concern for the analysis of imagery as well as its obvious mediational role in laboratory studies of paired-associates.

The analysis of imagery has forced psychologists to go back to the mnemonists in search of the variables that underlie learning. Psychologists have been forced to recognize what all mnemonists know and what some of them vigorously assert (Weinland, 1957): Aside from the techniques of pegs, linkage, and substitution, the memorizer must work rather intensively. He must exert himself in what the mnemonists call "original awareness," that is, he must pay the closest attention to the material and actively select the imagery that will work for him. The current reopening of interest in the area of attention can be credited to some degree to the mnemonists. The emphasis on active search and analysis can now be brought to the attention of students in a salutory manner. A simple classroom demonstration of the use of the 1-bun technique, resulting in the rapid mastery of a 10-item list shows students in the

most practical of ways how they can learn if they "pay attention." The student can no longer blame his failures on a "poor memory" because he can be shown so easily that his memory is in fact, superb. He can be told, with some convincing security, that if he actively engages in the learning process, scrutinizes the material, and makes suitable observing responses, he will learn quite automatically with the opposite consequences when he fails to do so.

Another psychological variable of considerable consequence has been generated from the study of mnemonic techniques. It is not commonly noticed or reported that most mnemonists are, especially in early stages before they have acquired considerable practice, slow and methodical in their work. They do not have photographic minds and do not take mental snapshots. They require time for the occurrence, appraisal, and selection of their associations. It takes the beginner between 4 and 8 seconds to find and select a suitable image by which he will remember: 8-gate-fountain pen. If he is rushed, his retention will be no better than that of the untrained person. All learning takes time. The curious practice of psychological laboratories of using memory drums which presented nonsense syllables at 1, 2, or 3 sec intervals could only have been designed to delay learning and obscure the process. It obviously was based on the now rejected hypothesis that simple repetition is the basic and sole principle of learning. This is not to say that repetition is without merit in all situations. For many kinds of learning repetition can be of value and needs no further defense here. The point to recognize is that time is of the essence, with no general schedule for every student for each kind of learning exercise. The mnemonist takes all the time he needs. Luria's subject took 3 minutes to learn ten 4-place numbers. Assuming that he took even 6 seconds to translate a number into a word, he still had perhaps 2 minutes to image the words in relationships with previously prepared pegs or to link the 10 words in a sequence. The stunt is remarkable only to the uninitiated.

The mnemonic techniques may be necessary to acquire and retain long lists of more or less unrelated materials, such as stock market symbols and the names of the companies they stand for. The question is not fully settled. Some unpublished and unreplicated work by Samuel

Renshaw at Ohio State University in the 1940s resulted in the creation of a group of mnemonists who used no system whatever beyond the activation of intense attention. Renshaw was able in a relatively short time—13 days or less—to get students to memorize 52 cards in sequence with 20-minute daily sessions. The students did nothing more than to try their best to memorize without using substitute imagery for the individual cards. They could also remember 50 words in two columns of 25 if they simply tried to visualize the words in the appropriately numbered blanks drawn and numbered on a page. Renshaw suggested the slogan: You are smarter than you think. The work, however, did not catch the fancy of psychologists then and continues to remain largely unknown. Replication of the Renshaw findings would find a more favorable psychological climate today. Renshaw, like the mnemonists, argued that the learning per se was automatic; that is, it occurred as the result of things falling into place, as into a pattern or structure. These words were used in the introduction and they are suitable in the closing. There appears to be no mystery in mnemonics. As with any other skill it takes effort. As with any other work, using a plan or system, an organization may facilitate production.

BIBLIOGRAPHY

LURIA, A. *The mind of a mnemonist.* New York: Basic Books, 1968.

MILLER, G. A.; GALANTER, E.; and PRIBRAM, K. H. *Plans and the structure of behavior.* New York: Holt, 1960.

PAIVIO, A. *Imagery and verbal processes.* New York: Holt, Rinehart and Winston, 1971.

RICHARDSON, A. *Mental images.* New York: Springer, 1969.

WEINLAND, J. D. *How to improve your memory.* New York: Barnes & Noble, 1957.

YATES, F. *The art of memory.* London: Routledge & Kegan Paul, 1966.

See also MEMORY: RETRIEVAL FROM LONG-TERM STORAGE; MEMORY: RETRIEVAL FROM SHORT-TERM STORAGE; MEMORY AND IMAGERY

B. RICHARD BUGELSKI

MODAL ACTION PATTERN IN ANIMAL BEHAVIOR

The concept of Modal Action Pattern (MAP) is an outgrowth of the concept of Fixed Action Pattern (FAP). Therefore one should first read the entry under Fixed Action Pattern to appreciate why it has become necessary to propose this new term, and to become familiar with some typical examples.

A MAP is a recognizable and repeated spatio-temporal pattern of behavior, including vocalizations. A given MAP is widely distributed in similar form throughout an interbreeding population of the species in question, thus ruling out idiosyncratic behavior. It may also occur in more than one related species. While environmental influence on the form of MAPs is not ruled out, it is necessary to preclude obvious cases of learning; this applies in particular to human behavior where many acquired stereotyped gestures characterize occupations, groups, or entire cultures. Universal patterned movements in humans, however, most likely qualify as MAPs, such as reflexive movements of infants and certain facial expressions.

MAPs have seldom been subject to quantitative analysis. The first such report, by B. Dane, C. Walcott, and W. H. Drury, appeared in 1959. They filmed and measured the duration of displays, and their components, in the goldeneye duck. Now similar film analyses have appeared for MAPs in clams, insects, crabs, chickens, doves, sage grouse, and sea birds, jackals, and especially lizards. Almost all the studies have been restricted to measuring duration. Phasic relationships or paths of movement have been described only for chicks of gulls and chickens, sage grouse, and for some lizards; generally only an example is given without statistical analysis. In only two studies, one on chicks and another on a lizard, has there been an attempt to affect the form of the MAP by altering the stimulus.

The reason there has been so little definitive research is obvious: Analyzing films is slow and laborious, and the analysis of the data is not easy. Furthermore, it is hard to film the animal such that the movements under study lie in the plane of the film. Otherwise, complex geometric corrections are necessary. They are now feasible with modern electronic equipment.

Vocalizations are the result of coordinated neuromuscular activity and may be considered as MAPs when they meet the criteria given above. Especially clear cases are the calls and songs of birds and frogs. They are readily analyzed, thanks to modern acoustic technology. There has not been much concern, so far, with vocalizations in relation to the concept of fixed or modal action patterns. The most important contribution here has been to the understanding of how experience does, or in some cases does not, enter into the development of birds.

BIBLIOGRAPHY

BARLOW, G. W. Modal action patterns. In T. A. Sebeok (Ed.), *How animals communicate.* Bloomington: University of Indiana Press, 1976.

KONISHI, M., and F. NOTTEBOHM. Experimental studies in the ontogeny of avian vocalizations. In R. A. Hinde (Ed.), *Bird vocalizations.* Cambridge: Cambridge University Press, 1969. Pp. 29–48.

See also FIXED ACTION PATTERN IN ANIMALS; TYPICAL INTENSITY IN ANIMAL BEHAVIOR

GEORGE W. BARLOW

MODAL PERSONALITY AND NATIONAL CHARACTER

Modal personality refers to the typical or most frequently found pattern of personality traits in any definitive adult population, usually a nation, society, or stratum thereof. It differs from similar conceptualizations, such as national character, social character, and basic personality type in its methodological requirement that the typical personality profile be constructed from the mode, mean, or median of assessments of *individuals* constituting a random sample of the population under consideration. Modal personality in contrast with stereotype incorporates emphasis on both uniformity trends and variability. The construct of modal personality is useful in efforts to identify and delineate distinctive personality traits of culture groups and to determine their antecedents, correlates, and consequences.

History

The term *national character,* which antedates modal personality, is associated with studies of the characteristic spirit or mentality of nations, usually without a standardized and replicable procedure. Travelers, missionaries, and historians have employed the national character approach. Cultural historians (Burckhardt, Spengler, and Huizinga) tried to show the unity in the arts, beliefs, and institutions of cultures. R. Benedict in *Patterns of Culture* (1934) followed their thinking in her anthropological field studies of primitive tribes. A. Kardiner (1939, 1945), cooperating with anthropologists in the study of mainly primitive cultures, formulated the construct *basic personality type* defined as the common denominator of personality traits in a culture group. According to his theory, basic personality is mainly determined by child-rearing practices of early childhood and is a major factor in shaping the secondary institutions and projective (belief) systems of a culture. The term *basic* refers to what is basic in the culture, not what is basic in determining individual personality. Instead, individual personality consists of deviations from basic personality.

During World War II and its aftermath, interest was focused on the national character of modern nations on account of its potential value in psychological warfare and in effecting the peace. Fromm (1941) used the term *social character* for the common personality traits of modern westernized man. He asserted that the stability of nations depended upon congruence between social character and social system.

The term *modal personality,* introduced by C. DuBois (1944) and R. Linton (1945), has largely replaced the term *basic personality.* The construction of a modal personality profile for the Tuscarora Indians from Rorschach protocols by A. F. C. Wallace (1952) exemplifies empirical and statistical features of the modal personality approach. Linton made explicit the importance of modeling and direct contact with culture objects, in addition to child-rearing practices, in the formation of modal personality.

Since the 1950s, social anthropologists have become disenchanted with the basic personality approach because of its overemphasis on child-rearing practices and simplistic application of psychoanalytic theory. Recognition of the lack of correspondence between national and cultural boundaries and of the complexity of even primitive cultures further alienated anthropologists from attempts to place national cultures under simple rubrics. Psychologists, on the other hand, found the empiricism of the modal personality approach appealing and have become increasingly interested in the culture and personality area, a specialty within anthropology, sociology, and psychology. R. A.

LeVine (1973), critical of the fragmentation and narrow range of topics investigated in the culture and personality area, has proposed a *population psychology* for the cross-cultural study of all psychological processes and characteristics.

Methodology

National character studies have used the following methods: study of a nation's history and examination of its existing institutions: anthropological field work with participant observation; interviewing; projective personality assessment techniques; and clinical case methods. The Sapir-Whorf hypothesis that language shapes thinking has stimulated studies of national mentality through analysis of language systems. Osgood considers his semantic differential to be ideal for cross-cultural studies, because it applies equally well to all language systems. Hall (1966) advocates the cross-cultural study of nonverbal communication, development of and preferences for sensory modalities, and perception of time and space. Demographic indexes (incidence of psychosis, suicide rate, caloric intake, and deaths from alcoholism) have been employed by Lynn (1971) as a basis from which to estimate anxiety levels in thirteen nations. Mead and Métraux (1953) recommend the following methods for studying cultures at a distance (inaccessible cultures): Interviewing refugees and immigrants, analysis of books, newspapers, periodicals, films, popular and fine arts, diaries, and letters from the culture in question.

The preferred approach today is a coordinated study of many nations by teams of investigators employing systematic and standardized procedures. LeVine and Campbell (1972) have developed a field manual for standardized interviewing in cross-cultural studies of ethnocentrism among nonindustrialized peoples. Psychologists are likely to use experimental laboratory procedures, personality assessment techniques, and attitude survey instruments in cross-cultural studies.

Selected Findings and Applications

In the course of a large-scale United Nations Educational, Social, and Cultural Organization (UNESCO) cross-cultural study of how nine na-

tions perceived one another, Buchanan and Cantril (1953) made the incidental finding that Americans and Australians were the most optimistic people and Italians and Mexicans the least. In a five-nation study on preferences for ways of living, Morris (1956) concluded that Americans were more activist, self-indulgent, less subject to social restraint, less open to receptivity, and lower in inwardness than Indians, Japanese, Chinese, and Norwegians. Almond and Verba (1963) found lower levels of social and interpersonal trust in West Germany, Italy, and Mexico than in Great Britain and the United States. Cantril (1965), in a thirteen-nation study, obtained ratings of self and country in regard to hopes and fears for the future, and concluded that the United States and West Germany were the most hopeful nations and India and Brazil the least.

Currently, there is great interest in applying the modal personality approach to studies of ethnic and regional subdivisions of large nations. Krug and Kulhavy (1973) used personality inventories in a study of six regions of the United States and found that the modal personality of each region was somewhat in agreement with the prevailing opinions about persons in that region, but much too complex to fit stereotypes. Kardiner and Ovesey (1951), on the basis of intensive interviewing and projective techniques, described the basic personality type of black Americans as centering around a core of injured self-esteem and rage, with defense mechanisms against these. A most pressing issue is the effect of massive immigration and extremely rapid cultural change on the modal personality of nations and the consequences of this for their stability.

BIBLIOGRAPHY

DuBois, C. *The people of Alor.* Minneapolis: University of Minnesota Press, 1944.

Duijker, H. C. J., and N. H. Frijda. *National character and national stereotypes: A trend report prepared for the International Union of Scientific Psychology.* Amsterdam: North-Holland, 1960.

Inkeles, A., and Levinson, D. J. National character: The study of modal personality and sociocultural systems. In G. Lindzey and E. Aronson (Eds.), *The handbook of social psychology* (2nd ed., Vol. 4). Reading, Mass.: Addison-Wesley, 1969. Pp. 418–506.

Kardiner, A. *The individual and his society.* New York: Columbia University Press, 1939.

Kardiner, A. (with the collaboration of R. Linton, C. Du

Bois, and J. West). *The psychological frontiers of society.* New York: Columbia University Press, 1945.

LeVine, R. A. *Culture, behavior and personality.* Chicago: Aldine, 1973.

Linton, R. *The cultural background of personality.* New York: Appleton-Century-Crofts, 1945.

Mead, M., and Métraux, R. (Eds.). *The study of culture at a distance.* Chicago: University of Chicago Press, 1953.

Wallace, A. F. C. The modal personality of the Tuscarora Indians. In *Bureau of American Ethnology Bulletin no. 150.* Washington, D.C.: Smithsonian Institution, 1952.

Philip M. Kitay

MODELING IN BEHAVIOR MODIFICATION

Modeling as typically practiced in behavior modification consists of a client observing another individual (i.e., a *model*) engage in behaviors the client wishes to develop. Without actually performing the observed behavior, the client can learn novel responses or can be induced to perform (or cease to perform) previously acquired responses. An essential ingredient in modeling appears to be covert or representational (verbal or imaginal) processes which code the modeled material (Bandura, 1970; Friedman, 1972). The representational processes are assumed to guide subsequent performance of the client when external modeling cues are no longer provided.

Although historically interesting examples of modeling can be culled from case studies in the literature, modeling as a behavior modification technique has been investigated more recently. Even now, relatively few investigations have evaluated the therapeutic effects of modeling independently of other procedures (e.g., reinforcement) with which it is sometimes combined (Bandura, 1971). However, a great deal of laboratory work, which began intensively in the early 1960s, has served as a source of information and empirical base from which therapeutic extrapolations have been made. Indeed, laboratory work on modeling has thrived in its own right and continues to investigate a number of important topics such as moral development in children, the effects of televised violence, and so on.

A number of theoretical interpretations of modeling or vicarious learning have been advanced to explain what is learned as well as why and how imitative behavior occurs after exposure to a model. Interpretations differ in the role accorded reinforcement of imitative behavior early in one's life, cue and stimulus control properties of modeled behavior, covert rehearsal of behavior, and symbolic events which mediate overt performance. Generally, different interpretations have not been contrasted in empirical investigations. Yet knowledge of the processes involved in modeling and of parameters which contribute to behavior change has advanced considerably.

Component Processes of Modeling

Although modeling requires exposure to a model, exposure alone does not necessarily result in modeling effects. Bandura (1970) has noted four processes which determine whether exposure to a model will influence an observer.

Attentional Processes. Obviously it is important for an individual to attend to the modeling stimuli to ensure that the events are registered at a sensory level (when visual or auditory cues constitute the modeling stimuli). Also, it is important for the individual to selectively attend to the relevant behavioral cues out of the total stimulus complex provided.

Retention Processes. In order to reproduce behavioral patterns which have been previously modeled, the individual must retain the modeled material, often for extended periods. Symbolic processes including imaginal and verbal representation of the events are required since external stimulus cues (i.e., a live or film model) may no longer be available when the response finally is performed by the observer.

Motoric Reproduction Processes. Overt performance of a modeled response by the observer contributes to, although it is not necessary for, modeling effects. Imitative responding by the observer in the presence of the model or in the actual situation in which the response is to be performed usually provides a closer approximation of the modeled behavior than does covert rehearsal alone. Overt rehearsal may be particularly significant when the modeled response is complex and includes several components which are not in the repertoire of the client. Motoric enactment of the response also provides proprioceptive feedback as well as self-imposed and externally imposed response consequences (e.g., reinforcement) which may contribute to subsequent performance in their own right.

Motivational Processes. Performance of modeled behavior by the observer depends upon external incentive conditions. Favorable consequences provided to the model increase, whereas aversive consequences decrease, the likelihood of observer performance of the modeled behavior. Incentives such as model reinforcement can influence other processes (e.g., attention to or retention of modeling stimuli) by increasing the salience of model behavior. Consequences presented to the observer rather than to the model, of course, directly influence performance of the previously modeled response.

Parameters Influencing Modeling

The effect of modeling on an observer can be enhanced by altering parameters which influence the processes mentioned above. Laboratory work indicates that modeling effects are influenced by cues of the modeling stimuli, characteristics of the observer, covert and overt client behavior during the modeling session, and model performance consequences.

Cues associated with the modeling stimuli can enhance modeling. Modeling effects are enhanced when the observer is exposed to several models who perform the behavior rather than a single model, models who are similar in age, sex, and other attributes or are high in status (e.g., prestigious, powerful, and competent), and models who receive favorable consequences for their performance.

Investigation of modeling in the treatment of avoidance behavior has revealed additional model cues which influence behavior. Clients who observe a model cope with anxiety-provoking situations (i.e., show initial anxiety followed by successful coping) show greater effects of modeling than those who observe a confident and fearless model. Also, indirect evidence suggests that elimination of avoidance is greater when the model engages in a graduated series of tasks progressing to increasingly arousing tasks than when he confronts the highly arousing situations alone. In addition, when the observer is trained to relax during the modeling sessions, modeling effects are slightly superior than when there is no relaxation.

Aside from attributes of the model, laboratory work has shown that observers differ in susceptibility to modeling stimuli. Observers who are low in self-esteem, feel incompetent, are highly dependent, or previously have been reinforced for imitative behavior are more susceptible to modeling influences. There is a paucity of research indicating the relevance of these dimensions for therapeutic efficacy.

Covert and overt behavior of the client during the modeling session can influence modeling. If the client symbolically codes the modeled stimuli by verbal labeling or vivid images of the model behavior, subsequent performance will match model behavior more closely than when such coding is not explicitly performed or is directly impeded. Overt enactment or rehearsal of the modeled behavior by the observer also enhances modeling and is superior to modeling alone.

The parameters which enhance modeling probably simultaneously affect different component processes of modeling. For example, attributes of the model and positive consequences following model behavior may influence both attentiveness to and subsequent retention of the modeling stimuli. The relative impact of different factors on modeling is not clear at the present time. Generally, preliminary evidence suggests that consequences (e.g., reinforcing) which follow model behavior outweigh attributes of the model or observer. However, this has not been firmly established in laboratory or clinical research.

Therapeutic Variations

A variety of modeling techniques have been evaluated in clinical research studies. Although the basic modeling paradigm requires that clients be exposed to performance of a model, it does not dictate the manner in which modeling stimuli are presented (Bandura, 1970). Generally, variations of modeling depend upon how the modeling stimuli are presented to the client.

Live and *film modeling* (i.e., observing a model or film of a model, respectively) constitute the most common techniques of presenting modeled information, both in laboratory and clinical research as well as case applications. As therapeutic strategies, live and film techniques probably offer different advantages and disadvantages. Live modeling permits flexibility in presenting the modeling cues so that a therapist can alter or repeat modeled behaviors as needed in therapy. Film modeling permits widespread administration of standard scenes across several clients (individually or in groups) which would be prohibitive to recreate as live modeling. Live and film modeling appear equally effective, although direct comparisons in therapeutic applications unconfounded by other variables are lacking.

A less commonly used procedure for presenting modeling stimuli is *audiomodeling*, where the client only hears the verbalizations of the model. This procedure often is combined with other procedures (e.g., overt rehearsal of the behavior) and, of course, is included in live and film modeling. Audiomodeling in behavior therapy has been limited largely to developing language patterns or social interaction skills where verbal repertoires play a particularly salient role.

Modeling has also been conducted as a "covert" procedure where the client imagines rather than actually observes a model engage in those behaviors the client wishes to develop (Cautela, 1971). Modeling stimuli are imagined by the client in response to verbal descriptions of modeling scenes given by the therapist. Although such *covert modeling* is quite recent, preliminary evidence attests to its efficacy and to its similarity to live modeling in its effects on behavior (Kazdin, 1974).

Another variation of modeling is distinguished not by how the modeling stimuli are presented but rather by the client's participation in the session. In the versions listed above, the client is exposed to the model in some form (live, film, audio, imaginal) but does not actually engage in overt behavior. The version of modeling referred to as *participant modeling* or modeling with guided participation does require overt client participation. (In the use of modeling to overcome avoidance behavior, participant modeling is also referred to as *contact desensitization*.) In participant modeling, the client usually views a live model (the therapist) and subsequently is encouraged to perform approximations of the modeled response. The therapist physically assists or guides the client in a graduated fashion (e.g., in approaching a feared stimulus) until the response can be performed without the therapist's assistance. Physical guidance by the therapist (rather than

mere verbal direction) and repeated remodeling of the response during the session appear to be important features of participant modeling. In general, participant modeling results in greater behavior change, more durable treatment effects, and greater changes in areas not directly focused upon in treatment than does modeling alone. The therapeutic effects of overtly practicing a behavior a client wishes to develop (behavioral rehearsal) or rehearsing the behavior in simulated situations (role playing) have been demonstrated in their own right in the absence of modeling stimuli (Friedman, 1972). Thus, it is no surprise that client participation augments modeling.

Range of Applications

Modeling has been used to alter a variety of behaviors, including fear and avoidance reactions (including fear of dogs, snakes, heights, water, and taking examinations), obsessions and compulsions, inassertiveness, social withdrawal, dependent behavior, interview behaviors, and others (Bandura, 1971; Friedman, 1972; Rachman, 1972). Clients treated with modeling have included adults, adolescents, and children in outpatient treatment as well as institutionalized psychotics, delinquents, and retardates.

By far, the majority of applications have been in altering avoidant behavior of individuals who fear small animals (e.g., snakes, dogs). A number of these studies include populations whose fear might be viewed as "subphobic." The generality of the findings with clinical populations with diverse behavioral problems who seek treatment without inducements (e.g., a free experimental treatment program) remains unclear. Modeling has been combined with other procedures, especially positive reinforcement, to alter a plethora of behaviors for therapeutic purposes, including language acquisition, imitative behavior, personal and adaptive skills (e.g., dressing in retardates), classroom behavior, and the elimination of bizarre behaviors in psychiatric patients.

In discussing the range of applications it is important to note that generalized treatment effects sometimes result from modeling. For example, in the treatment of avoidance behavior, modeling not only alters the behavior focused upon but also favorably affects attitudes and emotional arousal as well. Moreover, therapeutic effects of modeling have been shown to generalize to problem areas which have not been focused upon in treatment. The generalized effects appear to be particularly apparent in modeling with guided participation, but they are also evident with live, film, and covert modeling.

Areas of Research

Research investigations have successfully developed an effective "modeling package" which includes diverse elements such as variation of model cues, verbal mediation of modeling stimuli, guided participation, and other elements. Moreover, effective treatment variations (e.g., live, film, covert) lend credence to the potency of modeling as a general therapeutic strategy.

Various research issues remain to be explored. First, the generality of modeling effects across diverse therapeutic problems and populations is unclear. With few exceptions, the investigations have had a relatively narrow focus in terms of problems (e.g., avoidance). Second, the extent to which behavior changes achieved with modeling are persistent over time remains to be determined. Follow-up data, if obtained at all, usually are of short durations (e.g., a matter of weeks). Third, it remains unclear whether behavior changes would be evident or as robust using unobtrusive assessment procedures to evaluate treatment effects in everyday situations rather than measures associated with the clinical or research setting. Differential expectancies for behavior change across groups in the clinical setting remain a possible interpretation of the results of several studies. Fourth, the influence of several variables, including number or spacing of therapeutic sessions, amount of stimuli to which clients are exposed within a session, and optimal proportions of modeling and participation, remain to be determined. The efficacy of a single or a few sessions with short modeling sequences and little or no guided participation may attest to the potency of the technique or the ease with which responses selected for investigation can be altered. Finally, comparative studies need to determine the differential effectiveness of modeling and other behavior therapy techniques. A number of the above points certainly apply to a variety of therapy techniques rather than to modeling alone.

BIBLIOGRAPHY

BANDURA, A. Modeling theory. In W. S. Sahakian (Ed.), *Psychology of learning: Systems, models, and theories.* Chicago: Markham, 1970. Pp. 350–367.

BANDURA, A. Psychotherapy based upon modeling principles. In A. E. Bergin and S. L. Garfield (Eds.), *Handbook of psychotherapy and behavior change.* New York: Wiley, 1971. Pp. 653–708.

FRIEDMAN, P. H. The effects of modeling, roleplaying, and participation on behavior change. In B. A. Maher (Ed.), *Progress in experimental personality research* (Vol. 6). New York: Academic Press, 1972. Pp. 41–81.

KAZDIN, A. E. Effects of covert modeling and model reinforcement on assertive behavior. *Journal of Abnormal Psychology,* 1974, *83,* 240–252.

RACHMAN, S. Clinical applications of observational learning, imitation, and modeling. *Behavior Therapy,* 1972, *3,* 379–397.

ALAN E. KAZDIN

MODELING AND IMITATION

Imitation refers to the tendency of observers to exhibit responses matching those of models. The observer may be human or a member of a subhuman species. The *response* exhibited may be one that did not previously exist in the repertoire of the observer or one that did exist and was exhibited following observation of the model. The *model* may be live or symbolic—that is, presented through film media, oral instruction, or written material. There is unequivocal evidence from laboratory research and naturalistic observations that the provision of models markedly facilitates the acquisition of most social learning tasks and that some highly complex skills can be acquired solely by imitation of a model.

The early theoretical conceptions of imitation included instinctual interpretations (Tarde, 1903) and attempts to account for imitation in terms of associative principles (Humphrey, 1921). In 1941, the publication by Miller and Dollard of *Social Learning and Imitation* placed the concept of imitation in a behavior theory framework within the sphere of interest of learning theorists who showed little theoretical or research interest, the one exception being Mowrer (1950, 1960), who formulated a sensory feedback theory of imitation in 1950 and then revised and extended the theory in 1960.

Multiprocess Theory

More recently a major theoretical conception of imitation emerged with extensive empirical support: the *multiprocess theory* of observational learning formulated by Bandura (1969). This theory emphasizes the role of contiguous sensory stimulation and mediational processes. Stimulus contiguity is a necessary but not sufficient condition for observational learning. For observational learning to occur, stimulus contiguity must be accompanied by discriminative observation. An observer will fail to acquire matching responses if he does not attend to, recognize, and accurately perceive the behavior of the model. Two representational procedures are involved in the learning process: the verbal coding of observed events and the formation of images. After modeled stimuli acquired through a stimulus contiguity-learning process are coded into verbal symbols and images for memory representation, they function as mediators for subsequent response retrieval and reproduction of the modeled behavior. The contiguity-mediational sequence relates to the *acquisition* of imitative responses; the *performance* of these responses is strongly influenced by reinforcing outcomes to the model and observer.

Contiguous sensory stimulation and the coding of observed events into words and images do not in themselves ensure observational learning. Bandura has specified three component functions that may determine the level of observational learning: *attentional, retention,* and *motor reproduction processes.* A number of attention-controlling variables can markedly influence the occurrence of observational learning by eliciting strong attending behavior in the observer. Some of these variables relate to characteristics of the model. Attractive, competent, powerful, and high-status models are likely to elicit more attention than models who lack these qualities. There is also evidence that subject characteristics such as high dependency, low self-esteem, incompetence, and a history of positive reward for exhibiting matching behavior are associated with a tendency to be highly attentive to the behavior of others. In addition to these attention-directing variables, *stimulus input conditions* such as rate, complexity, and discriminability of modeling stimuli, as well as *incentive conditions,* will to some extent determine the level of observational learning.

Observational learning is often retained over long periods of time before the observer overtly exhibits the behavior. The retention of modeled events can result from efficient symbolic coding and covert rehearsal operations. Decrements in retention may occur when characteristics of the stimulus input, such as complexity, exceed the observer's capacity.

Observational learning of motor response patterns will depend partly on the availability of the essential component responses. Motor response patterns are most readily acquired when the observer already possesses the component skills and need only synthesize them into new patterns. Often modeled motor response patterns are successfully acquired in representational form but cannot be exhibited because of physical limitations of the observer.

The foregoing major components of modeling phenomena markedly influence the occurrence of observational learning. The failure of observational learning to occur following exposure to modeling stimuli may result from sensory registration difficulties, ineffective imagery formation, inability to code observed events, retention decrement, motor deficits, or unfavorable incentive conditions.

The rapidly accumulating body of research on observational learning has demonstrated the acquisition of complex response patterns following exposure to models, the modification of gross behavioral deficits such as autistic behavior through graduated modeling procedures, the vicarious conditioning of emotional responsiveness, the occurrence of inhibitory and disinhibitory effects as a result of observing response consequences to others, and the social facilitation of behavior patterns in groups.

In the basic observational learning paradigm used in this research, the subject is exposed to modeled behavior but is not instructed to attend to or learn the behavior. Later the subject participates in the same or similar setting, and measures are obtained of observational learning. Many variations of this procedure are possible—for example, the characteristics of the model, the use of reward, the period of exposure—while still maintaining the integrity of the principal components of the paradigm. One highly effective variation is the *modeling with guided participation procedure* in which the model leads a fearful or phobic subject up a hierarchy of increasingly difficult tasks (all of which involve the feared object) using demonstration, practice, and joint participation in the feared activity, all under optimal conditions, until the subject can successfully perform the desired response without fear.

Modeling procedures have been used with considerable success in diverse settings, including classrooms, hospitals, therapy groups, parent-child interactions, and vocational training programs. However, the potential and extent of applicability of this social learning theory has only begun to be realized. Bandura (1977) has specified the rationale and a general blueprint for the utilization of modeling principles in planned sociocultural change and has extended social learning principles to an analysis of transcultural modeling, which probably will be an increasingly important phenomenon with the development of global communication technology.

BIBLIOGRAPHY

BANDURA, A. *Principles of behavior modification.* New York· Holt, Rinehart and Winston, 1969.
BANDURA, A. *Social learning theory.* Englewood Cliffs, N.J.: Prentice-Hall, 1977.
HUMPHREY, G. Imitation and the conditioned reflex. *Pedagogical Seminary,* 1921, *28,* 1–21.
MILLER, N. E., and DOLLARD, J. *Social learning and imitation.* New Haven, Conn.: Yale University Press, 1941.
MOWRER, O. H. Identification: A link between learning theory and psychotherapy. In O. H. Mowrer, *Learning theory and personality dynamics.* New York: Ronald Press, 1950. Pp. 573–615.
MOWRER, O. H. *Learning theory and the symbolic processes.* New York: Wiley, 1960.
TARDE, G. *The laws of imitation.* New York: Holt, 1903.

SHEILA A. ROSS

MODELS AND METHODS
See COMPUTER SIMULATION OF INTELLIGENCE

MOEBIUS, PAUL JULIUS (1853–1907)

Paul Julius Moebius, born in Leipzig, stressed the psychological component of many mental diseases, and emphasized the psychological origin of hysterical symptoms to a greater extent than Charcot or Janet. In terms of classification, he included traumatic neuroses under the heading of hysteria and attempted a psychological explanation of this condition. He recognized the importance of the sexual driving force and noted that this was reflected in the beauty of nature. Mental disease was subdivided by him into exogenous and endogenous classes.

He was particularly interested in creativity and talent. Again, using psychological understandings in the examination of artists, he coined the term *pathographies* or psychopathologically-oriented biographies. From this work came his theories of the superior genera and he categorized himself as one. This approach was also seen in the works of others, primarily Lombroso.

In 1901 he published "On the Physiological Imbecility of Women," in which he described woman as being halfway between a child and a man on a scale of physical and mental attributes. Moebius's main studies are included in his *Neurologische Beiträge, Part 1: Über den Begriff der Hysterie und andere Vorwurfe vorwegend psychologischer Art* (1894).

LEO H. BERMAN

MOEDE, WALTHER (1888–1958)

Moede was a German psychologist who was one of the founders of applied psychology. In an area called "psychotechnique," he tried to relate psychological knowledge to technical, industrial, and cultural problems. He investigated the selection criteria for talented pupils, telephone operators, streetcar conductors, and automobile drivers. He further explored graphology, the dependence of individuals on group behavior, and the psychologist as court expert. He headed the Institute for Industrial Psychology of the Technische Hochschule in Berlin. His two major texts are *Experimentelle Massenpsychologie* ([Experimental mass psychology], Leipzig: 1920), and *Lehrbuch der Psychotechnik* ([Applied psychology], Berlin: 1930).

FRANK WESLEY

MONITORING AND VIGILANCE
See VIGILANCE AND MONITORING

MONOAMINE: NEUROCHEMICAL AND NEUROPHYSIOLOGICAL CHARACTERISTICS OF BIOGENIC AMINES

The terms *biogenic amine* or *monoamine* may be properly used to designate any primary ($R.NH_2$), secondary ($R_2.NH$), or tertiary ($R_3.N$) amine produced by living cells. Used in this fashion, the terms encompass a large number of physiologically unrelated substances. Within the neurological disciplines, however, the terms are used chiefly in reference to four pharmacologically active compounds which are proven or putative neurotransmitters: *dopamine (dihydroxyphenylethylanine), norepinephrine, epinephrine,* and *serotonin* (5-*hydroxytryptamine*). The first three substances are catecholamines; the fourth, serotonin, is an indolealkyl amine.

In mammals dopamine, norepinephrine, and serotonin are synthesized by neurons within specific central nervous system nuclei; epinephrine does not appear to be present in significant amounts in the mammalian central nervous system (CNS) with the possible exception of the olfactory bulb. Outside the mammalian CNS norepinephrine is formed in sympathetic ganglion cells; both epinephrine and norepinephrine are produced by chromaffin cells. In amphibians epinephrine rather than norepinephrine is the catecholamine produced by sympathetic ganglion cells.

Biosynthesis

The initial steps in the synthesis of dopamine, norepinephrine, and epinephrine are identical. The synthetic pathway begins with the conversion of tyrosine to DOPA *(dihydroxyphenylalanine)* by the enzyme tyrosine hydroxylase. DOPA is then decarboxylated by DOPA decarboxylase to form dopamine. This step is the end point of the pathway in those groups of neurons which specifically secrete dopamine (dopaminergic neurons). In the case of noradrenergic neurons or chromaffin cells the pathway is carried a step further with the hydroxylation of dopamine by dopamine beta-hydroxylase to form norepinephrine. Adrenergic mammalian chromaffin cells and

amphibian sympathetic ganglion cells contain phenylethanolamine-N-methyltransferase which converts norepinephrine, a primary amine, to epinephrine, a secondary amine by methylation of the amine group. The rate limiting step in catecholamine synthesis is the hydroxylation of tyrosine to form DOPA.

Although there is active and continuous turnover of catecholamines in neurons and chromaffin cells, the level of catecholamines in these tissues remains relatively constant. Axelrod and others have identified and elucidated long-term hormonal and short- and long-term neural mechanisms which regulate catecholamine synthesis. Hormonal regulation is operative chiefly in the adrenal medulla. Here, Axelrod has shown that glucocorticoids are necessary to maintain the normal activity of phenylethanolamine-N-methyl-transferase, the enzyme responsible for the formation of epinephrine from norepinephrine. The maintenance of normal activities of other catecholamine-synthesizing enzymes is influenced by ACTH.

The influence of neural activity on catecholamine synthesis has been observed in noradrenergic cells in the adrenal medulla, the sympathetic nervous system, and, in some cases, the brain. Short-term neural regulation of catecholamine synthesis involves the feedback inhibition of tyrosine hydroxylase activity by norepinephrine. In the absence of stimulation excess accumulation of norepinephrine is prevented by inhibition of tyrosine hydroxylase, the rate limiting enzyme in the pathway. With stimulation and release of norepinephrine, inhibition of tyrosine hydroxylase is reduced and the rate of norepinephrine synthesis increased resulting in the maintenance of normal or even slightly elevated tissue norepinephrine levels during periods of increased noradrenergic activity.

The long-term type of neural regulation which involves a transsynaptically induced increase in the formation of tyrosine hydroxylase, dopamine beta-hydroxylase, and phenylethanolamine-N-methyltransferase in response to neural stimulation has been demonstrated in the adrenal medulla. In regard to tyrosine hydroxylase and dopamine beta-hydroxylase, a similar response occurs in sympathetic ganglion cells. Only tyrosine hydroxylase synthesis appears to be enhanced in the brain as a result of neural stimulation.

The biosynthesis of serotonin has not been elucidated as fully as the biosynthesis of catecholamines. Serotonin is one of a group of compounds known as indolealkylamines which occur widely among plants and animals. Interestingly, certain fruits such as pineapples and bananas contain extremely large concentrations of serotonin. In mammals serotonin is synthesized by specific brainstem neurons. The bulk of the body store of serotonin is located outside the nervous system, principally in the enterochromaffin cells of the intestine and, to a lesser extent, in the blood platelets.

The formation of serotonin begins with the hydroxylation of tryptophan by tryptophan hydroxylase producing 5-hydroxytryptophan. This compound is decarboxylated by 5-hydroxytryptophan decarboxylase to form serotonin (5-hydroxytryptamine).

Storage and Release

The intracellular storage of catecholamines occurs in subcellular particles called dense core or granular vesicles. These structures range in size from 500–1,200 angstroms (Å) in diameter. They are composed of an outer limiting membrane and an electron dense core. In small diameter vesicles the core may be demonstrable only after fixation with potassium permanganate. The granules contain catecholamine and ATP in a molar ratio of 4:1, the enzymes dopamine-beta-hydroxylase and ATPase, and a characteristic group of soluble proteins, the chromogranins.

Two sizes of amine-containing, granular vesicles are present within catecholaminergic neurons: small granular vesicles (SGV) with a diameter of 500 angstroms and large granular vesicles (LGV) with a diameter of 1,000 angstroms. Particles lacking catecholamine but structurally similar to LGV may be seen in neurons which are not catecholaminergic. Within the catecholaminergic neuron the SGV are found chiefly in the axon terminals; LGV may be found in the cell body, axon, or axon terminal. In adrenal medullary cells catecholamines are stored in granular vesicles which range in diameter from 800–1,200 angstroms but are otherwise similar to those in catecholaminergic neurons.

Release of catecholamines from axon terminals or adrenal medullary cells is thought to occur by exocytosis. This process involves transient fusion of the vesicle membrane and the plasma membrane of the cell with extrusion of the soluble contents of the vesicle into the intercellular space. The evidence for catecholamine secretion by exocytosis is most definite with regard to adrenal medullary cells. Whether other mechanisms may be involved in the release of catecholamines from axon terminals is not certain.

It is believed that serotonin is also stored in granular vesicles similar to those associated with catecholamines. The evidence, however, for this form of storage is indirect and incomplete. Interestingly, dense core granules have not been demonstrated in pineal cells which are known to contain large amounts of serotonin. The only dense core granules within the pineal are catecholaminergic and are located within axon terminals derived from neurons in the superior cervical ganglion. Little is known about the mechanisms of serotonin secretion in neurons or pineocytes.

Degradation and Inactivation

In mammals two enzymes *monoamine oxidase* (MAO) and *catechol-O-methyl transferase* (COMT) catalyze the first steps in the degradation of dopamine, norepinephrine, and epinephrine. The principal end product of catabolism may vary according to the anatomic site or the specific catecholamine involved. In the sympathetic nervous system and adrenal medulla *vanillylmandelic acid* (VMA) is the principal metabolite of norepinephrine or epinephrine catabolism. In the central nervous system the major metabolite of norepinephrine is *3-methoxy-4-hydroxylphenolglycol* (MHPG). Measurement of urinary VMA is often used to assess sympathetic nervous system function or to detect tumors, such as a neuroblastoma or pheochromocytoma, which secrete catecholamines. Plasma levels of MHPG, however, do not provide a useful index of central noradrenergic activity. Most of the plasma MHPG, though only a minor metabolite of peripheral norepinephrine, is, nevertheless, formed in the sympathetic nervous system. The principal metabolite of dopamine metabolism is *homovanillic acid* (HVA). HVA levels in brain or spinal fluid are thought to reflect activity of dopaminergic neurons. The spinal fluid concentration of this metabolite is reduced in patients with Parkinson's disease.

The cellular localization of monoamine oxidase (MAO) and catechol-O-methyl transferase (COMT) within the nervous system is different. MAO is located in the membrane of mitochondria present within synaptic terminals. At this site MAO appears to degrade catecholamine which might leak from storage granules. COMT is believed to be located outside nerve terminals adjacent to the synaptic cleft where it could act before or after catecholamine has come in contact with its receptor.

The enzymatic activity of MAO and COMT results in both chemical degradation and pharmacologic inactivation of catecholamine released at synapses. Enzymatic catabolism, however, is not the only or even the principal means of in vivo pharmacological inactivation of catecholamines. This type of inactivation is accomplished chiefly by the reuptake of catecholamine by the axon terminals from which it was originally released. This process is distinct from the process involving storage of catecholamine in granular vesicles. The existence of this method of pharmacological inactivation was first suggested by J. H. Burn in 1933 and conclusively demonstrated by Axelrod in a series of experiments published from 1959 to 1961.

The degradation of serotonin involves deamination by a monoamine oxidase which appears to be similar to the enzyme involved in catecholamine metabolism. The resulting aldehyde may be oxidized by an aldehyde dehydrogenase to form 5-hydroxyindoleacetic acid.

Pineal alternate pathways involving the enzyme *hydroxindole-O-methyl transferase* (HIOMT) result in the formation of melatonin or 5-methoxytryptophol. This pathway has physiological significance. The activity of the pathway is affected by ambient illumination. HIOMT activity is markedly increased in rats raised in constant darkness. As a result of the increased production of either melatonin or 5-methoxytryptophol the incidence of vaginal estrus is reduced in these animals.

Function

The roles of norepinephrine as a neurotransmitter in the mammalian sympathetic nervous system and of epinephrine as a neurotransmitter in the amphibian sympathetic nervous system have been established. These two amines also function as adrenal medullary hormones. The function of norepinephrine, dopamine, and serotonin in the central nervous system has not been conclusively established largely because of technical problems. The available evidence points convincingly to their involvement in the chemical transmission of nerve impulses probably as neurotransmitters.

Because of the development of sensitive and specific histochemical methods for the identification and localization of monoamines and monoaminergic neurons, it has been possible to identify specific monoaminergic pathways in the mammalian brain. Nuclei, including the locus coeruleus, composed of noradrenergic neurons occur in the midbrain, pons, and medulla. Descending axons from these cells terminate in the spinal cord; ascending axons traveling chiefly in the medial forebrain bundle terminate in the hypothalamus and the cerebral cortex including the limbic system. Noradrenergic terminals are also found in cerebellar cortex. Dopaminergic nuclei giving rise to ascending fiber systems have been found in the hypothalamus and midbrain. The largest and best known of these pathways is the nigrostriatal tract which originates from the neurons of the substantia nigra and terminates in the caudate nucleus and in the putamen. Serotoninergic neurons make up the raphe nuclei of midbrain and pons. Tracts arising from these nuclei terminate in the hypothalamus, cerebral cortex, and cerebellum.

The functions of the monoaminergic systems in the regulation of behavioral phenomena such as mood, sleep, and perception are being intensively investigated. The possibility that monoaminergic systems are involved in behavioral phenomena is based in part on pharmacological evidence. Drugs such as iproniazid or reserpine which raise or lower CNS monoamine stores also produce neurophysiological and behavioral changes. Similar kinds of changes are produced by imipramine and chlorpromazine which alter the functional availability of the monoamine at central synapses through changes in membrane permeability or inhibition of monoamine uptake.

Pathophysiology

Alterations in monoamine metabolism have been described in a number of human neurological disorders and are reputed to underlie certain psychiatric disorders. In many of the neurologic disorders the disturbances are either of a secondary type or result from the inclusion of monoaminergic neurons or their processes in unselective lesions.

Other than tumors, the common human disease in which monoaminergic neurons are known to be selectively and exclusively affected is Parkinson's disease. The basis of this disorder is bilateral degeneration of the nigrostriatal pathways. In some cases the nigral neurons are destroyed in the course of an unusual type of encephalitis. In most cases the cause of degeneration is obscure. Whatever the cause, degeneration of the nigrostriatal pathway results in low levels of neostriatal dopamine and symptoms of Parkinsonism. Administration of DOPA ameliorates the symptoms. DOPA readily penetrates the blood-brain barrier and initiates catecholamine synthesis at a point beyond the rate limiting step. The therapeutic effect of DOPA is apparently the result of its conversion to dopamine and the subsequent accumulation of this substance in the neostriatum. In effect DOPA seems to provide a means of replenishing striatal stores of dopamine lost during the degenerative process.

BIBLIOGRAPHY

AXELROD, J. Noradrenaline: Fate and control of its biosynthesis. *Science,* 1971, *173,* 598–606.
COOPER, J. R.; BLOOM, F. E.; and ROTH, R. H. *The biochemical basis of neuropharmacology.* London: Oxford University Press, 1970.
SNYDER, S. Catecholamines and serotonin. In R. W. Albers, G. J. Siegel, R. Katzman, and B. W. Agranoff (Eds.), *Basic neurochemistry.* Boston: Little, Brown, 1972. Pp. 89–104.
USDIN, E. and SNYDER, R. (Eds). *Frontiers in catecholamine research.* New York: Pergamon Press, 1973.

JAMES S. NELSON

MONOAMINE OXIDASE

The monoamine oxidases catalyze the oxidation of monoamine groups, generally to aldehydes.

$$R \ CH_2NH_2 + H_2O + O_2 \rightarrow R \ CHO + NH_3 + H_2O_2$$

Some histochemical methods depend on the visualization of the aldehyde groups formed by enzymatic action, by the Schiff reagent. Difficulties have been encountered with respect to preexisting aldehydes, to the solubility of the enzymatically produced aldehydes, and their tendency to couple with other groups, such as amino groups, at sites other than those at which they are produced. Pretreatment of the tissues being studied with hydroxylamine hydrochloride or with hydrazine has served to block preexisting aldehyde groups. The presence of 2-hydroxy-3-naphthoic acid hydrazide has been utilized to effect the rapid precipitation of the enzymatically formed aldehydes. The hydrazine, however, reacts with some lipid to produce Schiff reactive substances. Tetrazolium salts have been substituted for the Schiff reagent, since some of the aldehydes formed enzymatically may reduce these to formazans.

Monoamine oxidase activity has been noted in the cytoplasm of neurons and in ependymal, choroid plexuses, and endothelial cells.

BIBLIOGRAPHY

ARIOKA, I., and TANIMUKAI, H. Histochemical studies on monoamine oxidase in the midbrain of the mouse. *Journal of Neurochemistry,* 1957, *1,* 311–315.
SHIMIZU, N., and MORIKAWA, N. Histochemical study of oxidase in the developing rat brain. *Nature,* 1959, 184, 650–651.

IRWIN FEIGIN
ABNER WOLF

MOOD

The word *mood* is an imprecise term both in common and scientific discourse. Both it and the term *emotion* are applied to temporary states or dispositions and their accompanying acts, thoughts, and feelings. However, these synonyms show some differences in denotation and connotation. The most frequent distinction is that moods are longer and less intense than emotions. A related and less common distinction is that mood is background for emotion, both as predisposing antecedent and as lingering consequent of an emotional occurrence. A related difference in connotation is that mood more frequently implies that the antecedent or cause of the temporary disposition is unknown, vague, and remote. These characteristics of longer duration, low or moderate intensity, and vague cause are often implied when the term mood rather than emotion or emotional state is used. Mood is a viable term as long as such distinctions are useful.

History of the Concept

Mood is an ancient idea, which is referred to in many languages with words and phrases having to do with temporary disposition, state of mind, emotional state, spirit, temper, humor, and the monitoring or measuring of one's changing self. However vague the general idea, common knowledge about mood and the control of mood is important and has influenced all professional thinking about mood. Aristotle's *Rhetoric* is a practical manual largely concerned with the induction of moods in listeners, written to help the forensic orator in the control of minds, feelings, and behavior. There are careful descriptions of how the speaker should first predispose his listeners in order to more effectively elicit certain desired emotional and other responses, such as an agreement to a verdict of guilty. His analysis depends on: (1) a distinction between that which predisposes and that which elicits the behaviors made more likely in that mood; and (2) the basic idea that, in fact, there is in mood a change in the probability of occurrence of certain behaviors. These two ideas are now assumed in most discussions of mood.

One of the important modern explications of the term is also based on common discourse. In several parts of his *Concept of Mind,* Ryle (1949) subjected to linguistic analysis many of the words related to mood, emotion, and feeling. According to Ryle, mood is a temporary disposition to exhibit certain learned actions and feelings. Since mood is disposition, each of

the behaviors toward which one is disposed in a mood may not occur unless strengthened or triggered by concurrent events. A mood is identified through inferences from behavior by an observer, or by the actor himself. An avowal of mood, such as the blurting of "I'm tired" with the intonations of tiredness, is one of the many things we learn to do in mood; as avowal it is a confession, not a description, and is to be judged for sincerity rather than accuracy.

The behavioral analysis of mood and emotion by Skinner (1953) parallels that of Ryle. Skinner also seems to make a distinction between mood as predisposition and emotion as disposition. It may indeed be useful to have a conceptual scheme (Broad, 1933) in which emotion (first-order disposition) varies with mood (second-order disposition), which in turn varies from person to person with temperament, an enduring third-order disposition.

Jacobson (1957), in her analyses of mood, independently pointed to the traditional ideas also delineated by Ryle, but as a result of her psychoanalytic studies of moods in individuals over long periods of time, added much new material on the psychodynamics of mood. Two of her more general important ideas have to do with the function and pathology of moods. She extended Freud's theory of the constructive function of normally protracted mourning to all those moods which follow experiences which are emotionally intense or frustrating and which produce tension which cannot, for various reasons, be readily discharged. The function of mood is a moderating of this surplus energy through reorientations and discharges. Mood is to be judged pathologic not so much on the basis of unusual prolongation, the usual criterion, but on the degree to which the mood-affected ego is crippled in its reality testing by distortions and denials of reality.

In addition to these accounts by Aristotle as naturalist, and by the linguistic analyst, the behavioral analyst, and the psychoanalyst, there is a singular treatise, fully focused on moods, by Heidegger (1927), which demonstrates the existential approach to fundamental moods and the phenomenological analysis of subjective experience. Arnold (1960) and Plutchik (1962) discussed mood vis-à-vis emotion, and a review of ideas about mood, together with original research relating mood to personality, was provided by Wessman and Ricks (1966).

Measurement of Mood

The measurement of mood is closely tied to the measurement of emotion; advances in the latter contribute directly to the former. Perhaps the only special trend in mood measurement, though also found in the study of emotion, is the growing use of tests based on responses to selected adjectives and attributive phrases which are found empirically to vary with mood. These adjectives have been learned in completing such sentences as, "I feel ___" or their equivalent. A mood adjective check list presents, in simplest form, a set of words, selected carefully after various empirical explorations, with instructions that each be checked for correspondence to momentary feelings at the moment it is read. Factors other than quality of textual response, some helpful, some interfering, always influence verbal behavior in such tests. Moreover, a check list of this kind is more useful in estimating change in mood from one time to another than in estimating differences in mood from individual to individual in a single administration, since individual characteristics unrelated to mood contribute much more to the variance in scores in the latter case. The most important characteristic of some of these adjectival responses is that when studied in the same individuals across a variety of mood-inducing situations, they tend to form small but reliable clusters. Such clusters are identifiable through the fact that in each cluster, test responses to these and only these few words vary consistently in intensity as mood changes from situation to situation. Moreover, the content of each of these small clusters is different from the clusters of synonyms found in the dictionary or through other semantic operations. The difference has at least two bases: (1) each word in a set of dictionary synonyms is often found to reflect more than one dimension of mood; and (2) some moods, such as concentration, activation, and depression, include a broader and more diverse set of dispositions than would ordinarily be encompassed in any set of synonyms.

Categories and Dimensions of Mood

Mood categories are more diverse than recognized in that special medical tradition which classifies all moods within one bipolar dimension; namely, elation-depression. They are, indeed, similar in range, diversity, and content to those of emotion, and include a few factors rarely identified empirically in even the most broadly based studies of emotion. In 1956, Nowlis and Nowlis hypothesized that moods were, in part, monitorings and appraisals of four important aspects of the general functioning and orienting of the person. They further assumed that bipolar factors would emerge from an analysis of responses to questions about four classes of feelings: How active? (activation-deactivation). How oriented socially? (positive-negative). How well in control? (organized control-disorganized lack of control). How appraised? (favorable, pleasant-unfavorable, unpleasant). Repeated factor analyses by Nowlis and Green (1965) of responses to a list of adjectives generated by these four hypotheses and tested in a variety of mood-inducing conditions failed to confirm the postulated bipolarities but did consistently yield up to 12 approximately orthogonal factors, each of which corresponds in part to the content of the originally hypothesized but now independent poles. The major factors were named as follows: vigor; fatigue; social affection; aggression; skepticism; egotism; concentration; nonchalance; anxiety; elation; surgency; sadness. Despite the fact that many other investigators have identified mood factors quite similar to some of the above, and usually but not always unipolar, the status of such factors is obviously that of imperfect, ongoing hypotheses, and require empirical explication in the future.

The persistent emergence of unipolar factors may be in part a result of format and instruction, but it suggests the continuing importance of a research design which does not preclude proper tests for the relevance of unipolarity and bipolarity. Dependence on formats with built-in bipolar scales ignores this point. Because of the dispositional nature of mood, it is in principle and in fact possible to have simultaneously high, or simultaneously equal as well as independently unequal levels of orthogonal mood factors ordinarily thought of as "opposites" and, thus, erroneously, as fully incompatible with or fully subtractive of each other. This means that as moods change, there can be simultaneous decreases or increases in "opposing" mood factors, such as vigor and fatigue, social affection and aggression.

Empirical Research

Common sense holds many beliefs about the antecedents and consequents of mood; there are practical rules about changing mood and expectancies about all the things one may do in this or that mood. The apparent antecedents fall into four overlapping classes: emotional provocations and counterprovocations; habitability and other features of the environment; drugs; and somatic and psychosomatic processes. The many research studies of how mood is related to factors in each of these four classes have yielded results which, though generally congruent with common sense, have helped to open a series of new questions about how such factors (e.g., drugs and environmental factors) interact with each other, as well as with long- and short-term characteristics of the person. There has also been research on how mood is related to various consequents, such as changes in feeling, thinking, and action. A current trend, largely in the area of experimental research in personality and social psychology, is the utilization of mood indexes for the investigation of hypothesized relations between other sets of independent and dependent variables.

BIBLIOGRAPHY

ARNOLD, M. *Emotion and personality* (2 vols.). New York: Columbia University Press, 1960.
BROAD, C. D. *Examination of McTaggart's philosophy.* Cambridge: Cambridge University Press, 1933.
HEIDEGGER, M. (1927). *Being and time.* New York: Harper, 1962.
JACOBSON, E. Normal and pathological moods; their nature and functions. *Psychoanalytic study of the child* (Vol. 14). New York: International Universities Press, 1957.
NOWLIS, V. On the use of drugs in the analysis of complex human behavior with emphasis on the study of mood (1956). In R. Glaser et al., *Current trends in the description and analysis of behavior.* Pittsburgh: University of Pittsburgh Press, 1958.
NOWLIS, V. Research with the mood adjective check list. In S. S. Tomkins and C. E. Izard (Eds.), *Affect, cognition and personality.* New York: Springer, 1965.
NOWLIS, V. Mood: Behavior and experience. In M. Arnold (Ed.), *Feelings and emotions.* New York: Academic Press, 1970.
NOWLIS, V., and GREEN, R. F. *Factor analytic studies of the mood adjective check list.* Springfield, Va.: National Technical Information Service, Catalogue no. AD 635 294, 1965.
NOWLIS, V., and NOWLIS, H. H. The description and analysis of mood. *Annals New York Academy of Sciences,* 1956, *65,* 345–355.
PLUTCHIK, R. *The emotions: Facts, theories and a new model.* New York: Random House, 1962.
RYLE, G. *The concept of mind.* London: Hutchinson, 1949.
SKINNER, B. F. *Science and human behavior.* New York: Macmillan, 1953.
WESSMAN, A. E., and RICKS, D. F. *Mood and personality.* New York: Holt, Rinehart and Winston, 1966.

VINCENT NOWLIS

MORAL DEVELOPMENT

The scientific study of moral development is one of the oldest and the newest activities in the social sciences. In the late nineteenth and early twentieth centuries there was considerable interest in this subject, as seen in the writings of William James, John Dewey, James Mark Baldwin, Emile Durkheim, and Sigmund Freud. This interest, however, died out in the early 1930s; its demise coincided with an enthusiasm for behaviorism, logical positivism, and "values free" social science then developing. As behaviorism's appeal waned in the 1960s the study of value-related psychological phenomena again seemed legitimate; the work of Lawrence Kohlberg was influential in reawakening serious scholarly interest in the subject.

Terminological confusions abound in the subdiscipline of moral development. The words *moral* and *development* in particular are used in contradictory ways by various writers. Three usages of each term can be identified:

Morality. (1) Social learning theorists, sociologists, anthropologists, and social psychologists tend to equate morality with the rules, norms, and values that prevail within a particular culture or society. Any action that a group holds to be good or right is also moral. This leads to *moral relativism,* the view that there are no universal moral principles, that right and wrong are entirely relative to each cultural context. Moral relativism has been supported by many influential writers (e.g.,

Durkheim, Freud, Piaget). To the degree that one adopts this view one can transcend ethnocentrism, provincialism, and loyalty to narrow regional ideologies. Nonetheless, moral relativism also leads to certain undesirable consequences. It requires, for example, that societies that practice slavery, cannibalism, or genocide be considered moral on their own terms, because what they do is right for them.

(2) Other writers, most notably Kohlberg and his colleagues, feel there are *universal moral principles,* applicable to all mankind, that have been known to careful thinkers from Plato to the present. These principles include respect for the value of human life, Kant's categorical imperative, and a particular view of justice defined as fairness. The notion that there are universal moral principles in terms of which all actions can be judged is a contrast to the facile moral relativism of many social scientists. Nonetheless, there are two problems with this universalistic view of morality. First, there is no agreement among philosophers or psychologists as to what counts as a universal moral principle. Second, even if it were true that, for example, people everywhere have always regarded human life as supremely valuable, it doesn't follow that human life ought to be considered valuable. Knowledge of what is the case can never tell us what ought to be the case.

(3) A third view of morality comes from a tradition that can be traced to Charles Darwin; it is exemplified in writings by D. Campbell, E. Erikson, and C. H. Waddington. This view holds that morality functions for people but instincts do for animals, that is, morality regulates conduct in a lawlike but relatively unconscious manner. The view assumes that certain actions (e.g., truth telling, loyalty, self-sacrifice) promote the survival of culture. Thus, morality is equated with a set of psychological dispositions required for the functioning of any society. The broad outlines of these dispositions, like the capacity for language, may be innate; like language, the specific form these dispositions take depends on particular environmental circumstances. This view leads to what might be called a *relatively absolute* perspective on morality; it assumes the existence of universal norms of conduct that are necessary for the functioning of any society. These norms represent what most people mean by morality.

Whether or not they are "truly moral" in an absolute sense, however, is seen as an unanswerable question that is also irrelevant for the study of moral development.

Development. (1) From a *learning* theory perspective development consists of the steady acquisition over time of specific response dispositions. Maturity means having more and better practiced responses available to deal with the exigencies of social life, that is, there is only a quantitative difference between maturity and immaturity.

(2) From the perspective of *cognitive-developmental* theory development proceeds in terms of a series of stages. Each stage is conceived as a *structured whole,* an organized system of thought, and movement from one stage to another entails a qualitative transformation in a child's thinking. These stages are typically regarded as forming an invariant sequence, and development is "forward," one stage at a time. Finally, stages are typically seen as hierarchically integrated; the higher stages incorporate and organize the lower ones.

(3) The *biological* perspective on development, best exemplified by Herbert Spencer, is defined by two themes. First, there are definable endpoints to development (in the case of moral development the endpoint is moral maturity) that are reached through a series of qualitative changes over time. Second, development is a never ending process reflecting the organism's (child's) efforts to adjust internal conditions to external demands. These adjustments are necessary because both the organism and the environment are constantly changing. Since change is the only certainty, any accommodation that a child makes to its environment will be at best temporary; no adjustment will be permanent.

The Study of Moral Development

Moral development is studied in three separate ways. These approaches are derived from social, developmental, and clinical psychology; they are quite distinct, and this reflects the increasing specialization of psychological research.

Social Psychology. The flavor of a social psychological approach to moral development is exemplified by the Character Education Inquiry of H. Hartshorne and M. May. A large number of children were tested in a variety of situations in order to examine the operation of a single trait, honesty or resistance to temptation. The findings—that honesty is a function of situational determinants (i.e., there is no general trait of honesty); that it is related to intelligence, social class, sex, peer group, and the possibility of being caught; that it is not related to age, personality, or temperament—are also typical of this approach; that is, the cumulative findings map the parameters of resistance to temptation, they are not used as elements in the formulation of a more inclusive theory of moral development.

Perhaps the most influential moral development research from a social psychological perspective is that of Bandura (1971) and his associates (social learning theory). For Bandura, all behavior, including moral conduct, is learned. Each specific form of moral conduct (e.g., telling the truth, keeping one's word, acting altruistically) must be learned separately, and this entails two consequences. First, for the social learning theorists there is no such thing as a generalized disposition to moral conduct or a good character structure. Rather, a child can perform only those moral responses it has learned, and only under circumstances similar to those in which its initial training took place. Second, conduct will be inconsistent across situations because there is no stable core to personality. Indeed, these writers regard the concept of personality itself as vague and indefinable.

Social learning theory is somewhat more general in its approach than the Hartshorne and May research in that it doesn't focus on the determinants of any particular trait. It analyzes how social behavior in general is learned; it relies primarily on a process called *modeling*. Bandura's research has taken two broad forms. On the one hand he has demonstrated the influence of modeling on virtually every aspect of social development. On the other hand he has spelled out rather carefully the variables that influence the modeling process. Generally speaking, some models elicit more imitation than others. This seems to be a function of the model's power and warmth (rewardingness), age, sex, and ethnicity. Some children are more willing to imitate models than others; and this seems to be related to a child's age, sex, reward history for imitation, and self-esteem.

The tradition of moral development research in social psychology has five distinct features. (1) It assumes that moral conduct is situationally specific. (2) It relies almost exclusively on the methodology of laboratory experimental psychology wherein (3) large numbers of children are studied to determine (4) the parameters surrounding the appearance of one specific behavior. (5) There is little attempt to place the resulting findings in a more inclusive conceptual or theoretical framework.

Developmental Psychology. The perspective of developmental psychology on moral development is best seen in the work of Piaget, most notably in *The Moral Judgment of the Child* (1964). This tradition focuses on children's moral thought and how it changes over time. The methodology consists of structured interviews, usually in a naturalistic setting. Piaget studied age-related changes in children's use of rules, theoretical moral judgments, and concepts of justice. His findings can be briefly summarized as follows. As to rules of games, young children seem to regard them as deriving from sacred authority (older children, parents, God) and therefore as unchanging and inviolable. Despite this, younger children alter rules as it suits them. Older children (above ten) believe that other children have invented the rules, that they are changeable, and that they have the practical consequence of making play possible. Furthermore, older children seem actually to comply with the rules.

Concerning children's judgments about hypothetical moral dilemmas, Piaget found that the younger ones take no account of an actor's intentions; rather they make judgments in terms of the amount of damage caused by a particular action. Older children continue to take account of the material consequences of an act, but their judgments primarily take the actor's intentions into account. Again, with regard to children's views of justice, young children think misdeeds should be followed by punishments, the type of punishment is irrelevant, and generally speaking, the more punishment the better. For older children punishment should fit the crime, and the goal of punishment is not expiation but education and reform—punishment should benefit the offender.

Piaget integrates these findings into a more general conceptual framework by defining two moral theories, one characteristic of younger, the other of older children, and these moralities generate the findings presented above. Younger children share a form of thinking called *moral realism,* characterized by the view that rules are handed down from divine authority, that rules literally exist and must be applied in a relentless manner without exceptions. Piaget described the older child's moral thought as a morality of cooperation; this is a more rational and desirable view wherein the child is aware of other perspectives and understands that moral rules grow out of and subsequently support social relationships. Piaget then described the transition from moral realism to a morality of cooperation in terms of two underlying processes. First, there is a natural decline in egocentric modes of thought that allows a child increasingly to view the world from perspectives other than his own. Second, over time a child's social relationships become less parent-centered (and therefore less authoritarian) and more peer-centered (and therefore more egalitarian). These changes in intellectual functioning and patterns of social interaction cause the child to replace moral realism with moral cooperation.

Kohlberg (1963) has further extended this approach to moral development. He studied the theoretical moral judgments of children from age ten to early adulthood, and identified six stages through which these moral judgments seem to evolve. At stage one, morality is defined in terms of the actions that adults reward or punish. At stage two, right and wrong are defined hedonistically, in terms of actions that bring pleasure or pain. At the third stage decisions are justified in terms of social praise and blame. At the fourth stage actions are justified by appeals to conventional morality as represented by the church, state, or government. Persons at stage five justify their actions in terms of social contracts, constitutions, and democratically accepted law. Persons at stage six justify their actions in terms of universal principles of moral conduct. Kohlberg regarded each of these stages as an ideal type; thus no one will precisely embody all the elements of a single stage. According to Kohlberg, each stage represents a more cohesive, logical, and moral view of the world than the preceding stage, and moral development consists of the successive acquisition and then abandonment of the first five of them.

The developmental perspective on moral development is conceptually richer and more sophisticated than the social psychological view. Nonetheless, it is liable to two potentially serious criticisms. First, there is little evidence to suggest that theoretical moral judgments are systematically related to real world behavior. Second, the methodology used to assess the level of children's moral judgments is statistically unreliable, and there is reason to believe that the reliable variance in these moral levels is confounded with IQ.

The work of Piaget and Kohlberg reveals the major themes of moral development research from the perspective of developmental psychology. (1) The methodology is structured interviews. The search is for (2) coherent patterns of thought, (3) consistent across situations. Temporal changes in these thought patterns are (4) described, and (5) these patterns of change are interpreted within a larger conception of cognitive development.

Clinical Psychology. The tradition of moral development research from the perspective of clinical psychology begins with the notion that moral conduct is a function of one's total personality. On this view moral development is only one aspect of personality development in general. Here the virtuous or vicious character structure rather than single virtues or vices is the subject matter. Two further themes distinguish this tradition from those presented above. First, character structure, the "real" determinant of moral action, is primarily unconscious—moral conduct is to a large degree unconsciously determined. Second, since moral development is but one aspect of personality development in general, this research focuses on the key social relations in a child's life; parents in particular are assumed to play an overwhelming role in shaping their children's character structure.

Peck and Havighurst's study of adolescent character development exemplifies this kind of research. Thirty-four children were studied in their community for over seven years using an extensive battery of interviews, written tests, peer, community informant, and staff ratings. Three general findings emerged from this research. First, Peck and Havighurst (1960) were able to identify five character types representing an ascending scale of maturity in terms of which all their children could be classified.

These character types were apparent by age ten, and were very well developed seven years later. Second, the behavior of any child in a given situation was more or less predictable in terms of its character type; thus character structure seemed to provide considerable consistency to behavior across situations.

Finally, each character type was associated with a relatively specific family history. The immature amoral types came from homes described as rejecting and chaotically inconsistent. Expedient types, who were conforming but lacked internalized values, had indulgent, child-centered parents whose rules were inconsistently enforced. The conforming types, who were rigid *rule* followers, had autocratic, consistent parents who exercised severe discipline. The irrational-conscientious children adhered rigidly to *principles;* their parents were very autocratic, very conscientious, and extremely severe in their discipline. Finally, the rational-altruistic children had parents who were consistent, strongly trustful and loving, and lenient in their punishment. As Peck and Havighurst (1960) noted, "When each adolescent is considered by himself, his personality and character are linked with . . . his family experience in an almost inexorably logical way."

The work of R. Hogan (1973, 1974) also reflects this clinical tradition. Hogan described moral development in terms of three problems that confront every developing child. The major dilemma facing an infant is to secure parental care and nurturance, and to make sense of the world. This is accomplished largely by allowing itself to be governed by adult rules. The parent-child variables that influence this process are well known, and the manner in which an infant adjusts itself to adult authority will have profound (and predictable) consequences for its later life.

Ultimately, however, each child must leave the exclusive care of its parents and make its way in a peer group. In the peer group a child must shed its infantile egocentrism and accommodate itself to a radically expanded set of social norms. This is facilitated by the development of empathy or role-taking ability, by a markedly heightened sensitivity to social expectations, social praise and blame.

By late adolescence a child is faced with the problem of establishing a life for itself. This requires reconciling the competing demands of its family and peer group and coming to terms with oneself; developing an autonomous life style. This is typically accomplished either through the development of an ideology that rationalizes one's intended life style, or through an identification with a "preferred character type," that provides one with an internalized standard for future behavior.

In this view, knowledge of how a person has handled these three problems will explain Peck and Havighurst's (1960) character types, and will permit a wide range of predictions concerning that person's conduct.

Five themes characterize the clinical approach to moral development. (1) Each person is studied in depth using an array of assessment procedures. (2) Moral development is seen as a portion of personality development broadly defined rather than a specific subject matter; (3) parent-child relations are considered to be crucial in the development of character structure; once formed, character structure (4) gives coherence to behavior across situations but remains relatively unconscious. Finally, (5) this tradition is very much concerned with placing the facts of moral development within a conceptual framework that takes into account the ontogenesis of personality as well as the cultural and historical circumstances in which the developing child lives.

BIBLIOGRAPHY

BANDURA, A. *Social learning theory.* Morristown, N.J.: General Learning Press, 1971.

CAMPBELL, D. G. Ethnocentric and other altruistic motives. In D. Levine (Ed.), *Nebraska Symposium on Motivation.* Lincoln: University of Nebraska Press, 1965.

HOGAN, R. Moral conduct and moral character. *Psychological Bulletin,* 1973, *79,* 217–232.

HOGAN, R. Dialectical aspects of moral development. *Human Development,* 1974, *17,* 107–117.

KOHLBERG, L. The development of children's orientations toward a moral order. *Vita Humana,* 1963, *6,* 11–33.

PECK, R. F., and HAVIGHURST, R. J. *The psychology of character development.* New York: Wiley, 1960.

PIAGET, J. *The moral judgment of the child.* New York: Free Press, 1964.

WADDINGTON, C. H. *The ethical animal.* Chicago: University of Chicago Press, 1967.

ROBERT HOGAN

MORALE AND ATTITUDE SURVEYS

The attitude survey is an instrument which can provide data as a basis for a highly reliable diagnosis of the human side of organization effectiveness. By going directly to the work force with a tool designed to measure what employees think, management obtains information that is unbiased, systematic, and representative of that organization's particular problems. Since the purpose of the attitude questionnaire approach is to provide the kind of accurate diagnosis that is the essential first step in effective action programs, careful attention must be given to the conceptual framework of the survey instrument, its administration, and the reporting of its results to both management and employees.

If the morale survey has been constructed within the proper conceptual framework—that is, to reflect utilization—(what the company gets from the employee) and equity (what the employee gets from the company)—then it is the administration of the survey that assumes next importance in assuring employee candor and employee commitment to both participation and utilization of the data received. Since the objective is to learn how the employees feel about their jobs, the survey instrument typically consists largely of some form of job satisfaction questionnaire.

The entire survey process, from interview through feedback stage, must be announced to the survey population. Employee frankness can be encouraged through reassurances that they will not be held personally to account for their answers. Since questionnaires are administered in large groups, on site, and during the regular workday, an exact administration schedule must be drawn up and announced to all managers and unit employees. The proper physical environment should be prepared (comfortable chairs, adequate light, pencils, answer sheets, etc.) and introductory remarks or guidelines given at the start of each administrative session. The actual completion time for the survey should be brief (under an hour may be ideal), and employees should find the experience enjoyable—a chance to state their views on the job itself, supervision, compensation, promotional opportunities, and the like.

Some employees may be unable to fill out the questionnaire within their scheduled time, and still other employee units may have a low rate of participation. Make-up sessions should therefore be scheduled, managers reminded as to their time and place, and arrangements made for administering the survey to any field population that exists. (These steps—and all the steps in smooth administration—are aimed at getting as high a rate of participation as possible.) Arrangements should also be made to send answer sheets on a regular basis for processing.

Clear, simple questions, answered truthfully, provide statistics from which a detailed analysis is drawn; the statistics are supplied by computer output. Three basic kinds of output have been used successfully. The first is *factor analysis,* a tool in which, through correlated methods, the basic dimensions measured by the questionnaire are generated. The second is the *response distribution* for the total survey population and for each subunit within it—a *subunit* being defined as a group (under the management of a single supervisor) small enough to be meaningful but large enough to protect individual identity. Response distribution also contains the number of valid and invalid responses, the mean, and the standard deviation. The third kind of output, *demographics,* divides the data by background variables, using the same measures for each category as were used for the total and for the subunits—the mean, the standard variation, and so on.

The diagnostician, having now drawn a quantitative picture of the strengths and weaknesses peculiar to the organization under study, has still not completed the task at hand —reporting the data in a fashion that will insure its full utilization. Utilization of results is the purpose of any industrial analysis, and it is best accomplished by reporting statistical data in three steps using a collaborative method (the involvement and input of both management and employees).

The management/supervisory level must next be trained in how to interpret the data and be shown the detailed data for their units before anyone else. An individualized computer printout can be prepared for each subunit manager/supervisor so that he may view his group's results in comparison with the organization as a whole. This "mirror image" of one's own practices is a powerful management development tool; managers themselves deal with their problems and report their plans for improvement upward.

Managers/supervisors now feed their unit results to their own employees, again having been trained in the proper feedback method. A very effective method is a written summary combined with an oral report in a departmental meeting.

Through the three-step method just described, the organization has the opportunity to proceed on two levels of action: companywide and unit level. As a final step, organization personnel may be trained in action techniques so as to provide in-house "key resources" for continuing action.

BIBLIOGRAPHY

SIROTA, D., and WOLFSON, A. D. Pragmatic approach to people problems. *Harvard Business Review,* 1973, *51,* 120–128.

DAVID SIROTA

MORAL ISSUES, MORALITY

MORALITY: HORNEY'S VIEW

Psychoanalytic consideration of moral behavior is based on a person's relation to himself and reflected in his relations with others. The basic nature of being human is the determinant of morality. If, as it often has been believed, man is evil by nature and there are innate life-destroying forces, then to live morally one must combat, repress, sublimate, or destroy such forces.

Some authors maintain that both good and evil are inherent in human nature. Therefore, to allow one to develop according to his nature is tantamount to perpetuating the basic moral split. The modification of natural tendencies would require that the bad be checked or transformed and the individual be guided toward constructive and good behavior. This is sought through the application of will, reason, and faith which are structuring rather than releasing energies and which are superimpositions on the self rather than being spontaneous expressions of the self.

If, however, as Horney (1950) believed, man has inherent evolutionary constructive forces which urge him to realize his inner potentials, then living morally means to encourage spontaneous growing and to seek no other goal than to become true to one's own nature. This is not only a prime moral obligation but also a prime moral privilege.

The task of therapy then is to help one become aware of, experience, grapple with, and outgrow those forces which oppose and retard healthy growth. However, to be able to choose right from wrong and to choose to strive for self-realization requires certain conditions: (1) One must be aware of the alternatives. Without alternatives, there is no choice, and also no morality. (2) One must have the ability to choose between alternatives. (3) Finally, one must be able to accept responsibility for the consequences of one's acts. The neurotic process by its very nature impairs one's ability to live morally.

Alienation and neurosis are an amalgam. As one is involved in trying to be what he is not, one loses touch with his true feelings, wishes, and beliefs. One is unaware of aspects of himself other than those which are directed toward the creation and maintenance of an *Idealized Image* and thus unaware of the alternatives. Moreover, rigidity, defensiveness, and the compulsive need to eliminate whatever conflicts with self-idealization create a powerful force which impairs one's ability to choose freely. Such neurotically driven behavior may disguise itself as dedication to high moral standards.

Since the neurotic, unaware of unconscious motivations, believes himself to be sincere, both he and those who observe him may be deceived. The neurotic strives for perfection and this goal is pursued through neurotic pride for the sake of maintaining unity, albeit a spurious one. Horney called these inexorable demands on one's self the *Tyranny of the Should* (1950).

If one externalizes his intentions and attitudes onto others and demands that others fulfill his neurotic needs, if he lives through others, and if he defends his neurotic pride at the cost of condemning and destroying whatever is imperfect in himself—then he is not capable of being truly responsible for himself.

The analyst cannot avoid considering moral values in both theory and therapy, since their distortion is a significant manifestation of the neurotic process and perpetuates neurosis. The analyst must consider whether the morality is compulsive and superimposed. The goals of therapy are to help the patient heal his inner dividedness, strengthen his inner autonomy, and foster his ability to relate directly to others without having to prove something. Through that process, moralistic tendencies are resolved and an authentic morality emerges.

BIBLIOGRAPHY

HORNEY, K. *Neurosis and human growth.* New York: Norton, 1950.

ARNOLD MITCHELL
HAROLD KELMAN

MOREL, BENEDICT AUGUSTIN (1809–1873)

Benedict Augustin Morel, born in Austria, was considered a leading French psychiatrist. He was a student of Falret and is remembered for his coining of the term *dèmence-precoce* which he used to describe the clinical course of a mental illness. Morel was a close friend of Claude Bernard and was influenced by the work of Darwin. At first he believed there was too much emphasis on organic aspects of mental illness and he urged the study of the emotional life. However he altered his views and later taught that external agents, such as alcohol and nar-

cotics, could operate in the deterioration of an individual. In 1850 when he intensively studied the condition he came to call *dementia-praecox*, he believed it to be a hereditary illness. He studied mentally retarded patients in the Maréville Asylum near Nancy, in regard to their hereditary background, illness in early infancy and the effect of poverty and miserable living conditions.

Morel also clinically described the "epileptic character," wrote on cretinism, goiter, medical-legal issues, and in his practice, secretly used hypnosis. His views were similar to those of the French school of organicists. He saw mental illness as part of the process of mental degeneration. The pathway was from neurosis to mental deficiency. This view greatly influenced Krafft-Ebing in Germany, Victor Magnan in France, Cesare Lombroso in Italy, Henry Maudsley in England, and psychiatrists of Latin America. One of Morel's main works is, with E. Lasègue, "Etudes Historiques sur l'Alienation Mentale" published in *Annales Medico-Psychologiques* (1844).

LEO H. BERMAN

MORGAN, CONWAY LLOYD (1852–1936)

Morgan was an English comparative psychologist. He was trained in geology, but was influenced by T. H. Huxley to pursue Darwinian biology. He contributed to the study of the evolution of the mind. He reacted critically to G. J. Romanes (1890). Morgan conducted systematic experiments in support of the experimental method, which he found superior to anecdotal information and the case study method. He offset the tendency to anthropomorphize when seeking the continuity between animals and man by stressing parsimony when assigning consciousness to animals. He influenced E. L. Thorndike's dissertation research (1898), which proximally initiated the modern experimental era in animal behavior research. Morgan was the first fellow of the Royal Academy of London to be elected for psychological work (1899).

J. WAYNE LAZAR

MORSELLI, ENRICO (1852–1929)

An Italian psychiatrist and anthropologist, Morselli's main contributions were devoted to epilepsy, traumatic neurosis, and aphasia. He was also the author of one of the first Italian textbooks on psychoanalysis (1926).

SILVANO CHIARI

MOSAIC TEST

The Mosaic Test, first introduced to psychology by Margaret Lowenfeld and later refined by Fredric Wertham and others, is a projective test with considerable apparent potential which has never been widely used by American psychologists.

The test materials consist of 456 plastic mosaic pieces of various colors and shapes and a wooden tray on which the subject is asked to make any pattern he wishes. The simplest procedure for recording the mosaic patterns made by the subject is to photograph them with color film.

A number of scoring systems for the patterns have been constructed. Some utilize detailed categories of shape and color; others are more global and deal with the mosaic patterns as a whole. The more global scoring systems seem to have been more successful.

Wertham (1950) elaborated 25 dimensions on which the design is evaluated, for example: number of designs, coherence of design, number of pieces used, choice of color, choice of shapes, emphasis on form or on color. Using such categories, Wertham as well as others claimed that the Mosaic Test is a useful clinical tool for differential diagnosis.

There is some disagreement among the users of the Mosaic Test as to the limits of its utility. Some find it to be a valuable test for a global assessment of personality with much the same kind of power as the Rorschach Inkblot Test. Others make more modest claims for it, suggesting that it is most valuable for differential clinical diagnosis and should be restricted to this function.

The Mosaic Test has also been used as a measure of organic brain damage, but the validity of the instrument as a psychological test of organicity is questionable.

BIBLIOGRAPHY

DORKEN, H. The Mosaic Test: A second review. *Journal of Projective Techniques*, 1956, *20*, 164–171.
WERTHAM, F. The Mosaic Test. In L. E. Abt and L. Bellak (Eds.), *Projective psychology: Clinical approaches to the total personality*. New York: Grove Press, 1950. Pp. 230–256.

PHILIP A. GOLDBERG

MOSSO, ANGELO (1846–1910)

Mosso was an Italian physiologist of worldwide renown for his study on fear (1884) and on fatigue (1891). To study muscular fatigue Mosso invented the ergograph which has been extensively employed not only by physiologists, but also by psychologists interested in how mental work affects physical capacity and whether mental fatigue is reflected in muscular fatigue. Another device for measuring blood supply is known as Mosso's balance.

SILVANO CHIARI

MOTHER

See FAMILY

MOTHER-INFANT INTERACTION

As early as the fourteenth century, the paintings of the Madonna and Child by Fra Angelico gave pictorial permanence to the maternal-child relationship. Not until the twentieth century, however, did mother and child receive noteworthy scientific attention. Two divergent theories of mother-infant bonds of affection were developed by two totally opposed schools. Rather than being antagonistic as one would expect, they are identical. Both schools, the behaviorist and the Freudian, assumed that infant-mother love was achieved by association of the maternal face and figure with breast and feeding.

Contact Comfort

Multiple experiments and years of effort at the Wisconsin Primate Laboratory have shown that the primary variable in infant-mother attraction and affection, surmounting the importance of breast feeding, is intimate bodily contact, known now as *contact comfort.* The experiments which demonstrated the statistical significance and fundamental importance of contact comfort employed the balanced breast phenomenon. Infant monkeys were given a chance freely to go to a mother of their choice. They had four choices, cuddly terrycloth mothers, half who nursed and half who did not, or wire mothers, half who nursed and half who did not. The babies not only chose the cloth mother over the wire mother when both mothers nursed but the nonnursing cloth mother was chosen over the nursing wire mother. Almost without exception, the infant chose the nonlactating cloth mother over the lactating wire mother and this learned reaction was achieved with rare rapidity and prodigiously perfect and persistent performance.

Along with contact comfort, infant love for the mother monkey was found to be influenced by other preferences, not as strong but still statistically significant. All important behaviors operate through multiple variables and not unitary factors. Infants prefer mothers who impart warmth, mothers with movement as well as mothers who give them sustenance. Together, the three secondary variables add their measure of confidence and love for the mother and increase the feeling of security and trust already engendered by the all important factor of contact comfort.

During the twentieth century, not only were theories tottering, but, soon after the mid-century mark, research results were rapidly revising the concept of the capacities and capabilities of the infant primate, human or subhuman. The baby emerged from the state of blooming, buzzing confusion to which he had been condemned for half a century by William James.

Harlow found that the neonatal rhesus monkey mastered simple discrimination learning problems as early as eleven days of age and that maximal facility on simple learning tests could be reached within a very brief length of time, comparable to that of much older monkeys.

Perceptual Differentiations

In 1958 Fantz led the way to utilizing the preferences of human infants to learn more about their capacities for perceptual differen-

tiations. An ingenious peephole made possible an examination of the reflections on the infant's retina, and the preferred targets of attention could be accurately recorded as to preferences of attention and time span.

From then on, confusion has been replaced by fast forming facts concerning what the babies can sense and perceive. Neonates will interrupt nursing in order to attend to a new sound or sight. If a desired view is obscured, the infant will wiggle and push to achieve a better posture for viewing. Even in the first few months, babies prefer patterns over solid planes and the most preferred patterns are those which resemble the human face. Aronson and Rosenbloom conducted an experiment which disclosed the fact that infants perceive within a common auditory-visual space. Infants were seated so that they directly faced and watched their mothers who were only 2 feet away but separated by a window and actually in another room. The mother's voice was directed by a loudspeaker to convincingly come from her face. After some minutes, the loudspeaker diverted the sound of mother's voice to seem to come from 90 degree angles to the right or left of the babies. Distress developed, the infants grimaced and writhed, some cried and most of them vigorously mouthed their tongues, a sign of sure stress. The infants could be distracted by a rattle, but violently opposed any attempt to get them again to look at mother with the displaced manner of speaking.

Communication

For many years it has been clear that mothers in many species, phylogenetically both more and less complex than the graylag goose, have in multiple, mysterious, and diverse ways communicated with their very young offspring. Baby monkeys ask maternal permission to leave the close contact of mother's body and learn to identify fierce, fearful faces from their experiences with mother's threats. Human mothers have also been aware of two-way communication systems with their babies. The scientific investigators remained unenlightened, however, until well into the twentieth century. It is now obvious that there are behaviors operating mutually through the visual, auditory, and gestural modalities between mother and child. These undoubtedly have unlearned components but are primarily the basis for learned and anticipatory forms of communication.

The extent of early communication between the mother and very young babies has been shown in many studies of eye-to-eye contact. There is no question that this contact plays a part in the development of early affectional relationships. Before the age of eight weeks, babies can follow the mother with their eyes when she leaves the room. At four months of age infants smile more to a face that smiles back at them. If a smiling face suddenly ceases to smile, baby not only loses interest but may actively attempt to avoid the sight. Mother's smile is of such importance that it has been used as a reinforcer in many experiments on attention. Mother's smile is the surest and soonest way to increase reciprocal frequency. This phenomenon works in two directions. Eighty-five percent of mothers do not feel any deep, warm affection for newborn infants until the baby is old enough to give the first emotional feedbacks through some communicative channel.

Love

Through maternal-infant interaction the infant learns to love and also what not to love, what to accept and what to fear. The mother first conveys security and trust to the infant through contact comfort, the warmth of her embrace, the lulling, rocking motion, and the soothing satisfaction of her nursing. Girded with this confidence, the infant rhesus gradually dares leave maternal protection to investigate the wondrous world. The monkey may stand with all four feet firmly founded on the terrycloth mother while he gingerly chews at a strange piece of cloth. His first longer safaris are usually interspersed with dashes back to mother to rub some maternal love from her body to his. To this very important extent the surrogate mother plays her role well. In training for fear situations, the real monkey mother shows some superiority. From birth on she plays the part of a stable, sure protectress against the dangers of the world. At the sight of a strange face she tightly holds the little one and expresses her total devotion by mean and menacing threat grimaces toward the intruder. When two- to three-year old mother-raised rhesus are placed in a strange, fearful situation facing a monster who emits sparks and horrible sounds and flails his arms and legs, they show less destructive fear than do surrogate-mother raised monkeys of the same age. They face the fear object and return threats by face and by posture, just as mother had done all of their lives.

The mother's love for the infant has been glorified for centuries but love of the infant for the mother was so thoroughly ignored that it was not even given a separate, specific name. Infant love for the mother is, however, without doubt the stronger and more persistent of the two. There is a very good underlying reason, as the mother can well survive in a feral environment without the infant.

The Battered Child

In an effort to unravel the history and the mystery of the battered child syndrome, motherless rhesus monkeys were studied at the Wisconsin Primate Laboratory. Females were raised in total isolation, without love from a mother or agemate friends. Eventually but with difficulty these females were mated and had babies. Not knowing love, they showed no loving care or attention to the baby. Contrarily, these mothers mimicked the mothers of the battered children. The creation of the cruel mother was complete, but another discovery was made in the course of the experiment. Although terrified, the baby returned time and time again to the mother, despite constant cuffing, repeated and violent rejection, and total threat. These persistent attempts at contact with the mother—the constant clinging and affectionate appeals of the infants—have been known to finally have therapeutic effect on her. For the sake of the average baby of a motherless mother, the experimenters do not recommend attempts to repeatedly replicate this research, but do advise that we never underestimate the power of an infant.

BIBLIOGRAPHY

Harlow, H. F.; Harlow, M. K.; Dodsworth, R. O.; and Arling, G. L. Maternal behavior of rhesus monkeys deprived of mothering and peer association in infancy. *Proceeding American Philosophic Society,* 1966, *111,* 58–66.
Harlow, H. F.; Harlow, M. K.; and Hansen, E. W. The

maternal affectional system of rhesus monkeys. In H. L. Rheingold (Ed.), *Maternal behavior in mammals.* New York: Wiley, 1963. Pp. 254–281.

HARLOW, H. F., and ZIMMERMANN, R. R. Affectional patterns in the infant monkey. *Science,* 1959, *130,* 421–432.

STONE, L. J.; SMITH, H. T.; and MURPHY, L. B. (Eds.). *The competent infant.* New York: Basic Books, 1973. Pp. 471–581, 990, 1076–1077.

HARRY F. HARLOW

MOTION PICTURES AND PSYCHIATRY

Dynamic psychiatry and cinematography belong to the twentieth century. At the time Freud was documenting cases of hysteria Charlie Chaplin appeared in his first movies, *Making a Living* and *Kid Auto Races at Venice* (1913). In 1927, *The Jazz Singer* with Al Jolson featured sound, and this first talking motion picture introduced an art form and new communication medium which has since influenced millions of people throughout the world.

The psychiatrist and the cinematographer both have great interest in man, and in his endless adventures, crises, conflicts, defeats, tragedies, courage, and transcendence. Both are interested in watching, seeing what is going on, observing the smallest detail of life, and grasping the enlightenment which may emerge. The psychiatrist has long pursued knowledge not only of the external realities, but also of the hidden processes of man, his thoughts, his fantasies, his feelings, and his instincts. The film-maker has also pursued the search for reality. Siegfried Kracauer writes, "Film . . . is uniquely equipped to record and reveal physical reality, and hence gravitates towards it." Thus, film more than any previous mode can capture the physical reality. In the faithful rendition of each motion and gestural nuance it can transmit human interactions and moments of intense emotion. But the film is more than just a photographic rendition of external realities. It is true that newsreels, cinema verité, and movies of therapeutic sessions may present material in real time and actual sequence, but creative cinema includes the director who selects not only the camera shots and angles, but whose editing makes the cinematic presentation. In this process the film's capacity to alter time and space dimensions, to leap past the

barriers of the physical realities to the level of fantasy, and quickly back again, augments its prime capacity as a recorder of realities.

It is in this total creative effort that the film makes a contribution to psychiatry, because no other communication form can so accurately and sensitively portray to other humans the inner fantasy life and the integration of personal experience. It is almost as if the director attains the capacity to project his own psyche so others can experience what he experiences. His dream becomes the viewers' reality, and the night fantasies of mental patients told from the couch can be exposed in their inadequacy. The director's artistic sensitivity often captures truths about the real world of human activity which ordinarily are obscured in the clichés of daily existence. Thus, when the film veers too far towards fantasy, the critics may complain. When it illumines too much social reality, the censors may appear.

The German psychologist Hugo Mauerhofer has elaborated other features of the "Cinema Situation" which further account for its compelling quality. He noted that a viewer may decide to enter a theater for entertainment or enlightenment, but that as soon as the lights dim profound psychological changes occur. In the isolation and anonymity of the darkened theater the viewer is cut off from other stimuli and his sense of time and space is altered. The hypnotic effect of the flickering screen has been noted, and Mauerhofer mentioned the affinity between the "Cinema Situation" on the one hand and daydreams on the other. He stated: "The position of the cinema is therefore that of an unreal reality, half-way between everyday reality and the purely personal dream."

Cinema in Psychiatry

Mauerhofer also described the *psychotherapeutic function* of the "Cinema Situation" which, he said, makes life bearable for millions of people as they salvage shreds of the films they have seen and carry them into their sleep. The cinema thereby offers compensation for lives which have lost a great deal of their substance. Aside from this effect of movies, it is not surprising that psychiatry should have sought to utilize motion pictures in the mainstream of its own deliberate efforts. In therapy direct utilization has been limited, but in training and research much wider application has developed.

Therapy. In 1954, J. Carrere et al. published results of using motion picture films in the psychotherapy of delirium in alcoholism. In 1960, F. Cornelison and J. Arsenian used motion pictures to confront patients with their own images. However, for such purposes the 16mm sound film has serious disadvantages. First, it is expensive, and secondly, there is of necessity a long delay between shooting time and the developing process. For both these reasons the widespread use of recorded data in therapy waited for the development of videorecording which emerged rapidly in the 1960s. Today it has wide application as an adjunct in many forms of psychiatric therapy.

Training. With the realization that the material of everyday life could be captured and preserved, workers in the field of psychiatry were no different from those in other fields in the attempt to "preserve the past." Such films have historic value, and home movies taken by Sandor Lorand of Freud and others in the early psychoanalytic movement still arouse excitement in audiences of modern colleagues.

The lessons gained in commercial moviemaking gradually were applied in the area of training films, as it was recognized that presentation of raw material was not enough to produce either good learning or good films. With the development of film production units in universities and large clinics, films of superior quality began to appear, and to fill an important role in the training of therapists. These and other production companies, often subsidized by government or private organizations, also served another field of education by the development of films for the general public, with subjects ranging from the problems of child rearing, to the problems of providing help to families with schizophrenic members.

Thousands of films are now available throughout the world, often at no cost, from university and public libraries. A sample would include *Marathon: Story of the Young Drug Users* (University of California, 1967); *The Kibbutz* (University of Indiana, 1966); *Group Therapy—The Dynamics of Change* (Abell, 1971); and *About Sex* (Scheidlinger, 1973).

A noteworthy effort was the production for professionals of the *Hillcrest Family Series*

(Audio-Visual Services, University Park, Pennsylvania). In this series four family therapists were filmed interviewing the same family.

Research. Therapeutic sessions which had been filmed (i.e., Hillcrest Family) gave promise not only of being useful in teaching, but also in research of underlying conflicts and psychodynamics and the study of the nature of the therapeutic process. Objections were raised that the very recording of the therapeutic process changed it so substantially that it was no longer the same phenomenon. Nevertheless, hundreds of hours of psychoanalytic sessions were filmed in Los Angeles, Chicago, and New York.

This problem of categorization and retrieval of data was somewhat clarified by the gradual development of new theories of human behavior. Earlier dynamic theories had been mainly intrapsychic. The advent of field theory, and general systems theory led to an interest in the context of behavior and interpersonal and group interactions. R. Birdwhistell, an anthropologist, made significant contributions in the development of kinesic analysis. The premise of his work is that one category of nonverbal behavior is really a culturally specific body language which plays a crucial role in the communication and behavioral control within any given group. Motion pictures proved the ideal way to isolate and identify minute bits of information, and important research evolved.

A. Scheflen, a psychoanalyst and behavioral scientist, used this method and in 1965 published an historic study on the contextual analysis of a psychotherapy session. Scheflen also outlined the advantages of motion picture recording over videotape for some research purposes. The moving picture film has higher resolution, and is more convenient for close study. Temporal measurements can be made more accurately. The researcher has perfect control over viewing material when using a hand-operated time-motion analyzer, which is essential for detailed dissection of movements. In addition, a pulse-driven stop motion projector is the best device for frame-by-frame analysis. With film, time can be expanded (fast speed during shooting), or contracted (shooting only one frame every few seconds). Finally, film is more stable than videotape, and less likely to be damaged during handling.

In 1967, E. Charny published a report on psychosomatic manifestations of rapport in psychotherapy, using the same research methods. He found that speech and body congruency of the patient and therapist were closely correlated, and concluded that congruent postural configurations in vis-à-vis psychotherapy are behavioral indicators of relatedness.

Some of the disadvantages of videotape have been overcome by the work of P. Ekman and W. Friesen who in 1969 reported the construction of a direct interface between a videorecorder and a small computer which allows digitized coded information on every body and facial movement to be placed on the videotape. This can then be read and interpreted by the computer. Material originally on film is first transferred to videotape by a film-to-video transfer chain. These developments give indication of the advances one can expect from new technology applied to evolving psychiatric theory in clinical settings.

Psychiatry in Cinema

As psychiatry has integrated the technology and phenomenology of film into its work, so has the cinema incorporated the developing field of psychiatry into its productions, both in the content of the films themselves, and in the concepts and values which are implicit in their creation. The area to be reviewed is so vast that some order may be brought into its consideration by noting briefly the portrayal of the psychiatrist in films; the handling of clinical case material in films; and the presentation in films of matters which fall in that vague dimension between psychiatric entity and social issue. The record runs from *The Cabinet of Dr. Caligari* (1921), a horror film, finally revealed to have been told by a madman, through *Secrets of a Soul* (1926), which was the first serious treatment of psychiatry on the screen, and for which the director, G. W. Pabst, had the professional advice of Hanns Sachs and Karl Abraham, right up to *A Woman Under the Influence* (1974). This was the portrayal of a woman having a breakdown under the stresses of her marriage.

Psychiatrists and Case Studies. The psychiatrist in his clinical role has been seen in the movies as dealing primarily with individual cases and psychopathology. Thus films from the 30s to the 60s typically portrayed the psy-

chiatrist in his special position as healer. The shifting attitude of less reverence towards the psychiatrist was documented, however, and during the 60s and 70s focus on social issues reflected the new awareness in psychiatric theory that individual behavioral disturbances are intimately related to social context.

Through the years all kinds of case material and clinical issues have been filmed. Split personality was the theme in *Madonna of the Seven Moons* with Phyllis Calvert in 1944; and in *The Three Faces of Eve*, Lee J. Cobb played a psychiatrist who did a fine traditional job of treating a "multiple personality." *The Snake Pit* (1948) was a deliberately unsensational study of mental illness. *The Lost Weekend*, and *David and Lisa* dealt with alcoholism and schizophrenia. In 1952 *Mandy* showed the teaching of a congenitally deaf child, and in 1963 *A Child Is Waiting* unveiled the world of the mentally handicapped.

Unvarnished case studies have been popular with audiences, including *El* in 1953 (paranoiac jealousy); *Pressure Point* (fascist tendencies); *Life Upside Down* in 1964 (withdrawal); *The Collector* (sexual obsession); *Repulsion* in 1967, and *The Boston Strangler* in 1969 (homicidal mania); *Bigger Than Life* (drugs); *Marnie* (frigidity); and *Morgan* (infantile regression).

A trend to move to larger issues appeared with Bergman's *Wild Strawberries* (1957) in which an old man shows the possibility of changing patterns of a lifetime. In 1964 *The Servant* explored the subtle way a dominant-submissive pattern can reverse, as the servant gradually comes to dominate his master. *The Killing of Sister George*, and *Sunday Bloody Sunday* in 1971 dealt with lesbianism and male homosexuality. Later, in *Diary of a Mad Housewife* (1972) and *Scenes From a Marriage* (1974), the effects of monogamous marriage in our society were shown. The same dilemmas were caught by *An American Family* (shown on TV in 1973, but originally filmed), and the Canadian film *A Married Couple*.

The portrayal of psychiatrists moved from the glib in *Dark Past* (1948), to *Harvey* (1950), showing that psychiatrists could be laughed at. In the 50s individual therapists were jibed at, while surface respect for the profession was maintained (*Mirage, The Group,* and *What a Way to Go*). In 1959 Rod Steiger in the British movie *The Mark* showed a more personal, relaxed, and human side of the psychiatrist. *Bob and Carol and Ted and Alice* (1969) in addition to laughing at "swinging," poked fun at the encounter movement, and also provided a spoof of the unresponsive therapist.

Finally, in 1975, Bergman filmed *Face to Face* with Liv Ullman, in which he explored the personal life of the psychiatrist beyond the professional role, and in which one character remarks, "Surely all psychiatrists are either insane, prestige-mad, or unwitted, or all three at once."

Social Issues. As psychiatry has moved more and more to include social context in its understanding of individual behavior, so the films have also reflected greater interest in the portrayal of current social forces and conflicts. *Easy Rider* (1969) revealed the lurking violence in America towards people who are different; while in 1970 Antonioni's *Zabriskie Point* depicted America's moral decay. The concern over ecology was satirically highlighted also in 1970 by *Brewster McCloud;* and social pollution and chaos was frighteningly envisioned by Jules Feiffer in *Little Murders.* Some attempts to portray black experience were *Lady Sings the Blues, Nothing but a Man, My Sweet Charlie,* and *Sounder.*

Violence and crime were underscored and exploited in *The Super Cops* (1974); *Godfather I and II; The French Connection I and II;* and films like *Kung Fu* (1973). Another dimension of films dating back to its silent beginnings is the pornographic movie. With changing societal mores and less censorship, hard-core porno is widely shown, as well as cleaned up versions such as *The Happy Hooker* (1975).

Brother Can You Spare a Dime (1975) is a striking portrayal of the 1930s depression with newsreel and old film montage; while *The Stepford Wives* (1975) is a horror film on the ultimate male chauvinism.

Commentary

Film has made possible a new experiencing and sharing of reality. Michael Roemer writes, "Only film renders experience with enough immediacy and totality to call into play the perceptual processes we employ in life itself." Other famous directors have tried to tell us what their creative experience is. Ingmar Bergman: "There is no art form that has so much in common with film as music. Both affect our emotions directly, not through the intellect." And he said further, "I try to tell the truth about the human condition, the truth as I see it."

Federico Fellini: "Part of the theme for all my films (is) . . . the terrible difficulty people have in talking to each other—the old problem of communication."

George Gerbner, professor of communications at the University of Pennsylvania, believes no change has had a larger direct impact on human consciousness and social behavior than the rise of communicational technology. Television is the ultimate in such technology, but the motion picture is another potent conveyor of modern myth. Gerbner noted that the Scottish patriot Andrew Fletcher once said, "If a man were permitted to write all the ballads, he need not care who should make the laws of the nation." Gerbner continued, "The ballads of an age are powerful myths depicting its visions of the invisible forces of life, society, and the universe. They inform as they entertain." He concluded, "Entertainment—the celebration of conventional morality— . . . has become the universal source of public acculturation."

Psychiatrists are also concerned with communication and are involved in promoting change, usually directed towards individuals, or small groups. The psychiatrist and the film maker have in common the socially-sanctioned roles and power to influence people. The psychiatrist is seen by some as an agent for social control, while the humanistic position views the true goal of the psychiatrist as promoting the fullest growth of each individual reflecting a value system that is genuinely human.

The cinema too can be seen as an agent of social control. It has been suggested that an underlying social regulator of the box-office smash *Jaws* (1975), is the message in these times of economic turmoil that people should not venture towards new environments, but should be satisfied with the status quo which is depicted as safe. Apparently the forces of mass communication, with their access to mass publics, and their capacity to alter attitudes and values is one of the most potent, and carefully guarded prerogatives in any culture. With such power mass communication, including the cinema, may no longer just reflect invisible societal forces, but may indeed become the conscious means of controlling entire nations.

BIBLIOGRAPHY

CHARNY, E. J. Psychosomatic manifestations of rapport in psychotherapy. *Psychosomatic Medicine,* 1966, *28,* 305–315.

EKMAN, P., and FRIESEN, W. VID-R and SCAN: Tools and methods for the automated analysis of visual records. In G. Gerbner (Ed.), *The analysis of communication content.* New York: Wiley, 1969.

GERBNER, G. Communication and social environment. *Scientific American,* 1972, *227,* 153–160.

HALLIWELL, L. *The filmgoer's companion* (Rev. 3rd ed.). London: MacGibbon and Kee, 1970.

MACCANN, R. D. (Ed.) *Film: A montage of theories.* New York: Dutton, 1966.

SCHEFLEN, A. E. *Stream and structure in communication: Context analysis of a psychotherapy session.* Philadelphia: Eastern Pennsylvania Psychiatric Institute Press, 1965.

THOMSON, D. *Movie man.* New York: Stein and Day, 1967.

See also AUDIOVISUAL TECHNIQUES IN PSYCHOTHERAPY

IAN ALGER

MOTIVATION, MOTIVE

MOTIVATION, DERIVED

In theories of motivation, it has long been recognized that appetitive (e.g., hunger) and aversive (e.g., pain) states, whatever their merits as explanatory constructs for lower animals or for young children, are insufficient bases to account for the persistence of motivated behavior in the human adult and for the acquisition of new information and skills in the years which follow early childhood. Possible solutions of the problem were advanced early. Woodworth, in his *Dynamic Psychology* (1918), proposed that a well-learned but not automatic skill "is itself a drive and capable of motivating activities that lie beyond its immediate scope." Gordon Allport (1937) suggested the idea of "functional autonomy," that is, that while an activity may have developed initially under the impetus of a biological drive it could become independent of this source and persist indefinitely as an autonomous motive. Neither of these proposals includes a theory of mechanism or process, and for that reason these ideas have been judged as not satisfactory.

However, attempts to specify and demonstrate the underlying processes of derived motivation have so far been either unsuccessful or lacking in general applicability and acceptance. An unsuccessful attempt used the concept of acquired drive. Still viable is the notion of incentive motivation. This idea rests on the proposition that desirable and undesirable objects and situations can come, through experience, to elicit arousal. The arousal then invigorates response tendencies of approach to a desirable object or situation and avoidance tendencies with respect to an undesirable object or situation. The arousal is nonspecific or nondirective with respect to what behavior is activated, but the cues of the situation in which the arousal occurs are presumably sufficient to control the specific forms of behavior the arousal potentiates. Anticipation of commerce with a desired goal object or of contact with an undesirable goal object is thought to be the basis for the arousal. Frustration and sometimes conflict may contribute to the arousal.

In a general way, the available evidence supports an incentive theory of motivation in the case of animal behavior, although many details remain to be worked out. Studies of fear, conditioned appetitive behavior, secondary or conditioned reinforcement, the predictive value of cues, and frustrative nonreward provide pertinent information.

With respect to the adult human being, however, detailed and systematic analyses in terms of incentive motivation have not appeared, despite considerable investigative work concerning such human motives as achievement, affiliation, aggression, anxiety, fear of failure, power, and others. In general, these motives have been conceived in terms of, first, a trait or disposition, which, second, is engaged in a situation but which, third, is only one of several factors deemed important in ensuing behaviors. Thus, for example, in achievement motivation, the motive is seen as a disposition in which individuals differ, that is, it is stronger in some people than it is in others. Measuring devices for the assessment of achievement motivation include procedures based on the Thematic Apperception Test. However, there are situations in which the motive will not be engaged, that is, those which the person does not perceive as related to achievement. While the motive is engaged in achievement-related circumstances, behavior, including choice and effort, depends also on judgments with respect to the probability that success will be forthcoming, and the value of success in the task or performance. Another motive, fear of failure, may also be engaged in the situation. People also differ with respect to the degree to which they possess this motive, and its role is also modulated by perceived probability of failure and the aversiveness of failure under the circumstances. The behavior that occurs is a consequence of a complex interaction of the motives engaged and the subjective probabilities and values just indicated.

There is a good deal in this account that refers to parameters of situations and tasks, and, of course, external cues are usually integral to accounts in terms of incentive motivation. But the factors involved in achievement, as adumbrated above, indicate both that achievement is a complex affair and that perceptual and judgmental processes, as well as the motive, are involved. Thus, a simple account is not easy to justify.

The complexity of such motivated actions as those related to achievement has led to emphasis on cognitive factors in motivation and to a relationship with the attribution theory of social psychology. It remains to be seen whether these developments can solve the problem of derived motives. Another theory, Solomon and Corbit's opponent processes theory of motivation, is also a candidate as a solution to the problem.

BIBLIOGRAPHY

ALLPORT, G. W. *Personality: A psychological interpretation.* New York: Holt, 1937.
BOLLES, R. C. *Theories of motivation* (Rev. ed.). New York: Harper and Row, 1975.
COFER, C. N., and APPLEY, M. H. *Motivation: Theory and research.* New York: Wiley, 1964.
WEINER, B. *Theories of motivation.* Chicago: Markham, 1972.

CHARLES N. COFER

MOTIVATION: HISTORICAL REVIEW

One may not ask the question "Why?" about physical events and expect a scientifically respectable answer. And yet that question is not inappropriately addressed to behavioral events, even within the framework of behavioral science. Physical objects are assumed to be subject only to physical influences; they do not have purposes; people, and presumably other animals, do. To ask "Why?" of an organism's behavior is to ask, broadly, about motivational processes—purposes, goals, incentives, drives, rewards, preferences, and so on, depending on the constructs used in a specific motivational theory. Of course, no explanation of some behavioral event is likely to be complete without reference to other processes as well (perception, learning, memory, and so on, again depending on the constructs employed in a specific behavioral theory).

Functions of Motivational Constructs

In general, motivational constructs are invoked to account for behavioral variation among individuals, or within a single individual from time to time, when apparently the variation cannot be attributed to changes in some other process or processes. That is, we typically are induced to ask "Why?" when reference to variation in ability or to processes such as perception and learning does not seem to supply a satisfactory explanation. Of course, in any particular instance, a motivational account may prove misdirected or gratuitous (as, for example, when it turns out that Johnny fails to answer questions in class, not because he is "unmotivated" or "resistant" or "intrapunitive," but because he can't hear them).

In systematic attempts to investigate motivational processes, special attention is paid to behaviors characterized by unusual persistence and vigor. Such behaviors often are initiated in the absence of some biologically significant commodity (e.g., food, water, a mate) and are terminated when the missing commodity has been encountered and, in some sense, consumed. Typically, as the interval increases between the onset of deprivation and access to the missing commodity, behavior becomes increasingly vigorous—at least until physical weakness, resulting from the deprivation, sets in.

Researchers of animal motivation and learning also find that along with a general increase in arousal level, deprived animals exhibit patterns of behavior that are specific to particular modes of deprivation. One way of considering what happens in the course of *learning* is that such motive-specific behavior patterns are modified; in particular, those behaviors which are successful in achieving the needed commodity become prepotent, while unsuccessful components of the initial pattern suffer a reduction in the likelihood of their occurring in the presence of that motive. Just how this transformation in the hierarchical organization of behavior patterns takes place is still a matter of considerable controversy. However, many theories of learning assign to the need-reducing or drive-reducing *(reward)* property of the consumed commodity the special role of strengthening or "reinforcing" learned behaviors. This is certainly so in the highly influential behavior theory of Clark L. Hull and its several derivatives.

In Hull's (1943) theory, the motivating process *(drive)* is a correlate of a state of physiological imbalance *(need)*. The reinforcement of learning is effected by the decrease in drive which accompanies a reduction in need level. In a variant of Hullian theory developed by Neal Miller (Dollard and Miller, 1950), the dependence of drive on need states is dropped; drive and reward are the crucial concepts, where a *drive* is defined as a strong stimulus and *reward* is simply a reduction in drive strength.

Some Historical Roots

Comprehensive behavior theories such as Hull's are, of course, the product of a long and multifaceted intellectual tradition. Historically, the importance of motivational constructs has waxed and waned in the course of psychology's development into an independent discipline. Broadly speaking, Western philosophers and theologians who addressed the issue of human nature, and who in that sense quite clearly are among the precursors of modern psychological theorists, assigned great significance to what would now be thought of as motivational constructs (Cofer and Appley, 1964). For example, the essence of the "good" life for Plato and Aristotle, and for their later Christian interpreters such as Augustine and Aquinas, involved in one variation or another controlling the passions, the sensual appetites, the animal instincts, or what have you through rational thought informed by knowledge and high moral principle. The word frequently used in reference to the controlling factor in human nature was *will*. It is in exercising "free will," or failure to do so, that one can be held accountable for one's behavior, here or hereafter.

Whatever the details of any specific philosophical or theological position (for example, will in Schopenhauer's philosophy was a force for evil, not good), it is clear that a predominant theme in Western thought for many centuries was that of a struggle between powerful inner contenders for determining the course of an individual's behavior. In modern terms, the outcome of that competition—that is, the person's short- and long-term choices, or more generally the *directions* his/her behavior takes—falls within the province of the motivational component of psychological theory.

Another historical source of motivational concepts, closely related to the philosophical-theological tradition, lies first in speculation and subsequently in research on animal behavior, and specifically behavior labeled *instinctive.* One result of this work was to introduce into systematic psychology—especially via the *functionalist* approach—a Darwinian-flavored concern for the pragmatic consequences of behavior. For example, within that framework, learning was viewed as a selection process (between successful and unsuccessful behaviors) rather than as a simple consequence of the repeated pairing of to-be-associated events (a position taken in Hullian theory, as mentioned above). Another product of work on animal behavior emerged from an eventual dissatisfaction with the instinct concept as being both teleological and lacking in true explanatory power. The term *drive* entered the jargon of psychology in the early decades of the twentieth century as a replacement for *instinct,* and as in Hullian theory, it was tied to specific states of physiological imbalance (or "tissue need"). The functionalist Robert Woodworth is usually credited with introducing the drive concept in his text *Dynamic Psychology,* published in 1918.

Motivational concepts in psychology derived from still another source, the psychoanalytic theory of Sigmund Freud, whose ideas were shaped by his clinical experience with disturbed patients as well as by his extensive reading in philosophy, anthropology, and literature—much the same works which, through other routes, also influenced psychological theory. Freud had considerable impact on the development of theories of motivation through his concepts, among others, of unconscious instinctual impulses *(Trieben),* defenses against conscious awareness of and direct behavioral expression of those impulses, and their resulting indirect expression in dreams, fantasies, and memory lapses, as well as in serious psychopathological symptoms. Freud, very much like his philosophical predecessors, saw the good life in the ever-increasing control of impulse by reason.

With all the emphasis on motivational constructs to be found in the several historical roots of modern psychology, it is a wonder that there could be a comprehensive psychological system devoid of a motivational component. Strictly speaking, there may be no such system, although some can be identified, such as the structuralism of E. B. Titchener and classical Gestalt theory, in which explicit motivational constructs played only a minor role, if any role at all. But this may not be surprising, considering that both structural psychology and Gestalt psychology were devoted primarily to describing properties of events in the sensory-perceptual-cognitive realm.

Some systems, rather than ignoring motivational variables, have deliberately excluded them as independent theoretical constructs, as for example when Edwin Guthrie (1952) treated drives, such as hunger and thirst, merely as cues. Thus, drive stimuli are simple components of the total stimulus complex present during the performance and/or acquisition of particular responses. In Guthrie's system, drive stimuli are no different in principle from other sources of stimulation, though they may be more intense and persistent, as well as more difficult for the individual to escape or avoid.

Contemporary Issues and Approaches

There are wide differences among systems which postulate a separate class of motivational variables. One major basis of disagreement has to do with whether motivation has a single or a dual function. In Hull's theory, as presented in *Principles of Behavior,* drive affects both the general arousal of and the specific directionality of behavior. In contrast, Donald O. Hebb (1949), in *The Organization of Behavior,* has articulated a position which takes behavioral arousal for granted, as a biological property of living organisms. Such single-function approaches pose only the directionality of behavior as the explanatory burden of motivational constructs: why this sequence of behaviors rather than some other? Hebb, in addition, made the case for considering as a motivational problem the directionality of covert cognitive processes—that is "trains of thought." In that respect, Hebb and Freud hold similar positions, since for Freud fantasies, dreams, free associations, and so on, as well as the more rational, "secondary-process" modes of thinking, are all influenced by, and hence revealing of, motivational factors (unconscious impulses, defenses, conflicts, and the like).

Theories of motivation differ also with respect to the presumed source(s) of motives. Both Freud and Hull exemplify biologically oriented theorists who assert that all motives stem directly or indirectly from innate drives, rooted in those biological mechanisms which, through evolution, assure individual and species survival.

A major thrust in contemporary motivational theory has been the development of models postulating autonomous perceptual-cognitive needs, or needs for behavioral competence, which are not derivatives of other "primary" biological drives (White, 1959). This "new look in motivation" focuses on curiosity, aesthetic reactions, needs for closure, understanding, variety, and so on (Berlyne, 1960; Dember, 1965). It views organisms as optimizers rather than minimizers of stimulation; further, it argues for the motivational centrality of the information value of stimulation, as opposed to the "goading" aspect emphasized in Freudian and Hullian theory and typified in Miller's definition of drives as strong stimuli. These emerging "cognitive" theories of motivation do not necessarily deny biology; if they do address the question of biology, they look centrally—in brain organization—rather than just peripherally for the locus of motivational processes (Dember, 1974).

BIBLIOGRAPHY

BERLYNE, D. E. *Conflict, arousal, and curiosity.* New York: McGraw-Hill, 1960.

COFER, C. N., and APPLEY, M. H. *Motivation: Theory and research.* New York: Wiley, 1964.

DEMBER, W. N. The new look in motivation. *American Scientist,* 1965, *53,* 409–427.

DEMBER, W. N. Motivation and the cognitive revolution. *American Psychologist,* 1974, *29,* 161–168.

DOLLARD, J., and MILLER, N. E. *Personality and psychotherapy.* New York: McGraw-Hill, 1950.

GUTHRIE, E. R. *The psychology of learning* (Rev. ed.). New York: Harper, 1952.

HEBB, D. O. *The organization of behavior.* New York: Wiley, 1949.

HULL, C. L. *Principles of behavior.* New York: Appleton-Century-Crofts, 1943.

WHITE, R. W. Motivation reconsidered: The concept of competence. *Psychological Review,* 1959, *66,* 297–333.

WOODWORTH, R. S. *Dynamic psychology.* New York: Columbia University Press, 1918.

WILLIAM N. DEMBER

MOTIVATION, HUMAN

Normal language treats the causal question of human behavior and experience with an amalgam of trait and motivational terms. Early writers addressing the question of the nature of man adopted an attributional strategy which emphasized the wants, desires, hopes, and fears of mankind. The Old Testament and classical writing provide a rich source of motivational explanations for the actions displayed by persons of every station (Burnham, 1968).

Presumably the ease with which such terms are used and understood testifies to the subjective fit between motives experienced and the observation of motivated action in others. Yet after more than thirty centuries of service, the beginning of the twentieth century saw a rapid discrediting of such language and a serious effort to recast the terms devoted to the analysis of motivated behavior for scientific purposes. With the advent of formal psychological science in the last half of the nineteenth century, questions of motivation were approached from an instinctive perspective with a constitutional bias toward emotional and appetitive states. So-called higher motives were developed from a combination of lower instincts in competition and concert. Social philosophers concerned with politics and economic policy made simplistic assumptions about wants and needs, leaving the study of refinements to folk psychologists. Jeremy Bentham (1843) was especially diligent in constructing a calculus of basic emotional needs to account for the strivings of mankind.

Holistic Theories

The peak of sophistication in the systematic delineation of instinctive motives appeared in the work of William McDougall (1916). In a parallel fashion, Freud was building a theory of personality function on a very narrow base of libido, aggression, and the capacity for anxiety. But when the reaction came, it was primarily against McDougall. The chief criticism was the dependence of instinct definition upon the goal state sought. This inability of independent explanation was condemned as obstructive of empirical definitions experimentally derived and as hopelessly uncontrolled.

Thus, as sociologist L. L. Bernard pointed out (1924), we could have an instinct for every goal sought. Behaviorism sought to reduce the energizing of action to the simplest drive base possible, and instinctoid motivational systems fell into disuse.

The continued acceptance of Freud's use of libido as the monistic driving force of behavior is instructive. Freud was concerned with personality function, and it has been the work of the personality theorists who followed him which have given us most of our motivational constructs. Not that all such theorists use motivational terms. At least one, Kelly (1955), has suggested a way to assume cognitive properties so that no motivational theory is needed at all. Throughout the period 1920–40 the general practice was to account for behavior, whether that of a rat in a maze or a phobic human being, with as simplistic a set of motivational characteristics as possible. Then in 1938 Murray's *Explorations in Personality* introduced a motivational system based on the *need* construct which attempted to portray the personality as a system of interlocking motives responsive to environmental stimuli having *press* quality. Whereas Gordon Allport (1937) chose to portray the richness of personality with a trait approach in the service of self-preserving and enhancing motivation, Murray, Maslow (1954), and Cattell (1946) chose motivational terms for the purpose.

Each of these three systemists assigned motive constructs a major role in personality function. For measurement purposes, Murray devised a projective technique, the *Thematic Apperception Test;* Cattell developed the *16-Factor Personality Inventory,* using factor-analytic techniques; and Maslow constructed elaborate case histories. In each instance the aim was to provide assessment devices designed to reflect the individual patterns of motivational dispositions.

Current Theories

A second wave of effort developed in the 1950s to research motivational questions at a less wholistic level. Mathematically modest statements of relationship for the prediction of behavioral tendency were developed by J. B. Rotter (1954) in clinical psychology, V. H. Vroom (1964) in industrial psychology, and

J. W. Atkinson (1957) for achievement motivation. These models had the advantage of confining the research to a limited number of variables whose study could generate an empirically derived "portrait" of the origins, functional dynamics, and expression of a particular motivational system. Since the 1960s most of this work has continued, as has the interest in more general theories. D. C. McClelland, whose preference is for sociohistorical analyses of the appearance and effect of particular motivational emphases, began to contrast the effects and interactions of the achievement, affiliation, and power motives. The latter has been subject to an exhaustive analysis by D. G. Winter (1973). The avoidance tendency associated with achievement motivation (fear of failure) has been researched by Heckhausen (1967) and Birney, Burdick, and Teevan (1969). Weiner (1972) has established linkage between attribution theory and achievement motive research.

More recent developments at the modeling level come from increased preoccupation with the role of incentives in guiding and releasing action. Irwin's (1971) work is a mathematically stated treatment whose full influence has yet to be realized. Korman's (1974) text presents an interesting attempt at a synthesis of motive theory, self theory, and consistency theory. The latter has emerged from studies of cognition which strongly suggest a basic tendency to resolve conflicting and contradictory information. The present literature displays a rich variety of systematic studies of socially important incentive classes which are just beginning to display certain shared characteristics of function.

BIBLIOGRAPHY

BURNHAM, J. C. *Handbook of personality theory and research.* Chicago: Rand McNally, 1968.

CATTELL, R. B. *Description and measurement of personality.* New York: Harcourt, 1946.

IRWIN, F. W. *Intentional behavior and motivation: A cognitive theory.* Philadelphia: Lippincott, 1971.

KELLY, G. A. *The psychology of personal constructs.* New York: Norton, 1955.

KORMAN, A. K. *The psychology of motivation.* Englewood Cliffs, N.J.: Prentice-Hall, 1974.

MASLOW, A. *Motivation and personality.* New York: Harper & Row, 1954.

WEINER, B. *Theories of motivation.* Chicago: Markham, 1972.

Winter, D. G. *The power motive.* New York: Free Press, 1973.

Robert C. Birney

MOTIVATION, INTRINSIC

The term *intrinsic motivation* refers to the motivational attractiveness or aversiveness of activities that are pursued or avoided because of characteristics inherent in the activities as such. Intrinsic motivation can be contrasted with *extrinsic motivation,* which refers to the motivational attractiveness or aversiveness of activities which are pursued or avoided as a means of reaching some goal or of preventing the development of some end state. Intrinsically motivated behaviors are sought or avoided for their own sake; extrinsically motivated behaviors are means to ends. Behavior that is determined primarily by intrinsic factors can be referred to as *autonomous* behavior; that determined primarily by extrinsic factors can be designated *instrumental* behavior.

Examples of activities that would ordinarily be considered intrinsically motivated are a boy playing with his dog, a man reading a novel, or a woman listening to a concert. Examples of behaviors that are presumably extrinsically motivated are a girl studying in order to pass an examination, a woman getting a job in order to make a living, or a man fixing the roof in order to keep it from leaking. Ordinarily, autonomous activities reflect ongoing behavior and have a process or "-ing" quality about them; instrumental activities, on the other hand, reflect the termination of given behavior sequences and have an "in order to" quality about them. The affect associated with the adequate functioning of an extrinsic motive appears to be one of satisfaction, whereas the affect associated with the effective functioning of an intrinsic motive seems to be a feeling of interest and zestfulness.

The distinction between intrinsic and extrinsic motivation is of course not always clear, since a given activity may involve some of each; this is presumably true, for example, of many of the jobs we hold. A person may enjoy a given activity as such (intrinsic motivation) and also carry it out in order to reach a given goal (extrinsic motivation), as when a professional tennis player is engaged in a match. Further, whether a given type of behavior by a given person is to be considered autonomous or instrumental may change over time, as when a man takes up golf in order to lose weight (instrumental) and comes eventually to play simply for the fun of it (autonomous). This would be an instance of what Gordon Allport referred to as the "functional autonomy of motives." The converse shift, from autonomous to instrumental, can also occur, as when a man playing tennis for enjoyment continues doing so, even after he becomes bored, in order to sell insurance to his playing partner.

The concept of intrinsic motivation has only in recent years become central in motivational psychology, but the idea itself is by no means new. Aristotle pointed out that people may do certain things for the pleasure of doing them. In the modern era, R. S. Woodworth, P. T. Young, E. R. Hilgard, Harry Harlow, and others noted that certain activities seem to be pursued for their own sake. A leading early exponent of this view was Allport who, as noted above, proposed (in 1937) the concept of functional autonomy. From the present point of view, Allport's suggestion, though it seemed rather drastic at the time, was in fact rather limited, since it included, in effect, only those instances of intrinsically motivated behaviors which had previously been extrinsically motivated.

The existence of intrinsic motivation is generally accepted today, interest being in the question of the underlying bases of autonomous behavior and the conditions under which it can be expected to occur. Though the matter is not yet fully clear, it appears that the efficacy of intrinsic motivation is in some manner associated with the fact that it seems to provide an optimal amount of novelty, change, and stimulus variability. Other areas of current research interest are individual differences in intrinsic motivation and interrelationships between extrinsic and intrinsic motivations.

BIBLIOGRAPHY

Day, H. I.; Berlyne, D. E.; and Hunt, D. E. (Eds.). *Intrinsic motivation.* New York: Holt, Rinehart and Winston, 1971.
Deci, E. L. *Intrinsic motivation.* New York: Plenum, 1975.

McReynolds, P. The nature and assessment of intrinsic motivation. In P. McReynolds (Ed.), *Advances in psychological assessment* (Vol. 2). Palo Alto, Calif.: Science & Behavior Books, 1971. Pp. 157–177.

See also Extrinsic Motivation; Functional Autonomy of Motives

Paul McReynolds

MOTIVATION: AN OVERVIEW

Motivation designates a class of factors thought to be central in the determination of behavior, but as Bolles (1967) has observed, it is not a fact of behavior or of experience. The psychology of an earlier day, for example, that of Ward, was primarily one of conscious experience. What we may now class as motivational was not ignored in that psychology, but the standpoint from which it was treated was experiential. Thus, experience was classified into the categories of cognition or knowing, feeling, and conation (will), the bipartite division derived from Aristotle being replaced by this tri-partite one, sponsored but not originated by Immanuel Kant. Feeling and conation refer to aspects of what we now mean by emotion and motivation; feeling connoted at least pleasure and pain, while conation (from Latin *conari,* to attempt) or will (from Latin *velle,* to wish) referred to choice, decision, purpose, desire, and striving. The actual movements, however, the consequences of conation or will, except as they affected conscious experiences, were not a part of psychological study. *Motive* is a term used in discussions of conation. It was a specific form of desire or craving.

Early Theories

The analytic study of conscious experience, it has been said, was directed to the identification and description by the method of introspection of what *is* in consciousness. The account just given is representative of this approach, though there were many variations on it. But events around the turn of the twentieth century were to overthrow this way of looking at the task of psychology, and in the consequent psychological systems, motivation achieved the status of a major conceptual category.

A first event was Sigmund Freud's development of *psychoanalysis.* Freud's views were strongly dynamic or motivational, and his work threw doubt on the value to be attained from the study of conscious experience, because he discovered the important role of unconscious factors in the symptoms and thoughts presented to him by his patients. Further, he could not take seemingly rational accounts of conduct at face value, because he found them often to disguise or distort the real reasons that underlay it.

A second event was the emergence, especially in the United States, of the *functionalist* position. Its advocates, including John Dewey, James R. Angell, and Harvey Carr, at Chicago, and E. L. Thorndike and R. S. Woodworth, at Columbia, asked "What is consciousness for?" rather than "What does it contain?" They were influenced by Darwinian evolution and saw consciousness as *functional* in the adaptation of organisms to their environments. They admitted work with animals and with children. Since neither of these groups could be trained in introspection, study of them necessarily was limited to their behavior. Further, in considering adaptations of organisms to their environments, the functionalists were concerned with such problems as intelligence and instinct (later transformed to drive), thus extending the range of psychological inquiry and, in the case of motivation, including the behaviors that mark the occurrence of states of deprivation, such as hunger, thirst, sex, and the like. William McDougall, an independent functionalist, proposed a theory of human conduct based on instincts and their associated emotions. McDougall's psychology placed motivation, as did Freud's, in center stage as the dominant factor in the causation of behavior and experience.

Since these developments, psychology has recognized motivation as a central theme. However, its theorists have not always agreed on the exact function the concept is to serve, and the functions proposed do not always correspond to the layman's view that the answer to the question, "Why did he or she do that?" is necessarily to be found in motivational terms.

A critical claim that is often made is that "all behavior is motivated." This assertion is made for perhaps two reasons: One is to express a deterministic view of action, that is, all behavior is determined, in some way, by motivational factors. The other, closely allied to the first, permits a reevaluation of personal responsibility for conduct. If one has acted from a strong motive, especially one that is unconscious, it is difficult to advocate personal accountability. This orientation, of course, has profound implications, especially in the areas of religion and jurisprudence.

Major Functions

Three major functions have, in one system or another, been assigned to motivation. One function is *arousal* or energization of behavior. In this use, motivation is seen as *activating* habits or innate tendencies which actually mediate the specific acts that occur. In other words, motivation lifts the organism from an inert state, but what behavior takes place in a situation is due to what the individual has learned to do there or to what innate endowment provides. A second function, closely related to the first, employs motivation to explain variations in the *vigor* with which behavior occurs; thus, when we respond very actively to weak stimuli or, alternatively, react mildly to strong stimuli, the source of the variation is sought in motivation. References to people as highly motivated or as lacking in motivation may exemplify in general what is meant here, though the reference is usually to specific behaviors in particular situations.

A third function assigned to the motivation concept is to explain the *direction* behavior takes, that is, why the organism does one thing rather than another. This orientation takes preference, choice, decision, goal, intention, and the like as the hallmarks of motivated behavior. It does not ignore arousal but tends to regard arousal in terms of emotion. Advocates of this function for motivation see its role very differently from the way those who espouse the first function regard that role.

Currently, the views of motivation are changing. There is dissatisfaction with prior theories, and emphasis seems increasingly to be placed on *cognitive* factors in situations involving motivation. This reorientation is perhaps more compatible with the third function than it is with the other two. The emphasis on cognition is not new but perhaps its resurgence marks a general trend in the field of psychology away from the functionalist-behaviorist tradition and toward a cognitive one.

BIBLIOGRAPHY

ATKINSON, J. W. *An introduction to motivation.* Princeton, N.J.: Van Nostrand, 1964.
BOLLES, R. C. *Theory of motivation.* New York: Harper, 1967.
COFER, C. N., and APPLEY, M. H. *Motivation: Theory and research.* New York: Wiley, 1964.
RYAN, T. A. *Intentional behavior: An approach to human motivation.* New York: Ronald, 1970.
WEINER, B. *Theories of motivation.* Chicago: Markham, 1972.

CHARLES N. COFER

MOTIVATION AS STIMULUS CHANGE

The concept of *stimulus change* refers to the special incentive properties of a simple change in a stimulus or an aspect of a stimulus in attracting attention or producing approach behavior. For a simple change in a stimulus to act as an incentive probably requires a degree of prior adaptation to a stimulus situation and a relatively low level of stimulation. Thus, it can be shown that if a person is shown a matrix of stimuli a number of times or for a single period permitting complete examination of the stimuli, and then on a subsequent exposure one element of the matrix is changed significantly, attention will be disproportionately devoted to the element which has been changed. Likewise, most laboratory animals will approach and examine an object introduced into a limited environment to which the animal has been exposed for some prior time. Stimulus change as an incentive thus presupposes a degree of boredom with the existing stimulus pattern, and the change in stimulation must provide a degree of novelty.

BIBLIOGRAPHY

FISKE, D. W., and MADDI, S. R. *Functions of varied experience.* Homewood, Ill.: Dorsey Press, 1961.

See also ATTENTION; BOREDOM; CURIOSITY

EDWARD L. WALKER

MOTIVATION THEORIES

In a general way, motivation is concerned with what has been referred to as the active, as opposed to the receptive or passive, functions of mind. Thus, motivation is concerned with movement in space and time, either actual or potential, or with precursors of such movement in experience. Theories of motivation, then, must be concerned ultimately with action, or, more properly, with the sources and precursors of action. But in the theories that have been advanced there are a number of differences. It is the purpose of this article to outline some of the issues to which the divergences among theories pertain. The issues are intertwined, a fact which obscures their delineation.

A fundamental distinction can be characterized by the terms *agent,* or one who acts, and *patient,* or one who is acted upon. Some theories view organisms as agents, others as patients. This distinction parallels, to a large degree, theoretical contrasts such as rational or cognitive versus irrational or mechanistic, conscious versus unconscious, growth versus conservative, intrinsic versus extrinsic or instrumental. The meaning of these contrasts will be specified as we survey the theoretical scene in motivation.

During the first half of the twentieth century, a substantial consensus appears to have developed on these issues, despite many differences among theories as to details. This consensus favored views that emphasized irrationality and mechanism, unconscious processes, conservative or equilibratory (homeostatic) tendencies, and the role of action as instrumental to the organism's needs. This consensus overturned many widely shared conceptions of the nineteenth century, for example, rationalism, but it was compatible with views of that century held, for example, by Schopenhauer and von Hartmann. It seems fair to say that this prevailing orientation has, since about 1950, begun to be abandoned in favor of alternative views with some resemblance to the rationalism of the last century.

Freud

The break with rationalism is marked most clearly in Freud and McDougall, who, independently, saw original human nature as composed of instincts. For Freud, these instincts were lodged in the id, "a cauldron of seething excitement," amoral, valueless, and without knowledge of good and evil. The instincts were sources of energy and tension, and their aim was to gain discharge of tension. Such discharge was deemed pleasurable and was achieved through neural mechanisms; the nervous system has "the function of abolishing stimuli" in order to reduce "excitation to the lowest possible level." But insofar as reducing stimulation was beyond the powers of the id, Freud had to postulate the ego, a structure which could be in contact with reality and control motor processes. The ego, then, had the responsibility of arranging for discharge of id impulses, but this discharge had often to be disguised because of the limitations and criticism posed by reality and the prohibitions of the superego. Anxiety was the means by which the ego was restricted from a too free and direct execution of id impulses.

However, Freud's theory required some measure of tension discharge, since his energy model was an hydraulic one, that is to say, tension, without discharge, would build up as does water flowing into a tank which has no suitable outlet. It should be added that normal development and psychoanalytic treatment, much of which was directed at unreasonable prohibitions by the superego, would enable the ego to develop acceptable means for discharge of the impulses of the id.

In Freud's theory, then, there is a clear emphasis on irrational forces, on the conservative or homeostatic nature of instinctive processes, on behavior as instrumental to the forces imposing themselves on the ego, and on unconscious processes. There is a parallel to Freud's model in the instinct theory of such ethologists as Lorenz and Tinbergen, for whom undischarged instinctual energy seems to build up, ultimately to express itself in displacement and vacuum activities. Freud's views are also represented in more or less direct form in conceptions of human motives like those of Henry Murray, whose method of measurement of motives, the Thematic Apperception Test, rested on the psychoanalytic principle that internal impulses and anxieties are projected onto people and into interpretations of events in the environment. Murray used pictures in his test in the expectation that stories told about the pictures would be revelatory of impulses and other concerns.

Drive Theory

Drive theory, being a descendant of McDougall's instinct theory, shares many of the characteristics of Freudian theory. It postulates sources of energy, tension or, in some versions, internal irritants, which arise, as Walter Cannon once said for hunger and thirst, "as powerful, persistent, and tormenting stimuli which imperiously demand the ingestion of food and water before they will cease their goading." Drive theory is homeostatic and sees behavior as instrumental to the body's needs. Since drive theory was developed largely in work with lower animals, it seldom made reference to conscious or unconscious process or to rationality-irrationality.

Later developments in psychoanalytic theory, ethology, and drive theory have altered some of these conceptions. Thus, it has been postulated that there are or can be ego functions which are autonomous, that is, free from origins in the id and in conflict. Drive and the hydraulic model in ethology have been found wanting by many ethologists; in general, drive theory has collapsed because most of the phenomena on which it rested can be given more plausible alternative conceptions (e.g., in terms of incentives).

Activation Theory

There are other theories which do not depend so directly as do Freudian, classical ethological, and drive theory on the hydraulic conception of the former two and the goading internal states of the latter. Among them is arousal or activation theory, whose main principles concern level of activation or energization and the relation of behavioral efficiency, reinforcement, tension seeking and reduction to levels of activation. The stress is on physiological arousal as indexed by measures like EEG, GSR, heart rate, and tension in the musculature. Arousal seems to be a nonspecific source of energization, much as was drive in the Hull-Spence theory. It is made to underlie the process of incentive motivation in such theories as the anticipation and sensitization invigoration mechanisms proposed by Cofer and Appley and in the similar proposals by Bindra. Solomon and Corbit's opponent processes theory of motivation rests, in complex ways, on arousal. While such views appear to treat the organism as patient and hold to a general homeostatic or balance process, they are usually noncommittal with respect to the other issues mentioned above.

Hedonism

The principle of hedonism is a very old one in human thought and took the position that choice is governed by anticipated pleasure or removal or reduction of pain. In modern representatives of this view, arousal seems to accompany the anticipation of pleasure, as in P. T. Young's theory, and of course pain is an aroused state to be diminished or avoided. The hedonic theory proposed by D. C. McClelland and his collaborators (e.g., John Atkinson) differs somewhat from a simple arousal theory. It holds that small deviations from a current adaptation-level will be pleasant and large deviations unpleasant. Deviations are motivating; cues which yield anticipations of pleasure will be approached, whereas cues anticipatory of pain or unpleasure will be avoided. Much of what Berlyne has said about curiosity, stimulus seeking, and hedonic reactions has some similarity to the McClelland theory, although Berlyne's view is in many respects closer to the notions of general physiological arousal than to adaptation level. These modern hedonistic approaches are applied across species and hence have made little commitment on some of the issues pertinent, for example, to Freudian theory.

Cognitive Theories

More cognitive current theories seem to stem largely from the work of Kurt Lewin and Fritz Heider, both strongly influenced by Gestalt conceptions. Although Gestalt psychology is not ordinarily accorded a place in treatments of motivation, it was a dynamic theory in the sense that it postulated that behavior and experience are products of forces operating in a psychological field. Lewin explicitly developed his notions of motivation around such concepts as the psychological environment, tension in components of that field, forces and valences. Lewin's views receive expression, in many respects, in Festinger's theory of cognitive dissonance, as well as in complex analyses of the factors involved in achievement-motivated behavior by Atkinson and his collaborators.

Lewin did not postulate drives, and he associated regions of tension with intentions and goals. Heider seems not to have postulated drives, either, but he developed balance theory in terms of relations in a triad, consisting of two persons and their attitudes to one another and to an object. In unbalanced triads, there is motivation for change. These views appear to see the role of the person as an agent, although to the extent that the person is unaware of his or her attitudes or intentions, for example, she or he may be subject to the control of forces without being able to control them. Attribution theory, a development from Heider's work, stresses the importance of perceived causality. How one perceives causality, whether, for example, as due to external or internal (a function of the person) factors, is important to what will occur. In Rotter's formulation, if one perceives accomplishment as due to good fortune, the expectancy of further accomplishment will differ from what it would be if the accomplishment is perceived as due to one's own skills and efforts. This kind of theory stresses the person's possible agentive role, while also emphasizing the way in which the circumstances are appraised or perceived.

Cognitive theories, generally, emphasize intentions, choice, goals, and preference by an agent who has some awareness of the factors involved. Drives are not stressed. Such theories postulate an originally active organism which does not have to be pushed or goaded into activity. Unfortunately, there do not seem to be considerations of individual development in the available literature, so that the growth of motivation in such systems cannot be specified.

Maslow

It remains to be said that there are other views of motivation. White spoke of competence motivation, an idea with strong relations to the higher motives in Maslow's hierarchical system of needs. Maslow viewed "lower" needs—physiological, safety, esteem, for example—as standing in the way of the expression of higher needs, such as self-actualization.

White seemed to eschew the classical drive and Freudian types of motivational factors, whereas Maslow, recognizing them, postulated that when adequately satisfied, they would be displaced by more individualized and creative motives. In his theory, Maslow's views have some relation to those of Fromm, Rogers, and Horney.

A theory proposed by Atkinson and Birch takes change of behavior as the motivational event. A complex and mathematical formulation of the factors producing and following from change is provided. This theory is at an abstract level and therefore it is not easy to place in the framework of this article.

Motivational theory in this century swung from the postulate of rationality to the postulate of irrationality and now seems, in some measure, to be swinging back to views akin to rationality. However, the current emphasis on cognition is not directed mainly to the analysis of the experience of action as it was in the nineteenth century. Rather, action as well as the experience of it, is in focus.

BIBLIOGRAPHY

COFER, C. N., and APPLEY, M. H. *Motivation: Theory and research.* New York: Wiley, 1964.
WEINER, B. (Ed.). *Cognitive views of human motivation.* New York: Academic Press, 1974.

CHARLES N. COFER

MOTIVE

The word *motive* means something that "moves or induces a person to act in a certain way; a desire, fear, or other emotion, or a consideration of reason, which tends to influence a person's volition; also often applied to a contemplated result or object the desire of which tends to influence volition." The word has long been used in psychology, originally as a part of the descriptive vocabulary of introspective study of consciousness or immediate experience. Despite the decline in description through introspection, the word has persisted in its usage. It seems now to designate human conditions (achievement, affiliation, power, for example), thought to provide impelling force to human behavior, broadly construed.

In many respects its use is similar to that of

drive, except that it has no readily identifiable physiological substrate, has deprivation or arousal conditions which are not easily specifiable, and is usually considered to be learned. Thus, we can refer to the achievement motive, the affiliation motive, or success motives and can speak of motives for work and for study, or of career motives, and the like.

See also DRIVE; MOTIVATION, DERIVED

CHARLES N. COFER

MOTIVES AND NEEDS AS TRAITS

The concept of motivation as an explanation of man's behavior goes back to antiquity. Early speculation about the causes of individual differences in behavior arose as a result of philosophical interest in the importance of knowledge and the issue of free will. Some of the early Greek theorists had attributed personality differences to variations in physique or physiology. The prevailing philosophical view, however, was that knowledge determined behavior, and Plato and Aristotle concluded that a concept such as *will* was an even more important determinant. Thomas Aquinas described animal behavior as motivated primarily by instincts and the senses, whereas man's behavior was more a function of rational insight into the relation between an act and its consequences. Descartes also formulated a dualistic system, arguing for physical determinants of animal behavior and a rational will for explaining human activity, but further postulated that the will was a function of other variables. Also important in the historical evolution of the concept of motivation are those philosophers who postulated specific motives of various kinds as crucial to the understanding of human behavior. For example, both Machiavelli and Hobbes proposed explanations of political leadership based upon such motives as egotism, fear, love, hunger, thirst, and sex. Although the doctrine of hedonism also goes back to antiquity, the concept was essentially an ethical one until Jeremy Bentham, in the early nineteenth century, formulated psychological hedonism as the basic determinant of human behavior.

By the mid-nineteenth century, the British associationist philosophers had established the principle that the content of the mind was a function of experience and learning. If mental content was understandable and predictable on the basis of an individual's previous experience, then the will, which determined behavior, was not free, but also explicable.

After publication of Darwin's theory of evolution, the concept of *instinct* became important as an explanation of complex patterns of behavior, which, since they were observed among lower animals, could not be attributed to "reason."

Freud

Before the end of the nineteenth century, Freud had published his evidence of the importance of irrational influences on human behavior, and the continuity between the behavior of animals and man was established. Basic to Freud's conceptualization of human behavior were the biological instincts (impulses). To understand an individual, one had to interpret his apparently contradictory behavior in terms of these underlying impulses. Since, for Freud, all behavior was determined, analysis of "unintentional" or unconscious behavior would reveal the organization of the personality around these repressed impulses. Situations were important chiefly insofar as they aroused unacceptable impulses and evoked anxiety. Personality traits were determined by the interaction of inherited dispositions and accidental experiences. More specifically, personality was shaped by the mechanisms which the individual adopted to cope with fear and anxiety. The mechanisms of identification and sublimation led to intellectual and moral development, while the *defense* mechanisms precluded growth and the acquisition of more adaptive behavior.

McDougall

The personality theory formulated by William McDougall around the same time had some similarity to Freud's, in that it also postulated instincts as determinants of human behavior and was based on motivation or purpose. McDougall stressed that behavior is often spontaneous and that goal-directed behavior persists for considerable periods after the initiating stimulus has disappeared. An instinct was defined, not by the kind of behavior it evoked, but rather by the nature of the goal, the change in the situation, in the object or in the organism's relation to it, toward which the instinct impelled the organism. Adult behavior consisted of learned modifications and combinations of instincts present at birth.

Lewin

Lewin (1938) departed from prevailing views in presenting an equation in which behavior was perceived as a result of the interaction between the person and his immediate psychological environment, $B = f(P,E)$. Motives were the resultant of forces within the psychological field. The strength and direction of these forces depended both on "the character and state of the person *P,* and upon the perceived nature of the object of activity" (p. 107).

Lewin believed that the investigation of motivation had been hampered by premature attempts to systematize needs into a small number of categories. In his own theoretical formulation, he also distinguished conceptually between motives as energizing behavior and motives as directing behavior. Lewin used the concept *need* for any motivated state.

Tension described the emotional state resulting from a need. *Valence* referred to the psychological property of objects to attract (positive valence) or repel (negative valence). Lewin also used the term *vector* to represent the forces impelling an individual toward or away from various areas of his psychological environment. This *life space* of the individual consisted of areas having boundaries of varying permeability. An arousal of a need led to unequal states of tension in the life space, or *disequilibrium.* The differential tensions among regions of the life space led to *locomotion* or movement toward a goal, the direction of the movement determined by the valence of the goal region. The finding that there tends to be much greater recall of uncompleted than of completed tasks (the Zeigarnik effect) provided the first empirical support for Lewin's theory of needs and tensions. Lewin's analysis of conflict situations was basic to later empirical studies. Lewin's conceptualization of *level of aspiration* as the result of a conflict situation involving forces toward success and away from

failure was elaborated into need for achievement theory.

Tolman

Atkinson (1964) has pointed out the similarity and complementarity of Tolman's views to those of Lewin. Both theorists sought to develop psychological rather than physiological explanations of behavior. Both viewed behavior as goal-directed, and as the result of interaction between characteristics of the person and the environment. Both took cognitive aspects of the person into account, Lewin in his concept of *perceived pathways,* and Tolman in his concept of *expectancy.* Tolman undertook the task of developing a theory of *purposive behaviorism,* in which the concepts could be stated and tested in terms of concrete, repeatable operations by independent observers. Tolman explained that what he had wanted was a behavioristic psychology which would be able to deal with real organisms in terms of their inner psychological dynamics. By introducing the concept of *intervening variables,* Tolman was able to relate observable antecedent events to observable consequences. For Tolman, mental processes were variables which intervened between the five independent variables of environmental stimuli, physiological drive, heredity, previous training, and maturity, on the one hand, and the dependent variable of behavior, on the other.

Murray

With some modification, Freud's psychodynamic interpretation of behavior became the framework of Murray's (1938) personality theory. Murray also proposed interpretation of behavior on the basis of underlying motives, but, influenced by Lewin's field theory, included in his systematic formulation both the concept of *need* and the concept of *press.* For Murray, all behavior is a function not only of internal needs, but also of environmental press. Thus Murray's basic unit of personality analysis is the *thema.* McDougall's definition of an instinct was basic to Murray's concept of a need as a force in the brain region which organizes behavior in such a way as to transform an existing, unsatisfying situation in a certain direction. Needs may be aroused by internal processes, but are more frequently activated by environmental forces. *Press* refers to the power of an object to affect the subject. A *thema* is a behavioral unit which includes the instigating situation (press) and the need that is operating. Needs may be viscerogenic or psychogenic; they may be overt, as well as covert (unconscious). Much of the current research on personality is based on Murray's complex and carefully detailed system of motivational constructs for classifying human behavior.

Perhaps the most influential application of Murray's theory has been in studies of need for achievement, defined as performance under conditions where an individual is aware that his performance will be evaluated by himself or by others in terms of some standard of excellence. Motivation to achieve, perceived as a relatively enduring personality characteristic, measured by scores on a modified version of Murray's Thematic Apperception Test, has been found to correlate with such personality characteristics as level of self-esteem and persistence, and with behavioral measures such as conformity and occupational choice. McClelland, Atkinson, Clark, and Lowell (1953) pioneered in need for achievement research, and considerable data have now accumulated, not only on achievement motivation, but also on other needs, such as power (Atkinson, 1964; Korman, 1973).

Allport

For Allport (1937), *traits* were the major motivational constructs. He conceived of traits as dispositions which initiate and guide behavior. Allport took strong exception to the psychoanalytic view that unconscious motives were the principle determinants of behavior in humans, stressing to an even greater degree than Murray the major role of conscious motivation in normal individuals. Allport also disputed behavioristic explanations which related human behavior to physiological needs, postulating instead a discontinuity between most adult motivation and childhood motivation, or the principle of the *functional autonomy of motives.* This principle states that, although behavior may have originated in the service of biological needs, it may be sustained because it has become an end in its own right.

Allport hypothesized that traits organize behavior by rendering many stimuli functionally equivalent.

The trait of *aggressiveness* has historically been treated as an innate drive, and this view prevails in both psychoanalytic and ethological theories today. Experimental studies by social-learning theorists have not supported this view of aggression as an innate trait.

Considerable research has been done on *fear,* or *anxiety,* as a motive. Questionnaires have generally been used to measure anxiety or fear, and scores have reflected significant individual differences on these scales. These differences have been found to correlate with performance on various tasks, but the results can not be unambiguously interpreted as relating only to anxiety. The conditions under which findings were obtained did not preclude the possiblity that other variables, such as fear of failure, may have been influential.

The status of *affiliation* as a motive-trait is also unclear, since measures have tended to confound it with other traits, such as anxiety and fear of failure. Need for affiliation, whether measured by projective methods or by objective behavior, reveals significant differences among individuals. Empirical studies have demonstrated that fear and anxiety may motivate affiliative behavior.

Approval motivation also has trait characteristics and is generally measured by questionnaires. Individuals high in need for approval choose socially-desirable responses. They tend to be high in social conformity, persuasibility, and failure-avoidance.

Festinger

Balance theory, particularly as elaborated by Festinger (1957) has generated countless experiments on the need for consistency. These experiments have generally followed the paradigm of inducing subjects to engage in behavior (or to commit themselves to engage in behavior) that is contrary to their attitudes. The results have tended to confirm the theoretical prediction that subjects will reduce dissonance by changing their attitudes in the direction of conforming with the induced behavior. Because many alternative ways of reducing dissonance are postulated, the theory can not be adequately tested. A number of variables appear to intervene in the experimental situation, including anxiety, self-concept, and expectations.

Cattell

Cattell (1946) has formulated a trait theory of personality based on motivational concepts developed through factor-analytic techniques. Cattell's concept of an *erg,* or motive, was derived from McDougall's definition of a motive as having the characteristics of spontaneity, specificity of sensation, and directedness. Ergs are innate drives or *constitutional traits,* identified through their emergence as factor-dimensions. It is the organization of and dynamic interrelationships among traits which determine behavior. The observable characteristics that tend to become encoded in common usage are defined as *surface traits.* The clustering or intercorrelation among terms used to describe individuals in ordinary language can be used to identify surface traits. *Source traits* are the underlying causes of the surface manifestations. Source traits, however, can be identified only by multivariate analysis of the underlying personality dimensions. Cattell distinguished three major trait categories. *Ability traits* determine an individual's effectiveness in achieving goals in complex situations. *Temperament traits* are primarily constitutional variables, such as tempo, excitability, and dominance. *Dynamic traits* are motives, interests, attitudes, and sentiments.

Dollard and Miller

Dollard and Miller (1950), in an effort to integrate Hull's (1934) learning theory with psychoanalytic concepts and findings from anthropology and sociology, concluded that social conditions tend, not only to obscure the role of innate drives, but also to emphasize *secondary* or learned drives. These secondary drives are learned in the process of socialization. Consequently, individuals are unique because each has learned different combinations of motives and values in the course of his particular life experience. *Fear* (in its repressed form, anxiety) is, for these theorists, one of the most important of the learned drives in influencing

behavior. Subsequent developments in social learning theory led to more extreme positions in which behavior was viewed as situation-specific, rather than the result of organized personality characteristics. Behavior was not to be interpreted in terms of underlying motivation or inferred traits, but to be studied as a function of the evoking stimuli and reinforcement history.

That behavioral consistency is a function of stable situations has been disputed by numerous investigators, who have argued that the behavior theorists typically attack an outmoded version of psychodynamic theory and that the methodology used by behaviorists in experimental research tends to underestimate the degree of consistency that does exist in the everyday behavior of individuals. More recently, social-learning theorists have placed increasing emphasis on the interaction between individual and situation, and on cognitive organization. Much of the controversy is caused by the exclusion from the definition of personality of any intellectual or cognitive characteristics, although current social learning theory leans heavily on cognitive influences on behavior.

Despite the evidence that intercorrelations among different measures of traits tend to be low, many personality psychologists believe in the existence of underlying personality structures. Earlier explanations for the discrepancies (usually citing the probability of errors of measurement) have not been supplemented by attributing inconsistent findings to *moderator variables.* A moderator variable is one that interacts with a predictor, resulting in differential correlation of that predictor with a criterion.

There is some empirical evidence that trans-situational consistency is itself a dimension of personality which can be used as a moderator variable in predicting responses across situations, and is meaningfully related to a variety of personality variables.

Chein

Chein (1972) has developed a metatheoretical system in which motivation serves as the integrating construct of personality. What is commonly referred to as *character* or *personal-*

ity is for Chein a stable, self-sustaining system of motives. These motivational systems are posited as the result of complex transformations of physiological drive states through the processes of derivation, perpetuation, and imbrication. *Derivation* refers to the hierarchical nested aspect of motives, so that the carrying out of a behavior may require a subsidiary behavior, which requires a subsidiary behavior, and another and another. Thus, "Behavior is a motive of the behaviors it includes" (p. 35). *Perpetuation* refers to the process by which some motives become continuing concerns, and consequently motivate other behaviors at times when they themselves do not need to be satisfied. By the *imbrication* of motives Chein meant the interpenetration of motives that results from the fact that the same behavior may be derived from a variety of motives and may, in different circumstances, motivate a variety of different behavior. For Chein, "motivation is not something that exists within our bodies. Motivation involves transaction between subject and object, transaction that requires commerce with mediating and intervening objects" (p. 85). Chein has argued that, since traits are patterns of behavior over time, to identify personality as an aggregate of traits implies that personality does not exist at any given moment. After a review of other shortcomings of trait theory, Chein concluded that "the concept of personality as an amalgam of traits is peculiarly sterile for scientific purposes" (p. 284).

The relative importance of motives, drives, and needs as explanatory factors in behavior has been declining since the mid-twentieth century for a number of reasons. Many theorists have abandoned these terms as meaningless in view of their application to diverse and inconsistent phenomena. In addition, there has been increasing dissatisfaction with traditional theories which posited underlying, relatively enduring personality traits. Different investigators tended to find different traits, and the predictive power of these theories across situations has been weak. Attempts to dismiss the need to postulate a dynamic personality structure in predicting behavior, however, have been moderated. Situationists place increased emphasis on the interaction between individual and situation, and on cognitive organization. One viable theoretical approach is that of *incentive* motivation. Incentive motiva-

tion posits both a physiological state of arousal (or central motive state) and incentive stimulation (presence of cues) as necessary to elicit a response. This theory is compatible with interactionist approaches and with evidence from ethology on *releasers*. It is also consistent with the findings in studies on particular motives, such as achievement, anxiety, and affiliation, where arousal stimuli are clearly implicated.

BIBLIOGRAPHY

ATKINSON, J. W. *An introduction to motivation.* Princeton, N.J.: Van Nostrand, 1964.

CATTELL, R. B. *The description and measurement of personality.* Yonkers-on-Hudson, N.Y.: World Book, 1946.

CHEIN, I. *The science of behavior and the image of man.* New York: Basic Books, 1972.

DOLLARD, J., and MILLER, N. E. *Personality and psychotherapy.* New York: McGraw-Hill, 1950.

FESTINGER, L. *Theory of cognitive dissonance.* Evanston, Ill.: Peterson, 1957.

KORMAN, A. K. On the development of contingency theories of leadership; some methodological considerations and possible alternatives. *Journal of Applied Psychology*, 1973, *58,* 384–387.

LEWIN, K. *The conceptual representation and the measurement of psychological forces.* Durham, N.C.: Duke University Press, 1938.

McCLELLAND, D. C.; ATKINSON, J. W.; CLARK, R. W.; and LOWELL, E. L. *The achievement motive.* New York: Appleton-Century-Crofts, 1953.

MURRAY, H. A. *Explorations in personality.* New York: Oxford University Press, 1938.

ABRAHAM K. KORMAN
MARGUERITE F. LEVY
WALTER REICHMAN

MOTORA, YUJIRO (1858–1912)

After receiving his Ph.D. at Johns Hopkins University, Motora became the first professor of psychology at Tokyo Imperial University in 1889. Motora introduced Wundtian experimental psychology to Japan and studies of somatosensory and visual perception. His later works were devoted to psychological and philosophical analysis of Oriental thought. He criticized the English associationistic view as being mechanical. He advocated the concept of an "active self" or a "dynamic psychic potentiality."

SHINKURO IWAHARA

MOTOR ABILITIES: AN OVERVIEW

People differ in how well they can perform various perceptual-motor activities and in how readily they can attain high levels of proficiency on these activities. What differentiates these skills from other human performances is that these skills involve movements of the body, limbs, or other body members (e.g., fingers) by action of striated muscles. The movements usually involve some spatial-temporal patterning and interaction of responses with sensory input.

This article is concerned with the ways in which people differ in the abilities (or aptitudes) which facilitate the learning of such motor skills. The article presents a conceptual framework for thinking about the dimensions of motor abilities, defines the different motor abilities, and describes tests which have been used to measure individual differences in these motor abilities. (The terms *motor, sensorimotor, psychomotor,* and *perceptual-motor* are considered interchangeable.)

A central concept in describing individual differences is the concept of "abilities." Abilities are defined by score consistencies among separate performances. The fact that individuals who do well in task A also do well in tasks B and C but not well in tasks D, E, and F indicates, inferentially, a common process involved in performing the first three tasks distinct from the processes involved in the performance on the latter three. To "account for" the observed consistencies, an ability is postulated. Once this has been achieved, further experimental-correlational studies are conducted to sharpen and define the limits and definition of this particular ability.

The Ability-Skill Distinction

The term *ability* refers to a more general trait of the individual which has been inferred from certain response consistencies (e.g., correlations) on certain kinds of tasks. These are fairly enduring traits, which in the adult are more difficult to change. Many of these abilities are of course themselves a product of learning and develop at different rates, mainly during childhood and adolescence. Some abilities (e.g., color vision) depend more on genetic than on learning factors, but most abilities depend on

both to some degree. At a given stage of life, they represent traits or organismic factors which the individual brings with him when he begins to learn a new task. These abilities are related to performances in a variety of human tasks. For example, the fact that spatial visualization has been found related to performance on such diverse tasks as aerial navigation, blueprint reading, and dentistry makes this ability somehow more basic.

The term *skill* refers to the level of proficiency on a specific task or limited group of tasks. Examples of skills are proficiencies in flying an airplane, in operating a turret lathe, or in playing basketball. The assumption is that the skills involved in complex activities can be described in terms of the more basic abilities. For example, the level of performance a man can attain on a turret lathe may depend on his basic abilities of manual dexterity and motor coordination. However, these same basic abilities may be important to proficiency in other skills as well. Thus, manual dexterity is needed in assembling electrical components, and motor coordination is needed to fly an airplane.

Abilities and Skill Learning

Implicit in the previous analysis is the important relation between abilities and learning. Thus, individuals with high manual dexterity may more readily learn the specific skill of lathe operation. The mechanism of transfer of training probably operates here. Some abilities may transfer to the learning of a greater variety of specific tasks than others. In our culture, *verbal* abilities are more important in a greater variety of tasks than are some other type of abilities. But in other cultures, *motor* abilities developed early may be more pervasive. The individual who has a great many highly developed basic abilities can become proficient at a great variety of specific tasks.

Abilities are relatively enduring traits of the individual. Unless he is subjected to marked environmental changes, a man's basic abilities are not likely to change much once he reaches adulthood. Thus, such abilities as numerical, verbal, and spatial abilities are fairly stable attributes of behavior over lengthy periods of time. This probably results from the fact that they have been learned, relearned, and practiced so many times during the individual's lifetime. The mechanism here is probably what is typically called overlearning. Thus, individuals may show no impairment of performance even after lengthy periods of time without practice. Probably man's abilities are stable because certain kinds of human performances have been practiced in varying degrees throughout an individual's lifetime and have become "overlearned."

Human adults, of course, show marked learning over time in practically any type of specific *skill*. However, according to this conceptualization, the rate of learning and the final level achieved by particular individuals in certain skills are both limited by the basic abilities of these individuals. The fact that these basic abilities are themselves fairly stable allows us to make useful predictions about subsequent performance in specific tasks. For example, knowledge about a person's numerical ability helps us predict his probable success later on in engineering training. Knowledge about the relevant motor ability components should help us predict performance in complex athletic skills. It is very clear that knowledge about basic abilities helps us predict subsequent more complex performances. Some abilities may be more important later in skills learning, while other abilities are critical earlier in learning (Fleishman and Hempel, 1954a, b). The idea that basic abilities place limits on later skill proficiency emphasizes the need to develop these abilities in preadult life.

Motor Ability Tests for Children

Early tests of mental functioning were largely sensorimotor. Galton (1883) identified such performance with "intelligence." Similarly, Cattell (1890) constructed "mental tests" which included measures of grip strength, rate of arm movement, and reaction time, along with simple sensory and memory measures. It was actually Binet who first concluded that tests of sensorimotor skills have little relation to "general mental functioning." Consequently, to Binet goes credit for separating out at least two gross classes of human abilities. Although the concept of "general intelligence" is still with us (less so in the United States than in certain other countries), few today are willing to postulate a general ability embracing both

psychomotor and intellectual classes of abilities.

Many "intelligence tests" for children, including the Stanford-Binet test, contain tasks which involve motor components. In fact, many investigators view tests for young children not so much as evaluations of intelligence as of general developmental level. Because the most observable developments in young children are in motor facility, these tests have included many motor skill types of items.

Thus, the Gesell Development Schedule (1940) includes among its tests at the 15-month age level: turns book pages, puts pellet in bottle, climbs stairs, initiates drawing stroke, places cubes in cups. Examples of items included in the 72-month level test are: jumping from a 12-inch height landing on toes, advanced throwing, standing on each foot alternately, walking the length of a 4-inch board.

The Merrill-Palmer Scale (Stutsman, 1931) contains predominantly sensorimotor items. Examples are throwing a ball, pulling a string, crossing the feet. The California Scale (ages 1 to 18 months) covers postural and motor development, manipulation of objects, perception, attention, naming objects, the motor items being predominantly in the lower ages.

A test developed by Oseretsky in Russia in 1923 received attention in various countries. The Oseretsky Tests of Motor Proficiency, edited by E. A. Doll in 1946 in the United States from a Portuguese adaptation, were designed especially for use with feeble-minded children and children with motor disorders and covered "all major types of motor behavior from postural reactions and gross bodily movements to finger coordination and control of facial muscles." There were six tests for each age which served as indices of "general coordination of hands," "motor speed," "simultaneous voluntary movement," and the "ability to perform without superfluous movements." Materials used included matchsticks, wooden spools, thread, paper boxes, balls, and sieves.

There are a number of other individual performance tests for children such as the Pittner-Patterson, Cornell-Cox, and the Arthur Point Scale of Performance. However, these performance tests are not tests of motor skill. They are essentially nonverbal scales of mental ability involving perceptual, spatial, or "insightful" behavior.

Adult Psychomotor Tests

As indicated above, earlier tests of psychomotor skills were of the simplest kind. Between 1920 and 1940 most of the research on motor skills remained confined to such tests. Laboratory investigations were conducted on such problems as the specificity of simple motor abilities, with some small-scale attempts to identify factors underlying individual differences in these abilities. Thus, studies by Robert Seashore and his co-workers (1940, 1942, 1951) indicated that in fine motor skills the sense employed is of moderate significance, the musculature employed is of slight significance, and the pattern of movement involved is likely to be the most important factor. Moreover, the investigators largely concluded that motor skill factors are relatively few and very narrow in scope. In general, these early studies showed simple motor skill tests to have low correlations with one another. This was largely a function of the choice of measures and restricted range of skills investigated. It remained for subsequent research to exploit these relationships more thoroughly.

With the possible exception of certain dexterity tests, test batteries of special aptitudes during this era seldom included motor skill measures. Seashore's pioneering attempt to develop a more comprehensive motor skills battery, the Stanford Motor Skills Unit (Seashore, 1928), contained six tests of representative types of motor performances: (1) the Koerth Pursuit Rotor, to measure accuracy in following with a stylus a small target moving rapidly in a circle; (2) the Miles Speed Rotor, to measure speed of rotary arm, wrist, and finger movements in turning a small drill; (3) the Brown Spool Packer, to measure precision in reproducing rhythmic patterns on a telegraphic key; (4) the Motor Rhythm Synchrometer, to measure precision in reproducing rhythmic patterns on a telegraphic key; (5) the Serial Discrimeter, to measure speed in making discriminating reactions to signals which change as fast as they are reacted to correctly; and, finally (6) speed of tapping a telegraph key. These tests were the forerunners of psychomotor tests dealing with more important types of psychomotor performances.

This era was characterized by an increasing number of validation studies of motor ability tests in field settings. A large number of these studies indicated zero or low correlations between proficiency in simple motor ability tests and more complex motor skills such as typing (Walker and Adams, 1934), machine shopwork (Seashore, 1951), and winding machine operation in knitting mills. High validities were found in a number of studies for simple steadiness tests in predicting rifle marksmanship. Finger and manual dexterities tests were shown on occasion to have some validity for watchmaking, electrical fixture and radio assemblies, coil winding, packing and wrapping, and certain kinds of machine operation. The United States Employment Service is one agency which employs simple motor ability tests in their comprehensive test batteries. Two of these, for manual dexterity and finger dexterity, involve pegboards and assembly-type tasks. Two others, purporting to evaluate motor coordination and motor speed, are paper-and-pencil tests (e.g., tapping in circles). Actually, research has shown that the latter tests measure neither "motor speed" nor "motor coordination" as such (Fleishman and Ellison, 1962).

The assumption underlying simple motor ability test development was that it should be possible to develop a battery of simple motor tests that indicated likelihood of success in more complex psychomotor skills. So strong was this belief that failures in prediction have often been attributed to faulty techniques, such as lack of reliability of the measures used, although in most cases the real cause was failure to sample the relevant psychomotor abilities.

World War II provided the impetus for developing a wide variety of tests of psychomotor ability. The most extensive program of this type was conducted in the United States Air Force psychology research program (Melton, 1947). Some of the most critical jobs in the Air Force depended upon psychomotor skills of a complexity never before investigated. Outstanding examples were the tasks of pilot, gunner, and bombardier.

The test apparatus employed varied in complexity from simple pegboards to complicated mechanical and electronic devices. The complex apparatus tests were shown to have substantial validity for predicting later proficiency in these jobs (Fleishman, 1956; Melton, 1947).

The Complex Coordination Test is one example. The examinee must make appropriate control adjustments of stick and pedal controls in response to successively presented patterns of visual signals (Figure 1). The task is to match the position of stimulus lights in each of three dimensions by coordinate movements of these controls. The score is the number of completed matchings in an 8-minute period. A validity coefficient of .45 was achieved for this test in predicting subsequent flying proficiency.

Another example is the Rudder Control Test, which also has been a consistent predictor of pilot success. The examinee sits in a mock cockpit arrangement. His own weight throws the seat off balance unless he applies correction by means of coordinated pedal adjustments. The score is the amount of time the apparatus is correctly aligned. The test takes 15 minutes to administer and has a validity of .40 for pilot selection.

Some have inferred that these tests are valid because they seem to represent a miniature job sample of certain aspects of the pilot's job. However, this is only a small part of the answer. Many tests thought to duplicate what seemed to be important aspects of the pilot's job failed to achieve any prediction.

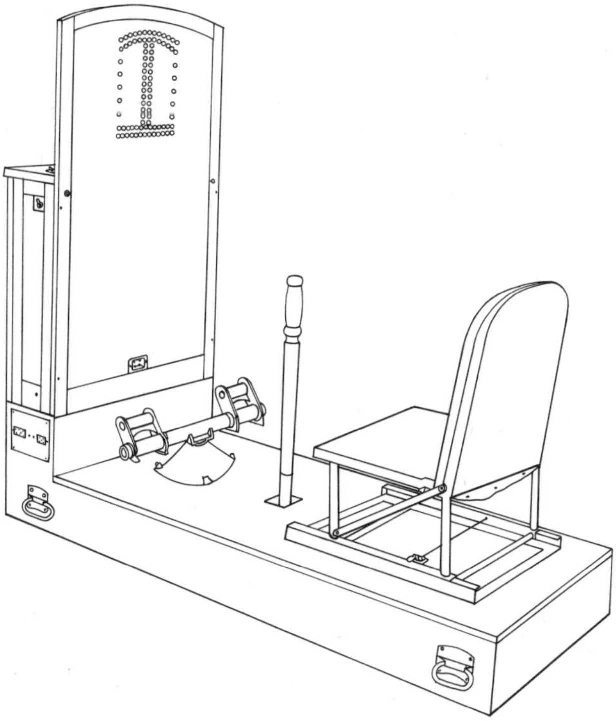

The reason the Complex Coordination Test and the Rudder Control Test are valid predictors is that between them they sample three of the underlying abilities which are crucial to pilot success (Fleishman, 1956). The resemblance of the task itself to the pilot's job is incidental to the fact that the Complex Coordination Test measures a spatial orientation factor and two psychomotor factors, while the Rudder Control Test measures these same two psychomotor factors. These factors have been identified as control precision and multilimb coordination (defined below).

Several other psychomotor tests found valid for pilots do not resemble the pilot's job at all. These tests tap the human abilities measured by the Rudder Control Test and the Complex Coordination Test. An example is the Rotary Pursuit Test, which was used in the U.S. Air Force Battery for over 10 years (Figure 2). The test apparatus resembles a phonograph turntable, with a disk revolving at a speed of 60 rpm. The examinee's task is to keep a stylus in contact with a small target embedded near the edge of the disk. The score is the amount of time the stylus is on target in five 20-second

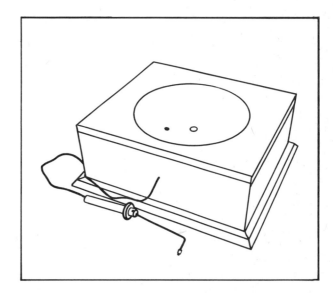

Fig. 1.   The Complex Coordination Test. (From Fleishman, E. A., "A Comparative Study of Aptitude Patterns in Unskilled and Skilled Psychomotor Performances," *Journal of Applied Psychology,* 1957, *41,* 263–272. © 1957 by the American Psychological Association; reprinted by permission.)

Fig 2.   Rotary Pursuit. (From Fleishman, E. A., "A Comparative Study of Aptitude Patterns in Unskilled and Skilled Psychomotor Performances," *Journal of Applied Psychology,* 1957, *41,* 263–272. © 1957 by the American Psychological Association; reprinted by permission.)

periods. The Rotary Pursuit Test does not resemble the task of an aircraft pilot, but it does measure the "control precision factor," which apparently accounts for its validity.

The Two-Hand Coordination Test is another example of a test which in no way resembles the pilot's task, but which is valid nonetheless, because it measures relevant abilities. In this test, one lathe-type control handle moves a target follower to the right and left, while the other control handle moves it to and from the examinee. By properly coordinated movements of both hands, the examinee can move the target follower in any direction. During the test he must keep the target follower on a visually perceived target as it moves along an irregular pathway. During World War II, scores on this test were found related to success in bombardier and flexible gunnery training as well as to pilot proficiency (Melton, 1947).

More recent research has investigated the *sources* of validity in such tests. A whole series of interlocking experimental factor-analytic studies, attempting to isolate and identify the common variance in a wide range of psychomotor performances, has been carried out.

Categories of Human Motor Abilities

It is perhaps not too extreme a statement that most of the categorization of human skills which is empirically based comes from such correlational and factor-analysis studies. This approach describes tasks in terms of the common abilities required to perform them. Tasks are specifically designed or selected to test certain hypotheses about the organization of abilities in a certain range of tasks. Other studies have introduced task variations aimed at sharpening or limiting ability factor definitions. The purpose is to define the fewest independent ability categories which might be most useful and meaningful in describing performance in the widest variety of tasks.

Studies have included analysis of fine manipulative performances (e.g., finger and manual dexterity) (Fleishman and Hempel, 1954a; Fleishman and Ellison, 1962) and gross physical proficiency (e.g., push-ups, chin-ups) (Hempel and Fleishman, 1955; Nicks and Fleishman, 1962; Fleishman, 1964). One study focused on positioning movements (e.g., reach-

ing, moving controls to specified positions) and "static reactions" (e.g., hand steadiness) (Fleishman, 1958a). The former concerns movements in which the terminal accuracy of the response is critical, and the latter primarily involves maintenance of limb positions. Another series of studies (Fleishman, 1956; Fleishman, 1958b; Parker and Fleishman, 1960) concerns "movement reactions," where the performance involves coordinated responses, or smooth responses, or precisely controlled movements, or continuously adjustive reactions.

Thus far several hundred different tasks have been administered to thousands of subjects in a series of interlocking studies. From the patterns of correlations obtained, it has been possible to account for performance on this wide range of tasks in terms of a relatively small number of abilities. In subsequent investigations, definitions of these abilities and their distinctions from one another have become more clearly delineated. Furthermore, it is now possible to specify the tasks which should provide the best measure of each of the abilities identified.

Some of the important individual difference variables that have been revealed in this series of investigations are listed below. Details on their definition and the devices which best measure them can be found elsewhere (Fleishman, 1954, 1958, 1962).

Control Precision. This ability is common to tasks which require fine, highly controlled, but not overcontrolled, muscular adjustments, primarily where larger muscle groups are involved. The ability extends to arm-hand as well as to leg movements. It is most critical where such adjustments must be rapid but precise.

Multilimb Coordination. This is the ability to coordinate the movements of a number of limbs simultaneously; it is best measured by devices involving multiple controls. The ability has been found general to tasks requiring coordination of two feet, two hands, and hands and feet.

Response Orientation. This ability factor has been found general to visual discrimination reaction psychomotor tasks involving rapid directional discrimination and orientation of movement patterns. It appears to involve the ability to *select* the correct movement in relation to the correct stimulus, especially under high-speed conditions.

Reaction Time. This represents simply the speed with which the individual is able to respond to a stimulus when it appears. There are consistent indications that individual differences in this ability are independent of whether the stimulus is auditory or visual and of the type of response required. However, once the stimulus situation or the response situation is complicated by involving alternate choices, reaction time is not the primary factor that is measured.

Speed of Arm Movement. This represents simply the speed with which an individual can make a gross, discrete arm movement where accuracy is not the requirement. There is ample evidence that this ability is independent of reaction time.

Rate Control (Timing). This ability involves the timing of continuous anticipatory motor adjustments relative to changes in speed and direction of a continuously moving target or object. This factor is general to tasks involving compensatory as well as following pursuit and extends to tasks involving responses to changes in rate. Research has shown that adequate measurement of this ability requires an actual response in relation to the changing direction and speed of the stimulus object, and not simply judging the rate of the stimulus alone.

Manual Dexterity. This ability involves skillful, well-directed arm-hand movements in manipulating fairly large objects under speed conditions.

Finger Dexterity. This is the ability to make skill-controlled manipulations of tiny objects primarily involving the fingers.

Arm-Hand Steadiness. This is the ability to make precise arm-hand positioning movements where strength and speed are minimized; the critical feature is steadiness.

Wrist, Finger Speed. This ability has been called *tapping* in many studies through the years. It has been used in a variety of different studies, primarily because these are in the form of printed tests which are quick and easy to administer. However, research shows that this factor is highly restricted in scope and does not extend to many tasks in which apparatus is used. The factor is best measured by printed tests requiring rapid tapping of the pencil in relatively large areas.

Aiming. This ability appears best measured by printed tests which provide the subject with very small circles to be dotted in as rapidly as possible.

Another large area of motor performance is that of *physical proficiency.* Experimental factor-analytical work indicates the following factors account for performance in tests of physical fitness (Fleishman, 1964).

Extent Flexibility. This is the ability to flex or stretch the trunk and back muscles as far as possible in either a forward, lateral, or backward direction (e.g., reaching tests).

Dynamic Flexibility. This is the ability to make repeated rapid-flexing movements in which the resiliency of the muscles in recovery from strain or distortion is critical (e.g., twist and touch).

Static Strength. This is the maximum force which a subject can exert for a brief period. In contrast to other strength factors, this is the force which can be exerted against external objects (e.g., lifting heavy weights, pulling against a dynamometer), rather than in supporting the body's own weight.

Dynamic Strength. This is the ability to exert muscular force repeatedly or continuously over time. It represents muscular endurance and emphasizes the resistance of the muscles to fatigue. The common emphasis of tests measuring this factor is on the power of the muscles to propel, support, or move the body repeatedly or to support it for prolonged periods (e.g., pull-ups, push-ups).

Trunk Strength. This is a second, more limited dynamic strength factor specific to the trunk muscles, particularly the abdominal muscles (e.g., leg lifts, sit-ups).

Explosive Strength. This is the ability to expend a maximum of energy in one or a series of explosive acts. This factor is distinguished from other strength factors in requiring mobilization of *energy* for a burst of effort, rather than continuous strain, stress, or repeated exertion of muscles (e.g., jumping, sprinting, throwing).

Gross Body Coordination. This is the ability to coordinate simultaneous actions of different parts of the body while making gross body movements (e.g., cable jump).

Gross Body Equilibrium. This is the ability

of an individual to maintain his equilibrium, despite forces pulling him off balance, where he has to depend mainly on nonvisual (e.g., vestibular and kinesthetic) cues. Although measured by balance tests where the eyes are kept open (e.g., rail walk), it is best measured by balance tests conducted with the eyes closed (e.g., one foot stand on rail).

Stamina (Cardiovascular Endurance). This is the capacity to continue maximum effort requiring prolonged exertion over time. (It is best measured by tests requiring a mile or more of running.)

Studies in the physical proficiency area clarified a great many measurement issues of what tests to use and under what conditions to achieve coverage of these factors. Nine Basic Fitness Tests developed to measure these factors most efficiently are described elsewhere (Fleishman, 1964). National norms and development curves based on 20,000 males and females from 45 school systems are available (Fleishman, 1964).

While the factors described here do not represent any kind of final list of individual psychomotor abilities, they do account for individual differences in a wide range of tasks. These categories have been useful in accounting for proficiency in practical skills (e.g., Fleishman, 1956, Parker and Fleishman, 1960). They have guided the development of batteries of laboratory tasks to examine the effects of such variables as drugs (e.g., Fleishman, 1972), noise (e.g., Theologus, Wheaton, and Fleishman, 1974), diet (Brozek, Fleishman, Harris, Lassman, and Vidal, 1955), and stress (Gorham and Orr, 1956) on different types of tasks. More recent research has used these ability categories as a basis for analyzing the physical requirements of jobs (Romashko, Brumback, Fleishman, and Hahn, 1974). From this kind of job analysis, which involves rating jobs in terms of their ability requirements, it is possible to match job requirements with the abilities of people to perform them.

BIBLIOGRAPHY

FLEISHMAN, E. A.   Dimensional analysis of psychomotor abilities. *Journal of Experimental Psychology,* 1954, *48,* 437–454.

FLEISHMAN, E. A.   Psychomotor selection tests: Research and application in the U.S. Air Force. *Personnel Psychology,* 1956, *9,* 449–467.

FLEISHMAN, E. A.   Dimensional analysis of movement reactions. *Journal of Experimental Psychology,* 1958, *55,* 430–453.

FLEISHMAN, E. A.   The description and prediction of perceptual-motor skill learning. In R. Glaser (Ed.), *Training research and education.* Pittsburgh: University of Pittsburgh Press, 1962.

FLEISHMAN, E. A.   *The structure and measurement of physical fitness.* Englewood Cliffs, N.J.: Prentice-Hall, 1964.

FLEISHMAN, E. A.   On the relation between abilities, learning, and human performance. *American Psychologist,* 1972, *27,* 1017–1032.

FLEISHMAN, E. A., and ELLISON, G. D.   A factor analysis of fine manipulative performance. *Journal of Applied Psychology,* 1962, *46,* 96–105.

FLEISHMAN, E. A., and HEMPEL, W. E., JR.   A factor analysis of dexterity tests. *Personnel Psychology,* 1954a, *7,* 15–32.

FLEISHMAN, E. A., and HEMPEL, W. E., JR.   Changes in factor structure of a complex psychomotor test as a function of practice. *Psychometrika,* 1954b, *19,* 239–252.

GAGNE, R. M., and FLEISHMAN, E. A.   *Psychology and human performance.* New York: Holt, 1959.

MELTON, A. W. (Ed.).   *Apparatus test.* AAF Psychological Program Report no. 4. Washington, D.C.: U.S. Government Printing Office, 1947.

ROMASHKO, T.; BRUMBACK, G.; FLEISHMAN, E. A.; and HAHN, C. P.   *The development of a procedure to validate physical tests.* Washington, D.C.: American Institutes for Research, 1974.

SEASHORE, R. H.   Work and motor performance. In S. S. Stevens (Ed.), *Handbook of Experimental Psychology.* New York: Wiley, 1951.

THEOLOGUS, G.; WHEATON, G.; and FLEISHMAN, E. A.   Effects of intermittent, moderate intensity noise stress on human performance. *Journal Of Applied Psychology,* 1974, *59,* 539–547.

EDWIN A. FLEISHMAN

MOTOR BEHAVIOR; MOVEMENT, PSYCHOMOTOR

MOTOR BEHAVIOR: SOCIAL FACTORS

Individual Motor Behavior

Little cognizance was given to the influence of the social milieu on motor behavior until the 1960s when a social psychology of motor behavior emerged. The social factors thought to influence individual motor behavior and thus receiving the most experimental attention included social facilitation, competition, observational learning or modeling, and social reinforcement. These social factors, however, habitually have not accounted for a large proportion of the variance in individual motor learning and performance. This is not unexpected, as many other factors are known to have pronounced influence on motor learning and performance. When other things are equal, though, these social variables acquire substantial importance in determining success or fail-

ure in skill acquisition and performance. Following is a brief review of when these four social variables are likely to become prominent factors in skill acquisition and performance.

The *social facilitation* phenomenon refers to both positive and negative effects on a person's behavior as a consequence of the presence of others. Early social facilitation research was equivocal, or so it seemed, until Zajonc (1965) applied drive theory to this body of research revealing considerable consistency in the findings. The theory is based on evidence that the presence of passive others is arousing and that arousal increases the probability of the dominant response being emitted. The dominant response tends to be the correct response in well-learned skills and the incorrect response in skills yet to be acquired. Thus, the presence of others impairs learning but facilitates performance of well-learned skills.

Motor behavior research supports Zajonc's theory in most cases for both speed and accuracy motor tasks. Additional research, including motor behavior research, has shown that the social facilitation effect is not caused only by the mere presence of others, but by the anxiety associated with the expectation of either positive or negative evaluation from the present others.

More recent social facilitation research with motor skills has examined how persons who differ in anxiety as well as in ability are affected by the presence of evaluative others, but results have been inconclusive. Current research continues to investigate a number of situational variables that may mediate the social facilitation effect. These variables include the social relationship between the performer and observers, number of observers, distance between the performer and observer, sex and age differences, and previous experiences in similar situations. Data are as yet too inconclusive to reach any generalizations about these potential mediating variables.

Another important social psychological process influencing motor behavior is *competition*. The effects of competition on motor performance have been investigated in over 25 experiments. Although generalizations are tenuous because of the diverse competitive situations studied, evidence indicates that competition facilitates performance on muscular endurance and strength tasks, as well as on well-learned and simple motor skills, but impairs performance on complex motor tasks that are not well learned. These findings are congruent with social facilitation effects on motor behavior and are imputed to the common element within both competitive and social facilitation situations—the presence of evaluative others.

One of the consequences of competing is that the person either wins or loses and the pattern of outcomes influences later performance. Several studies have shown that persons who win about 50% of the time perform better than those who win or lose considerably more. These findings, however, have been obtained only when manipulating the prior win-loss ratio for short periods. The consequence of various win-loss ratios over long periods is unclear, although given a choice consistent losers are frequently observed to quit.

Drive theory, which predicts a positive linear relationship between arousal and performance, adequately explains the performance results reviewed for both social facilitation and competition. A rival hypothesis is the inverted-U hypothesis (stemming from the Yerkes-Dodson law), which states that the relationship between arousal and performance is non-monotonic—that is, as arousal increases performance improves up to some point after which additional increases in arousal impairs performance. Common sense makes this hypothesis appealing, and several motor skills experiments, using both social and nonsocial stressors to elicit arousal, have supported the inverted-U hypothesis. At present both these positions explain different sets of experimental results. It remains to be seen if these conflicting positions can be integrated theoretically.

Observing a model demonstrating a skill is one of the fundamental means through which new skills are learned. Teachers of complex motor skills rely extensively on modeling as a means of communicating how to perform the skill. Because of the obvious importance of this mode of learning, it is perplexing that so little research has examined the effects of modeling on motor skill acquisition. Apparently because of the certainty that modeling helps in the acquisition of motor skills, the actual process of how modeling helps has not been examined until relatively recently.

According to Bandura (1969), whether or not observational learning occurs is dependent upon four processes: attentional, retentional, motor reproduction, and motivational. It is obvious that attending to the modeled stimuli and retaining the conveyed information is essential in skill acquisition. What is not obvious are those factors that affect the attentional and retentional processes when modeling motor skills. Research specific to this issue has not yet been done.

Of immense importance for motor skill acquisition is knowing how, if at all, a model facilitates learning. Indications are that modeling facilitates response selection through knowledge about the stimulus environment and the goal, but not the motor processes necessary to implement the planned movement. Thus, in the actual performance of a skill, modeling may facilitate knowing what to do, but only practice is likely to develop the motor processes necessary to produce the planned movement.

Bandura's final process, the incentive or motivational process, cannot be neglected in skill learning through the modeling modality. Although a person may have perceived and retained information about response selection and he may have acquired the motor processes enabling him to reproduce the skill, if he is not motivated he may select not to reproduce the modeled response.

One question in the modeling of motor skills is whether the skill should always be demonstrated correctly or whether observing an incorrect demonstration facilitates learning as well. Indications are that incorrect modeling impairs learning when compared to no modeling, but that correct modeling facilitates learning. This generalization is likely to be qualified by different task dimensions which further research will need to determine. A related question concerns what types of motor skills are better acquired through the modeling modality. Because modeling appears to be most helpful in response selection, those skills that demand difficult or complex response selection decisions should be assisted most by modeling. Those skills that have extensive response production demands must be acquired primarily through practice.

Social reinforcement, or nontangible reinforcement under the control of others, is an important modifier of a wide range of behaviors. Commonly social reinforcement is in the form of praise and reproof, smiles and sneers, and friendly and hostile gestures. Two features are essential for the successful use of social reinforcement: the reinforcer must be powerful, and the reinforcing event must be made contingent upon the desired behavior.

Substantial research has shown that social reinforcers are effective in modifying behavior on very simple motor tasks—for example, marble dropping and card sorting. Both positive and negative social reinforcers have been shown to facilitate performance on these tasks, but with positive social reinforcers having longer or more enduring facilitory effects. The influence of social reinforcement on simple motor tasks has been attributed to changes in motivational state.

Of greater interest is the function of social reinforcement on complex motor skill acquisition performance. Evidence has shown that social reinforcement has had little effect on skill acquisition when the motivational state of the performer was high and other, more specific sources of feedback about performance were available. In all studies examining the effect of social reinforcement on motor skill acquisition, knowledge of results and response-produced feedback were more specific sources of information available. Of two stimuli, the one more informative for the person has the strongest reinforcement potential. Because social reinforcement failed to provide nonredundant and more specific information, it lost its reinforcement potential.

For social reinforcement to be maximally effective, other sources of feedback should not convey the same information as social reinforcement, and the task should have low intrinsic motivational properties. Most complex motor tasks tend to elicit considerable intrinsic motivation. Hence, social reinforcement is unlikely to function as an important factor in the early acquisition of a motor skill. After learning has occurred, however, and intrinsic motivation begins to wane, evidence suggests that social reinforcers are motivating and facilitate performance to some extent.

In summary, social psychological research on individual motor behavior has sought to determine unitarily if social factors facilitate or impair learning and performance in terms of speed and accuracy. Current theory intimates that performance of well-learned skills is af-

fected primarily by social motivational factors and that skill acquisition is affected by both, although the informational component has primacy.

Group Motor Behavior

The study of group motor behavior has been limited because of the increased complexity of measuring group performance and the difficulty in determining individual contributions to the group product. The measurement of group motor behavior has consequently been less rigorous than the measurement of individual motor behavior. Rather than research using experimenter-designed motor tasks in laboratory settings, most small-group research has been done in the field using available measures of group productivity.

Small-group research has three interrelated parts: *group structure,* or the pattern of interpersonal relations; *group processes,* or the activities within the group structure; and *group products,* or the output from the group process. Group productivity is determined by task demands, individual and group resources, and the group process.

Task demands are the requirements imposed on the group by the task itself or by the rules under which the task must be performed. The *resources* consist of all the abilities, skills, and knowledge possessed by the members of the group. The *process* of the group involves intra- and interpersonal actions taken by the group to transform its resources into a product. A knowledge of task demands and of group members' resources indicates a group's potential productivity. Steiner (1972) has theorized that the discrepancy between the group's actual productivity and its potential productivity is a consequence of faulty social processes. These faulty processes consist of coordination losses between members of the group and motivation losses.

Group motor behavior research has lacked theoretical direction, but Steiner's (1972) *group task taxonomy,* which is based on the requirements the task imposes on the group, is helpful in organizing the findings and in providing direction for future study. The major task dimension consists of *unitary* tasks, which have no division of labor, and *divisible* tasks, which do. Within unitary tasks there are four different categories for how the members of the group may combine their individual efforts. When only one of the available individual contributions can be accepted as the group product and all others are rejected, it is a *disjunctive* task. When the product of the group is determined by the performance of the individual member who does least well, it is a *conjunctive* task. An *additive* task is one in which the group product depends on the sum of the individual contributions as they choose. In divisible tasks there are specialized subtasks to which individual members must be matched. Divisible tasks vary according to whether the subtasks and the matching of persons to the subtasks are specified or unspecified by the task.

Early research on group productivity was concerned primarily with the question of whether individuals perform more or less efficiently than groups. For additive motor tasks actual productivity never reaches potential productivity (the sum of individual group members), but the group is always able to do more than an individual. For example, using a rope-pulling task, the efficiency of performance decreased as the size of the group increased up to about three of four members, after which efficiency remained about the same as group size increased to six. Tasks lending themselves to a division of labor increases the probability that the group will be more productive because it is possible for the group to utilize its potentially greater resources. If the resources of the group can be implemented with minimum process losses, group performance will be superior. If the process losses are great, however, individuals may perform the task more efficiently alone. In terms of the speed-accuracy tradeoff, groups usually provide more accurate responses but require more time to complete the task than do individuals.

Group research has also focused on whether group performance can be predicted from knowledge about the ability of individual group members. The answer is dependent upon the nature of the interaction required or permitted by the task. On conjunctive motor tasks the least proficient member's performance best predicted team performance, while on disjunctive and discretionary motor tasks group performance was better predicted by the performance of the most proficient member of the group.

Group Composition. The productivity of a group in part depends on the characteristics of its members, independent of the role structure of the group. Abilities, personality characteristics, and motivational factors are three member properties that have been shown to influence group motor performance. It should seem obvious that groups with higher ability perform better, but this is not always the case. For simple tasks higher ability is superfluous. For divisible tasks a distribution of skills that is of sufficient range to deal with the task demands yields better performance than a narrower range of skills.

Increased heterogeneity of abilities establishes higher levels of potential productivity with disjunctive and discretionary tasks, lower potential productivity with conjunctive tasks, and is irrelevant with additive tasks. Group motor performance research has found no evidence that either homogeneous or heterogeneous grouping on ability facilitates either skill acquisition or performance, although homogeneous grouping is usually preferred by members of a group.

Group performance may in part depend on the personalities of the group's members. Individual differences affect group performance more when the role system of the group does not adequately guide collective action. Little evidence is available on individual differences as they pertain to group motor behavior, but some of the research with problem-solving tasks is likely to apply to motor behavior. For example, the more socially sensitive, the more dependable, the better adjusted, and the less anxious the group member, the more likely that he will be successful in helping the group achieve its goals. Ascendant persons, who are dominating and self-assertive in groups, generally facilitate group performance as well.

The extent to which homogeneity or heterogeneity of personality characteristics is desirable depends on the task demands. Heterogeneity has been shown to be desirable when task demands require the person to perform highly specialized roles. In this case, persons with different but complementary personality attributes are more compatible and hence more effective as a group. When the task demands require everyone to perform the same role, homogeneity is more desirable.

Group members' motivation is another composition variable that is important in understanding group motor performance, but this relationship is not yet well understood. One important distinction is knowing whether group members are motivated toward group goals or individual goals. The motivation toward group or individual goals is dependent upon the available reward pattern. Groups perform better as groups when they are rewarded as groups, particularly on divisible motor tasks. Thus, cooperative conditions rather than competitive conditions within a group promote group effectiveness for divisible tasks.

Group Structure. Several facets of group structure, or the patterned regularities among group members, have been shown to influence group performance. The communication structure, the affect structure or group cohesion, and the leadership structure are the three facets most studied.

It is not surprising that increased *communication* among all members of a group facilitates performance, particularly on divisible tasks. Communication is important in developing effective group social process; it is essential in developing and maintaining high levels of cohesiveness and in clarifying group goals to its members. Thus, the communication structure is important in group motivation. Emerson (1966) cited evidence obtained from a Mount Everest mountainclimbing expedition to support the theory that the communication in groups striving to achieve difficult and important goals tends to maximize and maintain uncertainty about the outcome through selective transmission of information. Communicated information tends to counteract the prevailing information provided in the environment, and communication feedback tends to counteract the information currently being communicated, thereby sustaining doubt and maintaining group effort.

Group cohesiveness is related to increased cooperativeness, better communication, and greater satisfaction within a group. These factors contribute to the general finding that cohesiveness and effective group motor performance are related positively. This generalization, however, must be qualified by the characteristics of the task. Research reveals that the positive relationship between cohesiveness and performance has been consistently observed for divisible tasks, those reliant upon group interaction for effective performance. For unitary tasks, however, the relationship has generally been insignificant and in some cases negative. The negative relationship may occur among groups who are too cohesive because efforts to maintain cohesiveness interfere with task performance.

The *leadership* requirements for effective group performance are also dependent upon the task demands. A task-oriented leader is more effective when the group-task situation is either very favorable or very unfavorable for the leader, whereas a relationship-oriented leader is more effective when the group-task situation is only moderately favorable or unfavorable for the leader. The task-oriented leader is thus more effective in existing high-cohesive groups, while the relationship-oriented leader is more helpful in low-cohesive groups.

BIBLIOGRAPHY

BANDURA, A. *Principles of behavior modification.* New York: Holt, Rinehart and Winston, 1969.

EMERSON, R. M.   Mount Everest: A case study in communication feedback and sustained group goal-striving. *Sociometry,* 1966, *29,* 213–227.

STEINER, I. D.   *Group process and productivity.* New York: Academic Press, 1972.

WOLMAN, B. B.   The impact of failure on group cohesiveness. *Journal of Social Psychology,* 1960, *51,* 409–418.

ZAJONC, R.   Social facilitation. *Science,* 1965, *149,* 269–274.

RAINER MARTENS

MOTOR BEHAVIOR IN INFANCY AND EARLY CHILDHOOD

The assessment of motor development has been incorporated into various tests of infant intellectual evaluation. Most investigators have concentrated on the first two to three years of life and have introduced examiner-determined tasks as the tools of assessment. As a result, it may be difficult to compare developmental schedules, since each assessor has some preferred tasks. It is the purpose of the following paragraphs to describe age-related motor development that is spontaneous and insofar as possible, little contaminated by observer intervention.

The First Year

The full-term newborn infant is not a very active creature, and spends much of its day asleep. Spontaneous motor activity is minimal unless the infant is stimulated by handling. Much spontaneous but rather reflexive activity is associated with crying such as the *Moro* and *asymmetric tonic neck reflexes*. If the infant is placed in the prone position, it tends to assume a flexed posture with the hips and knees flexed under the abdomen and the arms flexed and adducted alongside the head. The head may be raised slightly and turned laterally. When supine, the flexion posture persists but with the hips tending to be abducted as well. The infant's fingers are also flexed over a flexed thumb. Between two and four weeks of age, the prone infant will raise its chin high enough to clear the supporting surface. This ability to lift the head in the prone position increases so that by three months most infants can bring the head almost to 90 degrees from the horizontal. This is accomplished by gradual elevation of the chest. At 3–4 months, the arms are flexed and the weight of the trunk is carried by the forearms. By 6 months, the infant can raise its chest off the supporting surface with the hands by fully extending the arms, while the lower abdomen and legs remain in contact with the supportive surface. During this same 3-month period the infant acquires the ability to roll. Generally it commences from the prone position. By extending one arm and turning the head laterally toward that arm, the infant pushes itself onto one side. Between 3 and 5 months of age this action is completed, so that the infant can turn from abdomen to back. Between 5 and 7 months, rolling from supine to prone is accomplished. Some infants then use rolling over as a means of locomotion. Most infants will move about, however, using the forearms to pull them forward. This is termed crawling and is in turn succeeded by creeping about on the hands and knees in a quadripedal manner of reciprocal flexion and extension of limbs.

Most normal infants have passed through these stages by 11 months. Between 8 and 11 months, spontaneous sitting without assistance from an adult is achieved, although the ability to maintain the seated position if placed upright has been present from age 6 months. Sitting also passes through stages which are age related. It is first accomplished from the hand-knee creeping position. The infant rotates its rump to one side and down to the supporting surface, pushing the trunk erect with both arms. Somewhat older children will roll to one side whether prone or supine and then push erect with both hands. Even at age 3 years, this technique is employed, though only one arm is used in assuming the erect position. By 5 years, the assistance of the arms is no longer necessary. Having succeeded in sitting erect, some infants use scooting, that is, sliding either forward or backward in the seated position instead of creeping. Once the infant has learned to sit, pulling itself into a standing position follows. In general, this is completed by 10 months. Cruising, that is, holding on to the crib side or to furniture and side stepping precedes walking. While occasional infants have an accelerated maturation of locomotor skills and are walking alone as early as 8–10 months, most infants have acquired this motor milestone between 12–15 months. Some normal children may not walk before 18 months and occasionally not before 22 to 24 months. Often one may find similar patterns of walking in the families of such infants.

From One to Six

Once the child does walk unsupported, it does so with the legs apart in a wide stance. The beginning walker may at times revert back to creeping on hands and knees, doing so because it is a more efficient mode of ambulation. The toddler soon acquires skill enough to remain biped. Going up stairs though is continued on hands and knees as creeping until the upright walking position has become stable, around 18–24 months. The toddler then requires one-handed support either from the adult or from the handrail. Ascent is mastered first. The ability to independently descend a flight of stairs may not be achieved before 4–5 years of age. When the child does begin, climbing is done with one and the same foot, successively raised to the step and joined by the following foot before the next step is mounted. Alternating the feet in ascending stairs is in general accomplished at 3 years of age but not usually until 4–5 years when walking downstairs.

The skill of running also passes through stages of age-related development. The stable early toddler can ambulate quite rapidly but it does not represent true running. It is more of a waddling walk with feet turned outward and the arms held flexed at the elbows and partially laterally abducted. True running makes its appearance about 2½ to 3 years of age, and by 5 it has developed into the familiar pattern with appropriate associated alternating arm movements.

Hopping is another locomotive skill that children develop independent of adult intervention. Few children begin to hop on one foot by 3 years and then at most 2–3 times. But by 4 years, most children can do so on one foot. Adeptness of hopping with either foot is met in the 5–6 year old, with girls being successful sooner.

In their play activities, children can be observed to jump over, down, and onto objects. This activity also reveals an age-related developmental pattern beginning late in the second or early in the third year of life. The toddler tries by using one foot to step down. The next achievement is jumping a short distance downward with both feet from a low chair or from a stair soon after two years. Only when the child has mastered this can jumping up or over be acquired. The prekindergarten child has usually learned these skills.

Manual Skills

In this discussion, acquisition of manual motor skills has been arbitrarily separated from motor development primarily involving trunkal musculature. The former will be considered at this point.

For the first two months, the infant's hands tend to be held loosely fisted. Arm movement is random and jerky in action. By the third month, the fingers begin to move more freely. The infant now moves the arms more smoothly as well. The hand may be brought to the mouth to suck or may bat at objects held before the face, or both hands may be brought together at face level. By 4–4½ months, reaching out with both hands into the environment becomes purposeful, with the attained object brought to the mouth. Most normal infants can, by 6 months, use just one hand to reach out for objects. Voluntary grasping evolves stepwise from a

full-hand or palmar grasp in which all the fingers work together in prehension to a thumb and 2-finger grasp, and finally to a thumb and index-finger pincer grasp by 10–12 months.

As refined prehension is developing, the manner in which objects are manipulated is also evolving. Between 4 and 6 months, objects brought to the mouth by one hand are generally kept in that hand. Transferring objects from hand to hand appears with independent hand movement, around 6 months of age, though the mouth may remain the intermediary for the exchange. This is no longer the case in the 8–9-month-old infant who freely passes objects from one hand to the other. The infant has now acquired the ability to take and hold two objects, one in each hand. When a third is profferred, it is taken only after a held object is released. The 12-month-old, however, will pick up several objects and may on request give them up when the hand is extended toward the captive object. Despite the manual adeptness reached by the 12-month-old and the explorative activity using the fingers, the mouth continues to play a role in the investigation of objects in the environment. As a result, if allowed, the infant will begin finger feeding using its neat pincer grasp to do so. However, when utensils or even crayons or pencils are first incorporated into the child's armamentarium of manual skills, a fisted grasp reappears. Thus, the 18-month-old making strokes with a crayon holds it grasped in his palm, the hand midway between pronation and supination, and usually draws with the point on the ulnar side, while a spoon is grasped with the hand held pronated. The gradual assumption of the familiar mature prehension of these tools between thumb, index, and middle finger occurs over a period of 1–2 years and possibly may not be present until the child enters kindergarten at 5–6 years of age.

The act of throwing commences around the middle of the second year of life as the infant learns voluntary release of objects. The usual game between the infant and adult, to the pleasure of the former, is to drop objects from the chair or table for the adult to retrieve. Random unorganized flinging of objects appears at this time, too. As the child matures, so does the technique of this skill, from a stiff-armed pattern to a flexible arm movement with some trunkal participation to a throwing pattern which includes the trunk and shifting of weight from one foot to the other. The time course for this activity is approximately 2½–3 years, beginning at about 2½ years of age. Subsequently, with practice and the gradual appreciation of distance, and strength required to reach the target, adeptness is obtained.

The preceding paragraphs have reviewed in order of chronological acquisition the development of motor skills from infancy to 5–6 years of age, first considering those which primarily involve trunkal musculature and then those skills in which the limbs are essentially the musculature of action. Although it may be an artificial separation, it serves to point out that all children develop over a time base but do not necessarily develop the same skills at the same time.

BIBLIOGRAPHY

CRATTY, B. J. *Perceptual and motor development in infants and children.* New York: Macmillan, 1970. Pp. 31–65.
GESELL, A., and AMATRUDA, C. S. *Developmental diagnosis* (2nd rev. ed.). New York: Harper & Row, 1947. Pp. 23–90.
ROSENBLOOM, L., and HORTON, M. E. The maturation of fine prehension in young children. *Developmental Medicine and Child Neurology,* 1971, *13,* 3–8.
TOUWEN, B. C. L., and PRECHTL, H. F. R. *The neurological examination of the child with minor nervous dysfunction: Clinics in developmental medicine* no. 38. London: Heineman. Pp. 50–57.
TWITCHELL, T. E. Reflex mechanisms and the development of prehension. In K. J. Connolly (Ed.), *Mechanisms of motor skill development.* Developmental Sciences Series. London: Academic Press, 1970. Pp. 25–37.

JEROME S. HALLER

MOTOR CONTROL AND THE CENTRAL NERVOUS SYSTEM

The emergence of modern electrophysiology and reflexology in the latter part of the seventeenth century ushered in a natural scientific concern for motor control. With these early techniques, inferential insight into central neural activity was largely dependent upon observed variations in muscle contractile or tension output (myography) to a known stimulus. Concepts at this time centered around both the unitary behavior of nerve cells *(neuron doctrine)* and functional neuronal interlinkages via presumed excitatory or inhibitory synapses. In essence, central control over motor events was viewed simply as those interactions which preceded and governed synaptic convergence on alpha motoneurons (α-MN) or, in accordance with Sherrington's view, the "final common path," that is, the sole efferent route to extrafusal muscle. Brain function and supraspinal locations closely associated with this path were principally determined from evoked motor responses (e.g., as in cerebral *cortical mapping)* using crude electrical stimulators, animal lesion experiments, and clinical neurological evidence which involved analysis of dysfunctional behavior in patients suffering from severe motor deficits.

During this early period, Charles Sherrington contributed enormously to our knowledge of spinal reflexes using relatively crude instrumentation. However, experimental exploration of the motoric role of cerebral function was largely confined to the anatomical organization of what was then called the *motor cortex (precentral gyrus).* Functionally, two interpretations evolved. John Hughlings-Jackson viewed the motor cortex as nervous arrangements representing movements while Sherringtonian followers took the position that only specific muscles were connected to these cortical networks, that is, muscles were represented by "punctate localization." While there is evidence to support both positions, it is safe to say that contemporary and more sophisticated views concerning supraspinal and spinal integration of movement awaited further electronic and technological innovations, notably the oscilloscope and microelectrode recordings.

What, then, does the central nervous system (CNS) control with respect to spinal motor pathways? From where within this system is the control exerted? How is this regulatory function accomplished? Considering the first question, the "final common path" remains a useful notion; however, the neural circuitry at this level has been more fully explored. There are actually two modes of synaptic convergence which excite or inhibit impulse transmission to extrafusal muscle: (1) a direct route via direct supraspinal synaptic convergence on alpha motoneurons (α-MN), and (2) an indirect route involving convergence on fusimotor or gamma motoneurons (γ-MN) with subsequent activation of α-MN through a peripheral feedback loop. In either case, the final common path is employed, therefore its known functional characteristics are discussed more fully.

Human α-MN are known to innervate at least two populations of extrafusal muscle—*fast twitch-glycolytic* (FG) and *slow twitch-oxidative* (SO) muscle fibers. The possible existence of a fast twitch-oxidative and glycolytic (FOG) fiber type as seen in subhuman primates has not been firmly established. FG fibers are fast contracting, depend more on glycolytic metabolism than oxidative phosphorylation, and are believed to be anatomic linkages between larger α-MN and greater tension producing extrafusal fibers. Physiologically and metabolically, the reverse is true in SO units which presumably involve smaller α-MN innervating extrafusal fibers with lower tension capabilities. Whichever the case, the muscle fibers innervated by a single α-MN are homogeneous in their anatomic, physiologic, and metabolic characteristics.

All human muscles tend to be comprised of a mixed population of motor units having FG or SO muscle fibers. Whether the whole muscle tends to be fast or slow contracting or more dependent on one metabolic pathway than another depends on the frequency distribution of these motor units. This latter outcome appears to be subject to manipulation through either disease or, possibly, natural causes such as a long term change in exercise habits.

Hence, the CNS has at its disposal, through preferential recruitment and frequency coding of FG and SO motor units, the ability to mobilize tension rapidly (e.g., via the direct route), as seen in jumping and throwing movements, or more slowly (e.g., through the indirect or direct route), as evidenced in "postural setting" or repetitive movements such as jogging. Orderly recruitment of motor units for movement skills supported by gradual increases or steady submaximal muscle tension seems well explained by the *size principle* as postulated by Elwood Henneman. Stated simply, this means that recruitment is an orderly sequence beginning with discharge from the smaller, lower threshold α-MN followed by activation of progressively larger units having higher stimulus thresholds. However, recruitment or-der does vary from this often observed pattern depending upon the tension demands of the activity, needed velocity of contraction, amount of proprioceptive facilitation, and the pathological state of the CNS.

Adaptive Control System

The indirect route offers an important, additional control system allowing gain control of α-MN through a peripheral, negative feedback loop. This represents an *adaptive control system,* the functional properties of which have been elucidated largely in the works of R. Granit (1970) and P. B. C. Matthews (1972). To elaborate, the indirect route involves the recruitment of muscle spindle intrafusal fibers (lying parallel to extrafusal muscle) through gamma activation followed by excitation of spindle primary and/or secondary mechanoceptors embedded on these muscle fibers. The adequate mechanical stimulus, elicited by a change in intrafusal length, causes spindle afferents to discharge impulses back to α-MN through monosynaptic or polysynaptic pathways. This centrifugal-centripetal circuitry is often referred to as the gamma loop.

Indirect control through the gamma loop is further complicated by what appears to be a dual gamma system, in that, two populations have been identified on functional grounds: static γ-MN and dynamic γ-MN. Activation of static γ-MN will increase the static firing rate of primary and secondary afferents at the existing static length of extrafusal muscle. Static γ-MN have little effect on velocity responses of spindle afferents during ramp stretch of the muscle. On the other hand, excitation of dynamic γ-MN increases the velocity response of primary afferents to ramp stretch as well as their static response. This latter function serves to rapidly mobilize facilitatory input to α-MN given a sudden, external load disturbance to extrafusal muscle.

Through this indirect system, adjustment of feedback gain to α-MN may be provided throughout the operational range of muscle length with respect to joint movement. Furthermore, this alteration in gain control can be rapidly adjusted upward or downward depending upon the nature of the change in "load" placed on the muscle.

How then does the CNS make use of these

direct and indirect routes to skeletal muscle fibers? Contemporary research supports the view that both pathways are activated simultaneously (α-γ coactivation), thus assuring mobilization of tension without loss of possible background support and servoaction through the gamma loop. Supportive evidence for this coactivation has been found in mammalian respiratory movements, locomotor movements, jaw movements and, in human voluntary finger movements.

Furthermore, recent research suggests that static γ-MN are under greater supraspinal influence than dynamic γ-MN while the reverse seems true of spinal sensory regulation. With respect to known contractile properties of intrafusal muscle fibers and the discharge characteristics of primary and secondary fibers, this functional hierarchical division of gamma control seems reasonable if a variety of movements which vary in velocity is to be supported by the gamma loop.

While there is still much to be learned about descending control of integrative events at the spinal level, the following functional interactions have been observed in animal models. Motoneuronal discharge is, in part, transsynaptically self-regulated by α-MN recurrent collateral(s) which in turn are linked to Renshaw cell(s) forming "internal" feedback loops. The Renshaw cell may inhibit homonymous α-MN, γ-MN, other Renshaw cells, and the inhibitory interneurons that provide reciprocal inhibition to antagonistic muscles via activation from spindle primary afferents located in the prime movers. Superimposed on this network is supraspinal and other spinal segmental afferent convergence on the inhibitory interneuron. Through this mechanism α-γ coactivation appears to be linked to the control of reciprocal inhibiton, that is, the reciprocal inhibiton of antagonists is coupled to the excitation of agonists. This type of relationship is not obligatory, however, and reciprocal inhibition of antagonists may be withdrawn by removal of supraspinal excitation of the inhibitory interneuron or recurrent inhibition of same through the Renshaw cell thus allowing for a greater tendency toward cocontraction. The functional significance of other spinal afferent input (e.g., flexor reflex afferents) to interneurons shared by descending pathways seems to be to alter their functional "states," resulting in a greater variety of output signals to motoneurons. Hence, there is considerable laterality for tension control involving spinal integration through internal and peripheral feedback loops as well as through supraspinal convergence.

Descending Control

Thus far, only allusions to descending control of motor outflow have been made. The remainder of this discussion will deal more specifically with this concern. Where within the CNS is α-γ coactivation elicited and how is this control organized? Access to the direct and indirect motor pathways has been traced to essentially all hierarchial levels of the neuraxis, for example, evidence of monosynaptic or polysynaptic input to gammas and alphas exist for the corticospinal (pyramidal), rubrospinal, reticulospinal, and vestibulospinal tracts. Although more circuitous routes are taken by the cerebellum and basal ganglia or extrapyramidal system, much of this control is also transacted via the corticospinal and subcortical tracts previously mentioned.

Considering descending fibers and specific spinal motor linkages, a generalization that seems to hold is that any central nucleus which is known to directly influence movement will likely have access to the indirect route as well, that is, γ-MN. However, the theoretical notion of α-γ coactivation implies the existence of supraspinal pathways that exert parallel effects on both of these motoneurons, and, logically, also the reciprocal inhibitory interneuron which is linked to the gamma loop through respective primary afferents. Clear evidence of this is seen in the monosynaptic, vestibulospinal activation of hindlimb extensor α and γ-MN of a cat. A reciprocal acting system also seems to exist involving the reticulospinal tract. In the latter case, monosynaptic excitatory convergence is predominantly found on flexor α and γ-MN. In either pathway, there is evidence of facilitation to the appropriate reciprocal inhibitory circuit. This supraspinal organization might be viewed as a forerunner to the "final common pathway" which is more proximally linked to the output side of selected higher integrative circuits.

One of the most direct routes from the cerebrum to α and γ-MN can be traced to pyramidal tract neurons (PTN) located in the motorsensory and sensorimotor cortex (*pre-* and *postcentral gyrus,* respectively). Although the major portion of this corticospinal tract is made up of small, slow conducting fibers, some PTN, presumably the larger ones, gain rapid access to spinal motoneurons through parallel, monosynaptic pathways. These fast descending routes to α and γ-MN have become known as the corticomotoneuronal (CM) and corticofusimotor (CF) systems, respectively.

The frequency of CM linkages increases as the musculature investigated is more distally located; this system is well developed in the hand of primates. It is partly on this basis that the CM system has been functionally associated with fine coordinated movements such as those evidenced in the hand. The CF pathway appears to provide an important additional control over the gain of the system by coactivating the gamma loop. Potentially, this would offset the unloading of spindles in cortically evoked muscle contractions. In agreement with this scheme is the observation that movements most severely impaired following pyramidal tract lesions are those of the fingers.

In investigating cortically evoked inhibition or facilitation on functional groupings of spinal motoneurons, corticospinal input appears to preferentially inhibit α-MN which presumably would play a role in maintaining antigravity posture, for example, extensor α-MN innervating SO fibers. In contrast to this, greater facilitatory input is seen leading to motoneurons serving flexion responses in these postural support areas. These observations have been explained on the basis that for the motorsensory cortex to play a role in initiating volitional movements, tonic antigravity postural mechanisms must first be arrested.

Largely due to the employment of more sophisticated techniques involving cerebrocortical stimulation greater knowledge concerning "input-output coupling" between afferent inflow to cerebral structures and efferent discharge to spinal motoneurons has evolved. Relationships between spinal afferents from peripheral receptors and discrete motor colonies (PTN functionally linked to the same α-MN) have been studied in distal muscle of primates and cats using intracortical microstimulation. The basic method involves recording PTN activity associated with receptive fields of peripheral sensory receptors followed by stimulation of the same cortical area through the recording electrode to determine the potential "coupled" motor effects. To summarize these findings, PTN receive information closely tied to movements of the related joint and the afferents of the target muscle. Skin receptors likely to be excited by the cortically elicited movement also provide excitatory input to these PTN. A long-loop arrangement of this nature indicates that somatic sensory input can provide a direct modulating function of motorsensory output. This transcortical feedback loop may well represent the neurological substrate for sensory responses such as tactile placing and automatic grasping reactions seen in monkeys and humans. Furthermore, these reactions are known to depend on the integrity of motorsensory and sensorimotor cortex.

A major limitation in discerning the functional relationship between higher brain structures and spinal motor outflow has been the technological inability to monitor neuronal responses on a microscale during natural volitional movement. In fact, prior to the 1960s much of what was known about central motor control was based on evidence garnered from anesthetized, immobilized animals. While these techniques unquestionably sharpen our understanding of neuronal networks, the sine qua non is verification that such processes are operative in natural movement.

Numerous experiments have now been conducted in which isolated units in motorsensory cortex, cerebellar, and basal ganglia have been monitored during both slow and fast voluntary arm movements in primates. While the total number of units sampled represent only a small fraction of the large population of neurons found within each structure, many units in the cerebellum (Purkinje cells or deep cerebellar nuclei) and all units in the motor cortex can be shown to discharge "in relation" to either type of movements; that is to say, the unit discharges in temporal contiguity with parameters upon which the movement response is contingent (e.g., EMG or muscle force). A large number of neurons in the basal ganglia (e.g., putamen) seem to discharge preferentially during slow movements. "Movement-related" cells, in some cases, can be seen to anticipate EMG onset by 100 msec or less. Such observations have been loosely interpreted to mean that these cells might serve "movement-initiating" function.

Transcortical feedback loops have been investigated further using the above mentioned techniques. There is evidence to suggest that sensory input of a proprioceptive nature can generate reflexive output from motorsensory cortex in association with learned movements. Furthermore, these cortical reflexes appear to be "gated" on or off by the preparatory set or expectancy of the animal. These findings add further to our knowledge concerning the subtle integration between "willed acts" and what all too often has been categorized separately as "reflexive" behavior.

Cerebellum

With respect to other supraspinal input-output relationships, the cerebellar cortex has received considerable attention in recent years. In contrast to the cerebrum, the cerebellum is relatively a homogeneous anatomical structure whose efferent and afferent pathways have been reasonably well-defined, for example, there is only one efferent fiber projecting from cerebellar cortex, the Purkinje (or Purkyně) cells (PC), and its actions are solely inhibitory. While PC action on other systems is principally through connections with deep cerebellar nuclei (DCN), these cells do have direct access to the vestibulospinal tract. Afferent inflow is from two types of neurons characterized by their terminal endings as climbing fibers and mossy fibers. Climbing fibers are excitatory to PC and mossy fibers are excitatory or inhibitory depending upon the nature of the intracortical polysynaptic linkage employed.

One can identify three mainstreams of contemporary research dealing with cerebellar functions in motor control. These include the cerebellar control of: 1) ongoing limb movement, 2) oculomotor and vestibular interactions and 3) potential *engram* functions relative to the learning of motor events. The following discussion will deal only with cerebellar involvement in ongoing limb movements.

Since cerebellar effects on spinal motoneurons can be excitatory or inhibitory, excitatory influences of PC must be produced through some reversal of action as seen in, for example,

disinhibition or *inhibitory sculpturing*, selective inhibitions of a field of tonically discharging cells (DCN), thereby modulating the discharge of potentially excitatory inflow to spinal motoneurons. Such modulation of α and γ-MN has indeed been shown with reversible nerve blocking procedures applied to either the anterior cerebellar lobe or the DCN. In the former case, cooling of the anterior lobe in a decerebrated cat tends to cause gamma depression with a concomitant increase in muscular rigidity. It has been shown that DCN cooling *(dentate nucleus)* during the performance of continuous and discontinuous movements by monkeys causes disruption of intensity factors such as peak velocity, suggesting in this case, that the dentate nucleus is needed to insure the proper temporal control of force.

Granit has long proposed that the cerebellum performs a "neural switching" function by directing excitation or inhibition into the spinal motoneurons. In his words (Granit, 1970):

For many years the favourite hypothesis of the writer has been that the cerebellum is the main central "compensator" of deviations from a desirable mean of excitability of acting motoneurons, upwards or downwards as the case may be, serving somewhat like a "fly wheel" automatically governing the motor apparatus. It is for this purpose that it receives information, direct and "edited," from sense organs and from the central nervous system. (p. 239)

A leading proponent of this conceptual view is Sir John C. Eccles (1973). Eccles suggested that the command for limb movement is directed from the cerebral cortex. Collaterals from command pyramidal neurons automatically activate brain stem nuclei (e.g., *pontine nuclei*) which inform deep cerebellar nuclei (DCN) and Purkinje cells (PC) of the ensuing or ongoing movements. The movement itself produces a flow of information from various limb receptors to cerebellar hemispheres via spinocerebellar pathways. Hence, the cerebellum receives diverse subsets of information from receptors activated by the movement and from the cerebral cortical controlling centers. In this scheme, the function of the cerebellum is to refine the evolving movement by on-line processing and effect change through the appropriate efferent command either to the spinal cord, to the cerebral cortex through a thalamic relay, or both.

Here again one is impressed with the enormous amount of sensorimotor or motorsensory processing that seems to occur at all levels of the CNS. Furthermore, it seems reasonably established that central motor control is dependent on multiple representation of information, distributed computation, internal as well as peripheral feedback loops, and numerous sites whereby motor commands are potentially modulated. The multiplicity of the system no doubt accounts for much of the recovery of volitional movement evidenced in clinical settings.

Feedback

Interest has been renewed in central feedback modulation of sensory information. Studies of internal feedback mechanisms are characterized by three levels of concern: (1) What compensatory function is served by these circuits if peripheral sensory feedback is disrupted or abolished? (2) Do perceptual-motor adaptations to environmental changes depend on these internalized signals? (3) Do any of these circuits carry with them a perceptual component, such as a "sense of effort?" Attention here is drawn only to the first question.

Much of the renewed interest in internal feedback has arisen from observations of voluntary movements in deafferented primates, that is, they are deprived of all sensory inflow from the extremity. In general, these animals exhibit marked recovery of movements generally employed in locomotion; climbing, reaching, and grasping. Although there are usually considerable deficits in fine finger movements, they nevertheless can learn to control finger opposition and finger pressure as accurately as normals. Deficits seem more notable in extensor muscles than in flexors and there is an apparent inability to maintain constant activity or posture of the affected limb. While these animals appear very visual dependent, the recovered normalcy of their movements is not. Given these observations, one wonders if some other source of feedback which is localized within the CNS and tightly coupled to each motor response is utilized. Circuitry certainly exists in support of this speculation as seen, for example, in anatomical connections between PTN and dorsal column nuclei. Furthermore, PTN have been shown experimentally to exert considerable modulation of sensory information feeding into the lemniscal system.

However, interpreting research of this nature is fraught with difficulty. Alternative modes of cueing, divergent routes of sensory inflow (e.g., via ventral routes), and neural plasticity are only a few of the other suggested explanations accounting for this recovery of voluntary movements.

Historically, it has been the trend to talk of central "efferent" patterning of movement that is closely tied to peripheral feedback. Now neurophysiologists are much more cognizant of the potential sensory functions conveyed through motor pathways themselves. While such notions as centrally patterned movements without (presumably) feedback are not new, in the past they have been typically employed to explain motor functions of the autonomic nervous system or stereotypic acts of lower animals such as bird vocalizations and tail flipping actions of the lobster. Now we see, for example, even in higher order vertebrates that a viable model for locomotor control consists of intraspinal interneural networks which "generate" sequential activation of the appropriate muscles. Hence, whether or not motor control is dependent on, interdependent, or independent of sensory feedback seems largely an academic question.

BIBLIOGRAPHY

ECCLES, J. C. The cerebellum as a computer: Patterns in space and time. *Journal of Physiology,* 1973, *229,* 1–32.

EVARTS, E. V.; BIZZI, E.; BURKE, R. E.; DELONG, M.; and THACH, W. T., JR. Central control of movement. *Neurosciences Research Program Bulletin,* 1971, *9,* 1–170.

GRANIT, R. *The basis of motor control.* New York: Academic Press, 1970.

HUTTON, R. S. Neurosciences: Mechanisms of motor control. In R. N. Singer (Ed.), *The psychomotor domain: Movement behavior.* Philadelphia: Lea and Febiger, 1972. Pp. 349–384.

MATTHEWS, P. B. C. *Mammalian muscle receptors and their central actions.* Baltimore: Williams and Wilkins, 1972.

PAILLARD, J., and MASSION, J. Motor aspects of behavior and programmed nervous activities. *Brain Research* (Special Issue), 1974, *71,* 189–575.

See also MOTOR RESPONSES: SPINAL ORGANIZATION

ROBERT S. HUTTON

MOTOR DEVELOPMENT

Spontaneous motor activity appears at an earlier stage of development in embryos of lower animals than that evoked by sensory stimuli. The motor apparatus of the spinal cord begins to develop prior to the sensory apparatus and the ventral roots myelinate before the dorsal roots in the human embryo. Nevertheless, patterned movement apparently occurs only upon the application of external stimuli in the human fetus.

Prechtl criticized the earlier studies of the reflexology of the human infant, for reflexes were catalogued and often any possible relationship to later development of spontaneous or voluntary movement was left unclear. The notion of the newborn infant as a "brain stem preparation" persists to the present day and is clearly erroneous.

Yet the human infant is clearly more "reflexive" than the older child and adult. The question remains, are the responses obtained by stimulation in the infant clearly separate and distinct from his spontaneous or voluntary behavior, or is there some kind of interrelationship between these two? Thus we might consider the "reflexes" of infancy in another context. Such a reinterpretation may provide further understanding of motor development and give us some clues regarding the role that these elicited responses play in voluntary behavior.

Fetus

It is convenient to begin such an appraisal with the studies of evoked responses obtained in the living human fetus. Ingram and Brown have described certain aspects of fetal behavior. From these studies and those of Hooker and Humphrey, a number of principles of behavioral development emerge:

1. Movements appear initially in head and trunk.
2. Avoiding responses can always be elicited at an earlier stage of development than approach or pursuit reactions.
3. Local reactions emerge from a total pattern behavior, for example, turning of the head alone occurs initially as part of a total reaction involving the whole trunk, and the isolated avoiding responses of lips, tongue and extremities occur initially as part of a generalized reaction described below.

The human fetus becomes responsive to externally applied cutaneous stimuli at 7½ weeks of age. The receptive field then is appropriately around the "snout" (i.e., the perioral region). It then spreads to include the alae of the nose and chin and by 11½ weeks of age most of the trigeminally innervated area is stimulus sensitive. The palms of the hands appear to become receptive at 10 to 10½ fetal weeks of age and the soles of the feet a little later. These receptive fields continue to enlarge so that all of the skin is stimulus-sensitive by 32 weeks.

The earliest response from stimulation of the perioral region (using a fine hair stimulator) consists of a contralateral bending of the head and upper trunk away from the point of stimulation. The response soon enlarges so that more of the trunk is involved in this general bending away reaction and at 8½ fetal weeks this trunkal avoiding reaction may also include opening of the mouth and abduction of fingers and toes. (The significance of these latter reactions will be made clear later.) By 10½ fetal weeks the same head-trunk avoiding response follows perioral stimulation but now the face also turns away as part of this generalized reaction. At 11½ weeks the face may turn toward a stimulus but again only as part of a generalized or total response. The stereotypy of the generalized reaction begins to subside at 13–14 fetal weeks and at this time perioral stimulation may cause the face to turn away without concomitant elicitation of the generalized response. Isolated approach or pursuit movements of the face alone from a tactile perioral stimulus do not appear until around term (rooting reactions).

Thus, a primitive kind of avoiding reaction of head and trunk appears as the earliest elicited response in the human fetus. Head turning as an isolated response emerges from a generalized reaction and adversive movements of the face appear before pursuit or approach movements.

Aside from the isolated movements of the head, those of lips and tongue appear as the clearest examples of local reactions in the developing human fetus and their evolution follows a pattern similar to that of the head. Thus mouth opening and tongue retraction (along with finger and toe abduction) may appear first as part of the general head-trunk avoiding reaction. At 9½ weeks, stimulation of the lower lip may elicit mouth opening alone. At 12–12½ weeks the mouth will close following stimulation of the lips and by 17–22 weeks the lips will also protrude and purse. Retraction of the tongue alone may be elicited at 13½–14 weeks and protraction at 33 weeks. The emergence of lip and tongue movements again demonstrates the principles stated earlier, that is, local reactions develop from a total generalized response, and avoiding responses (mouth opening, tongue retraction) precede pursuit (lip pursing, tongue protrusion) movements.

Movements of the hands and feet as well as the extremities have also been elicited in the human fetus, but these will be discussed later.

Neonate

Haller has suggested a reflex mechanism for some of the early spontaneous behavior in the neonate and young infant. It does seem that the kinetic labyrinthine reflex responsible for the elicited Moro reaction may well play a significant role in the apparently spontaneous abductions and extensions of the arms. It often appears that movements of the head in relation to the body which are actively produced by the infant induce an obligatory posture of the extremities resembling the tonic neck reflex attitude. Reflex mechanisms requiring contact stimulation of the buttocks along with labyrinthine mechanisms certainly contribute to the ability to sit and both quadripedal creeping and later spontaneous standing and walking appear to require the integrity of supporting, placing, and hopping reactions. It is suspected that the early predominant flexion posture of the neonate and younger infant is considerably influenced by cutaneous input from the trunk. It must be reiterated, however, that although reflex mechanisms may play a significant part in the motor behavior of the young infant, it does not mean that his total behavior or indeed his motor behavior is integrated solely at a brain stem level, but rather indicates a greater receptivity and reactivity of the immature nervous system to external stimulation.

To return to the hand and development of prehension: Umansky has provided a concise review of the factors involved. The earlier notion of voluntary grasping somehow emerging from a primitive grasp reflex is clearly outmoded. Yet the infant does display a number of elicited responses of the hand which appear to contribute significantly to the development of voluntary prehension.

As noted above, stimulation of an 8½ week old fetus might result in a generalized head-trunk avoiding reaction associated with opening of the mouth and abduction of the fingers and toes. It is believed that this represents the earliest appearance of avoiding reactions of the extremities which again occur initially as part of a generalized total response. Older fetuses may demonstrate dorsiflexion and abduction of fingers and toes as local avoiding reactions following tactile stimuli of these parts. Flexion of the fingers associated with flexion of wrists and elbows also has been elicited in the fetus and probably is identical to the traction responses described below.

Grasping and avoiding responses of increasing complexity can be elicited in the human infant. Although they emerge in overlapping sequence as the infant matures, avoiding responses to tactile stimuli appear first and their increasingly complex forms antedate the appearance of their groping counterparts.

In the neonate, tactile stimulation of the hand elicits only an avoiding response. This consists of abduction and dorsiflexion of the fingers. By six weeks of age the response is more facile and then may be associated with some flexion withdrawal of the whole upper extremity. With maturation of the infant the response begins to show local signature so that at 12–20 weeks the hand may also pronate and supinate to actually "avoid" contact with the stimulus. Pronation appears first and is prepotent. By 24–40 weeks of age the instinctive avoiding reaction develops in which the hand and arm now make any kind of adroit movement to avoid the tactile stimulus. Visual control is not necessary for production of this reaction.

Grasping

Flexion of the fingers can also be elicited in the neonate. It appears as part of a proprioceptive reaction, the traction response, elicited by passive stretch of flexor muscles at any joint in the upper limb and appearing as a total flexion synergy of the upper limb. Thus, flexion of the fingers occurs along with flexion of wrist, elbow and shoulder.

This proprioceptive response is soon modulated by cutaneous stimuli so that when the baby is four to five weeks old, tactile stimulation of the palm will facilitate the flexion synergy. Eventually (8–20 weeks) a specific kind of tactile stimulus of the palm will trigger flexion of the fingers without evoking the entire flexion synergy. This new response is a true grasp reflex. It itself is further fractionated so that by 16–40 weeks tactile stimulation limited to the palmar surface of one finger will induce flexion of that digit alone. Further modulation of tactile grasping responses occurs at 16–36 weeks when the hand begins an approach orientation to a stimulus with supination being the prepotent movement. By 20–44 weeks an instinctive grasp reaction can be elicited. Visual control is not necessary for this response in which the hand will grope after a tactile stimulating object, adjust to, and finally grasp it.

What role might these reactions have for the development of voluntary grasping in the infant? One may suggest an apparent close relationship. For example, the closed fingers of the resting newborn infant may reflect a kind of postural bias induced by the predominant flexion synergy at that stage. The fingers begin to open more after a month or so when the tactile avoiding response of the hand is more readily elicited. Under natural circumstances the infant does not direct his hand toward an object in the environment until the grasp reflex has developed and his early grasping is contaminated initially by a pronate and later by a supinate approach which may reflect relative postural bias induced by the emerging tactile avoiding and grasping reactions at that stage of development. Isolated finger-thumb opposition does not appear until the grasp reflex itself can be fractionated and eventual dexterous manipulation and shaping of the hand occurs only toward the end of the first year after full development of instinctive grasping and avoiding reactions. The notion that these reactions have some role to play in the emergence of voluntary grasping is further strengthened when one compares the development of prehension in the normal infant with that of the infant or child with a congenital encephalopathy (cerebral palsy). Here the dexterity of voluntary grasp appears directly related to an underlying reflex mechanism; for example, if a traction response is the most complex form of elicited reaction, then his voluntary grasp also appears as a flexion synergy. If a grasp reflex can be elicited yet cannot be fractionated into isolated finger movements, then the child's grasp is limited to a crude palmar grasp with flexion of all fingers in unison.

Yet Bower (1974) has described precocious voluntary grasping in the newborn with direction of the hand toward an object and closure of fingers around it. He has also reported shaping of the hand to the size of the object and finger-thumb opposition in the newborn. Twitchell and others have been able to induce the amazingly complex and dexterous manipulative movements of the hand characteristic of the year old infant at three months of age by delivering tactile stimulation to the hand within the infant's intact visual field. Thus it appears that a combination of tactile and visual stimulation can induce advanced manual dexterity at a time when the infant is barely able to voluntarily direct his hand into the environment toward an object and when the sole reaction to tactile stimulation alone would be a tonic grasp reflex. These findings and those of Bower suggest that the motor apparatus for complex movement is present at birth and under natural circumstances requires some facilitator for its effectuation. This may be a function of the cutaneous pursuit reactions described above. Further evidence for this is suggested in an earlier study in children with hemiplegic cerebral palsy (Twitchell, 1965; 1970). These children were unable to flex a finger alone. When attempt was made to do so, all the fingers flexed in unison as part of a flexor synergy of the arm. The grasp reflex could not be elicited in these children. Yet they could quickly be taught to make these isolated finger movements by proprioceptive facilitation. Thus a different kind of facilitator was substituted for the missing tactile facilitator.

Bower's (1974) studies indicate an ability for the very young infant to project and shape the hand to an object in the environment. The infant at this age does not do it as readily as an infant of five or six months of age nor certainly as dexterously as an infant of 11 or 12 months of age. The newborn then is lacking the trigger or facilitator, one aspect of which appears to be a cutaneous-motor mechanism (the grasp reflex). The more dexterous manipulatory prehension and palpatory behavior of the older infant requires the development of more complex cutaneous-motor reactions (the instinctive grasping and avoiding reactions). Further evidence for the importance of cutaneous input in motor function may be found in the discussion by Umansky of experimental studies in animals of input-output relations and deafferentation.

If the cutaneous reactions we have described have something to do with triggering voluntary movement and refining its dexterity, they also may contribute to certain postural bias during certain stages of development. Thus the pronate approach and later supinate approach of the hand in the five or six month old infant may reflect contamination by the relative preponderance of oriented avoiding and groping responses at that stage. Some residual avoiding response postural bias in terms of slight overpronation of the hand is common in normal children up to five or six years of age.

If the normal infant is relatively more susceptible to stimulation from the environment, the patient with cerebral palsy is even more so. Exaggerated reflex mechanisms, often in conflict with one another, play a large role in the motor deficit. Ingram and Brown have commented on some aspects of this problem. For example, they describe strong extension of legs (supporting reaction) together with dorsiflexion of ankles and toes (avoiding response). Obligatory neck and labyrinthine reflexes may antagonize certain attempts at voluntary movement. Ingram and Brown do not mention, however, the important role of exaggerated avoiding responses lacking the usual balancing effect of their groping counterparts in the motor deficit in cerebral palsy. Thus the patient frequently has difficulty approximating the lips or protruding the tongue. Unopposed avoiding reactions of the hands cause the fingers to abduct too widely when approaching an object, and on contact the hand may bound away. In extreme cases the hand cannot even be extended toward a desired object. In the lower extremities exaggerated avoiding responses of the feet cause overflexion of hips and knees and the foot is not advanced enough. Athetosis appears as a conflict between disequilibrated avoiding and grasping responses.

So far the role of sensory input on behavior has been stressed. Yet the behavior of the infant itself may also affect the response to input. Prechtl has commented on the role of "state" in determining the facility for elicitation of different types of reflexes. We have observed a similar phenomenon in regard to avoiding and groping reactions. Avoiding reactions can be elicited more easily in the irritable and fussy infant, while groping responses are more easily obtained in the placid and contented infant.

Further examples of this input-output relationship at a higher level may be found in other descriptions of behavior cited by Haller and Prechtl. A novel situation may initially induce a more primitive response. Thus the walking infant may revert to quadripedal creeping on first climbing stairs. The older infant when first confronted with a crayon or spoon utilizes a more immature palmar grasp rather than the dexterous prehensile manipulation of which he is fully capable. When food is first offered on a spoon, the infant returns to sucking.

Kaplan's studies of the development of normal praxis appear to document this theme in older children. Here at a still higher symbolic level of function there appears to be an initial dissolution of the kind of motor ability of which the child is capable of using and does use in his natural enviroment. The evolution of praxis recapitulates the developmental sequence from body-bound limb movement to freely projected manual dexterity.

BIBLIOGRAPHY

Hooker, D. *The prenatal origin of behavior.* New York: Hafner, 1969.

Humphrey, T. Postnatal repetition of human prenatal activity sequences with some suggestions of their neuroanatomical basis. In R. J. Robinson (Ed.), *Brain and early behavior.* New York: Academic Press, 1969.

Twitchell, T. E.   On the motor deficit in congenital bilateral athetosis. *Journal of Nervous and Mental Disease,* 1959, *129,* 105–122.

Twitchell, T. E.   Normal motor development. *Journal of the American Physical Therapy Association,* 1965, *45,* 419–423.

Twitchell, T. E.   Reflex mechanisms and the development of prehension. In K. J. Connolly (Ed.), *Mechanism of motor skill development.* New York: Academic Press, 1970.

See also CEREBRAL PALSIES: DEVELOPMENTAL ASPECTS OF POSTURE AND MUSCLE TONE; MOTOR BEHAVIOR IN INFANCY AND EARLY CHILDHOOD; NEURAL MECHANISM IN INFANT BEHAVIOR; PREHENSION IN INFANCY

THOMAS E. TWITCHELL

MOTOR DEXTERITY: MEASUREMENT METHODS

It has long been recognized that the person who works well with his "head" does not necessarily work well with his hands. Accomplishments like shaping a fine piece of pottery, hitting a home run, or operating complex machinery have little to do with intelligence or formal school training. Tests of motor dexterity primarily are used for selecting persons for particular types of jobs or training programs, such as for aircraft pilots, dentists, and machine operators. Tests of motor dexterity usually are included in more comprehensive batteries of tests concerning mechanical aptitude in general.

Types of Motor Dexterity Tests

Among the oldest motor tests are the pegboards designed to measure arm, hand, and finger dexterity. A typical example is the *Stromberg Dexterity Test.* The first part of the test requires the subject to place 60 cylindrical blocks into holes as fast as he can. In the second part, the blocks are removed, turned over, and put back in the holes. Another widely used test is the *Crawford Small Parts Dexterity Test.* In the first part of the test, the subject uses tweezers to place pins in holes and then places a small collar over each pin. In the second part, he puts small screws in place with a screwdriver.

Some tests are designed specifically to test how well the individual can work with tools and small mechanical parts. A typical test of this kind is the *Bennett Hand-Tool Dexterity Test.* The test requires the subject to remove and replace nuts and bolts as quickly as possible.

More complex tests involving hand, arm, and leg coordination have been designed for particular jobs. One of the best known of these is the *Complex Coordination Test,* which the U.S. Air Force uses in selecting pilots. The test employs a partial replica of an airplane cockpit, complete with stick and rudder; lights on a control panel simulate the maneuvers of an airplane. The subject must use the stick and rudder to match the stimulus lights, much as he would steer an airplane.

Characteristics of Motor Dexterity Tests

Most tests of motor dexterity are highly dependent on speed. Consequently, they prove to be better predictors of jobs in which speed rather than quality is important. There are many jobs in which speed is only a minor consideration. The person who can saw a board quickly does not necessarily have the craftsmanship of the skilled cabinetmaker.

An important characteristic of motor dexterity tests is that few of them correlate highly with one another. When the testing task is changed even slightly, it is sometimes found that different abilities are required to master it. For example, the two parts of the Crawford Small Parts Dexterity Test correlate on the average less than .50. A correlation of only .57 was found between the two parts of the Stromberg Dexterity Test. Correlations between different motor dexterity tests usually are even smaller. Factor-analytic studies of motor dexterity tests have generally found few broad common factors. Tests in this area tend to be characterized by specificity.

Because of the small overlap between motor dexterity tests, there are no general measures of motor ability such as general intelligence tests supply for intellectual functions. Motor tests are thus of relatively little use in vocational counseling. They are most legitimately used in vocational selection where the job is simple, requires a definite set of motor skills, and is highly dependent on speed. Among jobs of this kind are those in production line work, sewing machine operation, and packaging.

Motor dexterity tests show at best only moderate predictive validity for most situations in which they are used. However, if they are used in conjunction with other ability tests, they often add a small but important increment to the overall validity of the battery. Motor tests tend to be more valid when they are made to resemble the actual machine or instrument featured on the job. Tests designed in this way are called *job miniatures.* If the job is that of lathe operator in a machine shop, the best motor test would employ a miniature lathe with the same kinds of dials, handles, and controls that appear on the real lathe. During World War II the Army Air Force used a variety of motor tests for the selection of pilot trainees. The Complex Coordination Test, which resembles most closely what the pilot actually does, generally proved to be one of the most valid instruments.

BIBLIOGRAPHY

ANASTASI, A. *Psychological testing* (3rd ed.). New York: Macmillan, 1968.
CRONBACH, L. J. *Essentials of psychological testing* (3rd ed.). New York: Harper & Row, 1970.
THORNDIKE, R. L., and HAGEN, E. *Measurement and evaluation in psychology and education* (3rd ed.). New York: Wiley, 1969.

See also MECHANICAL APTITUDE: MEASUREMENT METHODS

JUM C. NUNNALLY

MOTOR LEARNING THEORIES

Early research on motor behavior was largely directed by the needs of the time, and as a result the turn of the twentieth century witnessed both applied and atheoretical investigations on such problems as the learning of telegraphic language, typewriting, and the related issue of distribution of practice. This work served to identify a number of fundamental problems and constructs in the motor behavior domain, but provided little input for a unifying theoretical interpretation of motor learning. It was not until the 1930s and 1940s that learning theories emerged to provide goals and guides for motor skill researchers. The classical learning theories generated during this period tended to be all encompassing by accounting similarly for animal and human learning. Consequently, the earliest theoretical accounts of motor learning had to be inferred from rather general descriptions of learned behavior.

Thorndike's Theory

Initial motor learning theorizing rested most heavily on the traditional S-R association theories of learning, which assumed that separate discrete responses and their stimuli are linked for performance either by reinforcement or contiguity. The pioneer of the associative position was Thorndike, whose principle tenet, the *law of effect,* postulated that an S-R bond was automatically strengthened or weakened as a function of whether the response was followed closely by a rewarding or punishing state of affairs. Thorndike's research interests included motor learning, and in 1927 he employed the motor task of drawing a line a criterion distance, to conduct a crucial test of his law of effect. Only persons receiving verbal reinforcement reduced error in relation to the target, and Thorndike interpreted the results as evidence for a connection being strengthened as a result of its consequences. Thorndike subsequently modified his views of learning by playing down the role of punishment in the law of effect and by abandoning the *law of exercise* (the effect of mere practice alone). The theoretical rationale behind the law of effect continued to be criticized, particularly regarding the interpretation of reinforcement's role in learning. However, the empirical law of effect remained, and provided a platform for a number of later motor learning studies on knowledge of results. Thorndike emphasized the specific nature of the connection between the stimulus and response, but his postulation of identical elements as a necessary condition for transfer of training was never thoroughly examined in the context of motor skills.

Hull's Theory

The other principal proponent of reinforcement theory was Hull (1943) who developed a sophisticated theoretical system, with a series of postulates to explain components of the learning process. Hull assumed that when an organism developed a need it became in disequilibrium with its environment, producing a drive within itself. When that need was met, drive reduction or drive stimulus reduction occurred. It was the reduction of drive which was reinforcing to the organism, and caused the response or habit to be learned. Thus for Hull learning resulted from need reduction which was dependent upon contiguity of stimulus and response closely associated with reinforcement. Of the sixteen postulates formulated within Hull's theoretical framework, it was the constructs of *reactive inhibition (Ir)* and *conditional inhibition (sIr)* that appeared most relevant to motor learning. According to Hull, mere evocation of any response generated reactive inhibition and the strength of this state was a direct function of the number of contiguous repetitive responses. Reactive inhibition reduced the likelihood of a particular response being repeated, and stimuli associated with the cessation of a response themselves became conditioned inhibitors. Hull's theoretical framework provided considerable impetus for research in motor learning during the 1940s and 1950s. Most of the pertinent studies employed the continuous response demanded by the pursuit rotor apparatus and the research focused primarily on the topics of distribution of practice, reminiscence, warm-up decrement, and the distinction between learning and performance variables.

Although Hull's predictions from theory could be put to the test, owing to the specific nature of his postulates, the theoretical assumptions were still rather general in terms of motor behavior. Later researchers attempted to refine Hull's postulates, notably Ammons (1947) who advanced a miniature theoretical framework similar to Hull's but designed specifically for human motor learning. Ammons's theory never received much attention but the gist of his formulations implied inhibition to be a performance rather than a learning phenomenon. Subsequent research suggested that almost all the performance benefits of distribution of practice could be accounted for in terms of the single inhibitory factor *Ir,* leaving *sIr* to play a negligible role in motor behavior. The majority of constructs emanating from Hull's theory were cast aside by motor behavior researchers in the 1960s, in favor of variables and constructs more directly related to the viewpoint that man operates as an information processor. However, Hull's contribution to motor skills research was substantial.

Guthrie's Theory

In contrast to Hull and Thorndike, Guthrie (1935) found no place for reinforcement in his theory of learning. Guthrie's one law of learning was based on the principle of contiguity, which posited that a combination of stimuli which have accompanied a movement will on their recurrence tend to be followed by that movement. Once the connection had been made by contiguity, no further practice or repetition would strengthen the association. In essence, Guthrie advocated one trial learning but this was misleading as he considered a learning situation to contain a multiplicity of S-R bonds. Repetition or drill was therefore necessary to enable the performer to connect all the bonds in the situation. It was Guthrie's interest in the pattern of movement itself, rather than the response outcome, that had direct implications for the field of motor learning, but his theory provoked little research in an area which tended to be overshadowed by the reinforcement positions of Hull and Thorndike.

The behavioristic associative tradition produced more theoretical positions than those outlined above. Theories with a more limited scope emerged during this early period, notably the Wheeler and Perkins (1932) maturation and stimulation hypothesis and the Snoddy (1926) two-opposed process hypothesis, both related to the distribution of practice problem. Motor learning researchers, however, took few cues from these theories and relied mainly on the formulations of Hull and Thorndike for a theoretical framework. This period was the time of the all encompassing theory, and S-R psychology in providing a number of examples became the backbone for motor learning theorizing.

Tolman's Theory

The other influential school of learning during the 1930s and 1940s posited the S-S cognitive position. This gave a perceptual emphasis to learning, conceptualizing it in terms of the organization of the subjects perceptual systems into a single unit. The main American proponent of perceptual organization as a construct in learning was Tolman (1932). Combining many Gestaltian concepts, he maintained that behavior was goal directed since the organism used environmental supports as guides or cues in achieving a goal, developing a general movement pattern rather than a specific response to a set stimulus. Some years later Tolman anticipated present day theorists by suggesting that one theory may not be able to adequately account for all forms of animal and human learning. As a result he outlined six types of learning, designating the domain of motor learning as fundamentally reflecting the study of motor patterns.

Associationism and Cognitivism

The period 1930 to 1950 produced a number of comprehensive theories of learning, which have been dichotomized under the school of Associationism and Cognitivism. Of the two positions, S-R theory undoubtedly made a more significant contribution to the area of motor learning. It stimulated considerable empirical research in addition to providing starting points for some recent theoretical formulations. However, the S-S cognitive position had more relevance to motor learning than was realized during the period of its inception. Tolman's emphasis on the development of maps or plans for the initiation of a response, and his nonacceptance of the S-R position that a set response is elicited from a specific stimulus, is consistent with modern theorizing. The cognitive influence in the motor learning domain has merely been latent.

An important distinction between the learning schools that has particular relevance for motor learning is their conceptualization of the role of feedback in responding. S-R psychology gave feedback, particularly proprioception, a prominent place in learning, viewing feedback as another stimulus to which responses became conditioned and ultimately learned. This was the basis of James's (1890) response-chaining hypothesis, but it is a position also found in the later associative theoretical formulations. Additionally, proprioception was given secondary reinforcing powers making feedback a powerful learning construct within the S-R framework. In contrast, the S-S position said that once a cognitive map had initiated a motor command, the movement sequence was run off without the requirement of feedback from the periphery. Thus both the *Associative* and *Cognitive* Schools were centralist or open loop in character. Neither gave response-produced feedback a place in controlling *ongoing responding,* and this became a growing criticism. S-R psychology emphasized the role of feedback in learning, but the stimulus response chaining role was very different to that given it by closed loop conceptions of behavior.

Information Processing

Current accounts of motor learning are predominantly closed loop in that they contain the essential ingredients of feedback, a reference mechanism to evaluate the feedback, together with mechanisms for error detection and response correction. The closed loop position originated with cybernetics and grew in status with the development of an engineering psychology domain around the time of the Second World War. This field imported concepts from engineering and communications regarding man as a machine or information processor, who receives information from a variety of sources and processes it to produce a response peculiar to the situation though still lawful to the stimulus present. The basic features common to all information processing models include a series of functional processes with information entering a receptor system, being filtered and coded before being passed to a limited central decision making mechanism which initiates a response through an effector system. Response-produced feedback has a key role within the model, being the basis for the regulation of ongoing movements.

The information processing theorists' major criticism of traditional learning theory was the latter's persistent attempts to account for behavior simply in terms of an association between a particular stimulus and a specific response. They argued that man is not a passive reflex machine springing into operation as a result of previously formed associations or reinforced S-R bonds. Rather, knowledge of results is information which the performer actively processes prior to purposely selecting and initiating the next response. Learning within the closed loop framework is generally associated with more efficient receptors, coding, and response selection mechanisms. How these mechanisms increase their efficiency and develop the capability to elicit and control learned movements, however, has not been the primary research thrust of information processing theorists, despite their original concern for it. Thus the closed loop model provided a framework for systematic investigation of motor performance, but to the exclusion of constructs and variables more commonly associated with motor learning.

Since the early 1960s, researchers in the motor behavior domain have had less cause to borrow or extend theories of learning developed in other research areas because several attempts have been made to construct specific theories of motor learning. These have extended the *closed loop model* by incorporating some elements essential for theory per se, and a theory of motor learning in particular. The Russian influence (Anokhin, 1969; Bernstein, 1967; Sokolov, 1969) has been particularly germane, but like the other closed loop theories generated (Laszlo, 1967; Smith, 1961), the theoretical formulations have been rather ambiguous making operationalization of constructs difficult. The result has been that these theories have no more explanatory power for learned motor behavior than the cybernetic closed loop models.

Adams's Theory

A refreshing exception has been Adams's (1971) closed loop theory of motor learning. This theory is grounded in the large body of data pertaining to discrete linear positioning movements and its theoretical constructs are open to operationalization and empirical test. Extrapolating from ideas originally expressed for verbal learning, Adams postulated motor learning to be the product of two independent states of memory labeled the memory trace and perceptual trace. The memory trace acts like a modest motor program selecting and initiating the response, and its strength is seen as increasing through stimulus response contiguity over practice trials. After the response has been initiated, the perceptual trace operates as a reference or recognition mechanism evaluating response produced feedback from the movement for error detection and correction purposes. This mechanism is defined as a representation

of feedback stimuli obtained from past movements and its strength is a function of the exposure to, and amount of, those feedback stimuli. Over acquisition trials with knowledge of results, the motor response generally becomes more accurate and consistent leading to the development of a dominant or model trace which represents the feedback stimuli associated with the correct movement. At this stage of learning the subject can maintain or even improve performance without knowledge of results because he has learned to associate response feedback with response outcome.

Adams's theory has stimulated more empirical studies on motor behavior than all the other *closed loop theories* of motor learning combined. This is in large part due to the specific and operational nature of the theoretical constructs postulated. However, a theory grounded in data is generally narrow in scope and the advantages gained by this approach are sometimes seen as limitations by theorists who are anxious to develop broader, but more speculative, theoretical positions. This has been the case with the Adams's theory and several attempts have already been made to extend his theoretical postulations for linear positioning to the response class of rapid timing movements. More importantly, the fundamental tenets of the closed loop view of motor learning have themselves been challenged, and the concepts more commonly invoked in this respect are *motor program, efference copy* and *schema*. All of these abstract notions have some empirical history in psychological research, but it is only very recently that they have been shaped formally into a theory of motor learning.

Motor Program and Efference Copy

The concepts of *motor program* and *efference copy* both deny the functional contribution of feedback in motor learning and performance. The motor program hypothesis assumes that a prestructured set of muscle commands can determine the full extent of a movement sequence uninfluenced by response-produced feedback from the periphery. To account for error detection and correction, motor program advocates appeal to the concept of efference copy, which postulates that a higher central system monitors the efferent motor commands issued to a muscle group. Thus von Holst's

(1954) traditional interpretation of efference copy has been extended from merely checking that an eye movement occurred to one of a central mechanism responsible for detecting erroneous response selection. The evidence supporting the motor program and efference copy positions is persuasive but not conclusive, and their advocates rely primarily on the indirect and preliminary findings that animal learning can occur in the apparent total absence of feedback, and that humans can initiate response correction faster than known reaction times.

Schema

The concept of *schema* challenges the way in which a movement command and its sensory consequences are stored and chosen, rather than the way in which a movement is controlled. The traditional learning theories and more contemporary closed loop theories all have specific movement commands and consequences uniquely stored in the brain. In contrast, the schema notion suggests it is generalized abstractions of individual movement sequences and their goals that are stored. Again there is little direct evidence for this position, particularly with respect to motor behavior, but logically it would reduce the storage capacity required of the brain and account for much of the transfer between novel learning situations experienced in every day activities.

Pew (1974) integrated the schema notion of storage representation with all the different modes of movement control to form a multidimensional process oriented model of human perceptual-motor performance. This model showed that different levels and approaches to movement analysis can be integrated, at least on a conceptual level, to form a compatible unified system. Pew considered that such an approach was necessary if a general theory of skill learning was to emerge.

However, as with the earlier models of human performance, Pew's general model lacks many of the elements essential for a theory of motor learning. This void has now been filled by Schmidt (1975) who combined many of the strong features of Adams's closed loop theory of motor learning with the basic concepts of Pew's model to form a schema theory of discrete motor learning. Schmidt organized the movement control concepts of feedback and

motor program with the schema notion of storage representation to form a comprehensive theory of motor learning. The formalization of the schema concept into a theory of motor learning was Schmidt's unique contribution. He postulated that four kinds of information relating to a movement are required to be stored: initial conditions, program specifications, response outcome and sensory consequences. After several movements of the same type have been made, the performer begins to abstract and store the relationship among those forms of information to form a schema or generalized plan. With increased practice under appropriate feedback conditions, the schema becomes stronger and more refined.

BIBLIOGRAPHY

ADAMS, J. A. A closed loop theory of motor learning. *Journal of Motor Behavior,* 1971, *3,* 111–150.

IRION, A. L. A brief history of research on the acquisition of skill. In E. A. Bilodeau (Ed.), *Acquisition of skill.* New York: Academic Press, 1966. Pp. 1–46.

PEW, R. W. Human perceptual-motor performance. In B. H. Kantowitz (Ed.), *Human information processing: Tutorials in performance and cognition.* Hillsdale, N. J.: Erlbaum, 1974. Pp. 1–39.

SCHMIDT, R. A. A schema theory of discrete motor skill learning. *Psychological Review,* 1975, *82,* 225–260.

KARL M. NEWELL

MOTOR MEMORY: LONG-TERM

Long-term memory is memory for events presented days, months and even years ago. Since events are usually rehearsed, reinforced and organized into meaningful material, the capacity of this system is thought to approach infinity (Adams, 1967). Retention intervals are often quite long, where control of learning and interpolated activity is practically impossible. It is fair to say that theories that explain forgetting have been derived from studies of verbal behavior, and have then been applied to motor behavior without much success.

Long-term retention of motor skills has a long history and there have been a number of reviews (Schmidt, 1972) which summarized the relevant literature and traced its theoretical development. The most striking feature of the long-term retention research is that motor skills are well retained. The prevailing opinion is that memory lost is very rapid in verbal learning but that retention lost is minimal in motor skills.

Apparatus and Procedures. The typical procedure in motor retention studies is to have a group of individuals learn a psychomotor task for either a fixed number of trials or to some criterion level. At this point a retention period is introduced during which no practice is allowed. This interval is followed by a retention test which may consist of one or two trials or of some longer designated series. Retention scores indicate the degree of originally learned skill that is remembered or recalled as a function of elapsed time, and these scores can be of two basic types: absolute retention, mean performance level after the retention interval; and relative retention, performance changes from the learning period to the retention period. These methods have been used in the past and have caused some confusion because they have often been used interchangeably.

The type of tasks utilized in motor retention has been extremely varied and consists of such types as the Complex Coordinator, Mashburn, Bachman ladder, pursuit rotor and the rho test. The requirements of these tasks generally stress some form of hand-eye coordination in which precise motor control is developed. Skilled behavior is expressed in numerical values such as correct responses, error percentages, speed of movement, rate of response and time on target. Performance scores during the retention test are then analyzed with alterations in motor memory reflected by changes in means, variances and correlations.

Explanations of Forgetting

Much of the work in motor retention has been concerned with the mechanisms of forgetting and involve tests of the two theories of forgetting: (1) the "trace decay theory," and (2) the "interference theory." The trace decay theory states that losses in memory occur spontaneously as a function of time and are not affected by other learning. On the other hand, interference theory explains forgetting through the interaction of other learned habits which disrupt memory representation. As such, forgetting is a dynamic process and may be of two types: proactive, from items learned prior to criterion learning and retroactive, from items interpolated between criterion learning and recall. Regardless of the type of interference, disruptive stimuli may come from either experimental or intraexperimental events. In both the interference and trace decay theories, competition between traces at the time of recall accounts for memory loss. It is only how the memory representation has been changed that distinguishes between these theories.

Trace Decay. The study of long-term memory has centered on trace decay and interference interpretations to account for memory loss, and inspection of the relevant literature reveals many contradictory findings. For example, investigators using a three-dimensional tracking task, a Bachman ladder, and a pursuit rotor, have all reported findings that indicate nearly no forgetting with retention intervals over one year (Stelmach, 1974). Other investigators have used tasks like a rho test or stabilometer and found evidence that motor skills are moderately retained. On the other hand, several investigators using a procedural task, with and without tracking components, have found that these skills were poorly retained (Schmidt, 1972).

The few studies which found at least moderate amounts of forgetting with no interpolated activity should be considered as in support of the decay theory. Moreover, in the studies where interpolated activity was not explicitly a variable, it can be assumed that motor activities in daily life are potentially interfering acts and may have caused forgetting. Nevertheless, most recall evidence indicates that trace decay has little explanatory power in motor forgetting.

Interference. If one is familiar with the vast verbal memory literature, it would be expected that many studies have been performed which have examined interference theory in motor skills. This certainly is not the case. Most of the experimental data on memory, and the theory derived from it, comes from verbal behavior studies. There have been few studies that have manipulated potentially interfering variables in motor retention. A series of experiments performed by Don Lewis and his associates at the University of Iowa sought to determine the extent to which retroactive interference was the cause of motor forgetting (Stelmach, 1974). In the first of three studies, they varied the amount of original learning on a Mashburn apparatus and then gave varying amounts of interpolated learning trials. In absolute performance terms, forgetting was found to be positively related to the amount of practice on the interpolated task. Subsequent studies by these authors have produced similar findings. It would be somewhat tenuous to generalize the viability of the interference theory based on these findings; particularly, since some of the above interpretations can be altered by plotting retention scores in the mean decrement form. Schmidt (1972) gave several examples of variations in retention measurement that can lead to equivocal interpretations.

The study of proactive interference in motor skills has been even more sparse. Duncan and Underwood (1953) conducted one of the two published studies on proactive inhibition in motor skills. They used a manual task which involved moving a lever to one of six slots and required learning specific sequential pairings. Despite considerable forgetting, no proactive inhibition was found. Schmidt (1968) questioned whether the Duncan and Underwood experiments met the basic conditions of proactive interference and followed his criticism with a proactive interference study and found no evidence of proactive interference. As should be clear from the foregoing studies, interference does not have much more support than the trace decay as an explanation of motor forgetting.

Discrete versus Continuous Tasks

It appears that consideration must be given to the type of task being studied if one wants to explain some of the differential forgetting found in the motor skill literature. Motor skills may be classified in many different ways: fine or gross, simple or complex, and discrete or continuous. Of particular interest for retention is the discrete versus continuous task comparison since it appears to be one factor which determines the amount of forgetting. When a task is discrete (e.g., characterized by a recognizable beginning and ending) compared to one which is continuous (repetitive movements with no definite beginning or ending), differences in retention loss become apparent. Analysis of these tasks revealed that those which are well retained seem not to be dependent upon cognitive decisions concerning what to do in a given

stimulus situation, but rather are concerned with making a well-defined movement correctly or quickly (Schmidt, 1972).

The high resistance of continuous motor behavior to forgetting processes has been thoroughly documented in the laboratory. An experiment by Fleishman and Parker (1962) in which subjects performed on a three-dimensional tracking task nicely demonstrates that the forgetting of complex motor behavior is negligible for intervals up to 24 months. The foregoing findings are not unique. Motor retention literature contains other instances to support this generalization. For example, Bell (1950) found high retention for pursuit rotor performance after one year, and Ammons et al. (1958) found very excellent retention of tracking performance for intervals up to two years. There appears to be no exceptions in the literature to the generalization that continuous motor responses are very well retained for long periods of time.

On the other hand, discrete motor responses appear to be forgotten much more readily and completely than continuous motor responses and are similar in character to the forgetting patterns observed in verbal skills. Duncan and Underwood (1952) used a six-unit discrete motor task that had six colored stimuli and six slots into which the subject moved a lever. The subject had to learn which slot was associated with the stimulus color, and the task was to be performed as rapidly as possible. For performance measured in terms of number of correct responses on a trial, they found forgetting to be a large 82% over a 14 month interval. Similar findings have been reported on discrete tasks like the rho test, lever positioning and in learning sequential operations (Schmidt, 1972).

What explanation can be given for the rapid forgetting of discrete motor responses compared to continuous ones? One intuitive possible reason is the degree of learning. Like verbal responses which are also discrete, the level of original learning for discrete responses may be low relative to continuous motor responses (Adams, 1967). A discrete response with its relative short duration and finite beginning and end probably receives only a very few reinforcements in a given trial. On the other hand, subjects that practice on continuous tasks such as a pursuit rotor may produce up to three responses per second. A second potential explanation is the interference theory of forgetting. It is defensible to consider that discrete motor responses have a verbal component. If so, they would be subject to the same interference sources in the everyday environment as verbal responses (Adams, 1967). A third reason may be that well-learned continuous motor responses like tracking and balancing develop memory traces that are relatively resistant to the forgetting process, and at recall the initial motor movements may fully reinstate appropriate cues.

A methodological reason for the differences has been raised concerning the measurement of error during a trial. In a continuous task, many response errors may occur at recall, but if of short duration, they make relatively little contribution to the total error score for that trial. In a discrete task, the slightest deviation will have a pronounced effect on the recall score. Finally, it has been postulated that continuous tasks are conceptualized to a greater degree so that there is greater "meaningfulness" associated with the movements which enable the subject to rely upon very well-learned principles and relationships (Schmidt, 1972).

Amount of Learning

The concept that increased exposure (practice) to a task will strengthen its memory representation and prevent it from decaying has been postulated for years. This classical reinforcement idea has been incorporated into a number of retention experiments. Ammons et al. (1958) investigated retention of two different motor tasks following different amounts of initial training. After five or thirty trials and rest intervals which ranged from 1 minute to 2 years they found extended practice to be a variable that reduced forgetting. Retention lost was very substantial in both groups with the most forgetting occurring in the group that learned the least. Interestingly, the groups with 30 training trials took longer to regain their lost skill even though their percent loss was less than for groups having only five training trials. A higher level of original training pays off in higher recall level but that which is forgotten is not easily regained when the skill is highly developed. Other studies that used the pursuit rotor, also found recall to be positively re-

lated to the amount of practice (Stelmach, 1974).

When studies vary the amount of practice, the degree of learning is usually left uncontrolled, which can create spurious interpretations due to differences in learning. Recognizing the need to equate subjects in terms of performance levels, Hammerton (1963) utilized two experimental conditions in which all subjects within a group had to achieve certain criterion performance levels. The results of this study indicated that performance achievement was a factor in preventing forgetting. Similar findings have been reported elsewhere in the motor retention literature (Stelmach, 1974). Such studies have utilized several experimental conditions in which subjects had to achieve a designated performance level and comparisons of forgetting revealed that increased performance level reduced forgetting.

Overlearning. Related to studies which have varied the amount of practice are those that examined overlearning. The essential difference between them is that in overlearning studies, a specific criterion performance level is specified and the amount of practice after reaching that criterion is then varied. The extended practice is expressed in terms of percent of overlearning. Evidence from stabilometer performance which examined memory lost for 0, 50, 100, and 200% overlearning conditions found retention, as measured in absolute terms, to be positively related to the amount of overlearning. When retention was calculated using a relative index, only the 200% overlearning condition was found to be resistent to forgetting. Similar studies by others found essentially the same results. Melnick, Lersten, and Lockhart (1972) attempted to determine the effects of overlearning on subjects classified as fast and slow learners over a seven day period and found no recall difference between them using absolute recall scores and mixed findings using a relative difference index. The mixed findings are difficult to interpret due to the potential confounding of amount of practice, level of learning, and ceiling and floor effects.

Ability Levels. In a recent investigation, Carron and Marteniuk (1970) examined the hypothesis that differential forgetting would be evident among subjects differing in initial ability levels. Three layoff intervals were examined (1, 7, 14 days) and there were no differences among the high, average, or low ability groups following the one or seven day layoff. However, a significant difference was present following the 14-day layoff. Inspection of the data revealed that the difference was a result of a slight improvement (reminiscence) in the high ability group combined with a forgetting effect for both the low and average ability groups. In a following study, Carron (1971) examined the high, low, and average subjects of the previous study after a retention interval of two years. After two years the high ability subjects demonstrated less forgetting than the average or low ability groups.

Research

The study of motor retention is not a highly developed research area. Motor research has had a strong alliance with applied psychology and often has asked questions about applied problems rather than basic law and theory; as a result the research has been mostly empirical and nontheoretical. Because of the general opinion that motor skills are not readily forgotten, researchers have not been attracted to this area because they feel there is no theoretical issue to study. As of 1976, there were only a few investigators working in this area and there have only been a few published studies. Nevertheless, psychologists generally agree that psychomotor behavior is best remembered when overlearning is high, interference is low, reinforcement is optimal, and no interpolated activities are present.

BIBLIOGRAPHY

ADAMS, J. A. *Human memory.* New York: McGraw-Hill, 1967.

AMMONS, R. B.; FARR, R. G.; BLOCK, E.; NEWMANN, E.; DAY, M.; MARION, R.; and AMMONS, C. H. Long-term retention of perceptual motor skills. *Journal of Experimental Psychology,* 1958, *55,* 318–328.

BELL, H. M. Retention of pursuit motor skill after one year. *Journal of Experimental Psychology,* 1950, *40,* 648–649.

CARRON, A. V., Effect of ability level upon retention of a balance skill after two years. *Perceptual and Motor Skills,* 1971, *38,* 527–529.

CARRON, A. V., and MARTENIUK, R. G. Retention of a balance skill as a function of initial ability level. *Research Quarterly,* 1970, *41,* 478–483.

DUNCAN, C. P., and UNDERWOOD, B. J. Retention of transfer in motor learning after 24 hours and after 14 months. *Journal of Experimental Psychology,* 1953, *46,* 445–452.

FLEISHMAN, E. A., and PARKER, J. F. Factors in the retention and relearning of perceptual-motor skill. *Journal of Experimental Psychology,* 1962, *64,* 215–226.

HAMMERTON, M. Retention of learning in a difficult tracking task. *Journal of Experimental Psychology,* 1963, *66,* 108–110.

MELNICK, M. J.; LERSTEN, K. C.; and LOCKHART, H. S. Retention of fast and slow learners following overlearning of a gross motor skill. *Journal of Motor Behavior,* 1972, *4,* 187–194.

SCHMIDT, R. A. Proactive inhibition in retention of described motor skill. *Proceedings of the International Society of Sports Psychology.* Washington, D.C., Oct. 1968.

SCHMIDT, R. A. The psychomotor domain. In R. Singer (Ed.), *Movement behavior.* Philadelphia: Lea and Febiger, 1972.

STELMACH, G. E. Retention of motor skills. *Exercise and Sport Sciences Reviews,* 1974, *2,* 1–31.

GEORGE E. STELMACH

MOTOR MEMORY: SHORT-TERM

Short-term memory (STM) is the memory of events that have just been presented; the capacity of this system is thought to be limited. Recall is usually in a matter of seconds and seldom exceeds a minute. Characteristically, information presented in meaningless and rehearsal processes are prevented. The methods employed usually allow strict control of learning periods, intertrial intervals, and difficulty of interpolated information processing. Short-term motor memory (STMM) began about 10 years ago with the overriding theme of making direct comparisons to verbal memory; since that time, STMM has emerged as an area of experimental psychology, that possesses its own theoretical orientations, methodological problems, and empirical controversies.

Adams and Dijkstra (1966) were the first to show that in simple motor movements there was rapid forgetting over short periods of time (0–90 sec), and that increasing the number of reinforcements (1, 6, or 15) reduced forgetting. After it was shown that motor movements demonstrate forgetting with brief delays, interest developed in the basic laws underlying motor memory. Such questions were asked as: What are the causes of forgetting, what movement cues are encoded, and how is this information stored and retrieved?

It is generally agreed that information enters the memory system from one or more of the sensory modalities and is then transformed into some internal code. In the case of movement, stimuli that develop into an internal code may be primarily kinesthetic, as such information may come from joint or muscle receptors. In addition, a record of motor outflow from the brain may be retained. These three sources of information may be further fractionated into various movement characteristics that may be stored in STMM and later used to aid in movement reproduction. Movement characteristics, such as distance, location, direction, rate, and muscular effort are but a few possible examples.

Apparatus and Procedures

Typically, in an STMM experiment, a subject makes a movement with a knob, lever, or a linear slide to a defined target location or through a defined extent. The movement is stopped by some device inserted by the experimenter that coincides with the designated target or extent. After remaining at the target for a brief time (usually 2 sec), the subject returns his arm to the original or some other starting position. After a variable period of time, the subject is then asked to reproduce the original movement extent or target with the device that stopped the previous movement removed. The time between termination of the original movement and the beginning of the reproduction is called the retention interval, which usually ranges from 0–90 sec. On the reproduction movement, the mismatch between the original and the reproduction movements is recorded in deviation units (inches, degrees, etc.). This deviation score is taken to represent the amount of forgetting that has taken place over a given retention interval. Since an STMM experiment usually consists of many trials, the movement apparatus used is designed to provide a variety of different movement amplitudes and target locations.

Dependent Measures

Unlike the recall of verbal items, in which errors are recorded on an "all-or-none" basis, the recall of a movement is recorded in degree of accuracy. The recall movement is compared to the criterion, and the difference between them is recorded. This procedure allows the researcher to utilize one of several types of scores to index forgetting. The recorded deviation scores can be analyzed in the form of either unsigned errors (absolute error), signed error (algebraic error), or within-subject variation (variable error). Inspection of the STMM literature will reveal that each of these dependent measures has been utilized, frequently leading to equivocal interpretations. Since changes in absolute error can arise from changes in constant error, variable error, or a combination of both, it is essential to analyze at least two types of dependent scores to interpret the nature of the forgetting. Much debate has focused on which of the three types of scores it is best to analyze (Schutz and Roy, 1973). One of the perplexing problems in choosing the appropriate dependent measure is that for a given set of data, the types of scores are in complete disagreement.

Very short movements have been known to yield overshooting response characteristics, whereas long movements reveal undershooting characteristics. This reproduction phenomenon has been labeled "range effects" and has been found in a variety of movements. Range effects were first observed in STMM by Pepper and Herman (1970), and since that time they have been found repeatedly in motor memory research.

Range effects appear to have some explanatory power in accounting for some of the conflicting findings between dependent measures. When there is a shift in constant error as a result of delay or interpolated activity, it is essential to know the response set of a given task or movement. A shift in recall error in a positive manner will yield smaller error if the response set was originally negative (undershooting), or it will increase if the response set was originally positive. Thus, if range effects are not considered before interpreting recall error, forgetting scores can be quite misleading.

Explanations of Forgetting

Trace Decay. There have been three main explanations of forgetting that have been utilized to explain forgetting in the STMM. Decay theory assumes that when a criterion act is made, a memory trace is formed which decays spontaneously over retention intervals, thus less discrimination between traces is possible. As a result, there will be greater error at recall.

Because of spontaneous decay, activity prior to learning or interpolated between learning and recall is assumed to be independent of forgetting. In STMM research, it has been found that with unfilled retention intervals, recall gets progressively worse. Due to the type of errors that are generated in movement research, decay interpretations can be fractionalized into two main interpretations: (1) shrinking with time, producing increased undershooting of the recall attempt (Adams and Dijkstra, 1970), and (2) "fading" with time, producing increased variability at recall (Laabs, 1973). Although the evidence is not convincing, it appears that a number of studies have found evidence to support a trace decay interpretation.

Interference. Interference theory views forgetting to be a result of competing responses learned either before or after a criterion item that somehow disrupts memory representation. The interference theory is an active theory, because it is based on the dynamic process of experiencing interpolated events and should be contrasted with the passive decay theory (Stelmach, 1974). The influence of interference theory on motor memory research is easily seen if one inspects the type of paradigm that has been most prominent.

Proactive paradigms. In verbal skills, it is well known that items learned before the presentation of a criterion item can disrupt recall. In STMM, it has been difficult to demonstrate proactive interference, and most studies that have examined prior trials effects have found no proactive interference. The exception is several studies that found proactive interference within a given trial. These studies required subjects to make either 0, 2, or 4 prior responses before making a criterion movement, and then to recall them in the reverse order of presentation. Proactive interference was generated in both the 2 and 4 response conditions and absolute and variable errors increased as a function of the number of prior responses (Stelmach, 1974). These studies demonstrate that proactive interference can be found within a trial under specific experimental conditions. Just what the nature of this interference is and how it operates must await further research.

Retroactive paradigms. The vast majority of studies in STMM have used some form of interpolated activity as an experimental variable. The aim of this research was to document the type of interpolated activity that causes increased forgetting, and the findings have been quite variable. Some studies have shown that interpolated motor activity causes increased absolute error at recall. Others have demonstrated changes in constant error, while still others have found increases in the variability, and some investigators have been unable to demonstrate interference with interpolated motor activity. While an overall interpretation is difficult, it appears that increasing the amount of interpolated activity which is similar to the criterion generates more forgetting. This forgetting generally manifests itself in the form of increased variability (Stelmach, 1974).

Response biasing paradigms. Some interpolated movements that deviate from the criterion response have been shown to produce sizable directional shifts in constant errors at recall. If an interpolated movement is of a greater extent or intensity than the criterion, recall error is influenced in a positive direction. In a similar manner, if an interpolated movement is of lesser extent or intensity, constant error is shifted in a negative manner (Pepper and Herman, 1970).

Directional error shifts at recall have been found by varying the amplitude of the interpolated movement. Other studies have shown that the longer one stays at an interpolated target and the later an interpolated movement is introduced in the retention interval, the greater the error shifts (Stelmach, 1974). It has also been shown that response biasing can be reduced by increasing the number of repetitions and by augmenting the feedback of a criterion movement.

Two views have been expressed to account for this phenomenon, which rely to some extent on the concept of assimilation. Pepper and Herman (1970) have postulated a trace interaction theory in which the memory traces of the criterion and interpolated movements interact to yield a memory trace that is a combination of both. The criterion recall response is therefore made with reference to the altered trace representation, and the directional shift at recall is seen as an assimilation effect. Laabs (1973) views the reproduction of the criterion as being made in reference to an "average" movement and to the criterion trace. Changes in the average movement that result from interpolated movements are seen as responsible for shifts in recall errors. With forgetting, more emphasis is given to the average movement and that there will be an assimilation toward a central distance or location.

Response biasing effects have also been explained in terms of the relative decay state (memory trace strength) between movements. This trace interaction view states that the weaker a given trace is relative to a stronger one, the more response biasing will occur. On the other hand, the stronger a trace is compared to a weak one, the less response biasing will occur (Stelmach, 1974). In data from studies that have manipulated time at an interpolated target, the temporal occurrence of an interpolated movement and the feedback associated with it have generally been in support of this explanation of response biasing.

While response biasing has been observed many times, it is not known what its localization is. Existing theory provides some broad insight into response biasing, but does not pinpoint the mechanisms involved. Of the three theories postulated to explain response biasing, there are few if any differential predictions between them. Current research is beginning to provide better insight into response biasing, and future research will hopefully discriminate between existing theories.

Limited Processing Capacity. The fundamental assumption behind this view is that there is a limit to the amount of information that can be processed in the short-term system. When the amount of information processed exceeds the system's capacity, items are displaced and are lost, because they cannot be transferred to permanent memory. Procedures are used that attempt to occupy the available capacity by requiring performance on the second task.

Posner and Konick (1966) were the first to utilize a channel-processing model in a STMM paradigm by varying interpolated task difficulty. Digital pairs were presented in which the subject had to record, add, or classify pairs into high or low, and odd or even categories. Forgetting was not found to be a function of interpolated task difficulty. Similar findings have been obtained in other studies that employed interpolated movements when task difficulty was varied between 2.3 and 10 bits/sec without finding it to affect STMM.

Some studies have attempted to isolate the information cues utilized in motor memory

and document their information-processing requirements. The procedures utilized made either distance or location information unreliable and then required movements to either a terminal location or to a certain distance. Using these procedures, it has generally been found that location information does not decay unless information-processing activity is introduced during the retention interval. In contrast, distance information research is equivocal. Some studies show distance is not as accurately recalled and demonstrates rapid forgetting over short periods of time without processing activity (Laabs, 1973), whereas others show findings identical to location information (Stelmach, Kelso, and Wallace, 1975).

The foregoing findings of Laabs (1973) led him to propose a two-component model of STMM to account for differences in recall accuracy between distance and location information. He proposed a kinesthetic memory code for distance information that is subject to spontaneous decay, and a central memory code for location that is subject to forgetting only when rehearsal is blocked. Of the research in STMM some has supported Laab's view of separate modes of storage while some has not (Stelmach, 1974).

Information Cues that Underlie Control. As STMM research began to develop some conceptualization, it became obvious that if motor memory was to be understood, it was imperative to examine how movement information was stored and retrieved. This orientation led investigators to attempt to isolate movement cues, so that their retention characteristics could be examined.

Distance versus location cues. Of the potential cues, end location and distance moved have been the most commonly manipulated. At issue in these investigations was to pinpoint the type of kinesthetic cue that is encoded by the subject and later used at recall. The original striking feature of these experiments was the finding that distance and location cues yielded differential retention characteristics. Location cues were well retained and it was only when information-processing activity was introduced that forgetting did occur. In contrast, distance information tended to yield larger errors and decayed spontaneously over retention periods regardless of whether information-processing activity was present. In addition, some studies have shown that when distance plus location cues were present, recall was not any better than when just location cues were available (Marteniuk, 1973).

Active versus passive. Another source of movement information, not generally included in the study of movement retention, arises from the efferent command to the muscles. One way of studying the contrast between properties of efferent and afferent codes is to compare the retention of movements that are actively and passively presented to subjects. In these types of studies, active conditions require subjects to actively move to a designated point or until the movement is stopped. In the passive condition, the subjects allow the to-be-remembered movement to be completed without their voluntarily contributing to the movement. Such studies (Marteniuk, 1973) have shown that active movement not only results in better immediate reproduction, but that it is also retained better than passively induced movement. These results have been interpreted as meaning that codes resulting from efferent information are more precise and have superior retention characteristics than those codes arising from afferent information.

Feedback. Presumably, to accurately recall a movement requires a memory trace about a past movement and immediate ongoing feedback from the responding limb. The strength of a given trace is thought to be a function of the amount of feedback and the exposure to it. Adams, Goetz, and Marshall (1972), using various combinations of augmented feedback (vision, audition, and heightened proprioception), demonstrated that forgetting in STMM is related to the amount of feedback available. Augmented feedback yielded smaller recall error at immediate recall, and reduced forgetting over periods of delayed recall. Similar data have been found in other studies, and support the view that a strong trace provides accurate recall and is relatively more resistant to forgetting. While the foregoing studies support the view that augmented feedback markedly reduces error, they do not delineate the relative contributions of each modality to trace strength. The data do indicate, however, that vision is relatively more important in strengthening the movement trace than either increased auditory cues or heightened proprioceptive cues.

Recognition Paradigms

In some experiments, investigators have not asked subjects to recall movements but rather have asked them to make a forced choice as to whether the second movement differs from the first. This procedure has been categorized as a recognition paradigm, since the subject has to recognize a movement rather than produce one. Typically, the second response varies from the first by either ±5, ±10, or ±15 degrees, and the recognition score is recorded as a percentage of correct choices given. The results have shown that recognition error increases over time as with the reproduction method, but that the amount of forgetting is much smaller (Adams, Goetz, and Marshall, 1972). Employing identical procedures, others have examined the effects of feedback and practice on the subject's ability to recognize and correct movements. Both were found to be effective in error detection and correction, provided that vision was one of the feedback channels. These results compare favorably with reproduction measures. While recall and recognition procedures require different behavior on the part of the subject, there appears to be little discrepancy between them, suggesting that they may have identical retention characteristics.

BIBLIOGRAPHY

ADAMS, J. A., and DIJKSTRA, S. Short-term memory for motor responses. *Journal of Experimental Psychology,* 1966, *71,* 314–318.

ADAMS, J. A.; GOETZ, E. T.; and MARSHALL, P. H. Response feedback and motor learning. *Journal of Experimental Psychology,* 1972, *92,* 391–397.

LAABS, G. J. Retention characteristics of different reproduction cues in motor short-term memory. *Journal of Experimental Psychology,* 1973, *100,* 168–177.

MARTENIUK, R. G. Retention characteristics of motor short-term memory cues. *Journal of Motor Behavior,* 1973, *5,* 249–259.

PEPPER, R. L., and HERMAN, L. M. Decay and interference effects in the short-term retention of a discrete motor act. *Journal of Experimental Psychology,* 1970, *83* (2, part 2), 1–18.

POSNER, M. I., and KONICK, A. F. Short-term retention of visual and kinesthetic information. *Organizational Behavior and Human Performance,* 1966, *1,* 71–86.

SCHUTZ, R., and ROY, E. A. Absolute error: The devil in disguise. *Journal of Motor Behavior,* 1973, *3,* 141–154.

STELMACH, G. E. Retention of motor skills. *Exercise and Sport Sciences Reviews,* 1974, *2,* 1–26.

GEORGE E. STELMACH

MOTOR PERFORMANCE: ATTENTION DEMANDS

Theorists have adopted an information processing framework for the study of human movement (Keele, 1973; Pew, 1974). The intent is to explain performance with general principles that deal with central processes—for example, memory storage and retrieval—as opposed to peripheral task-specific findings. The type of questions asked about motor control often focus on central phenomenon such as the coordination of internal codes, the time-course of preparation, and the operation of motor programs. This approach contrasts with task-based analyses and with the learning theory approach to movement developed in the 1930s. The *information processing* perspective is an outgrowth of study begun near the end of the nineteenth century. In this period, for example, psychologists utilized *reaction time* to isolate stages of mental processing, explored the nature of voluntary movement, and studied man's ability to perform two tasks simultaneously. However, these interests were brushed aside early in the twentieth century and were not again pursued actively until the end of World War II. Then, in the 1950s and 1960s, experimental psychologists turned to mathematical information theory as a possible framework for describing the time needed to respond to external signals. The notion that man possesses some type of central system with limited capacity was advanced to explain man's frequent inability to respond independently to more than one external signal. As a consequence, locating and characterizing decision bottlenecks became a major concern. Attempts to use *information theory* to specify a fixed human information processing capacity proved unsuccessful. However, the conceptual and methodological advances made with the information processing perspective have fostered more detailed and sophisticated study of internal cognitive processes.

Within the information processing approach, the human performer is viewed as an adaptive information processing system (Posner and Keele, 1973). Operations for such a system may be described both by *time limitations* and by *demands for processing space* within some central mechanism of limited capacity. Time lags in performance are well-documented and,

in addition, given experience with the complicated machinery of our times, relatively intuitive. We are aware, for example, of the time needed to press the car brake in response to a traffic signal. The focus here is on the demands for processing space—commonly labeled attention demands—associated with human movement. Although attention demands may seem less intuitive than time demands, we are aware of the difficulties involved in performing two tasks together and may question the possibility of timesharing specific skills (e.g., walking and chewing gum). Operations which require attention may be equated with "conscious" operations.

The first section of this article considers methodological issues in measuring attention demands. The next two sections review the extent and nature of attention demands during two different subsets of movement: (1) single movements and (2) continuous movements. The final section discusses practical applications.

Measuring Attention Demands

Since two tasks which simultaneously require access to the limited capacity system often interfere with one another, leading to degraded performance on one or both tasks, interference techniques provide a convenient means for measuring attention demands. Although there is some evidence that attention demands may be indexed by physiological measure (Kahneman, 1973), emphasis will be placed on behavioral measures. Some studies require simultaneous performance on two different continuous tasks. Here performance on both tasks is often degraded in relation to control performance on each task performed individually. However, it is usually possible to pinpoint attention demands more exactly when one task, designated the secondary task, is employed specifically to measure attention demands during another primary task (Kerr, 1973). If secondary task performance measured during a primary task is poorer than control performance on the secondary task alone, the primary task is said to require attention. If secondary task performance during the primary task is equivalent to control performance, the primary task is said to be automated. Performance on the secondary task may be used to compare attention demands for the different components of a primary task—for example, comparing demands during initiating as opposed to terminating a movement to a target. In addition, performance on the secondary task may be used to compare two levels of difficulty for a primary task—for example, comparing demands for driving a car in shopping and residential districts.

Continuous tasks such as tracking, discrete tasks such as pressing a key in response to a tone, and signal detection tasks such as detecting a specific letter in a brief visual display have been used as secondary tasks. Choice of secondary task depends upon the type of primary task to be measured. The secondary task should not influence performance on the primary task. Ideally, scores on the primary task in the dual task setting should equal scores in a control situation without the secondary task so that the secondary task scores measure attention demands during *normal* primary task performance. For this reason, payoff strategies favoring the primary task are often used to encourage subjects to give priority to the primary task. In addition, secondary tasks that interfere structurally with the primary task should be avoided. Structural interference is thought to occur whenever two tasks place incompatible or excessive demands on specific perceptual, memory, or response systems. Obviously, it is unreasonable to ask subjects to respond to two different signals with the same limb. However, it is probable that more subtle forms of structural interference occur. For example, tasks requiring the visual system and tasks requiring spatial representation are known to interfere. In general, two highly similar tasks appear more apt to interfere structurally than two dissimilar tasks.

Attention Demands During a Single Movement

A number of movements involve merely the displacement of a limb from one position to another. For example, lifting a cup from the table to one's mouth, pushing a brake pedal, and moving a stylus from a center target to a side target are single movements. A single movement to a target endpoint has two distinct component phases: (1) the reaction time phase between the signal to respond and response

initiation and (2) the movement phase between response initiation and actual contact with the target endpoint. As a rule, attention demands prove higher during the initiation phase and first portion of the execution phase than during the final portions of the execution phase. However, demands may increase toward the end of the execution phase if the movement requires a controlled termination, such as a landing. Attention demands during the initiation phase vary with the number of possible alternative targets and prove independent of precision requirements in the ensuing movement. However, during the execution phase, attention demands are independent of the number of choices at initiation and vary with the precision requirements. Moving to a narrow target proves more demanding than moving to a wide target. In some cases, a movement into a physical stop (no precision requirement) proves to be automated. Automation occurs when the movement itself is constrained by the apparatus so that the subject's task is merely to execute force until reaching the stop. However, unconstrained movements to a stop may require attention. Even a single forward armswing takes attention. It appears that few movements are automated but that it is not movement per se that requires attention. Attention demands during movement may be related to the monitoring and correction procedures required to maintain movement along a prescribed path and/or to terminate movement at a precise location (Keele, 1973).

Attention Demands During Continuous Movements

Many skills involve an ongoing continuous movement or patterned sequences of discrete movements. However, both the difficulties inherent in identifying commonalities among these tasks and the problems in identifying and isolating component stages within these tasks have hampered study in this area. Three categories of continuous movements are discussed briefly. Some continuous skills utilize movement patterns or sequences that are repeated periodically; walking, swimming, and bicycling are common examples. While some may argue that well-learned skills of this type are automated, the evidence available is largely anecdotal. The question remains to be tested experimentally.

A second category of continuous skill involves patterns of discrete movements made in response to a series of discrete signals. Sight-reading music, typing from a manuscript, and pressing keys in response to a series of lights are examples of such continuous patterns. Attention demands in these tasks reflect the number of possible signals and the time-pressure for responding. Another consistent finding is that attention demands are lower in tasks with signal redundancy or sequential dependencies than in tasks with completely independent signals. In fact, a secondary task may force differences between redundant and nonredundant primary tasks whose scores prove equivalent without the secondary task (Welford, 1968; Kahneman, 1973). It is likely that tasks with predictable events require less attention than tasks with unpredictable events because subjects are able to access information about subsequent events without interfering with the response in progress (Keele, 1973).

A third category of continuous skill includes visually guided behaviors such as driving a car and pursuit tracking, which require monitoring a changing visual display and making appropriate motor corrections. Manually tracking itself proves attention-demanding and demands reflect task difficulty. For example, tracking with aided-acceleration control is less demanding than tracking with unaided-acceleration control. In tracking-monitoring situations, one may react both to expected (anticipated) and unexpected (unanticipated) events. Surprisingly, expected changes may prove more demanding than unexpected ones. This suggests that it is possible to focus or direct attention for expected signals. If a person knows he must make a signal-dependent movement change, his attention is directed toward receiving the necessary information and he may be slow to direct attention to another signal (Klein, 1976).

Practical Questions

A recurring theme in the study of attention demands is automatization. Does the skilled machinist automate all or part of his movements in order to work more efficiently? Does the skilled athlete automate movement patterns in order to devote more attention to other aspects of performance, such as analyzing an opponent's position and formulating strategy? The answer is largely unknown. A limited subset of movement, constrained movements to a stop, have proved to be automated. In addition, we know that both skilled pianists and typists may timeshare performance under special circumstances in which stimulus-response pairs are highly compatible and stimuli do not share a common input modality (Shaffer, 1975). However, advancing our understanding beyond task-specific findings will require insight into both (1) the degree to which specific components of executing, monitoring, and correcting movements require attention and (2) the mechanisms responsible for allocating attention in performance (Kahneman, 1973; Keele, 1973).

Does the actual learning of a new skill demand attention? One study raises the interesting possibility that performance on a second task may interfere with performance, but not learning, for a primary task. Eysenck and Thompson (1966) found that pressing a foot pedal in response to a secondary signal interfered with concurrent pursuit rotor performance. However, subsequent rotor performance was not impaired. This result is consistent with the finding (Pew, 1974) that subjects may learn a pattern without being aware they are learning. However, it would be premature to conclude that, in general, learning fails to require attention.

One principle in designing equipment is to minimize attention demands for the human operator. Attempts to find a *single* secondary task suitable for serving as a "yardstick" for comparing attention demands across different primary tasks have often been unsuccessful because the secondary task interacts differentially with different primary tasks as the result of different structural limitations (Kahneman, 1973, chap. 10). However, specific results have concrete applications for establishing display panels and manual controls to minimize attention demands in military and industrial tasks (Welford, 1968). In addition, consideration must be given to the operator's ability to work efficiently. Both the ability to shift the focus of attention quickly when necessary and the ability to combine secondary task performance with a primary task may serve to predict future success in skills such as driving a car and flying a plane.

Application in sport suggests (1) minimizing the attention demands for one's own performance and (2) attempting to maximize demands placed on one's opponents. Presumably, skilled performers have learned to minimize their own attention demands by taking advantage of redundancy and sequential dependencies within a game itself and a specific opponent's style of play. They also generate high attention demands for opponents by minimizing predictability in their own play.

BIBLIOGRAPHY

EYSENCK, H. J., and THOMPSON, W. The effects of pursuit rotor learning, performance and reminiscence. *British Journal of Psychology*, 1966, *57,* 99–106.

KAHNEMAN, D. *Attention and effort.* Englewood Cliffs, N.J.: Prentice-Hall, 1973.

KEELE, S. W. *Attention and human performance.* Pacific Palisades, Calif.: Goodyear Publishing, 1973.

KERR, B. Processing demands during mental operations. *Memory and Cognition,* 1973, *1,* 401–412.

KLEIN, R. M. In G. E. Stelmach (Ed.), *Motor control: Issues and trends.* New York: Academic Press, 1976.

PEW, R. W. Human perceptual motor performance. In B. H. Kantowitz (Ed.), *Human information processing: Tutorials in performance and cognition.* Hillsdale, N.J.: Erlbaum, 1974.

POSNER, M. I., and KEELE, S. W. Skill learning. In R. M. Travers (Ed.), *Handbook of research on teaching.* Chicago: Rand-McNally, 1973.

SHAFFER, L. H. Multiple attention in continuous verbal tasks. In P. Rabbit and S. Dornic (Eds.), *Attention and performance V.* London: Academic Press, 1975.

WELFORD, A. T. *Fundamentals of skill.* London: Methuen, 1968.

See also MOTOR PROGRAM; REACTION TIME AND CHOICE; SKILLED MOTOR PERFORMANCE: ANTICIPATORY TIMING

BETH KERR

MOTOR PERFORMANCE: MOTIVATION

What "moves" people to select the motor activities they do, and to engage in them with vigor and persistence is a question of the field known as the psychology of motivation. This field examines factors within the individual that initiate activity and determine the long- or short-range goals to which the activity is directed.

Therefore, motivation is defined as an internal factor that arouses, directs, and more importantly, integrates a person's behavior. Motivation, like other psychological constructs, is not observed directly but, rather, is inferred from goal-directed behavior or may even be assumed to exist to interpret behavior. Motivational constructs, whether they be called drives, needs, or motives, are assumed to underlie behavior, for without them, behavior would either not occur, or if it did, it would be random or purposeless. As with other behaviors, motivation is implicitly assumed when learning motor skills. Many contend that motivation determines the extent of learning, and in turn may be a product of learning.

The behavioral focus of the present review is primarily confined to human motor performance. The approach will be to review relevant material located within the various theoretical frameworks of motivation. The first three behavioristic theories encompass most of the research done to date in the area; the last, a cognitive theory, has a limited research base, but represents a growing research interest.

Learning Theory

The study of motor performance has long been influenced by the behavioristic tradition. Terms such as drive, activation, and arousal are behavioristic constructs used to describe the intensity dimension of behavior. Many definitions for these terms can be found, but the commonalities among them have led motor performance investigators to use the terms interchangeably. However, these terms take on more specific meanings, if for example, the drive contains a particular goal, or if drive reduction is assumed to be rewarding.

Within the framework of learning theory, specifically the punishment paradigm, a series of response-time experiments were undertaken in the early 1950s in the research laboratory of Franklin M. Henry. A drive was created in some of these experiments by the administration of a noxious stimulus or *stressor,* such as electric shock, loud noise, or bright lights. The onset of the drive stimulus was relevant to the stimulus-response-reinforcement contingencies. The empirical *law of effect* recognizes that reduction of noxious stimulation following a response is reinforcing; such may be the case when no electric shock is applied if the subject's responses are faster than his own average. Subjects motivated in this way demonstrated significant gains over control groups on a variety of speed of movement tasks. Although all groups improved in performance, these gains were always greater when the stressor was contingent upon performance than when stressors were unrelated.

The effects of motivational transfer were investigated in another series of experiments. Subjects first practiced a coordinated movement, then subsequently practiced a simpler, but different movement, and finally were retested on the original coordinated movement. The experimental group differed from the control group in that a stressor was administered for slow responses on the simpler intermediate movement. This manipulation resulted in enhanced performance for the experimental group, while controls failed to exhibit any significant transfer. Motivational transfer was in some cases retained by subjects up to seven weeks before retrogressing toward their initial speed of movement.

Drive Theory

Although these early response-time experiments were designed to manipulate drive strength, its relationship to the directional aspect of behavior was not clearly specified. The direction of behavior, referred to by the theoretical construct of habit strength, enabled investigators to overcome this deficiency by permitting a priori predictions as to the direction in which the response would occur. As expressed in Hull's formula:

Behavior = Drive Strength X Habit Strength

The theory postulates that although the individual may be motivated to act (high drive), he may not act unless the habit is sufficiently well established though numerous associations of contiguous S-R connections. Any strong stimulus, the reduction of which is reinforcing, should increase the probability of the dominant behavioral response at the time. Early stages of skill acquisition presumably contain dominant responses that are incorrect, whereas later, as the skill is mastered through

practice, the dominant response becomes the correct response. Therefore, a positive linear relationship should exist between drive and performance when the correct response is well established. The exact relationship is less clear, however, when the incorrect response is dominant. In this case, heightened drive may not further impair performance, but it may suppress the rate of skill acquisition. Studies examining arousal effects during learning as compared to the performance of a motor task have reported findings that are sometimes conflicting (Martens, 1974). Elsewhere, Martens (Cottrell, 1972) has shown substantial support for drive theory predictions by finding that arousal induced by an evaluative audiences' observation of subjects' performance significantly impaired learning, but facilitated performance of a coincident-timing motor task.

In the motor performance literature, the most prevalent procedure for manipulating drive strength has been to determine the subject's emotional responsiveness, measured on the Manifest Anxiety Scale, and then compare the motor performance of high-anxiety and low-anxiety subjects. In reviewing this area, Martens (1974) was unable to muster definite experimental support for the drive theory hypothesis. The inconsistent support for drive theory is not surprising, particularly where obvious methodological inadequacies were apparent in many of the studies reviewed.

Another drive theory approach has been to examine motor performance on the same task, with intervals ranging from several hours to several days interpolated between original practice and recall. Using an achievement drive aroused by task instructions, Eysenck conducted several studies (Martens, 1974) and found that high-drive subjects showed greater reminiscence than low-drive subjects on mirror-tracing tasks, but not for reaction-time tasks. *Consolidation theory* has been used to explain the greater reminiscence of high-drive subjects. This theory maintains that high drive during practice will result in a more "robust" activity trace, resulting in greater long-term memory. Although not examining reminiscence per se, Sage and Bennett (Martens, 1974) have shown support for consolidation theory when subjects were retested one day later on a pursuit rotor. These results and those of other investigators have consistently been obtained only when the administration of electric shock was related or contingent upon past performance.

The inconsistent support for drive theory is understandable, since there have been few attempts to provide manipulation checks for the occurrence of drive, and even more serious has been the complete absence of a priori specification of habit strength for a given task. The determination of habit hierarchies for motor tasks may be impossible at present for continuous-type tasks which involve a sequence of often unidentifiable responses. Habit-strength determination for other types of motor tasks is possible, but as Hunt and Hillery (1973) have shown, motor tasks need to be redesigned and measures operationalized in terms of drive theory predictions. These less complex tasks include serial and discrete tasks involving speed and/or power of motor responding (Hokanson, 1969), or a single qualitative response to a goal or target (e.g., archery). Further research into the determination of habit strength for different motor tasks is needed before recommending that investigators abandon any further examination of drive theory predictions for human motor performance.

Activation-Arousal Theory

The most popular motivational framework in which to examine motor performance has been arousal-activation theory. Activation is the degree of energy release of the organism, which varies on a continuum from deep sleep to high excitement. This energy can be measured centrally by means of an electroencephalogram, but is more commonly inferred from peripheral measures of arousal, such as muscle tension or heart rate. Whereas many drive theorists assume that behavior is aroused and directed to achieve drive reduction, activation theorists assume that behavior is aroused and directed toward some kind of "balanced" or optimal state. For a given organism at a given time or setting, their past experiences have determined an *activation level* that is optimal, and the organism will be motivated to maintain that state. The degree of deviation from this optimal state will effect the degree of activation and its direction; and hence, should lead,

ceteris paribus, to an inverted-U-shaped relationship between arousal and task performance, a variation of the Yerkes-Dodson law. If activation is too low, as in a drowsy or less alert state, performance will be poor; likewise, if activation is in excess of the individual's optimal state, ineffective performance also occurs. This deterioration in performace is perhaps due to overcompensatory actions or to a narrowing of the range of cue utilization. Support for the hypothesis is shown in studies reviewed by Hokanson (1969). These studies indicated that maximum performance on a tracking task, and the fastest reaction-times were found at intermediate levels of arousal which was inferred from muscle action potential and skin conductance.

Yet another approach to this problem has been to examine motor performance on a variety of motor tasks as a function of *trait anxiety.* Martens' (1974) review indicated that the findings were equivocal, perhaps because trait anxiety only indicates a predisposition to respond with greater arousal, provided the situation encountered is stressful. For example, Martens and Landers (Martens, 1974) examined the tracking performance of boys selected from three different trait anxiety levels, and exposed to three levels of a situational stressor. The *inverted-U hypothesis* was supported separately for trait anxiety and situational stress—moderate groups made fewer performance errors than their respective high and low extremes. Surprisingly, each effect was independent of the other. Manipulation checks indicated three distinct levels of situational stress were created, but neither questionnaire nor physiological measures substantiated the creation of three distinct levels of trait anxiety. The difficulty in finding clear support for individual differences in laboratory studies has prompted some investigators to examine more extreme forms of stress found in naturalistic settings. Epstein's (Martens, 1974) field experiments of experienced and novice sport parachutists is a case in point. Epstein found that before a jump, heart rate and respiration rate rose steadily, but a few minutes before the jump, the more proficient, experienced jumpers, more so than the novice jumpers, began to reduce their arousal level to a more moderate level. Hence, a moderate arousal level was more predictive of subsequent performance, which was rated technically correct.

A third paradigm in which the inverted-U has been examined are studies manipulating levels of *induced muscular tension (IMT)*. This is done by requiring subjects to squeeze a hand dynamometer at varying levels of intensity while performing a motor task with their dominant hand. In general, these studies fail to show clear support for the inverted-U hypothesis. Exemplary of these studies is a 1968 study by Marteniuk (Martens, 1974). In this study, subjects with the fastest responses on a reaction-time task were observed at a tension level intermediate among the five varied. However, movement-time did not indicate a curvilinear relationship between IMT and performance; instead increasing tension levels resulted in a linear trend toward slower movement-time. Marteniuk's results, and others like them, suggest that important task characteristics may mediate the arousal-performance relationship. This possibility has been suggested by Fiske and Maddi (Martens, 1974), who argue that the range of optimal arousal is much broader for performance of simple tasks than for complex tasks. The task factor has yet to be examined for human motor performance, but some support is noted in the animal literature. After the introduction of a stressor, the speed with which rats swam through mazes of varying difficulty showed support for Fiske and Maddi's supposition (Broadhurst, 1957). Other investigators (e.g., Naatanen, 1973) reconcile the inconsistent IMT findings by arguing that the relationship between arousal and performance is a positive linear function, and the downward slope of the inverted-U curve "is an artifact of relatively uncontrolled behavioral direction, as well as the ecological unrepresentativeness of such experiments" (p. 155). Thus, it was suggested that the additional demands of squeezing a dynamometer, rather than the increase in the level of activation caused by it, may have contributed to the performance decrements.

Other studies by Levitt and Sjoberg (Gutin, 1973) have also found that intermediate levels (e.g., heart rate of 115 and 145 bpm) of *exercise-induced activation (EIA)* produced faster responses, regardless of whether the task was simple or choice reaction-time. However, comparisons between studies prompted Gutin (1973) to conclude that motor steadiness tasks requiring considerable inhibition are performed at very low levels of EIA, whereas disinhibition tasks (e.g., arm speed) are performed best at very high levels. Although these and other motor task parameters have been advanced as post hoc explanations of some of the disparities in tests of the inverted-U hypothesis, at present these explanations are not testable. That is, they lack the conceptual clarity necessary for a priori specification of the conditions under which the inverted-U relationship will or will not occur.

Expectancy-Value Theory

The conceptualization of motivation as limited to an intensity and directional component was not sufficient for some theorists. They found it necessary to explain the conditions under which the original impetus to or arousal of behavior develops. They employed cognitive intervening variables, such as expectations, goals, and values, to explain behavior in terms of what the organism wanted, and what he *expected* to find. Similarly, individual differences in response to antecedent conditions could be explained by different expectancies resulting from the organism's genetic makeup, as well as his prior learning experiences.

The application of the *cognitive orientation* to motor performance was first seen in the *level of aspiration* literature. Locke and Bryan (1966), for example, found that subjects with high aspirations did better on a complex coordination apparatus than those subjects who were simply told to do their best. Cognitive variables have since permeated the previously mentioned behavioristic paradigms which, as originally conceived, were devoid of nonphysicalistic constructs. For example, Cottrell (1972) has modified the drive theory explanation of social facilitation by stipulating that arousal, created by the presence of others, is dependent upon the subjects' expectations of positive and negative outcomes. The amount of effort expended on gross motor tasks has also been shown to be a function of subjects' expectancies. Nelson and Furst (1972) found that the outcome of arm wrestling matches was more closely related to expected strength of their opponent than to their own objectively determined strength.

Perhaps the most lucid and applicable formulation of expectancy-value theory for motor performance is in the area of achievement motivation. Atkinson and Feather (Healey and Landers, 1973) have proposed that the environments in which motivation to achieve will be greatest will differ for two theoretical types of individuals: persons predominantly motivated to achieve success (Mas) and those motivated mainly by the fear of success (Maf). Accordingly, the behavior of Mas individuals is said to be a multiplicative function of expectancy for success, incentive for success, and habit strength on the particular task. Comparison of the motor performance of Mas and Maf subjects have supported predictions of achievement motivation theory. For instance, Mas subjects prefer intermediate levels of task difficulty and perform better than Maf individuals in a competitive situation, but the reverse is noted for the noncompetitive situation. These differences are most pronounced in the early stages of learning and dissipate as practice continues. As this research indicates, behavior is a function of expectancy of value attainment and its availability in a particular environment at a particular time.

BIBLIOGRAPHY

BROADHURST, P. L. Emotionality and the Yerkes-Dodson Law. *Journal of Experimental Psychology,* 1957, *54,* 345–352.

COTTRELL, N. B. Social facilitation. In C. G. McClintock (Ed.), *Experimental social psychology.* New York: Holt, Rinehart and Winston, 1972. Pp. 185–236.

GUTIN, B. Exercise-induced activation and human performance: A review. *Research Quarterly,* 1973, *44,* 256–268.

HEALEY, T. R., and LANDERS, D. M. Effect of need achievement and task difficulty on competitive and noncompetitive motor performance. *Journal of Motor Behavior,* 1973, *5,* 121–128.

HOKANSON, J. E. *The physiological bases of motivation.* New York: Wiley, 1969.

HUNT, P. J., and HILLARY, J. M. Social facilitation in a coaction setting: An examination of the effects over learning trials. *Journal of Experimental Social Psychology,* 1973, *9,* 563–571.

LOCKE, E. A., and BRYAN, J. F. Cognitive aspects of psychomotor performance: The effects of performance goals on level of performance. *Journal of Applied Psychology,* 1966, *50,* 286–291.

MARTENS, R. Arousal and motor performance. In J. H. Wilmore (Ed.), *Exercise and sport science reviews* (Vol. 2). New York: Academic Press, 1974. Pp. 155–188.

NAATANEN, R. The inverted-U relationship between activation and performance: A critical review. In S. Kornblum (Ed.), *Attention and performance IV.* New York: Academic Press, 1973. Pp. 155–174.

NELSON, L. R., and FURST, M. L. An objective study of the effects of expectation on competitive performance. *Journal of Psychology,* 1957, *54,* 345–352.

DANIEL M. LANDERS

MOTOR PERFORMANCE OF LIMBS

Historical Background

If we wish to make movements accurately, we make them slowly. If we wish to move quickly, we run the risk of being inaccurate. The relationship between speed and accuracy was quantitatively studied for the first time by R. S. Woodworth in the last years of the nineteenth century. Research since the 1950s has revealed much more about the mechanisms underlying the relationship.

Woodworth (1899) asked his subjects to aim repeatedly, in time with a metronome, at targets on a piece of graph paper, or alternatively, to reproduce repeatedly a line of given length. He found that, in both cases, and in the medium range of speeds between 40 and 120 movements per minute, accuracy decreased as speed increased. Below 40 and over 120 movements per minute, accuracy was unaffected by speed, showing an upper and a lower limit to the accuracy of movement.

Woodworth fitted the equation

$$E = S^n \qquad (1)$$

to his data, where E is a measure of error, S is speed of movement, and n is an exponent less than unity. Perhaps more illuminating is the descriptive account which he gave of his results, since this description contains the germ of much later theoretical work. He distinguished the "initial adjustment" of movement, which was independent of speed, from the "current control," which was intermittent and was only possible during slow movements. At higher speeds, current control became progressively important until it ceased altogether at 120 movements per minute.

In the 1920s and 1930s there was a considerable amount of research of a descriptive nature into limb movements. Gilbreth analyzed skilled manual movements into sixteen different types of action which he called "therbligs" from the reverse spelling of his own name. Therbligs are such things as "select," "grasp," "release," and "lift." By attributing a minimum time to each therblig and by working out the minimum number required for any repeated cycle of industrial work, such as bricklaying, Gilbreth was able to achieve considerable improvements in speed.

During the Second World War, psychologists began to work with engineers in designing man-machine systems. From this liaison, psychologists learned about, and made use of, two contemporary theoretical advances in mathematics applied to engineering. These were information theory and control theory or cybernetics.

Application of Information Theory

The first modern formulation of the relationship between the speed and accuracy of movement was that of Paul Fitts. Although his formulation, based on information theory, has been largely superseded by others based on control theory, it makes use of concepts which must still be taken very seriously. These concepts are derived from the mathematical theory of information (largely the work of Claude Shannon), which in essence specifies the relationship between the length of a coded message and the number of alternative messages which could be sent by the same length of message. The measure of information is the logarithm of the number of alternative messages, and it is demonstrable that, in optimally coded systems, the length of the message is proportional to its information content.

Information theory has been particularly successful in accounting for the relationship between response time (T) and the number of alternative responses (N) which the subject might be required to make. At about the same time (1952–1953) Hick in England and Hyman in the United States suggested that the observed logarithmic relationship

$$T \propto \log N \qquad (2)$$

could be explained on the assumption that log N represents the information content of the signal to which the subject responds (see Welford, 1968).

Fitts (1954) worked with a situation very like Woodworth's, but instead of allowing the speed to dictate the accuracy, he varied the size of two targets and instructed his subjects to hit them alternately as rapidly as possible. He found that the equation

$$T \propto \log \frac{2A}{W} \qquad (3)$$

fitted his data very well, where T is the movement time, A the distance between the centers of the targets, and W the width of the targets. Fitts assumed that the more accurate movement required more time because it took longer to specify the precise movement to be made. On this assumption $2A/W$ is the number of possible movements of accuracy W and mean amplitude A. By this reasoning, Equation (3) is equivalent to Equation (2), and in this case also the movement time is determined by the information content of the message.

Crossman and Goodeve (unpublished but summarized in Welford, 1968), derived a logarithmic equation, very similar to that of Fitts, from the mathematics of control theory. However, most applications of control theory have led to rather different equations which will be described in the next sections.

Application of Control Theory

At about the same time that Shannon was elaborating information theory, Norbert Wiener coined the term *cybernetics* to describe the mathematical study of control systems and other reactive systems. The behavior of the simplest of these systems can be fully described in terms of its amplitude of response and phase lag at different frequencies. For linear systems the response to complex waveforms can be predicted by treating the waveform as the sum of a series of sine waves (Fourier analysis) and adding together the expected response to each of these.

During the Second World War, there was a great upsurge of interest in control systems, which were important in the engines of war, and in their interaction with the human beings who controlled them. Since these engines could be treated as linear systems, it was reasonable to attempt to describe the behavior of the human operator in the same way, since this would allow the behavior of the total system to be described and optimized by matching the characteristics of the machine to that of the man controlling it. After the war many researchers hoped to use the same mathematical techniques to discover how we control our own movements (Stark, 1968). These psychological applications of control theory have had some success, but have also run into very serious difficulties, mainly because the assumptions on which the mathematics are based are violated in so many ways (Licklider, 1960).

The earliest work of Craik, Taylor, and others suggested that control was not continuous, as in most mechanical and electrical systems, but intermittent, with samples taken every half-second or perhaps every tenth of a second. This was most clearly revealed in responses to discrete stimuli, such as step functions in manual tracking of a moving target. When the track to be followed required two large movements in rapid succession, the response to the second was delayed. This was similar to an effect observed in 1931 by Telford, who found that the response to the second of two auditory stimuli was delayed relative to the response to the first, provided that the two stimuli occurred within half a second. Since this effect is found in responses to many different types of stimuli, it is sometimes called *central refractoriness* and may be the main cause of intermittency in control of movement. Most theories of "refractoriness" assume that it is concerned with the organization and monitoring of movement and that until the first movement has been adequately organized and checked, the response to the second stimulus cannot begin to be processed (Welford, 1968).

Although human tracking performance breaks down at frequencies above 2–3 Hz (hertz, or cycles per second), it does so in ways fundamentally different from the way even a relatively complex reactive system would do so. Above the natural frequency, reactive systems attempt to follow the frequency of the stimulus but are unable to maintain the amplitude. Human subjects usually maintain the amplitude but get the frequency wrong, either underestimating or overestimating it (Licklider, 1960).

The subject seems to be attempting to predict the characteristics of the stimulus. It has been shown that for unpredictable stimuli, the normal reaction time results in a lag, while for predictable stimuli the lag may be zero. In this respect the hand is rather different from the eye, since the eye is less able to make use of advance information (Stark, 1968). Although the eye movement system has a lower reaction time than the hand, it is less able to follow high-frequency sine waves, perhaps because of this inability to predict. Since, when we are tracking with the hand, our eyes usually follow the moving target, this difference between the eye and hand control systems may be highly significant.

However, the major difficulty in applying control theory to the control of human limbs is the very great variation in the characteristics of the system. The assumption of linearity is violated because a simple sine wave can be tracked without lag, while its combination with other waves results in a lag. Similarly, the characteristics of the response depend on the relationship of the movement to the display. "Stimulus response compatibility" has a large effect on simple and choice reaction times. Fitts, Vince, and others have shown that it also affects tracking. Control systems can involve position, velocity, or acceleration control, or the display can be of the position of the target or of the current error in tracking. More or less advance information may be given. All these factors affect the characteristics of the man as a control system so that no simple description of his performance can be given in control theory terms (Licklider, 1960).

However, recent experimental work within this tradition has shed new light on the old problem of the relationship between speed and accuracy, but without making much use of the mathematics of control theory.

Variable Error and Speed of Movement

If accuracy is measured at right angles to the direction of movement, we find that constant errors are very small while the variable errors can become very large at high speeds of movement. If the illumination is switched off as soon as the movement is started, then the constant errors remain small, while the variable error is large, virtually independent of the speed of movement and linearly proportional to the length of the movement. This suggests that these movements have a characteristic angular error which is independent of speed. (This is what Woodworth called the "initial adjustment.") When we can see the target and our hand, then error on target seems to depend on the distance away at which the last correction is made. This has been confirmed by switching off the light when the hand is at varying distances from the target. Howarth, Beggs, and Bowden (1971) used these observations as the basis of a new description of the dynamics of limb movements. They measured the trajectory of the hand as it approaches the target. They found that the last decelerating phase could be fitted by the equation

$$d = kD\left(\frac{t}{T}\right)^n \qquad (4)$$

where d is the distance of the hand from the target, t the time away from the target, D the total length of the movement, T the total movement time, and k a constant required to subtract the initial accelerating phase of the movement. The exponent n has a value of between 1.2 for naive subjects and 1.8 for very highly practiced subjects. There is a body of descriptive data from many sources showing that these changes in the nature of the movement, as the subject becomes more familiar with it, are due to the subject's better understanding of the task, leading to an improved strategy in performance. In this case, the higher values of n reflect the subject's ability to slow down his movement as he approaches the target, so that the final adjustment can be made with the hand very close to the target. In more complex movement the elimination of unnecessary elements of movement (therbligs) and increased smoothness and better timing of the movement may also be involved.

Howarth and Beggs assumed that the last correction would be made when the hand was, on average, one corrective reaction time away from the target. At that moment, the hand will be a distance (d_u) away from the target, which can be calculated from Equation (5). If d_u is then multiplied by the angular error of aiming (σ_θ), which can be separately estimated from the experiment in which the movement is made in the dark, then the error on target (σ_E) can be predicted. It was found empirically that even when d_u was zero, errors were still made due to the irreducible tremor of the hand (σ_0).

Since these two sources of error are independent, the theory predicts

$$\sigma_E^2 = \sigma_0^2 + (d_u\,\sigma_\theta)^2 \qquad (5)$$

By putting together Equations (4) and (5), Howarth and associates were able to account very fully for the observed relationship between speed and variable error. Although these equations are rather more complex than the information theory equations, they contain no arbitrary constants. All of the terms in Equations (4) and (5) can be estimated in more than one way. Among other things, the equations account for the upper and lower limits to accuracy observed by Woodworth. At low speeds, accuracy is limited by the tremor (σ_0). At high speeds, no corrections can be made, so that d_u is the same as the total length of the movement (*D*).

Constant Errors and Variable Errors

By specifying the width of the target, Fitts was unable to distinguish between variable and constant errors. While the latter were negligible in Howarth and Beggs's task, they are large and dependent on speed in the situations used by Fitts and Woodworth. This is because they measured accuracy in the direction of movement and therefore the accuracy of stopping. In both situations, variable errors seem to be well described by the Howarth and Beggs equations, but when constant and variable errors are confused, the data may be well fitted by Fitts's equation.

A Second Look at Tracking

The assumption of a constant angular error of aiming, which is independent of speed, also accounts in a very simple way for the relationship between speed and accuracy of unpaced tracking (Beggs, Sakstein, and Howarth, 1974). If we assume that errors in tracking can be detected easily and almost instantaneously, but that they cannot be corrected in less than a corrective reaction time, then most of the error will be that which develops before it can be corrected. If d_c is now the distance moved before a correction is made, then, as before,

$$\sigma_E^2 = \sigma_0^2 + (d_c \sigma_\theta)^2$$

But in this case

$$d_c = s t_c$$

where t_c is the correction reaction time and s is the speed of movement. Putting the two equations together, we get

$$\sigma_E^2 = \sigma_0^2 + (s t_c \sigma_\theta)^2$$

If speeds are high enough for the tremor term to be negligible, we get

$$\sigma_E = s t_c \sigma_\theta \qquad (6)$$

In 1959 Rashevsky showed that an equation very like Equation (6) described the relationship between speed of driving a car and road width. However, he did not distinguish between constant and variable errors. In 1971 Drury produced an equation even more like Equation (6) and showed that it applied to the driving of forklift trucks and to drawing a pencil line between curved or straight parallel lines. Drury pointed out that relationship depended on the level of error the subjects were prepared to risk. Beggs et al. (1974) showed that Equation (6) applies to the speed at which people can walk along a narrow beam, as with other aiming and tracking tasks. Unfortunately, σ_θ is not a constant for an individual, nor is there any correlation between the values of σ_θ obtained from different tasks.

The simple theory embodied in Equation (6) has only been tested for unpaced movement along simple tracks with complete advanced knowledge of the shape of the track. The tracking movements studied by Craik and others were paced and more complex, and involved little advance information. We do not yet know if Equation (6) can be applied to such situations.

There has been little systematic study of intermediate situations, but it is clear that advance information, which allows anticipatory planning of the movement, is a very great help. (The work of Leonard, Poulton, Gibbs, and others was described by Welford in 1968.) In addition, the amount of practice may fundamentally change the nature of the control (Keele, 1968).

Taking anticipation and practice into account, the dynamics of activities such as playing a new piece of music on a piano, or reading aloud, or driving a car, or playing a ball game, are considerably more complex than our present theories can cope with. For example, there has been very little work on the dynamics of interacting movements of different parts of the body. We now know quite a lot about simple repetitive movement, about the control of simple predetermined movement, and about the interaction of simple discrete movements. However, there is a great deal we do not understand about more complex activities.

BIBLIOGRAPHY

BEGGS, W. D. A.; SAKSTEIN, R.; and HOWARTH, C. I. The generality of a theory of the intermittent control of accurate movements. *Ergonomics,* 1974, *17,* 757–768.

FITTS, P. M. The information capacity of the human motor system in controlling amplitude of movement. *Journal of Experimental Psychology,* 1954, *47,* 381–391.

HOWARTH, C. I.; BEGGS, W. D. A.; and BOWDEN, J. The relationship between speed and accuracy of movement aimed at a target. *Acta Psychologica,* 1971, *35,* 207–218.

KEELE, S. W. Movement control in skilled motor performance. *Psychological Bulletin,* 1968, *70,* 387–403.

LICKLIDER, J. C. R. Quasi-linear operator models in the study of manual tracking. In R. D. Luce (Ed.), *Developments in mathematical psychology.* New York: Free Press, 1960.

STARK, L. *Neurological control systems: Studies in bioengineering.* New York: Plenum, 1968.

WELFORD, A. T. *Fundamentals of skill.* London: Methuen, 1968.

WOODWORTH, R. S. Accuracy of voluntary movement. *Psychological Review* monograph supplement 3, 1899.

C. I. HOWARTH
W. D. ALAN BEGGS

MOTOR PROGRAM

The idea that human movement is controlled by centrally stored, prestructured sets of muscle commands has been with us for a long time, but the first strong evidence for this position was presented by Karl Lashley in 1917. Lashley tested the movement accuracy of a patient who had suffered total deafferentation of the lower limbs via a gunshot wound in the lower back. The patient could move his lower leg to specified positions with an accuracy not unlike that of a "normal" subject. The fact that the patient could make these movements without any sensation from the responding limb led Lashley to conclude that movement was controlled centrally, via prestructured muscle commands that do not require response-produced feedback. This *centralist* (or "open-loop") idea has been restated many times since Lashley's original observation, and the controlling agent has been recently termed the *motor program* in direct analogy to the commands that drive the electronic computer.

The major rival hypothesis with which the motor-program notion has had to compete is the *peripheralist* view, which states essentially that the subject makes use of his response-produced feedback in producing movement. One version, the *response-chaining* hypothesis, holds that the subject "triggers" the next action in a sequence with response-produced feedback from an earlier action. But a more popular notion says that the subject uses feedback to determine the extent of his movement error, and then operates to reduce this error to zero. This latter idea was made popular by the recent application of the thinking regarding servomechanism control to human movement, and is usually referred to the "closed-loop" model for movement.

A simple statement of the closed-loop notion is that the subject monitors the difference between the output of his motor system with respect to its achievement of the specified environmental goal. For example, if the subject's task is to move his hand for a distance of exactly 30 cm, the closed-loop model says that the subject determines the difference between the limb's location and its desired location (30 cm away) as he travels along the path, making a number of corrections to reduce the actual-desired deviation to zero. To the contrary, the open-loop model assumes that all of the decisions about the path and end point of the movement are made in advance, with movement being controlled by the motor program.

Closed- and Open-Loop Control

There are a number of lines of evidence that provide difficulty for the closed-loop notion, but the most important has been the fact that responding to feedback (or error) stimuli requires a great deal of time, making it doubtful that feedback can be used *within* a movement, especially if the movement is a rapid one. A signal presented to the subject requires from 120 to 200 msec (one "reaction time") in order that the subject *begin* a response to it. Thus, if

a signal that the movement is not achieving the environmental goal is presented during the movement, he cannot begin to respond to it until at least 120 msec later. In addition, errors in achieving the goal do not usually occur in only one way, and the subject must prepare himself for a number of different types and directions of errors. But reaction time is known to increase markedly with the number of stimulus alternatives increasing the time required to respond to one of a number of possible error stimuli within a movement. Further, when two stimuli (or errors) are presented close to one another in time, the response to the second stimulus is markedly delayed (termed the *psychological refractory period*) thus increasing reaction times to stimuli (or errors) presented sequentially. Taking all of this together, perhaps the strongest evidence against the closed-loop idea is that a subject can initiate a hand movement and bring the hand to a stop 20 cm away, all in 100 msec. If it is assumed, as do closed-loop theorists, that the instructions about stopping the movement were initiated by a stimulus arising during the movement, the movement would be terminated before this instruction could *begin* to have an effect.

Some additional lines of evidence, related to the above arguments, also provide difficulty for the closed-loop model. For example, Henry and Harrison (1961) had subjects make a rapid, horizontal arm swing as quickly as possible after a stimulus. Occasionally, however, a second stimulus would occur from 100–400 msec after the first, indicating that the subject should inhibit his response, or stop it if the movement had already started. Even when presented 100 msec prior to the movement's beginning, second stimuli could not be responded to, and the subject carried out the movement seemingly uninfluenced by the "stop" instructions. While providing difficulty for the closed-loop view, the data suggest that the motor program's action cannot be inhibited for 200 msec once it is set in motion.

Slater-Hammel (1960) had subjects watch a sweep timer (1 revolution/sec) begin from *0* and lift their finger from a key when the timer reached *8*, 800 msec later. Occasionally, the timer would stop before reaching *8*, in which case the subject was to inhibit his finger movement. If the clock stopped 168 msec or more before reaching *8*, more than 50% of the subjects could not inhibit their movements. These data suggest that the program is initiated about one reaction time before the movement is to begin, and that initiating the program causes movement to occur even if information is presented in the environment suggesting that it should be inhibited or changed.

The essential conclusion from these data is that the response to peripheral stimuli, which include stimuli about the correctness of the movement pattern, require approximately one reaction time for a response to begin. This fact makes it unlikely that performers monitor stimuli from their moving limbs, initiating corrections if errors in meeting the environmental goal should occur, especially if the movements are rapid (e.g., less than 200 msec). Of course, these temporal limitations do not preclude the possibility of making feedback-based corrections in movements that are far longer in time, such as in positioning responses or in tracking; indeed, it is in these classes of movement that closed-loop models appear to have their best predictive power.

Because of these temporal limitations in responding to peripheral stimuli, the open-loop view appears to have explanatory power for the control of (at least) rapid movements. In addition, the idea has been extended and modified somewhat to account for performances in tasks having longer movement times, and even to continuous tracking tasks. Here the individual is assumed to execute a short (e.g., 300 msec) motor program, then monitor the response-produced feedback, then execute another motor program. This *intermittancy* view postulates open-loop control while the program is being executed, with closed-loop control between programs. These separate programs, with the "aid" of inertia from the responding limbs, produce the smooth movements commonly seen in tracking tasks.

It should be pointed out that the motor program argument is primarily a "default" argument, in that it holds because the alternative view of motor control (closed-loop) seems unlikely in humans. However, there are data from subhuman species that provide additional support for the motor program view. For example, Wilson (1961) deafferented the wings and related musculature of locusts and showed that electrical stimulation of a ganglion near the head caused movements of the wings resem-

bling flying, the movements continuing well after the stimulation had ceased. The fact that the movements occurred without the involvement of feedback supports the program view, but these findings have been limited in applicability to humans because the movements are probably *innate*. Also, Taub and Berman (1968) showed that monkeys deafferented from the neck down can learn to squeeze a bulb with the hand to avoid a shock; feedback from the responding limb was probably not mediating learning and performance of this task, again supporting an open-loop interpretation.

Role of Feedback

There is strong evidence, taken by some as contrary to the conclusions drawn above, that feedback can have a role in movement control, with latencies far shorter than the 150–200 msec mentioned earlier. Briefly, the evidence shows that when sudden abberations are introduced into a movement pattern, there can be increased electromyogram (EMG) activity in the correcting musculature within 30–50 msec. These changes are probably related to the muscle spindle. Other findings suggest that additional feedback loops compensate for unexpected variations in the joint angle (e.g., Merton, 1974), with the loop times being somewhat longer (60–80 msec); these are perhaps mediated by the cerebellum. Closed-loop theorists incorrectly point to these findings to suggest that feedback can operate sufficiently rapidly to provide a basis for a closed-loop view of motor control. However, these loops operate to correct for unexpected variations in the resistance presented to the movement, unexpected fatigue states, or "noise" in muscular output, and thus provide a means for the accurate production of the movement *actually programmed*. However, if something in the environment suddenly indicates that the movement will not achieve its environmental goal (e.g., the batter sees the ball curve unexpectedly), there is no evidence that these loops can provide rapid corrections for this type of error. To the contrary; these loops seem to provide insurance that the now-inappropriate movement is executed faithfully.

Because of the role of spinal feedback control of motor output, it is probably incorrect to define the motor program as carrying out movement without the involvement of feedback. Rather, the program should be seen as a set of prestructured commands that, when executed, are capable of carrying out all of the movement details, with signals from the environment or moving limb indicating that the pattern of movement chosen should be changed if ineffective, until the program has run its course. Even though the evidence points strongly to a motor-program interpretation, the issue of closed-versus open-loop control of movement has not been settled, and a number of theories (Adams, 1971) hold that learning is the development of more effective references of correctness against which feedback is compared during the movement.

Characteristics of the Motor Program

Program Running Time. From the research cited above, there is reason to believe that a program must run its course for at least one reaction time (or until a very fast movement is completed). This is an ideal minimum, however, and a more realistic minimum is somewhat longer. First, a signal from the environment indicating that the movement pattern should be changed will usually require that enough of the movement has been completed so that an error can arise, lengthening the minimum to one reaction time plus the movement time necessary to produce the error (perhaps as much as 400 msec). In addition, errors can occur in more than one way, and thus the time to react to one of many signals is substantially greater than the reaction time to a single alternative, again increasing the estimate of the minimum program time.

In regard to the maximum running time for a program, the evidence is not so clear, but one could imagine that a program could guide motor activity, without any signal to change the "intended" pattern of movement, for as long as a few seconds. A common point of view is that many well-learned movements with 1- or 2-second movement times may be entirely programmed, freeing the attentional requirements of the subject to perform other tasks. However, if something happens in the environment that indicates that the "intended" movement will not meet the environmental goal,

feedback can be used to execute another program that corrects the error.

Response Factors. Research has asked which movement variables (e.g., movement speed, distance, load, time) are important determiners of the extent to which a movement is programmed, or alternatively, the extent to which feedback can be used during the movement to guide behavior toward the environmental goal. It seems obvious that any factor that increases the movement *time* tends to decrease the possibility of feedback involvement and thus increases the extent to which the movement is programmed; variables such as movement distance, movement load, and movement speed can all affect movement time, and thus are important determiners of programming. However, when the movement time is held constant, speed per se does not have any effect on the extent to which a movement is programmed; that is, for a 200 msec movement, performances at two different speeds (with different movement distances) are programmed to the same extent (Schmidt, 1975).

Program and Learning. Early thinking about motor programs usually conceptualized them as being associated with only one motor response, with a separate motor program needed for every movement one wishes to make. This view has been challenged, suggesting that programs may be more "generalized," subserving a rather narrow class of movements (e.g., throwing in various ways), with parameters needed in order to specify how the general program is to be run off (e.g., with great force, rapidly, etc.). Some research has indicated that timing is one of the important parameters, and it appears that the individual predetermines the speed with which the entire program is to be run (Brooks, 1974). Others have suggested that the force characteristics are another parameter, so that the movement sequence can be carried out under various loads using the same motor program (Schmidt, 1975).

BIBLIOGRAPHY

ADAMS, J. A.   A closed-loop theory of motor learning. *Journal of Motor Behavior,* 1971, *3,* 111–150.
BROOKS, V. B.   Some examples of programmed limb movements. *Brain Research,* 1974, *71,* 299–308.
HENRY, F. M., and HARRISON, J. S.   Refractoriness of a fast movement. *Perceptual and Motor Skills,* 1961, *13,* 351–354.

Keele, S. W.   Movement control in skilled motor performance. *Psychological Bulletin,* 1968, *70,* 387–403.

Lashley, K. W.   The accuracy of movement in the absence of excitation from the moving organ. *American Journal of Physiology,* 1917, *43,* 169–194.

Merton, P. A.   The properties of the human muscle servo. *Brain Research,* 1974, *71,* 475–478.

Schmidt, R. A.   A schema theory of discrete motor skill learning. *Psychological Review,* 1975, *82,* 225–260.

Slater-Hammel, A. T.   Reliability, accuracy, and refractoriness of a transit reaction. *Research Quarterly,* 1960, *31,* 217–228.

Taub, E., and Berman, A. J.   Movement and learning in the absence of sensory feedback. In S. J. Freedman (Ed.), *The neuropsychology of spatially oriented behavior.* Homewood, Ill.: Dorsey Press, 1968.

Wilson, D. M.   The central nervous control of flight in a locust. *Journal of Experimental Biology,* 1961, *38,* 471–490.

See also Reaction Time and Choice

Richard A. Schmidt

MOTOR RESPONSES: SPINAL ORGANIZATION

Man produces a wide range of highly coordinated movements under a variety of conditions. This ability normally requires the integration of central motor commands and peripheral sensory signals at motor pools of the anterior horn. Much of this interaction depends on an extensive network of interneurons which surround the pools at each spinal segment. This review is concerned mainly with organization of motor units and the intrapool and interpool organization provided by various segmental mechanisms.

Organization of Segmental Motoneurons

Motoneuronal Pools.   The cell bodies of skeletomotor and fusimotor neurons are located in distinct cytoarchitectural areas called lamina IX of Rexed (Fig. 1). Both types of motoneurons are intermingled in the motor pool of their specific muscle. Each pool extends through one to three spinal segments, and motoneurons contained within are responsible for the innervation of one to three synergistic muscles. The most medial pools innervate the proximal musculature, while the most lateral pools govern the distal musculature (Fig. 1). The large cells of skeletomotor neurons give rise predominately to *alpha fibers* (α-MN)

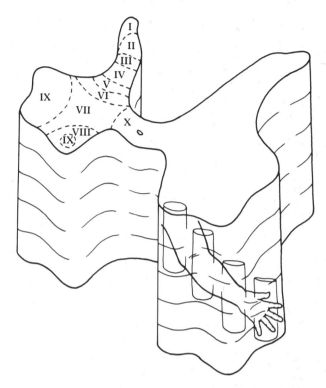

Fig. 1.   A schematic illustration of the Rexed laminae and the motor pool organization of segments C_5–T_1 are shown.

whose diameters range from 12μ to 18μ and innervate only large extrafusal fibers, while the smaller cells of fusimotor neurons give rise predominantly to *gamma fibers* (γ-MN) whose diameters range from 2 to 8μ and innervate only intrafusal fibers of the muscle spindle. Intermediate size cells give rise to *beta* (β) fibers (8–12μ) which may innervate either extrafusal or intrafusal or both (skeleto-fusimotor).

Dendritic Bundles.   Within each motor pool approximately 80% of the dendritic branches of α-MNs form closely packed bundles of 3 to 10 shafts. Dendritic bundles extend rostrocaudally over several millimeters and frequently include dendrites of α-MNs from more than one pool as well as dendrites from propriospinal neurons. The extent to which dendrites of γ-MNs participate in the bundles is not known.

Within each individual bundle, membranes are packed so tightly that electrotonic coupling between adjacent dendrites is possible. The level of excitability of bundled fibers is determined by a series of postsynaptic and electronic interactions which allow for extremely fine modulations. Electrical synapses also provide for the synchronization of groups of neurons involved in the production of highly synchronous volleys. It has been shown, for example, that MNs of the abducens nuclei in cats are coupled electronically. These are motor command nuclei in which synchronization plays an important role, in the quick phase of nystagmus or in saccadic eye movements.

Dendritic bundles, at least in the hindlimb of cats, begin to develop after birth, and they do not appear fully developed until the fourth or fifth postnatal month. Full development of these dendritic bundles is coeval with reciprocal sequencing of flexor and extensor muscles, suggesting that bundles may serve as intrapool and interpool organizers which are prerequisite to synchronous and reciprocal activity of hindlimb muscles during locomotion and weight bearing. Dendrites or forelimb motor pools show considerable evidence of bundle formation at birth. Since alternate treading motions of the forelimbs associated with suckling appear almost immediately after birth, it is likely that dendritic formations support the segmental organization required for reciprocal activity of muscle pairs.

Recurrent Collaterals. As the single axons of α-MNs emerge from the motor pool, recurrent collaterals may branch off and reenter the anterior horn. There is a roughly linear relationship between the incidence of such collaterals and the distance of the motoneuron (MN) soma from the anterior horn exit zone. Axons of cells in the lateral MN pools generally have at least one and may have as many as 5–6 collateral branches, while axons extending from the medial pools seldom have more than one collateral and most usually have none.

Recurrent collaterals enter Rexed's layer VII and synapse with a particular type of inhibitory interneurons called Renshaw cells. Inhibition provided by Renshaw cells helps to limit the frequency maxima of the collateral's parent cell and other motoneurons (MNs) in the pool including γ-MNs by a process called recurrent inhibition (Fig. 2). Whereas small α-MNs are subjected to a more effective recurrent inhibition than large α-MNs, Renshaw cells are triggered predominantly by the latter. Thus Renshaw cells may play an important role during fast movements by suppressing the influence of small α-MNs which innervate slow-contracting fibers.

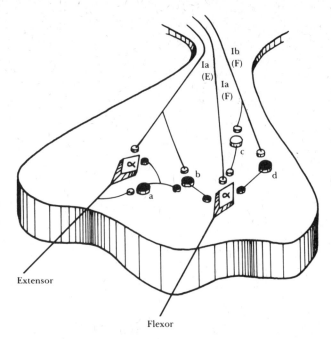

Fig. 2.   Interneuronal circuits influencing Ia and Ib reflexes of extensor *(E)* and flexor *(F)* muscles are shown. Filled circles indicate inhibitory synapses, while open circles indicate excitatory synapses. Interneuron *"a"* is a Renshaw cell; *"b"* is a Ia inhibitory neuron; *"c"* is a "presynaptic" interneuron and *"d"* is a Ib inhibitory neuron.

The Renshaw cell is more than an intrapool organizer, for its axonal branches may extend a few millimeters along the rostrocaudal axis of the segment, but they do not decussate. It has been demonstrated that Renshaw cells inhibit each other monosynaptically. Mutual inhibition of Renshaw cells is arranged intersegmentally and can be produced by collaterals of motor axons innervating different muscle groups. In addition, Renshaw cells inhibit anterior horn interneurons which are monosynaptically excited by group Ia muscle afferents (see Fig. 2). Mutual inhibition and inhibition of Ia interneurons both could contribute to the phenomenon of recurrent facilitation of spinal MNs.

Muscle Units for Skeletomotor and Fusimotor Neurons

Extrafusal fibers innervated by each α-MN are dispersed through a large portion of a single muscle. Each muscle fiber of the motor unit has identical mechanical and metabolic profiles, and in most mammalian muscle three types of extrafusal fibers can be identified although the percentage of each type may vary considerably muscle to muscle.

Slow-Twitch Oxidative (SO) Motor Units. SO fibers are innervated by small α-MN with average conduction rates of 85 m/sec. The units are characterized by slow twitch contraction times (58–110 msec), small tetanic tensions, and they are extremely resistant to fatigue during repetitive stimulation. The muscle fibers are generally small in diameter and have histochemical profiles suggesting high oxidative enzyme capacity, high mitochondrial density and low myofibrillar ATPase activity. Type SO motor units seem well suited for sustained, but relatively low tension contraction, such as may be required for postural support, walking and many maintenance tasks such as feeding, grooming and the like.

Fast-Twitch Glycolytic (FG) Motor Units. FG fibers are innervated by large α-MNs with average conduction rates of 100 m/sec. Type FG motor units have the shortest twitch contraction times (20–47 msec), the largest tetanic tensions and are very susceptible to fatigue with only a few hundred contractions. The muscle fibers are generally large in diameter and have low oxidative enzyme capacity and low mitochondrial density, but exhibit high capacity for anerobic glycolysis and high myofibrillar ATPase activity. FG units can produce very high tension and quick contractions, but they fatigue rapidly, presumably because of their dependence on anaerobic glycolysis and intrafiber glycogen stores. FG units seem specialized only for brief and intermittent activity, characteristic of sprinting, weight lifting and maximal efforts seen in jumping and throwing.

Fast-Twitch Oxidative, Glycolytic (FOG) Motor Units. Type FOG units, common in laboratory animals, but seldom identified in human muscle, have relatively short contraction times (30–55 msec), produce moderate tension in fused tetani and are more resistant to fatigue than FG units, but less so than type SO units. The muscle fibers of FOG units resemble those of FG units, except that they are smaller in diameter and have considerably greater oxidative enzyme capacity and mitochondrial density. The FOG units combine the advantages of quick contraction and reasonably high tension, plus resistance to fatigue. Endurance activities such as bicyling, long distance running and swimming may depend on these motor units, and athletes trained for endurance activities have a significantly greater number of extrafusal fibers with both high oxidative and high glycolytic capabilities.

Fusimotor Units. Gamma (γ) and more rarely beta (β) motoneurons innervate the striated poles of the diminutive intrafusal fibers of muscle spindles. Although intrafusal fibers represent usually less than 5% of the total muscle mass, over 40% of the motoneurons in the ventral root are fusimotor neurons. It is estimated that each fusimotor neuron innervates only a few poles, and some γ-MNs activate only one pole per spindle. Generally the polar regions of nuclear chain and nuclear bag fibers are governed independently, however a substantial proportion of γ-MNs (25–30%) control poles of both types of intrafusal fibers, while many β-MNs control both intrafusal and extrafusal fibers.

The slow contraction of intrafusal fibers does not add appreciably to gross muscle tension, because intrafusal fibers are few in number and small in size compared with extrafusal fibers. Contractions of the polar regions stretch the equatorial region of the intrafusal fibers, thereby deforming and depolarizing the sensory endings. The influence of fusimotor neurons on gross muscle contraction is conducted indirectly by reflex connections of the gamma-loop (Fig. 3).

Segmental Reflexes and Their Influence as Intrapool and Interpool Organizers

Autogenic Excitation and the Gamma-Loop. The gamma-loop includes one γ-MN, the spindle endings it biases and the synaptic influence the sensory endings exert on homonymous and heteronymous α-MNs. The gamma-loop serves as an intrapool and interpool organizer because spindle afferents (Ia and II) facilitate homonymous α-MNs (autogenic facilitation) and inhibit antagonistic heteronymous α-MNs (Fig. 2, 3). Slow-contracting motor units (SO) receive the greatest amount of γ-loop excitation and inhibition, while fast-contracting units, especially α-MNs of FG fibers, are rarely influenced by this regulated reflex.

Alpha-gamma coactivation by motor command centers insures that spindle afferents of

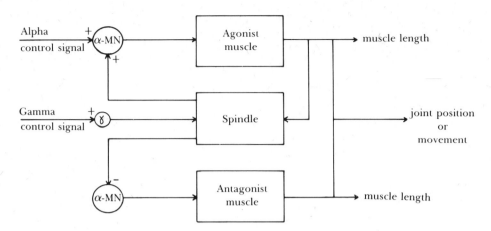

Fig. 3. A schematic illustration of α-γ coactivation shows that the γ-MN controls autogenic excitation of the agonist α-MN and reciprocal inhibition (the Ia inhibitory neuron is not shown) of the antagonist α-MN.

the contracting muscle will not be silenced by gross muscle shortening. For a number of naturally occurring movements, both reflex and volitional, it has been possible to demonstrate a coactivation of α- and γ-MNs so balanced that the sensory discharge from spindles actually increases during muscle shortening. The coactivation of alpha and gamma motoneurons has been termed a "servo-assisted" rather than a "servo-controlled" method of producing movement. Other names such as γ-α linkage and conditional feedback have been used also. The main advantage of servo-assisted motor control, as opposed to control by either α-MN or γ-MN alone, is that the motor system is less sensitive to changes and non-linear properties of muscle fibers and receptors.

Autogenic Inhibition and the Tendon Organ. The Golgi tendon organ, located predominantly at musculotendinous junctions and less wholly within the tendon, signals longitudinal tension created by muscular contraction and more rarely by muscle stretch. The Ib afferents of tendon organs have synaptic contact with inhibitory interneurons in area VII, and they govern autogenic inhibition of the contracting muscle (Fig. 2). The recruitment and rate coding of α-MNs is limited, therefore, by two segmental mechanisms, recurrent inhibition of the Renshaw cells and autogenic inhibition of the Ib afferents. These two inhibitory mechanisms, coupled with autogenic excitation provided by the gamma-loop, serve to regulate

the muscle's stiffness under varying conditions.

Flexor Reflex Afferents. Flexor reflex afferents (FRA) are afferents, which in the spinal animal, evoke the classical flexor reflex: excitation of ipsilateral flexors and inhibition of ipsilateral extensors. FRAs are generally identified as high threshold muscle, joint and cutaneous afferents whose axons are classified as group II or III. Quick withdrawal motions, orchestrated by FRAs are targeted specifically for the fast-contracting motor units of flexor muscles, while slow-contracting units of the muscle are inhibited. Both α- and γ-MNs are influenced by FRA reflexes.

Cutaneous Reflexes. When the skin is stroked lightly, iced or heated, muscles directly underneath the skin will contract or relax depending on the type of stimulus. Cutaneous reflexes have not been mapped out in detail, but it is generally agreed that these reflexes exert reciprocal control of muscle pairs through segmental and propriospinal interneurons which regulate α- and γ-MNs.

Interneuronal Organization of the Anterior Horn

Interneurons are located in Rexed layers VII and VIII (Fig. 1). All interneurons have a multibifurcating axon whose branches take diverse paths including participation in propriospinal fasciculi. There are no short Golgi II axons in the anterior horn which serve exclusively as intrapool organizers. It is estimated that several hundred cells receive contact from one interneuron, and that each internunical cell receives converging signals from an equal number of terminals.

Convergence on Single Interneurons. Segmental afferents from identical receptors generally converge on single interneurons. This convergence is usually spatially specific, but sometimes afferent fibers from receptors located in heterologous sites converge on a single cell. Convergence of segmental primary afferents is not limited to homogeneous receptors, however, for many interneurons receive monosynaptic excitation from muscle and cutaneous afferents. For example, inhibitory interneurons excited by Ia fibers of extensor spindles also receive excitatory actions from ipsilateral FRA fibers, while Ia inhibitory interneurons impinging on flexor MN are facilitated by contralateral FRA. The later circuit is used in the crossed-extensor pattern, while the former is used during ipsilateral withdrawal reflexes.

Interneurons also integrate supraspinal signals with segmental signals. The inhibitor Ia interneuron provides excellent examples of this process. Facilitation of Ia reciprocal inhibition from corticospinal and rubrospinal tracts has been demonstrated for flexor as well as extensor MNs with long segmental latency indicating a polysynaptic linkage. Brief latency facilitation of Ia inhibitory neurons to motoneurons (MNs) supplying hindlimb flexors, following volleys in the vestibulospinal tract, have indicated a monosynaptic excitatory action of Ia inhibitory interneurons.

Presynaptic Interneuronal Interaction. Many terminals of segmental afferents have their reflex potency decreased by interneurons synapsing upon them and giving rise to presynaptic inhibition. Golgi tendon afferents (Ib) are particularly effective at eliciting presynaptic inhibition especially those from flexor muscles which strongly decrease the effectiveness of Ia fibers from flexors (Fig. 2) and Ib fibers from extensors. Ia fibers have weak presynaptic actions reserved primarily for other Ia fibers, while FRA fibers decrease the synaptic efficacy of FRA and Ib fibers.

Presynaptic patterns, however, are not invariant, and their role in reflex control of muscle depends on various supraspinal and segmental inputs. For example, activation of reticulospinal fibers can alter the presynaptic pattern of FRA afferents from a presynaptic inhibition of FRA and Ib fibers to a presynaptic inhibition of Ia fibers.

Postsynaptic Interneuronal Interaction. Interneurons have postsynaptic contacts with other interneurons, and this network provides circuitry for interpool organization and the generation of patterned movements. The Renshaw cell, for example, inhibits the active MNs as well as the Ia inhibitory interneuron (Fig. 2). Recurrent inhibition of the Ia inhibitory neurons may serve as a segmental autoregulatory mechanism that prevents α-γ linked reciprocal inhibition from becoming excessive during increased activity in agonist α-MNs.

Locomotion, a complex patterned movement, is now thought to be organized by an intraspinal interneuronal network, which generates the sequential activation of different muscles in the step cycle of individual limbs. The nature of this central interneuronal network or generator is at present unknown; two main alternatives have been proposed: (1) an oscillator arranged with two reciprocally organized interneuronal half-centers and (2) a closed chain of interneurons. Although the network is influenced by both segmental and supraspinal inputs, it is genetically coded to provide the organizing array of signals to motor pools which participate in locomotion.

Movement Without Segmental Sensation

Recovered motor function following dorsal root transection has been studied extensively in the past decade. Primates deprived of segmental cutaneous and proprioceptive signals lack normal reflex and γ-loop support. In spite of these losses, blind infant monkeys, deafferented soon after birth, are capable of using the affected limbs for support, walking, climbing and picking up objects. From these reports, it appears that some motor programs may be coded genetically and do not require segmental or visual monitoring.

Adolescent and adult monkeys also have shown marked recovery after dorsal rhizotomy. Immediately after surgery, however, reaching movements of the forelimb are extremely ataxic and appear to be directed from the shoulder as an overhand fling. Grasping is absent and the monkeys merely strike at the viewed objects. After a two-month recovery period and considerable practice the monkeys are able to extend their arms and grasp objects, even when the arm is hidden from view.

The possibility that some limb sensation is available to deafferented animals has been suggested by the presence of unmyelinated sensory fibers which were discovered recently in the ventral root. In fact, it is estimated that nearly 30% of the axons in L_7 and S_1 ventral roots (cat) are unmyelinated and extend from soma located in dorsal root ganglia. These unmyelinated fibers appear to be activated by visceral stimuli such as rectal and bladder distentions. None of the unmyelinated ventral root afferents examined, to date, have had cutaneous or proprioceptive fields.

Summary

Organization of motor responses at the segmental level depend on intrapool and interpool mechanisms which regulate α- and γ-MNs: dendritic bundles, α-MN collaterals, interneuronal circuits and the converging influence of signals from descending and spinal afferent fibers. The spinal cord is an intricate, integrative organ, and there is now evidence to suggest that complex movement patterns, such as locomotion, are programmed at segmental levels and rely minimally on reflex and supraspinal modulation.

BIBLIOGRAPHY

BOSSOM, J. Movement without proprioception. *Brain Research,* 1974, *71,* 285–296.

CLIFTON, G. L.; VANCE, W. H.; APPLEBAUM, M. L.; COGGESHALL, R. E.; and WILLIS, W. D. Responses of unmyelinated afferents in the mammalian ventral root. *Brain Research,* 1974, *82,* 163–167.

GRANIT, R. *The basis of motor control.* New York: Academic Press, 1970.

MATTHEWS, P. B. C. *Mammalian muscle receptors and their central actions.* Baltimore: Williams and Wilkins, 1972.

STEIN, R. B.; PEARSON, K. G.; SMITH, R. S.; and REDFORD, J. B. (Eds.). *Control of posture and locomotion.* New York: Plenum Press, 1973.

See also MOTOR CONTROL AND THE CENTRAL NERVOUS SYSTEM

JUDITH L. SMITH

MOTOR SKILL LEARNING AND PERFORMANCE: METHODOLOGY

The bulk of research in psychology is concerned with describing motor performance in terms of outcomes rather than process. Emphasis is placed on *which* response was made rather than on *how* it was executed. For the most part, motor (and verbal) responses are counted and classified into a predetermined and limited set of categories which reflect the immediate interests of the researcher. Often there are only two categories: correct responses and error responses. The focus is on the question of which response alternative the subject selected and whether his choice was right or wrong. Thus, two simple indicants of performance are available in the typical study—namely, the number of correct responses and the number of error responses.

While it is true that skilled performance is frequently described in terms of response outcomes (e.g., a basketball player's shooting percentage or a baseball player's batting average), research on motor skills is primarily concerned with the *execution* of responses rather than their selection. By *execution* is meant the temporal-spatial pattern of the behavior as it is organized along the dimensions of direction, amplitude, rate, force, duration, and the like. In this case, performance cannot be assessed by classifying responses as correct or as errors, but rather must be described in terms of the magnitude of error—that is, the amount by which response output is discrepant from some criterion or desired output.

The implications of this position for motor skills methodology are rather straightforward. Tasks which require motor responses but which do not reflect in the performance criteria some aspects of the precision with which those responses were executed do not constitute motor skill studies. Studies which require button pressing, toggle switching, or head nodding may well assess cognitive or perceptual skill, but not motor skill. Motor skill tasks should permit the subject to vary his responses continuously along one or more dimensions and should measure the precision with which he does so, relative to some performance criterion.

While description and evaluation of the execution of responses has been emphasized in the preceding paragraphs, motor skill research is concerned with response selection, not among qualitatively different response alternatives, but rather among *motor programs* which control and determine quantitative differences in response execution. In this sense, the basketball player who misses the basket can be said to have chosen the wrong response, inappropriate with respect to direction, parabolic arc, force, or some combination of these characteristics. The selection of an appropriate program in these terms is quite different from selection among distinct response alternatives, such as shooting, passing, dribbling, or holding the basketball.

Performance Measures: Discrete or Serial Responses

When a task requires essentially single biphasic movements between a starting point and a target position, or a series of such discrete movements, primary concern may be with indicants describing the distribution of responses or the error distribution with respect to amplitude. If, for example, the task is to move a slide 10 inches along a track and to repeat that movement a number of times, the actual lengths of the movements can be recorded and plotted as a frequency distribution. The arithmetic mean of this distribution minus the true target distance (10 inches, in this example) describes the *constant error* (CE), while the standard deviation of this distribution describes the *variable error* (VE) of performance. These two indicants are statistically independent, but may be observed to be significantly related, since practice (with knowledge of results) may be expected to reduce both types of errors, and skilled performance tends to be both accurate (low CE) and consistent (low VE). The average *absolute error* (AE), or the modulus mean error, describes the deviations of the responses from the target without regard to the sign of the error. This indicant reflects both constant and variable error to the extent that these are present; at the same time it confounds these two types of error and is therefore ambiguous as to the performance it describes. Like the standard deviation, the root-mean-squared (rms) error averages the squared deviations of observations as measured from a fixed value; however, rather than from the mean of the response (or error) distribution, deviations are computed from the

point of zero error. Thus, rms error will be discrepant from the standard deviation of the error distribution to the extent that the mean of that distribution differs from the target value—that is, to the extent that there is constant error (CE) in the performance. While CE and VE are statistically independent, rms error and AE are related measures. Furthermore, both of the latter two measures are related to and reflect both CE and VE.

The example presented above used response amplitude as the dimension along which skill level was evaluated, and a number of indicants of the performance were described. The dimension might as readily have been any one of those along which temporal-spatial organization of responses can vary—for example, duration, direction, force, or rate. In any case, it might be asked whether one indicant is more appropriate than another. The answer depends, in part, upon the hypothesis and the independent variables being considered. Generally, no one measure provides as complete information as some combination of measures. A treatment or variable may affect one without any substantial effect on another. For example, practice without knowledge of results appears not to affect CE for drawing lines of a specified length, but the same practice tends to reduce the variability of responses (VE). Naturally, such a performance change would be reflected in AE and rms error (unless the CE was extremely large), but the interpretation of the performance change would not be completely clear from either of these latter measures. As Poulton (1974) has pointed out, these measures can be ordered with respect to how well they meet the distribution assumptions for parametric statistics. With this criterion, CE is preferred, followed by rms and VE, AE, and finally by mean-squared error. On the other hand, CE is often the least interesting and informative measure.

Frequently, it is convenient to record responses automatically, using counters or other devices, or simply to define target zones as in a "bull's-eye" target. To the extent that these target bands are sufficiently fine-grained and the distributions of responses do not depart drastically from normal, the above indicants are appropriately applied. However, at the extreme only two zones are defined: "on-target" and "off-target," in which case one is again dichotomizing responses into "correct" and "error" categories. While "percentage hits" may provide a performance criterion, it may be relatively insensitive to experimental effects and unanalytical of changes in motor behavior.

Response Information. Simple biphasic responses can be described within the framework of information measurement, not in the usual sense that the choice of one of four discrete and equally probable responses (e.g., pushbuttons) convey $\log_2 4$ or 2 bits of information, but rather in terms of the terminal accuracy requirements relative to the amplitude of a movement. Fitts (1954) described the *index of task difficulty Id* as

$$Id = -\log_2 \frac{Ws}{2A} \text{ Bits/response}$$

where *Ws* is target width and *A* is the average amplitude requirement of the task. Using this metric, Fitts had a rational basis for equating three rather diverse performance tasks in terms of requirements for movement precision. The same rationale can be used to describe the average information per response (or the rate of information in a serial or repetitive task), given a mean amplitude and a distribution of responses. Response information has also been described for continuous tracking tasks (Crossman, 1957).

Performance Measures: Continuous Response Tasks

In tasks requiring continuous adjustment of response, such as continuous control or tracking tasks, additional indicants of performance can be identified. Overall performance reflects both temporal and spatial precision, and it is of some interest to assess these sources of error independently. The spatial and temporal characteristics of any continuous signal can be specified completely with an amplitude distribution (which describes the frequency of responses of different amplitudes) and a power-density spectrum (which describes the relative power of responses for each of a number of frequency bands, much as a spectral analysis of sound or light frequencies). These distributions describe, respectively, the spatial (amplitude) and temporal (frequency) characteristics of a continuous response function. As Bahrick and Noble (1966) noted, other response indicants re-

flect characteristics of either or both of these distributions. These distributions and other indicants may be used to describe either the response function or the error function. The difference, as compared with discrete responses, is that with a continuous task the criterion (target) value is changing so that response and error functions cannot be related to one another except through knowledge of the input, or target course, of the task.

In some cases it may be quite informative to compare the amplitude distribution (and/or the power-density spectrum) of the response function with that of the input function.

However, while the amplitude distribution and power-density spectrum summarize a continuous response (or error) function in the spatial and frequency domains, they indicate very little about the strategies of the subjects for predicting and coping with signal events. Furthermore, obtaining these analyses from analog signals requires either special analog processors, analog-to-digital (a-d) computer facilities, or boundless energy for the hand-scoring of oscillographic records. For the record is continuous and the data are infinite; thus, a-d conversion with or without a hybrid computer involves obtaining a finite sample of measures of the error function adequate to reflect both its amplitude and frequency characteristics.

Overall Measures of Error. The measures discussed as indicants of performance in discrete tasks apply as well in continuous tasks, whether discrete values are obtained by a-d conversion or analyses are performed in the analog mode. As Poulton (1974) indicated, these are taken with regard to algebraic sign (CE and standard deviation—SD—error) or as absolute measures (AE and rms error). In addition, one may either summate the absolute values of error obtained at some discrete sampling rate or integrate the area under the error curve. The latter is readily obtained in an electronic-tracking system where target and follower are represented by comparable voltages. The error function is obtained as the absolute difference between these two functions and integrated over time by means of a few operational amplifiers. Such scores, taken over trials of fixed deviation or converted to error per second, provide meaningful summary indicants of performance. They can serve as criteria of overall performance for the testing of hypotheses and for the evaluation of response strategies which can be revealed only by more fine-grained analyses of the continuous records. Some of the indicants which may reveal these strategies will now be described.

Amplitude Errors: Overshoots and Undershoots. Oscillographic records on which the track and the response can be compared directly can be scored for amplitude errors at those points at which the target reverses direction. (At other points the discrepancy between target and response functions confounds amplitude and timing errors.) When the peak amplitude of the primary response exceeds that of the target, it is labeled an *overshoot error;* when it falls short of the target, it is an *undershoot error.* It follows that these can be combined into an error amplitude distribution from which the distribution measures, described earlier, can be obtained. A constant error would indicate an average tendency to overshoot or undershoot the target. Poulton (1974) has alerted us to another sort of constant error, a systematic bias in which the subject overshoots right-to-left reversals but undershoots left-to-right reversals. The mean of the amplitude distribution might well be zero, and *S* could be faithfully reproducing the spatial pattern, but with a systematic shift along the scale (this could signal an error in calibrating target and follower to the same values).

Timing Errors: Leads, Lags, and Phase Angles. With track and response superimposed on the same graph and with time as the abscissa and amplitude as the ordinate, lead and lag values may be obtained on any line drawn parallel to the abscissa, as long as both functions intersect the line. This latter condition will not always hold near the extreme amplitudes if there are amplitude errors (overshoots and/or undershoots). At this range, one also must be careful that the two points being compared are on the same side (temporally speaking) of the reversals, that is, in the same phase of the cycle.

When the response function reaches the line first, the subject is leading the target; when it arrives after the target function, the subject is lagging behind the target. Coding lead and lag durations as plus and minus values, one may again describe a distribution of timing error. The algebraic mean (CE) of this distribution would indicate whether the subject tended to lead or lag behind the target. Naturally, the

other indicants (VE, AE, SD, rms) would be appropriate (to the extent that assumptions about the distribution were not seriously violated by the data) and could be meaningfully interpreted. The sample could be taken from a single horizontal line, which in the case of simple sine-wave tracking might be the mean of the track course, from a number of parallel lines representing different amplitudes or at a fixed time rate (e.g., every 0.25 second).

Any continuous function can, as we have seen, be analyzed into its component frequencies. Complex tracking inputs are frequently constructed by combining sine waves of different frequencies and amplitudes. However, when the composition is unknown, as in the case of a response function, the components can be estimated rather accurately. This is accomplished electronically by passing the signal through a number of narrow band-pass frequency filters. With both target and response functions filtered in this way, they can be compared at each frequency band as to their *phase relationships.* If, for example, the frequency of a particular component is 2 Hz (hertz, or cycles per second) and phase lag is 0.25 sec, then the target and response functions are out of phase by 180° at this frequency. At other frequencies the phase lag may be different. However, one way of describing the phase relation between two complex functions (i.e., combinations of two or more frequencies) is in terms of the *average phase angle lag* (or lead) in degrees. This value may be converted to mean lead or lag time, with reference to the fundamental, or primary, frequency (see Trumbo, Noble, and Baganoff, 1965). Actually, the average phase angle between signal and response cannot be translated directly into lag time, since it is a composite of different lags at different frequencies; but an interpretation relative to the fundamental frequency is probably not seriously misleading. An analysis of the error in phase taken only at the fundamental frequency might be a reasonably good indicant of the temporal error of performance.

The phase angle at any frequency band is determined by the method of *cross-correlation.* This may be performed in the analog mode by what is essentially a cross-multiplier of the two functions, or in the digital mode by familiar correlation methods. Cross-correlation of two functions which have been digitized begins with a simple product-moment correlation. Then the values representing one function are displaced with respect to the other (usually by one sampling interval) and the correlation is repeated. This process is continued until a maximum relationship is found between the two functions. This coefficient describes the relationship between the two functions when they are "in phase," and the number of displacement steps (sampling intervals) necessary to reach this maximum indicates the time lag between the two functions. The relationship between phase angle scores obtained by analog computer methods and mean lead-lag scores obtained by hand-scoring or step-function tracking at 2 samples/cycle is a positive and relatively high value, but not a perfect relationship, as shown by Trumbo and associates (1965). An alternative method, but one which Poulton classified as "not recommended," is obtained by cross-correlation values taken at a fixed sampling rate from the entire track and response functions, rather than separate from the different component frequency bands. Poulton's objection was essentially that an overall analysis may be misleading, since the time lags at reversals may be significantly larger than time lags at the points of reflection, for example. On the other hand, in the case of simple sine-wave tracking where the fundamental is by far the predominant frequency in both target and response functions, a simple cross-correlation may give an estimate of the phase relationship between signal and response which is not seriously biased.

Poulton (1974) also classified as "not recommended" (1) overall estimates of high frequencies in the response or (2) in the error function obtained by counting reversals and determining the excess number relative to reversals in the track; (3) frequency analyses of the error function and the phase relation of error to the track; (4) the autocorrelation function of the error (obtained as in cross-correlation, but where a function is correlated with itself, rather than with another function, then repeatedly displaced in time by some sampling unit and recorrelated, yielding a picture of the periodicities in the error function); and (5) time-on-target scores. Each of these indicants was rejected by Poulton because it may give either misleading results or artifacts of some sort. Of particular interest, because it is so much a part

of the tradition in motor skill research, is the *time-on-target score* (TOT). The TOT is the measure normally obtained from the pursuit rotor, or rotary pursuit, a standard laboratory apparatus for the study of motor skills for a number of decades. The pursuit rotor is essentially a phonograph turntable with a target near the perimeter of the disc which the subject attempts to track with a stylus as the table turns. When he is successful and the stylus point is in contact with the target, a standard electric clock or other time measurement device operates. Thus, the score obtained is the total time on target, which is evaluated relative to a fixed trial period of, say, 30 or 60 seconds. Major limitations of TOT scores were first cited by Bahrick, Fitts, and Briggs (1957). Like dichotomous scores used in nonskill studies, TOT divides the time course of a trial into two values: the time on target and, by subtraction, the time off target. Within these two categories no consideration is given to variability of response within the target range or outside that range. Thus, with a large target, performance would be seen to improve rapidly until the score approximated 100% of the time on-target, then the indicant would be insensitive to further changes in performance. Nevertheless, analysis of the subject's total response distribution, as measured from the center of the target, might well show a continued reduction of rms error. Similarly, a very small target might well be relatively insensitive to large changes in rms error early in the development of tracking skill. These nonlinear relations between TOT and changes in the error distribution (rms error) could lead to misinterpretations of the effects of independent variables on rate of learning, as Bahrick and his colleagues have shown. In this connection, Bahrick and his associates (1966) offer an appropriate summary for this section on the measurement of skill:

The principal danger in using response indicants is not the loss of information. . . . Frequently investigators are interested in certain aspects of performance that are adequately reflected by a given indicant, and the neglect of other potentially available information is justified by the purpose. The danger lies in the arbitrary choice among indicants reflecting somewhat different characteristics of the underlying distribution without detailed knowledge of the nature of these differences. Such arbitrary choice, coupled with the failure to recognize the consequent selectiveness of the obtained information, may lead to apparent conflicts of results from studies using different indicants as well as to significant misinterpretations of data. (p. 650)

Experimental Methods

While this review has focused on measures and indicants which serve as dependent variables in studies of skill, there remain a number of other considerations with respect to both experimental and correlational research which should be acknowledged, however briefly.

Independent Variables. For the most part, studies of motor skill have been concerned with three classes of independent variables: organismic, procedural, and task variables. Procedural variables, those conditions which define the learning situation such as length of trial, work-rest intervals, instructions, and the like dominated research on motor skills prior to World War II. These studies were concerned with testing theoretical issues emanating from general learning theories, such as questions of reactive inhibition, massed versus distributed practice, and transfer of training. Little consideration was given to analyzing or describing skilled performance, emphasis being on readily assessable outcome scores reflecting overall efficiency of learning (or performance) under the various procedural treatments.

After World War II, with the growth of engineering psychology and concern with human performance in man-machine systems, emphases shifted to task variables, including, for examples, the physical properties of the control, the coherence of the stimulus, display amplification, control-to-display ratio, and configurations of stimulus and response elements. At times research on task variables has been concerned with effects on the skilled motor performance of the operator, but perhaps more often attention has been focused on measures of system performance rather than of human performance. Taylor (1957) first sounded the alert that systems research might well tell us something about systems behavior but little about the behavior of the human operator. Systems performance measures rather hopelessly confound man and machine components. Thus, to use Taylor's example, the fact that a boy-plus-bicycle system will win a race against a boy-plus-pogo-stick system reveals very little about the relative skill level of the two boys or

about the task conditions which affect skilled performance. Nor are the implications of this example limited to complex systems or simulators, as Taylor noted. Whenever we place a control in a subject's hand and record the performance of a piece of laboratory apparatus to which that control is attached, we measure the performance of a system. Change the control, the display, or whatever, and the resulting change in system output is a confounding of effects on man and machine. Taylor's message is simple, but it is perhaps the most fundamental issue of all for those who would study skilled performance.

Organismic variables are concerned with internal states and changes brought about by such factors as aging, sleep loss, drugs, prolonged continuous performance, or unusual environmental conditions. Actually, as these examples suggest, organismic variables may be more appropriately seen as intervening rather than independent variables. Thus, if one considers the drug or the sleep loss as the treatment, the effects of which depend upon changes in an organismic state (e.g., "arousal"), then that state is an intervening variable.

Tasks. There is no universally accepted schema for classifying tasks used in motor skills research. The scheme used thus far in this article has been based on stimulus and response continuity leading to the three classes: discrete, serial, and continuous movements. Other schemata have been based on the extent of muscular involvement ("gross" and "fine" coordinated movements), the type of muscular contraction ("isometric" and "isotonic"), the extent of control by antagonistic muscles ("slow tension" versus "ballistic" movements) and the type of feedback information available ("visually guided," "blind," etc.). Fleishman (1966) has continued to refine a taxonomy of skilled performance tasks based on eleven factors identified through correlational and factor-analytic techniques. Fitts, Noble, Bahrick, and Briggs (1959) suggest a taxonomy based on the concept of *response constancy.* These authors describe the concept as follows:

The term "response constancy" describes the fact that an individual is able, on successive occasions, to select from among a large family of response patterns a particular one which will permit him to achieve a uniform outcome. As an illustration, an individual is able to throw a ball through a variety of trajectories and with a variety of throwing motions and yet hit a target consistently. (pp. 1.12–1.13)

Tasks can be classified into four categories based on this fundamental characteristic of skills, depending on (a) whether the body is in a stable relationship with the environment just prior to response initiation, and (b) whether external stimuli are fixed or changing during the execution of the response. Type I response constancy ("a self-initiated response following preparation") permits preparation from a stable position with responses made in relation to a fixed environment (throwing darts, hitting golf balls). Type II ("stimulus-initiated response sequence following preparation") assumes a stable body position but a changing stimulus, as in throwing darts at a moving object, attempting to hit a baseball, trapshooting. Type III ("a self-initiated response sequence without preparation") assumes a changing body position and a stationary environment, as in running shots in basketball or the infielder throwing to first base on the run. Type IV ("a stimulus-initiated response sequence without preparation") describes skilled performance where both the body position and the relevant environment (target) are dynamic, as when the basketball player passes on the run to a running teammate, or the quarterback, fading back, passes to the receiver angling across the football field. This taxonomy, based as it is on a fundamental property of motor performance, would seem to be a useful one, though it has received little notice. The bulk of research in skill appears to deal with Types I and II response constancy—that is, where responses are initiated from a stable body position.

Specification of Task Conditions Affecting Anticipation and Timing. Skilled motor performance is possible because people can anticipate future events and time movements to coincide with them, thereby overcoming the reaction time handicap. Poulton (1957) identified three types of anticipation, based on the kind of foreknowledge available. *Effector anticipation* refers to response readiness or preselection on the basis of foreknowledge about the amplitude, force, direction, or rate required. As an example, in a task which always requires responses of a fixed or restricted range of amplitudes, the subject can be preset to make such responses and not others. Knowledge of the control, the control-display ratio, the limits of the display, and so on will benefit effector anticipation. *Receptor anticipation* concerns the operator's opportunity to read ahead and "see" what responses will be required in the immediate future. The main determinant of receptor anticipation is *preview* of coming events, as when one can see the highway ahead and anticipate necessary control operations. *Perceptual anticipation* depends upon prior experience with the task and on its coherence—that is, redundancies, periodicities, and limits. It refers to anticipation based on an accurate cognitive model of the task and its deterministic or probabilistic properties. Thus, for example, the driver on a familiar highway is prepared for certain curves, stops, or turns because he knows when to expect them.

Perceptual anticipation, in particular, is aided when the regularities of the track are readily detectable. This accounts, in part, for the general superiority of *pursuit* over *compensatory* displays in tracking task. With pursuit tracking the target is presented as one of two dynamic elements in the display and runs its course independent of the control actions of the operator. Similarly, the control actions are faithfully represented in the second element (the follower) of the display. By contrast, compensatory displays have a single dynamic element, the second element being a fixed null indicator. The deviations of the dynamic element from the null position (the error) comprise a joint function of an external program and the operator's attempts to compensate, that is, to keep the error nulled. Pursuit tracking thus provides unconfounded information about the track course and unambiguous feedback about the effect of control movements on the controlled element (i.e., the follower); consequently, visual and kinesthetic feedback data can be coordinated.

Timing. Effective utilization of advance information (obtained through preview or prior learning) depends on timing. Anticipation implies responding in advance of or simultaneously with some environmental event. The ability to do so depends on accurate estimation of the passage of time following some prior event. The temporal coherency, the frequency properties, and the rhythmic patterning of the task affect timing accuracy; furthermore, there is evidence that kinesthetic feedback provides cues for timing behavior. Whether the decaying kinesthetic memory trace from the prior response (Adams and Creamer, 1962) or the level of kinesthetic activity during the interresponse interval (Ellis, 1969) is more critical for timing is controversial. Nevertheless, specification of the dynamic properties of the control affecting kinesthetic information as well as the amplitude, rate, and acceleration requirements of the task would appear to be important in predicting and understanding the timing performance.

Specification of Task Conditions Affecting Movement Control. Task conditions described in the previous section affect kinesthetic feedback which may provide information important for timing. Such information also may be relevant to the control of movement amplitude, rate, and acceleration, as Bahrick (1957) suggested. Essentially, Bahrick assumed that control dynamics which provide discriminable changes in force cues relevant to a dimension of movement control will benefit performance on that dimension. Thus, a spring-damped control provides a gradient of force which varies with the *amplitude* of movement, while a viscous-damped control has a force requirement which varies with *rate* of movement, and control mass determines the gradient of force which varies with acceleration. It seems reasonable that precision in the control of movements along any dimension would be facilitated by discriminable and relevant force cues. Conditions affecting such cues should be considered in designing research in motor skills and should be specified in reporting results.

Correlational Methods

The methods of correlation and factor analysis have been used in a number of ways to study motor skills. Most prominent have been studies identifying factors in skilled performance and the change in factor structure which occur as skill is acquired. Early attempts in this direction utilized intertrial correlation matrices for a given task. Woodrow (1938), noting that correlation coefficients decrease as a function of the distance between trials but that coefficients between successive trials increase from early to late practice, speculated that abilities which are initially important for performance fall off as practice continues and that other abilities, important for refinement of skill, assume greater importance. Jones (1966), citing similar data, concluded that the process governing the effects of practice on performance is *simplification,* the dropping out of more general factors as practice proceeds, leaving factors specific to the criterion task. Fleishman (1966) agreed in general, but argued that more general abilities also play a role and interact with level of learning. He cited, for example, evidence that while spatial-visual abilities tend to drop out as predictors of skill performance, kinesthetic abilities show an increasing importance (Fleishman and Rich, 1963). Seashore (1951) used correlations and factor analyses to evaluate the role of sense modality, muscle system, and movement patterns in skill performance. He concluded that performance was seldom limited by sensory or effector mechanisms, but primarily by inadequate patterning or sequencing of movements.

Fleishman (1966) made extensive use of factor analyses to identify the ability factors in performance. His taxonomy of eleven factors and the refinement of reference tests to measure each factor represents the most systematic work in this area.

Finally, correlational and factor-analytic methods have been used to provide the sort of information about the relationships between performance indicants called for earlier in this article. Here the procedure is to correlate different measures and indicants taken from the same task, rather than scores from different trials or different tests. Fitts, Noble, and Bahrick (1959) reported on the factor analysis of 17 indicants of performance on a compensatory tracking task; 6 of 8 factors extracted could be meaningfully interpreted, providing insights into the components of the criterion performance.

BIBLIOGRAPHY

Bahrick, H. P.; Fitts, P. M.; and Briggs, G. E. Learning curves: Facts or artifacts? *Psychological Bulletin,* 1957, *54,* 256–268.

Bahrick, H. P., and Noble, M. E. Motor behavior. In J. B. Sidowski (Ed.), *Experimental methods and instrumentation in psychology.* New York: McGraw-Hill, 1966.

Fitts, P. M. The information capacity of the human motor system in controlling the amplitude of movement. *Journal of Experimental Psychology,* 1954, *47,* 381–391.

Fitts, P. M.; Noble, M. E.; Bahrick, H. P.; and Briggs, G. E. *Skilled performance.* Wright-Patterson Air Force Base,

Ohio: United States Air Force, Wright Air Development Center Final Report, 1959.

FLEISHMAN, E. A. Human abilities and the acquisition of skill. In E. A. Bilodeau (Ed.), *Acquisition of skill.* New York: Academic Press, 1966.

JONES, M. B. Individual differences. In E. A. Bilodeau (Ed.), *Acquisition of skill.* New York: Academic Press, 1966.

POULTON, E. C. *Tracking skill and manual control.* New York: Academic Press, 1974.

SEASHORE, R. H. Work and motor performance. In S. S. Stevens (Ed.), *Handbook of experimental psychology.* New York: Wiley, 1951.

TAYLOR, F. V. Psychology and the design of machines. *American Psychologist,* 1957, *12,* 249–258.

WOODROW, H. The effects of practice on test intercorrelations. *Journal of Educational Psychology,* 1938, *29,* 561–572.

DONALD A. TRUMBO

MOTOR SKILLS: TECHNIQUES OF TRAINING

The Systems Approach

The training process may be conceived as a system involving an interconnected set of decisions and procedures carried out within the context of a set of given resources and constraints imposed by the realities of the specific situation. The system may be thought of as having an overall goal, such as achieving a specified level of performance in the trainee population within specified time and cost limits. The principal decisions include the definition of post-training (or transfer) performance criteria, decision about precisely what is to be learned, and decisions about the choice of training media and techniques. The procedures include methods of defining performance goals and deriving the training content, procedures for controlling and scheduling practice, and procedure for evaluating training outcomes. The constraints include the characteristics of the trainee population, the cost of training media and in many instances either the total time available or some target date, such as the commissioning of a plant or even a crucial football fixture. Thus, the systems approach focuses on methods of analyzing training problems and not just on recommendations about the efficiency of particular techniques, for each training problem is to some extent unique.

Task Analysis

Methods of analyzing training problems are legion (Duncan, 1972). The essential difficulty is that there is no generally agreed taxonomy of human performance. One of the best known is that of Gagné (1965), but Miller's work (1953, 1962) is perhaps more relevant to motor skills, with attempts to describe different sorts of performance required of the skilled operator in terms of processes such as scanning and search, detection of cues, identification of cues, short- and long-term retention of information, interpretation and decision making. To be of practical use, any taxonomy must specify a set of categories which are mutually exclusive and exhaustive; moreover, they must be unambiguous to any reasonably well-trained task analyst. If these stringent conditions are not met, then it is hardly possible to test the generality of prescribed training techniques. Existing taxonomies, though useful in a general way, can often be faulted in this respect.

A given task can be described at a variety of levels, and some aspects of skill can be described more adequately than others. A task such as piloting an airliner clearly involves a complex of knowledge, procedures, strategies, and perceptual skills. Gross statistical analyses, such as critical incident technique, can sometimes point to aspects of performance which might be modified by training or better engineering design. At the other extreme, routine assembly skills have been described (e.g., Seymour, 1966) by methods similar to those used in work study as a step by step list of cues and actions. There is, perhaps, no one descriptive system which is suited to all cases.

Annett and Duncan (1967) have proposed a practical approach to the problem of analysis at different levels, and this consists essentially of a series of increasingly detailed redescriptions of the task. Any task can be thought of as having goals and being comprised of actions aimed at the attainment of these goals and requiring various kinds of input information, some externally provided and some being feedback for previous actions, which is needed to control activity. The task is described as a hierarchy of subtasks, each of which is redescribed until a level is reached at which a specific training solution can be proposed that will achieve the desired performance level. This turns out to be useful in practice, since it is often possible to identify the "gaps" in knowledge or skill which training must fill without proceeding to the sensorimotor level of analysis.

Skill Acquisition

In reviews by Fitts (1964) and Annett (1971), the process of skill acquisition is divided into three overlapping phases. In the *cognitive* phase, the trainee acquires job knowledge, learns rules and strategies, and can generally be helped by a variety of procedures including verbal instruction. In the second *associative* phase, actual practice of the task predominates, and the trainee learns association between inputs and between actions and their results directly through his own experience. In the third *autonomous* phase, further changes are thought to occur which increase the efficiency of information processing within the nervous system and which are characterized by reduction in the degree of conscious control of perception and movement. The trainer has available to him a battery of techniques, which include verbal instruction and demonstrations, control over task difficulty and various forms of guidance, the scheduling of practice trials and rest pauses, the provision of error corrective feedback, and evaluation comment. We will now discuss these techniques in relation to the Fitts scheme of skill acquisition.

Cognitive Training

Even simple motor skills depend heavily on what the operator *knows* about the situation. In the more complex skills typified by the aircraft pilot, knowledge of the dynamic properties of his machine and of procedures cannot be clearly separated from the actual skills of flying. Knowledge of principles have been shown to affect perceptual judgments, and rules and strategies relevant to the skill can be learned. Not all "theory" is however relevant or helpful, as has been shown with troubleshooting tasks. Knowledge of electronic theory is less effective than having a useful search strategy, and it has been shown that experienced troubleshooters forget basic theory while becoming more proficient at the actual task. In general, it would seem that for the learning of motor skills, ver-

bal instructions can guide behavior or at least eliminate some trial and error, but the verbal principles must be clearly relevant to that aim. Verbal instructions in the form of "coaching tips" may, however, play a significant role when, for instance, the performance can be held together by the use of strategy, and that strategy is capable of verbal encoding. Coaches often give verbal instruction in analogical form. For example, in hockey, "Imagine there is a nail sticking out of the side of the ball and hit it," or in piano playing, "*Love* that top E!" Such instructions are designed to elicit behavior which at least approximates the desired performance. Keele (1973) has argued that the development of skill depends on the formulation of a set of motor programs. While practice with feedback is necessary to the final adaptation or selection of motor programs, verbal description or their model performances may be the first step. If this is so, it clearly depends on a fundamental process of imitation, that is, the ability to translate a visually or verbally encoded sequence of actions into at least approximately adequate motor programs.

Verbal instruction may also be a means of sensitizing the trainee to relevant cues, that is, as a method of controlling attention. Where a skill depends critically on a sensory discrimination, the presentation of labelled instances and noninstances seems to be effective. Often a trainee may know in some sense what to do without knowing exactly what things should look like when the performance is adequate.

In general, verbal instruction seems to have at least three main functions—first, as a means of generating approximately the desired performance; second, as a means of controlling attention to relevant cues; and third, as a means of identifying relevant cues, which may then be stored in memory for later use as "templates" against which to match potential action and feedback signals.

Guidance

The role of verbal instruction or modeling in generating motor programs may also be fulfilled by other forms of guidance, such as mechanically inducing the appropriate action or preventing error. Guidance techniques have a long history (Holding, 1965; Annett, 1969). Mechanical guidance has been used in learning sequences (mazes), positioning and tracking, and perceptual learning (where it is usually termed cuing or prompting). A general conclusion from many studies is that guidance is only effective if it is used early in training where it can effectively reduce random trial and error, but transfer to unguided tasks can be poor, especially in situations where guidance provides a cue and/or crutch upon which performance depends.

Associative Learning and Practice

The second phase of associative learning is characterized by progressively improved speed and accuracy of responses which have at least in principle been learned by repeated practice. The extensive literature on massed versus spaced practice with simple skills is described elsewhere, but generally recommends spaced practice as superior. Part/whole training has similarly long history, and nowhere is the need for a definitive taxonomy more obvious. The problem is how to define a "part" skill and how to classify "parts" with different characteristics. Naylor (1962) classified tasks according to their difficulty along two dimensions, "organization" and "complexity." Organization refers to their difficulty, presumably measured by error rate or amount of practice needed to reduce error. From the fourfold classification of tasks on these two binary dimensions, two empirical generalizations are: that with a task high in organization, an increasing task complexity favors the use of whole methods, while with tasks of low complexity, increasing low organization, increasing complexity favors part methods.

Annett and his associates (1971), using their *task analysis method,* proposed four ways in which a part of any task is related to its superordinate whole. The whole may be made up of a sequence of relatively simple operations (in which case whole methods will capture this sequence), or it may be made up of relatively unrelated subroutines, where whole and part methods are equivalent. Where any subtask forms part of a strategy (one test in a troubleshooting sequence), whole training which emphasizes the decision rules should be superior. Where two or more tasks are time shared in the accomplishment of the whole, the decision whether to use part or whole methods depends on the degree of interference between these subtasks, and this may in turn depend on the level of skill achieved. Thus, part training may be necessary before the whole can be practiced without performance breakdown, but this must be followed by practicing the whole.

Information Feedback

It is generally agreed that information feedback is the most significant factor in skill training (Bilodeau, 1969; Annett, 1969; Holding, 1965). The crux of the matter is not so much what kind of artificial feedback is possible, but when and how to withdraw it. Additional feedback introduced by an instructor or a training device may be to no avail if transfer to the real situation (without intrinsic or training feedback) leaves the trainee bereft of the necessary information to execute the task, since it is generally found that the removal of KR usually produces performance decrement. In practical terms, it is important that the trainee should be able to use intrinsic task feedback. During practice with both augmented and intrinsic feedback, learning might occur by a simple associative process by which the intrinsic feedback takes on the characteristics of the augmented feedback, but this cannot always be guaranteed in situations where the extrinsic cue is used to control performance.

Extended Practice

In the final autonomous phase, the supposed underlying process is one of decreased dependence on external and kinesthetic feedback. After extensive practice, a repetitive motor skill is thought to be run off by a motor program. For a simple motor skill, such as aiming at a target, Crossman (1959) suggested that evidence of changes in the distribution of response patterns may mean that less effortful responses are selected by feedback. Keele (1973) proposed that effective motor programs may not need extrinsic feedback. The efferent signal is accompanied by a matching pattern, which is used as a kind of internal check somewhere in the peripheral nervous system. Whatever is the case, it seems likely that feedback processing demands are progressively reduced by repetitive practice. At this stage, where performance may continue to improve indefinitely, rather little is known about optimal training conditions. However, the progressively reduced load on central information processing may result in boredom which might be relieved by introducing more demanding targets or by adding secondary loading tasks.

Training Devices and Simulators

The justification for many training devices is partly economic and partly pedagogic, with consideration of the safety of trainees and equipment and often technological factors taken into account. Practice on a realistic simulator can be cheaper than, say, flights in a jumbo jet, by many orders of magnitude, and this is often the overriding consideration when complex civil and military hardware is involved. The question of safety to the trainees and instructors is also important, since many flying accidents occur on training flights.

The pedagogic reasons lie in the control over the learning situation which a device can permit. For example, exercises may be repeated at will and rest pauses taken as necessary in a way which may not be possible in the real situation. In particular, infrequently occurring situations, such as emergencies, can be produced at will. A training device will often incorporate performance recording which may not be possible in the real situation, and these performance records can be used for selection testing and training evaluation or to provide augmented feedback to the trainee. Typical of these uses are the flexible gunnery trainers used in World War II, which used filmed target planes and direct tracking and ranging measurements.

Another compelling reason for the use of a simulator is, as in the case of space flight, the technological difficulty of producing "real" experience. As a preliminary to the space program, a number of attempts were made to simulate weightlessness, including the use of water tanks, drop-towers, and centrifuges, and even extending to flying aircraft in a parabolic trajectory to produce up to 30 seconds of true weightlessness.

The design of simulators typifies one of the essential and recurrent problems of training, namely, what differences between the training trials and the criterion trials are desirable and justifiable to produce the best results in terms of cost and transfer in a given situation.

Osgood's (1949) theory of transfer and interference is of limited value, predicting as it does, that transfer is proportional to stimulus and response similarity, and predicting interference when stimulus similarity is high and response similarity is low. His two-dimensioned transfer surface points to the desirability of realism, but complete realism is often either undesirable on other grounds or is technically difficult or too expensive to achieve. A more detailed theory is required, but empirically, excellent transfer can often be attained with gross departures from superficial realism. In flight trainers, displays and controls are relatively easy to simulate, but motion cues can only be simulated expensively and inadequately, in the event it may often be necessary to discover by experiment whether a particular cue in a particular form is necessary for positive transfer.

Adaptive Trainers

The advent of the computer has added a new and potentially valuable dimension to the design of training devices, namely, the possibility of adaptive training. Adaptive trainers typically vary task difficulty as a function of ongoing performance. One of the earliest was the Solartron Automatic Keyboard Instructor (SAKI) designed by Pask (1960). The task is to translate a set of numbers into key punch responses, and both response latency and errors were used to modify the presentation rate or the type of material presented. Adaptive tracking trainers have been described by Hudson (1964) and Kelley (1962). It is possible to vary the forcing functioning and display and control gains, and so hold the trainee's tracking error constant at all stages of practice. Adaptive training is found to be clearly superior on training on some fixed difficulty level, especially either very high or very low difficulty relative to the level of the criterion task. Kelley makes the interesting suggestion that adaptive tasks may have a use not only in directly training difficult vehicle-control skills, but also to provide secondary loading tasks to aid the acquisition of fixed difficulty skills.

BIBLIOGRAPHY

ANNETT, J. *Feedback and human behavior.* London: Penguin, 1969.

ANNETT, J. Acquisition of skill. *British Medical Bulletin,* 1971, *27,* 266–271.

ANNETT, J.; DUNCAN, K. D.; STAMMERS, R. B.; and GRAY, M. S. *Task analysis, training.* Information Paper 6. London: Her Majesty's Stationers Office, Department of Employment, 1971.

BILODEAU, I. McD. Information feedback. In E. A. Bilodeau and I. McD. Bilodeau (Eds.), *Principles of skill acquisition.* New York: Academic Press, 1969.

DUNCAN, K. D. Strategies for the analysis of the task. In J. Hartley (Ed.), *Strategies for programmed instruction on educational technology.* London: Butterworth, 1972.

FITTS, P. M. Perceptual-motor skill learning. In A. W. Melton (Ed.), *Categories of learning.* New York: Academic Press, 1964.

HOLDING, D. *Principles of training.* London: Pergamon, 1965.

KEELE, S. W. *Attention and human performance.* Pacific Palisades, Calif.: Goodyear, 1973.

NAYLOR, J. C. Parameters affecting the relative efficiency of part and whole practice methods: A review of the literature. *United States Training Devices Center report 950–1,* 1962.

See also MOTOR LEARNING THEORIES; TRANSFER OF TRAINING

JOHN ANNETT

MOURNING: PSYCHOANALYTIC THEORY

Freud's Theory

Sigmund Freud's *Mourning and Melancholia* (1917), first drafted in 1915, went beyond the clinical explanation of the mechanism of grief and its resolution as compared to the pathological condition of melancholia. Freud called mourning an affect. Since the German word *Trauer,* the term Freud used in the title of his paper, can be translated as either "mourning" or "grief," an affect having outward manifestations as well as internal contents, one can view Freud's contribution as one to affect theory as well as to clinical mourning theory.

Pollock (1961) proposed that mourning is an adaptational process, having sequential phases and stages, phylogenetically evolved and present as a reaction to loss, but not solely to object loss. Freud (1917) already noted that grief is the reaction to the loss of a loved person or to the loss of some representation in the abstract of a meaningful object—for example, one's country, liberty, or an ideal. Freud reaffirmed that grief or mourning is not to be regarded as a patholog-

ical condition, not to be treated medically, and is overcome after a certain lapse of time. Freud noted that any interference with normal mourning is either useless or potentially harmful. Behaviorally and psychologically the mood of mourning is painful and is accompanied by a loss of interest in the outside world, a loss of capacity to invest in a new love object or ideal, and a turning away from any activity unconnected with the loss.

Although reality indicates that the loved object or ideal no longer exists, the mourner initially is unable to withdraw his love or attachment from that which is lost. Instead, a counterreaction may ensue—namely, the mourner may turn away from reality and cling to the lost object or ideal through denial or even through a hallucinatory wishful psychosis that keeps the absent object or ideal alive. Normally reality is the victor, although not at once. As Freud (1917) wrote, reality gradually predominates

at great expense of time and cathectic energy, and in the meantime the existence of the lost object is psychically prolonged. Each single one of the memories and expectations in which the libido is bound to the object is brought up and hypercathected, and detachment of the libido is accomplished in respect of it. . . . When the work of mourning is completed the ego becomes free and uninhibited again. (p. 245)

Thus, we can suggest that an object or ideal loss is transformed into an ego loss, which utilizes the adaptational process of mourning to "heal itself." Mourning processing, like "working through," is internal work to restore psychic equilibrium.

If one considers the mourning process with its eventual phase of freedom and noninhibition in relation to ideals, thought, or artistic, scientific, or creative activity, then one can recognize this fundamental and universal process as the adaptation to loss and change with an outcome of resolution, gain, creativity, and/or investment of psychic energy in new areas or objects. The mourning process, an example of the utility of the economic or quantitative point of view, is not, as Freud noted earlier, only the reaction to object loss or bereavement, which is a subclass of the mourning process. It is a universal adaptation, goes on throughout the life cycle of the individual, is found in all cultures, and when ritualized can be found throughout man's existence in his religious, social, and cultural practices.

Other Psychoanalytic Theories

Various researchers have written about the mourning process after Freud's major contribution to this area. Melanie Klein (1940) saw mourning as a phase of disorganization and subsequent reorganization of both the inner and outer world of the mourner. Further, she indicated that one's way of responding to the loss of a loved object in later life is patterned on the way he responded to similar experiences which he may have had in infancy and early childhood. Klein argued that our mode of reorganizing our object relations will be in large part determined by the means utilized in earlier experiences. Not all psychoanalysts accept Klein's theoretical conclusions, especially her equation of early life loss and grief with adult mourning. Further, her approach to mourning was mainly through the study of depressive illness. This latter may be an outcome of abnormal mourning, and hence may not be the same as the mourning process as seen by others.

Lindemann's (1944) observations on symptomatology, the course of normal grief, and deviations from the normal were important contributions to the understanding of acute grief. Bowlby (1961) and Pollock (1961) called attention to the occurrence of mourning behavior in animals.

Bowlby (1961) believed that grief is an amalgam of anxiety, anger, and despair following the experience of what is feared to be an irretrievable loss. It differs from separation anxiety in that anxiety is experienced when the loss is believed retrievable and hope remains. Bowlby described three phases of mourning: (1) the urge to recover the lost object, (2) disorganization, and (3) reorganization. In an earlier paper Bowlby (1960) demonstrated the reality of grief in very young children, from six months onward, and the intimate relationship that grief has to separation anxiety. Bowlby described the sequence of responses to be observed when young children were removed from their mothers and placed with strangers in three phases: protest, despair, and detachment. Protest is associated with separation anxiety, despair with grief and mourning, and detachment with defense through lack of attachment.

Pollock (1961) viewed mourning as an adaptation process consisting of an acute and chronic stage, each having various substages or phases and the resolution of the process heralded by the investment in new objects.

Parkes (1970) studied the reactions of widows to the deaths of their husbands for 13 months after the loss. In this fashion, he empirically gathered data about the process of grief and its changes over time. In earlier work Parkes reported increased mortality among widowers after the deaths of their wives.

Pathological Mourning

Pathological mourning reactions have frequently been equated with depression and, in the older terminology, melancholia. However, the distinction between these two conditions —pathological mourning and the depressive states—may be psychologically and perhaps biologically significant. In pathological mourning we may see various manifestations of defense against mourning; Deutsch (1937), for example, described the absence of grief, and Fleming and Altschul (1959) described the activation of the mourning process during psychoanalytic treatment. Somatic reactions, symbolic acts, and affective states may also indicate abnormal mourning. Among the psychological reactions, we may observe denial, hallucination, thanatophobic behavior, survivor guilt, and even suicide. Further research may increasingly assist us in making meaningful differentiations as well as comparisons between these two pathological entities: abnormal mourning and pathological depression.

Freud (1917) suggested that the object representations lose their libidinal energy when loss occurs and mourning begins. The withdrawal of libido, however, cannot be accomplished in a very short time, if what is lost was meaningful to the mourner. Hence the explanation for the gradual and relatively long, drawn-out process. Although Freud questioned whether the process begins simultaneously at several points or follows some form of fixed sequence, in psychoanalysis it frequently becomes evident that first one and then another memory becomes activated. In the minimourning process, the acute grief work always sounds similar; however, each lament is derived from some different source and the process repeated microscopically, over and over again, albeit with shorter durations. If the loss does not possess great significance for the ego, a significance reinforced by many links, then the loss will not be of such quality as to evoke the characteristic mourning process that is usually seen in losses following more intensive involvements.

Pollock's Theory

Pollock (1962) attempted to study four loss situations in an attempt to more fully understand the mourning process: (1) adults who had lost one or both parents through death during childhood, (2) adults who had lost one or more siblings through death during childhood, (3) adults who had lost one or more of their children through death, and (4) adults who had lost one or more spouses through death. His findings confirmed the universal phases and stages of the bereavement category of the mourning process; however, he found that with some losses mourning could never be totally completed—for example, a mother's loss of her child.

Pollock's research also clarified the differentiation of the mourning process from the effects of the object loss, especially in childhood, on subsequent personality development. Grief and mourning seemingly can occur during childhood and adolescence, although some psychoanalysts believe that mourning cannot occur until adolescence, while others believe that mourning can occur in young children. Perhaps these differences can be reconciled if one considers the mourning process with its phases as having different developmental times when they first appear. In young children and higher mammals, we may observe the earliest phases of the process, but psychic immaturity may preclude total mourning processing. In adolescence, where the personality becomes much more coherent and integrated, the fuller process may be possible. Further clinical studies will be needed to provide data that can convincingly answer this important issue.

Uncompleted Mourning

The question of uncompleted mourning as compared to pathological mourning also has great clinical significance. Obviously many childhood losses are traumatic without being pathogenic. When there has been a childhood loss through death, one may observe an object "extirpation" which may then give rise to compensatory mechanisms designed to handle the possible resulting psychic deficiencies. These mechanisms need to be distinguished from defensive operations, which are utilized to handle intrapsychic conflicts. Therapeutic and technical handling of individuals with these difficulties may be different depending upon the type of loss, when it occurred, the preloss relations with the object, the stage of development at the time of the loss, and the type of mourning process that occurred. Was there an arrest in the mourning process, a fixation in the process, or a pathological deviation of the process? In children and adults, repeated observations have been made of anniversary reactions which are indications either of an uncompleted mourning process or in some instances of serious somatic illness or suicidal tendencies, all indications of serious pathological mourning reactions.

Conclusion

In summary, the mourning process seems to be a universal adaptive process to change and loss with an outcome of gain and freedom once the process has been completed. Bereavement, the specific reaction to the death of a loved object, is a subclass of the mourning process. The mourning process is a means of reestablishing equilibrium intrapsychically, interpersonally, socially, and culturally. As such, it is intimately connected with religious belief systems and especially ideas of the "afterlife" (Pollock, 1975).

The mourning process has evolved from lower forms of adaptations and may be seen in higher mammals. Socioculturally the mourning process is intimately involved with the rites of passage. One can observe a phylogenetic sequence in the emergence of the process, the initial phases being the ones that can be observed earliest in young children, whereas later phases of the process seemingly appear in older children and adults. Mourning process resolution and outcome can be freedom, revitalization, and, in gifted individuals, creative products. If there is an arrest of the process at a particular stage or if a component is fixated at a particular phase, clinically one must determine why this occurred, under what conditions it occurred, what are the distinctive manifestations of the arrest, fixation, or regression, what resolutions occurred, what interventions are possible to affect outcome, and what can be done preventively. The identification of high-risk vulnerable individuals is a significant task to be undertaken. Recent preliminary biological studies (Hofer, Wolff, Friedman, and Mason, 1972) suggest biochemical and possible neurophysiological alterations that vary during the various phases of the mourning process. These approaches, integrated with clinical observations, may assist our further understanding of this adaptation to change.

As we become more aware of the various adaptations man must make during the life cycle, the importance of the mourning process for various stages of the life cycle will take on additional significance. Current research studying these issues cross-culturally, in various socioeconomic groupings and in various age categories, indicates that successful mourning adaptations facilitate life processes.

BIBLIOGRAPHY

BOWLBY, J.   Grief and mourning in infancy and early childhood. *Psychoanalytic Study of the Child,* 1960, *15,* 9–52.

BOWLBY, J.   Process of mourning. *International Journal of Psycho-Analysis,* 1961, *42,* 317–340.

DEUTSCH, H.   Absence of grief. *Psychoanalytic Quarterly,* 1937, *6,* 12–22.

FLEMING, J., and ALTSCHUL, S.   Activation of mourning and growth by psychoanalysis. *Bulletin of the Philadelphia Association for Psychoanalysis,* 1959, *9,* 37–38.

FREUD, S. (1917).   Mourning and melancholia. *Standard Edition.* London: Hogarth Press, 1957, *14,* 243–258.

HOFER, M. A.; WOLFF, C. T.; FRIEDMAN, S. B.; and MASON, J. W.   A psychoendocrine study of bereavement, parts I and II. *Psychosomatic Medicine,* 1972, *34,* 481–504.

KLEIN, M.   Mourning and its relation to manic-depressive states. *International Journal of Psycho-Analysis,* 1940, *21,* 125–153.

LINDEMANN, E.   Symptomatology and management of acute grief. *American Journal of Psychiatry,* 1944, *101,* 141–148.

PARKES, C. M.   The first year of bereavement. A longitudinal study of the reaction of London widows to the death of their husbands. *Psychiatry,* 1970, *33,* 344–467.

POLLOCK, G. H.   Mourning and adaptation. *International Journal of Psycho-Analysis,* 1961, *42,* 341–361.

POLLOCK, G. H.   Childhood parent and sibling loss in adult patients: A comparative study. *Archives of General Psychiatry,* 1962, *7,* 295–305.

POLLOCK, G. H.   On mourning, immortality, and utopia. *Journal of the American Psychoanalytic Association,* 1975, *23,* 334–362.

GEORGE H. POLLOCK

MOVEMENT PERCEPTION

Detection of movement is a fundamental capacity of even the most primitive of visual systems. It is important not only for the detection of moving objects, which might be predator or prey, but also for the accurate estimation of the organism's own movement with respect to the environment. The primitive nature of the ability to detect motion is reflected in the fact that it can exist in the absence of ability to analyze form. The frog, for example, will starve to death even if surrounded by unmoving flies; it responds to and consumes them only if they are in motion. The periphery of the human retina can be taken as another example of a system which sometimes requires movement of an object for its detection; a small object held in the periphery of vision can be invisible unless it is moved.

The ability to navigate using visual signals as information about the motion of the organism with respect to stationary objects also seems to exist even in primitive visual systems. All rapidly flying insects, for example, must use vision to avoid collisions. It has been suggested that the necessary information is contained in the pattern of expansion produced by the "looming" of the pattern in the visual field (Gibson, 1968). Avoidance reaction in response to such optical "looming" appears to be a reflex present in many lower animals and has also been shown to be present in the human infant at ten days of age (Bower, Broughton, and Moore, 1970).

Motion Detectors

Since motion had been considered a higher-order phenomenon by many earlier investigators, its existence in primitive forms presented something of a paradox. An apparent resolution of this paradox has been achieved recently by discoveries in neurophysiology. Using newly developed techniques which allow recording from a single neuron, investigators have found what seem to be motion-detecting units (sometimes called directionally sensitive units) in the visual systems of a wide variety of both vertebrate and invertebrate species. These units may respond to a stimulus moving over the retina in one direction but not another. They are thus able to signal the presence of a stimulus motion of a particular direction. While these simple motion-detecting units seem to provide the necessary physiological mechanism for motion sensitivity in lower animals, the extent to which they underlie human motion perception is not clear and is currently one of the key issues in the field.

One classic phenomenon which seems particularly susceptible to explanation in terms of motion-detecting units is the motion aftereffect. This is seen after viewing an area with continuous motion, such as a waterfall or rotating spiral. After viewing such a moving pattern for 30 seconds or so, a stationary surface will be seen to move in the opposite direction. This illusion can be explained by assuming that motion detectors are arranged in opponent pairs which normally antagonize and "balance" each other. Fatigue of one member of the pair would result in an "imbalance" and an illusion of motion. The motion aftereffect is specific to a particular area of the retina, which seems to localize it at a fairly early stage of visual processing. It is similar in this respect to the color aftereffect.

In its simple form, the motion detector will be triggered when two separate areas of the retina are stimulated in the proper sequence. This implies that any motion percept mediated by these motion detectors would coincide with the motion of an optical image with respect to the retina. The assumption of the coincidence of perceived motion with motion of the image with respect to the retina can be called the "image/retina hypothesis." While the motion aftereffect seems to offer some support for this hypothesis, there are many other phenomena of motion perception which seem to be counterexamples.

Induced Motion

One counterexample to the image/retina hypothesis is the phenomenon of induced motion. This can be observed when the moon is seen through moving clouds; the moon appears to move in the opposite direction to the clouds, even though its image may be stationary on the retina. This phenomenon can be explained in terms of motion-detecting units with the assumption that they respond at some level to a motion *difference.* If so, the units would respond to relative motion, that is, motion of one part of the image relative to another part, rather than image motion with respect to the retina.

The assumption that perceived motion is basically relative motion is, of course, not new; it was fundamental to the Gestalt theory. This assumption requires that, at some later stage, the sensed relative motion is attributed to one or the other (or perhaps both) of the moving objects. Gestalt theory postulated some rules which govern this process, among them that an enclosing object tends to be the frame of reference for the motion of the enclosed object.

Induced motion can be considered analogous to simultaneous brightness contrast, that is, a gray patch looks darker against a white background than against a black background. Simultaneous brightness contrast has been explained by the assumption that the visual system responds to the ratio of the brightness of adjacent areas, rather than the absolute brightness level. Units which are sensitive to such differences, that is, contour-detecting units, are known to exist in many visual systems. Units which respond to differences in motion would similarly account for induced motion. Such units have, in fact, been discovered recently in the cat (Bridgeman, 1974).

Motion Analysis

Another counterexample to the image/retina hypothesis is closely related to the phenomenon of induced motion; this is the phenomenon of "motion analysis" (Johansson, 1975). In one demonstration of this phenomenon, a wheel rolls in a dark room with one illuminated point at its rim; this point describes a cycloidal path, and this path is perceived. If now a light at the hub is added, the cycloidal motion is perceived as two distinct components: a circular motion of the rim point as it rotates about the hub and a translatory motion of the whole rolling wheel. The generally accepted explanation of this phenomenon is in terms of the Gestalt "frame of reference" (Wallach, 1959). The "common" motion of the moving points (in the case of the rolling wheel, the common motion would be the horizontal translatory component) is somehow extracted, and then this common motion, or some system possessing this common motion, is used as a frame of reference for the "remaining" motion. While the mechanics of this frame of reference are generally left undefined, the phenomenon seems clearly to involve some more complex process than motion-detecting units.

An entire class of counterexamples to the image/retina hypothesis occurs when eye movements are considered. One such counterexample occurs when the eye makes saccadic movements. (These are rapid "flicking" movements from one stationary fixation to another; they are distinct from the much slower pursuit movements which involve fixation of a moving object.) The "hopping" of the image over the retina produced by the saccadic eye movement does not lead to a motion percept. This perceived stability during saccadic eye movements is sometimes called "position constancy."

One line of explanation for this perceived stability is to simply reject the assumption that image/retina motion is ever responsible for the perception of object motion (Gibson, 1968). In terms of motion-detecting units, only the output of the "relative motion units" would ever produce the percept of a moving object; since an eye movement shifts the entire field at once, no relative motion, and, thus, no object motion would be seen, and perceived stability would result. However, though the lack of relative visual motion must be at least part of the explanation of perceived stability, it cannot be the entire explanation. If one eye is closed and the other rocked to and fro by gently pulling at the corner of the eyelid ("passive" eye movement), a rocking motion of the entire visual world can easily be seen. This must be due to the unitary motion of the visual image over the retina. The classic explanation of the difference in perception between the passive eye movement and the saccade is sometimes called the cancellation theory. It was first suggested by Helmholtz over 100 years ago but remains the generally favored explanation today. According to the cancellation theory, image/retina motion does produce a motion signal, perhaps mediated by motion detectors. However, this motion signal can be "cancelled" by a second, antagonistic, signal, called the "extraretinal signal," produced somewhere in the oculomotor system. This extraretinal signal is assumed to be proportional to the "command" signal from the brain to the eye muscles; it would thus be present during the saccade but absent during the passive movement. The command signal, when present, is assumed to be accompanied by an "extraretinal signal" which cancels just the amount of image motion expected to be produced by the commanded eye movement.

Another related counterexample to the image/retina hypothesis is the well known fact that a luminous moving object, in an otherwise dark room, can be seen to move even though the eye pursues it so as to completely eliminate image motion with respect to the retina. This is true even if the "object" is an after-image, thus completely ruling out any possible image/retina motion. This motion percept must also be due to an "extraretinal signal" of some kind which arises somehow from the oculomotor system. This extraretinal signal would presumably be generated whenever the eye is sensed to move relative to some perceptually stable frame of reference, such as the room in which the observer stands.

Cancellation Theory

The perceived stability of the world during saccadic eye movements and the perceived motion of a pursued object both seem to involve a "taking into account" of eye movements along with image/retina motion to produce a veridical percept. The cancellation theory assumes that the same process is responsible for both phenomena; this process would involve a "subtraction" of the extraretinal signal produced by the oculomotor system from the image/retina signal. Thus, the image/retina signal would give rise to a motion percept in the case of a really moving object with a stationary eye, or in the case of passive eye movement. The extraretinal signal would give rise to a motion percept in the case of a pursued object. But, with normal active eye motion, the two signals would "cancel," and perceived stability would result. Further evidence for this "cancellation" theory comes from the study of patients who have a paralyzed eye muscle. Attempts on the part of the patient to move his eye produce a perceived motion of the world in the direction of the attempted movement, presumably mediated by the extraretinal signal.

While the eye-movement evidence almost certainly requires the postulation of some sort of extraretinal signal in addition to the "retinal" signal from the motion-detecting units, it is not clear that the two signals add to each other algebraically, as the cancellation theory assumes. One problem with this assumption is that it requires a highly precise prediction of the extent of eye movement if complete cancellation is to result. This precision seems unlikely considering the inexactness of the saccadic eye movements themselves. Another problem is that, in the case of pursuing an object against a stationary background, the background *can* be seen to move in a direction opposite to the object—the Filehne illusion—(Stoper, 1973). This background motion can be seen even in a normally illuminated environment, though, for many observers only with difficulty. This difficulty is in part due to the paradoxical nature of the motion involved; the background seems to move, yet in another sense it seems stationary. In the terminology of Gibson, it is motion of the visual "field" rather than of the visual "world." The perceived background during pursuit can be contrasted with that during a saccade. In both cases, the visual "world" is stationary, but the visual "field" motion of the background is not seen during the saccade. One explanation for the difference in perceived motion between saccade and pursuit is that there are two different types of extraretinal signals. One would be capable of generating motion of an object which is stationary with respect to the retina but would not cancel any image/retina motion. The other, which would operate only during the saccade, would simply inhibit the image/retina signal. This assumption of inhibition of motion detectors during the saccade is consonant with the findings of several investigators that the threshold for displacement detection rises during the saccade. A simple demonstration of this momentary decrease in motion sensitivity is the fact that one's own saccadic eye movements are invisible in a mirror, while a second observer can see them easily.

The assumption that the extraretinal signal which occurs during pursuit does not cancel the retinal signal suggests a possible mechanism for motion analysis. Thus, if there is ocular pursuit of "common" motion of a complex display, the retina itself would serve as a frame of reference for the "remaining" motion. When the eye follows the translatory component of a rolling wheel, the points at the rim will describe a circle relative to the retina. The circular component would thus be carried by the retinal signal, while the translatory component would be carried by the pursuit extraretinal signal. Since they do not cancel each other, both these components would remain distinct in perception.

Illusory Motions

Other examples of phenomena which seem explainable only by invoking an extraretinal signal are the autokinetic effect and the oculogyral illusion. The autokinetic effect refers to the illusory motion of a small point of light in a completely dark room. This illusory motion can occur even with an afterimage, showing that image/retina motion is not necessary; its source is most likely the extraretinal signal which operates during pursuit. Somehow the visual system erroneously "assumes" that the eye is moving. Some recent experimental evidence indicates that an image-retina signal due to eye drift might be involved in this erroneous assumption (Matin, 1964).

The oculogyral illusion occurs commonly after the head is spun about a longitudinal axis; the world seems to spin the other way. It can also occur with alcohol or barbiturate intoxication or various pathological conditions. The illusion is sometimes explained in terms of vestibular nystagmus; this nystagmus is assumed to produce image/retina motion, and thus illusory motion. However, the oculogyral illusion occurs even in the absence of observable nystagmus (Howard and Templeton, 1966). It can best be understood by noting that the vestibular system normally functions to produce compensatory eye movements which keep the retina more or less stationary with respect to the real world, even in the presence of head and body movement, and even in the absence of visual input. An object moving with respect to the real world will thus move with respect to the retina, and its motion will be sensed by means of the resulting retinal signal. If this object is fixated, the motion of the object would be sensed by means of the pursuit extraretinal signal. The magnitude of this signal would be proportional to the oculomotor activity necessary to maintain fixation, above and beyond the compensatory motion. The aftereffect of vestibular stimulation can be seen as producing an erroneous compensatory motion, which results in image/retina motion even with stationary objects and thus illusory motion. Even if the stationary objects are fixated, the additional oculomotor activity necessary would lead to a spurious pursuit extraretinal signal, and thus, once again, illusory motion.

Stroboscopic Motion

Another phenomenon of motion where no image motion over the retina exists is *stroboscopic motion* (also known as phi phenomenon, apparent motion, beta motion). This is the apparent motion that occurs with sequential presentation of stationary stimuli. The motion perceived on a moving-picture screen is stroboscopic, since each frame is really a stationary picture. In the laboratory, two spatially separated stimuli are presented separated by some time interval. If this time interval is too short, the two stimuli are seen stationary and simultaneous. If too long, they are seen stationary and in succession. At some intermediate range of interval, between 50 and 200 msec, depending on distance, one object is seen moving between the two locations. This was a key phenomenon in the development of Gestalt theory, which explained it in terms of a "fusion" of the cortical excitations produced by the stimuli. This fusion was likened to a cortical "short circuit," and the resulting flow of current was assumed to be the physiological correlate of apparent motion (Koffka, 1935). Gestalt physiology has been discredited by several experimental findings (that is, stroboscopic motion can take place across a scotoma produced by a cortical lesion even though no "current" can conceivably flow across this lesion). It cannot be said, however, that motion detectors provide a satisfactory substitute physiological mechanism.

There is no particular difficulty in accounting for the simple occurrence of stroboscopic motion in terms of motion detectors; these respond to discrete sequential stimulation as well as to continuous motion. One oft-cited argument against motion detectors as mediators of stroboscopic motion is based on the evidence of Rock and Ebenholtz (1962). These investigators showed that, if stimuli are flashed at locations A and B, but an eye movement occurs between the flashes so that A and B excite the same retinal locations, stroboscopic movement will nevertheless result. This movement cannot be due to motion detectors, since they would require disparate retinal excitations. They also showed that a stimulus flashed twice in the same physical place, but with eye movement causing spatially disparate retinal excitations, will be seen as stationary. They conclude that it is disparity in phenomenal, rather than retinal, location which is the necessary condition for apparent motion. An alternative explanation, however, is that image/retina motion is normally necessary for apparent motion but that the extraretinal signals occurring during eye movement must also be taken into account.

Other facets of stroboscopic motion are not so easily explainable in terms of relatively simple motion detectors and extraretinal signals. One of these is the fact that motion is obtainable over huge angular separations (as much as 180° if long-duration stimuli are used). No detectors with receptive fields anywhere near this size have yet been discovered. Another facet of stroboscopic motion is its high susceptibility to so-called "higher-order influences" such as set, configuration, and various "intelligence factors" (Sigman and Rock, 1974). It is difficult to see how these factors could exert their influence on low-level motion detectors. For example, the Gestalt laws of "grouping" seem to govern which of several possible motion percepts will occur. In the arrangement shown, a stimulus A is followed by both B and C, with B closer than C. If B is not present, motion from A to C will be seen. But with B present, *only A to B* motion is seen; C is seen stationary, simply flashing on and off. A motion-detector hypothesis might explain this by "inhibition" of one detector by the other. But what seems to contradict such an explanation is that no inhibition occurs if stimulus D is included in the dis-

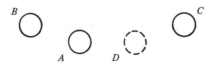

play and flashed at the same time as *B*. Now, both *A* to *B* and *D* to *C* motion can be seen simultaneously. Despite the evidence against Gestalt physiology, its concepts of attraction and fusion between excitations seem to be the most plausible explanations of such phenomena. In this particular case, the fusion of *A* to *B* would decrease the attraction between *A* and *C* and thus prevent motion from *A* to *C*.

Other facets of stroboscopic motion which seem to be more readily explained in terms of Gestalt concepts concern the phenomenal observation that perceived motion is motion of an *object*. Thus, in the case of optimal time interval between stimuli, only one object is seen in motion even though two stimuli are presented. This object is seen to smoothly change location, and if conditions are optimum, can clearly be seen in intermediate locations (Kolers, 1972). Such facts seem to require that an adequate theory of motion perception be somehow integrated with a theory of object perception. At present, though tantalizing, the existence of motion dectectors can be seen as at best only a very partial explanation of visual motion perception.

BIBLIOGRAPHY

BRIDGEMAN, B. Visual receptive fields to absolute and relative motion during tracking. *Science,* 1974, *178,* 1106–1108.

GIBSON, J. J. What gives rise to the perception of motion? *Psychological Review,* 1968, *75,* 335–346.

HOWARD, I., and TEMPLETON, W. *Human spatial orientation.* New York: Wiley, 1966.

JOHANSSON, G. Visual motion perception. *Scientific American,* 1975, *232*(6), 76–88.

KOLERS, P. A. *Aspects of motion perception.* New York: Pergamon, 1972.

KOFFKA, K. *Principles of Gestalt Psychology.* New York: Harcourt, Brace, 1935.

MATIN, L., and MACKINNON, E. G. Autokinetic movement: Selective manipulation of directional components by image stabilization. *Science,* 1964, *143,* 147–148.

ROCK, I., and EBENHOLTZ, S. Stroboscopic movement based on change of phenomenal rather than retinal location. *American Journal of Psychology,* 1962, *75,* 193–207.

SIGMAN, E., and ROCK, I. Stroboscopic movement based on perceptual intelligence. *Perception,* 1974, *3,* 9–28.

STOPER, A. Apparent motion of stimuli presented stroboscopically during pursuit movement of the eye. *Perception and Psychophysics, 1973, 13,* 201–211.

WALLACH, H. Perception of motion. *Scientific American,* 1959, *201,* 56–60.

ARNOLD STOPER

MÜLLER, GEORG E. (1850–1934)

Müller was a German psychologist, who produced considerable research in the areas of attention (doctoral dissertation), psychophysics (invented method of right associates—*Treffermethode*), vision, physiological psychology, and memory (developed memory drum with F. Schumann). Müller conceived of learning and memory as a more active process than had Ebbinghaus, such that the learner consciously organizes and groups material, finding meaning even in nonsense syllables. Müller's group at Göttingen entertained ideas later considered basic to Gestalt psychology.

PATRICK J. CAPRETTA

MÜLLER, JOHANNES (1801–1858)

A German physiologist, Müller formulated the doctrine of specific nerve energies (in *Handbook of Physiology,* 1833), stating that sensation consists of awareness of properties of sensory nerves themselves, and that each sensory nerve has its own characteristic energy or quality. Müller's was the first systematically presented alternative to the age-old image or emanation theory of sensation. Müller conducted empirical research in sensation showing, for example, the relation between the anatomy of the ear and acoustics; that gases could also be tasted; and that mechanical stimulation might elicit tastes. Müller prompted his student Helmholtz to devise a technique for measuring the speed of neural impulse by his own insistence on instantaneous conduction of such action.

PATRICK J. CAPRETTA

MULTIDIMENSIONAL SCALING

Taken in its broadest sense, multidimensional scaling is the simultaneous representation of a set of *n* objects with respect to a set of *k* scales. If this representation is numerical, the result is a set of nk numbers. A particular number can be indicated as x_{im} where *i* is the index of the object and *m* is the index of the scale. Alternatively, the representation may be graphical, in which case each object is plotted as a point in a space whose dimensions or axes correspond to the scales. Such a graphical representation can be translated into a set of numbers by using x_{im} to refer to the projection of the ith point on the mth dimension.

An enormous range of data analysis techniques could be described in this way, but multidimensional scaling usually refers only to techniques designed for measures of either similarity or dissimilarity for a set of pairs generated from the set of objects. Thus, multidimensional scaling can be compactly described as similarity analysis and the key concept which must be analyzed is the notion of nearness or closeness which similarity denotes. Although our language favors the use of terms such as *similarity, proximity,* and *nearness,* it is in fact somewhat more direct to analyze the inverse of these and thus subject the concept of dissimilarity to careful scrutiny. However, the term *difference* will be avoided because of the danger of confusion with the arithmetic operation.

Univariate Dissimilarity

If one denotes a measurement of the dissimilarity of two things i and j by d_{ij}, then it seems essential to require this measurement to satisfy the following simple restrictions: (a) $d_{ij} = d_{ji}$ (b) $d_{ij} = 0$ if the objects are identical with respect to the scales in question and $d_{ij} > 0$ otherwise. If the scale values of these objects are x_i $(i = 1, \ldots, n)$, then a simple example of a function of the scale values which meets these requirements is

$$d_{ij} = |x_i - x_j|$$

Dissimilarity can be thought of as a univariate continuum in its own right which has a lower bound naturally indicated by zero, no intuitively obvious upper bound, and has a symmetric relation to the two objects whose scale values are x_i and x_j.

An important question is whether dissimilarity is additive. That is, is there some order preserving function f such that the combination of two dissimilarities $d^{(1)}$ and $d^{(2)}$ can be represented algebraically as $f^{-1} [f(d^{(1)}) + f(d^{(2)})]$? All multidimensional scaling techniques in use at this time assume that this is so. This assumption implies that dissimilarity is

what is referred to in psychophysics as a prothetic continuum.

Univariate similarity is clearly some order reversing function of dissimilarity which shares the properties of symmetry and nonnegativity. Although it is easy to produce a pair of things having zero dissimilarity, this is not quite so easy for similarity. The upper bound for the similarity scale can be set at either infinity or some positive number such as one. Two obvious examples of similarity functions are $1/|x_i - x_j|$ and $\exp(-|x_i - x_j|)$.

Composite Dissimilarity

Since in most contexts ascertaining how dissimilar two objects are is helpful even when a number of properties or aspects of the objects must be taken into account in arriving at this information, dissimilarity in a multivariate context must be viewed as some form of composition or concatenation of univariate dissimilarities. Aside from this consideration, there does not seem to be any reason to suppose that this kind of dissimilarity differs in any essential respect from its univariate counterpart. That is, it still remains a univariate, nonnegative, and possibly additive continuum which has a symmetric relation to its components. It is only multivariate insofar as more than a single property is involved in its specification.

In considering the precise way in which a composite dissimilarity is derived, the assumption of additivity becomes quite critical and has not been seriously challenged. By far the most popular composition rule has been

$$d_{ij} = [\sum_m (x_{im} - x_{jm})^2]^{1/2} \qquad (1)$$

which is the assumption of a root-sum-of-squares rule for combining the k univariate dissimilarity functions $|x_{im} - x_{jm}|$. The more narrowly additive

$$d_{ij} = \sum_m |x_{im} - x_{jm}| \qquad (2)$$

also suggests itself as a possible composition rule and, more generally,

$$d_{ij} = [\sum_m |x_{im} - x_{jm}|^p]^{\frac{1}{p}} \qquad (3)$$

where the parameter p is to be specified or even estimated from the data. Which, if any, of these rules is to be employed is a matter for which there are no clear guidelines, although computational convenience heavily supports the use of **1**.

If a composite dissimilarity rule satisfies the additional restriction $d_{ij} \leq d_{ik} + d_{kj}$, known as the triangle inequality, then it can be called a distance formula and can be said to specify a metric for the set of points. General rule **3** is a distance provided $p \geq 1$. Rule **1** is the familiar Euclidean or straight line distance, **2** is referred to as the city-block metric, and **3** is referred to variously as an L_p metric, a Minkowski p-metric, or a power metric. Traditionally, composite dissimilarity rules have been thought of as distances, although there seems to be no a priori reason to restrict them to satisfy the triangle inequality.

Although corresponding composition rules for similarity readily suggest themselves (such as using $p \leq -1$ in the right side of **3**), existing techniques either presume that the data are dissimilarity measures or provide internal rules for translating similarity measures to dissimilarity measures rather than attempting their direct analysis.

Since the main goal of multidimensional scaling analysis is the estimation of the scale values x_{im} from composite dissimilarity measures, it is important to query any specific composition rule concerning how far these scale values can be estimated even in principle. The use of $|x_{im} - x_{jm}|$ as a univariate dissimilarity function immediately implies that any constant can be added to each scale value for a particular scale and the resulting dissimilarity will remain unchanged. Thus, the origins of the resulting scale values are arbitrary and can be set, for example, at their mean so that $\sum_i x_{im} = 0$.

The commonly used rule **1** implies an even broader class of transformations of the x_{im} which leave the composite dissimilarity unchanged. If a new scale value is formed from a weighted sum of the old as follows:

$$y_{im} = \sum_q x_{iq} t_{qm} \qquad (4)$$

and the weights satisfy the two relations

$$\sum_m t_{qm} t_{pm} = \begin{cases} 1 & \text{if} \quad q = p \\ 0 & \text{if} \quad q \neq p \end{cases} \qquad (5)$$

(which is to say that the weights are orthonormal), then the dissimilarity of a pair of things will be exactly the same if calculated on the basis of the scale values y_{im} as if the original x_{im} are used. In graphical terms, transformations of this sort correspond to a rotation of the axes and imply the familiar rotational invariance of Euclidean *straight-line* distance. This feature of rule **1** can be either viewed as very troublesome if it has no intuitive justification in terms of the underlying scales or as a realistic feature of the model if it expresses a conceptual invariance.

Indices of Similarity or Dissimilarity

The scaling of the degree of similarity or dissimilarity displayed by a particular pair of objects is a univariate scaling problem and, in general, the advantages and limitations of the various techniques developed for this purpose apply here as well. Thus, one might employ rating scales, magnitude estimation, or confusability indices, to mention only a few possibilities. However, it should be noted that dissimilarity has a natural zero point and that some multidimensional scaling techniques implicitly require that the dissimilarity measures relate to this zero point. That is, the solution may not be invariant with respect to change of origin in the dissimilarities. For this reason, univariate scaling techniques which yield interval scale results may not be suitable in some situations.

A complication in any univariate scaling situation is the frequently observed nonlinear relationship between measures obtained by different techniques or even by the same technique applied with different standards. Thus, the possibility should always be entertained that the dissimilarity model being used will fit some nonlinear transformation of the dissimilarity measures substantially better than the original measures.

Fitting Dissimilarities

The heart of multidimensional scaling is the technique for converting a sample of dissimilarity measures into scale value estimates. Currently available techniques divide into two groups, the first of which analyzes the derived quantities:

$$b_{ij} = \tfrac{1}{2}(d_{i.}^2 + d_{.j}^2 - d_{..}^2 - d_{ij}^2) \qquad (6)$$

where $d_{i.}^2$, $d_{.j}^2$, and $d_{..}^2$ are the averages of the ith row, the jth column, and the entire array of an $n \times n$ matrix of squared dissimilarities, respectively. The advantages of this transformation is that, in the case of Euclidean distance rule 1,

$$b_{ij} = \sum_m x_{im} \, x_{jm} \qquad (7)$$

so that b_{ij} is a scalar product. Principal components analysis of the array of b_{ij}s yields the desired scale value estimates. This is the earliest approach to multidimensional scaling (Torgerson, 1952) and is sometimes referred to as a metric technique because of the strong assumption that the dissimilarity data are Euclidean distances.

An alternative approach is the approximation of the dissimilarities themselves. In order to express this, let d_{ij}^* denote the approximation by the model and d_{ij} denote the actual observation being approximated. The quality of the fit for some particular set of scale value estimates x_{im} is typically defined by specifying a badness-of-fit or loss function $L(d_{ij}, d_{ij}^*)$ which is minimal when $d_j = d_{ij}^*$. This loss function can be chosen to satisfy a variety of conditions which seem important to the data analysis, scale invariance the most common example. On the other hand, numerical minimization techniques involving a certain amount of expense and unreliability are required in order to determine the values of the x_{im}s which will minimize $\sum L(d_{ij}, d_{ij}^*)$. Nevertheless, the flexibility offered by defining the estimation problem in this way more than offsets this disadvantage.

A paper by Shepard (1962) provoked intense interest in defining a loss function $L(d_{ij}, d_{ij}^*)$ which was invariant with respect to any order-preserving transformation of the data, d_{ij}. This interest was due in part to the hazards of univariate scaling of dissimilarity mentioned earlier and in part to the desire to analyze data having an unknown but monotonic relation to a particular dissimilarity model. As a result of this work, the range of data suitable for multidimensional scaling has been greatly broadened. For example, similarity measures can be readily analyzed by employing any order-

reversing transformation and using a dissimilarity model such as Euclidean distance. This family of techniques is referred to as nonmetric because of the weaker assumptions made about the relation of the data to the model.

The essential step in nonmetric multidimensional scaling is the definition of a second function $T(d_{ij}, d_{ij}^*)$ which creates a set of numbers having two characteristics: (a) they are ordered in the same way as the data d_{ij} and (b) they are as close as possible in some sense to the approximations d_{ij}^*. One obvious illustration of such a transformation is a simple permutation of the d_{ij}^*s wherever necessary in order to make their ranking conform to that of the d_{ij}s. Guttman (1968) refers to this method as the *rank image* approach while Kruskal (1964) employs a somewhat different procedure termed *monotone regression*. A loss function $G[T(d_{ij}, d_{ij}^*), d_{ij}^*]$ is then specified and some numerical procedure employed to minimize its sum. In short, two loss functions are defined, one an intermediate function T which defines the degree of rank order conformity, and the second a global function G which defines the degree of fit of the approximations d_{ij}^* to the "nearest" order preserving transformation of the data defined by T. Combined, they determine a single loss function L which is sensitive only to the ordering of the observations d_{ij}.

Let $\hat{d}_{ij} = T(d_{ij}, d_{ij}^*)$. Then the loss function

$$S = \left[\frac{\sum(\hat{d}_{ij} - \hat{d}_{ij}^*)^2}{\sum \hat{d}_{ij}^2} \right]^{\frac{1}{2}} \qquad (8)$$

is called stress in the multidimensional scaling literature while the goodness-of-fit function

$$K = \left[\frac{(\sum \hat{d}_{ij}^2)(\sum d_{ij}^{*2}) - (\sum \hat{d}_{ij} \, d_{ij}^*)^2}{(\sum \hat{d}_{ij}^2)(\sum d_{ij}^{*2})} \right]^{\frac{1}{2}} \qquad (9)$$

is referred to as the coefficient of alienation.

A great deal of practical experience along with several comprehensive Monte Carlo studies of nonmetric multidimensional scaling algorithms can be summarized as follows: (a) various nonmetric approaches produce rather similar results, (b) they are less sensitive to certain kinds of error in the data than metric techniques, (c) they should be employed only when $n/k > 4$, and (d) there is a serious danger that nonmetric algorithms will converge to solutions which do not give the lowest possible minimum of the criterion, so that a variety of starting approximations should be employed. Shepard (1974) has reviewed the literature on the performance of these nonmetric techniques.

Individual Differences in Multidimensional Scaling

It is typical in experiments employing dissimilarity or similarity judgments to collect data from several respondents. The dissimilarity models described so far imply that replications of a dissimilarity measure d_{ij} will be across essentially equivalent units. In fact, this is seldom the case where more than one subject is involved; two people are almost certain to view the objects before them in fundamentally different ways. Consequently, there have been a number of attempts to write some form of interindividual variation into the dissimilarity model.

Let the rth observation of dissimilarity for objects i and j be indicated by d_{ijr}. Carroll and Chang (1970) proposed the following very simple modification of Euclidean distance:

$$d_{ijr} = [\textstyle\sum_m w_{mr} (x_{im} - x_{jm})^2]^{1/2}$$

This model permits individuals to vary in the relative importance that they attach to the k scales, and this is indicated for the mth scale and rth individual by the weight w_{mr}. As it happens, this extension of the Euclidean model removes its rotational invariance. The x_{im}s then define a set of scale values which indicate the group perception of the objects.

This model can be thought of as allowing for a differential stretching of the dimensions of the group space but with no variation in the directions which are differentially stretched. One step in generalizing this scheme would be to permit individuals to vary in the k directions which are differentially weighted but require that these directions be orthogonal.

More generally, individuals might differentially stretch the group solution along any k noncoincident directions. This latter model has been investigated by Tucker (1972).

BIBLIOGRAPHY

CARROLL, J. D., and CHANG, J. J.   Analysis of individual differences in multidimensional scaling via an N-way generalization of "Eckhart-Young" decomposition. *Psychometrika*, 1970, *35*, 283–319.

GUTTMAN, L.   A general nonmetric technique for finding the smallest coordinate space for a configuration of points. *Psychometrika*, 1968, *33*, 469–506.

KRUSKAL, J. B.   Multidimensional scaling by optimizing goodness of fit to a nonmetric hypothesis. *Psychometrika*, 1964, *29*, 1–27.

SHEPARD, R. N.   The analysis of proximities: Multidimensional scaling with an unknown distance function. *Psychometrika*, 1962, *27*, 125–140, 219–246.

SHEPARD, R. N.   Representation of structure in similarity data: Problems and prospects. *Psychometrika*, 1974, *39*, 373–421.

TORGERSON, W. S.   Multidimensional scaling: I. Theory and method. *Psychometrika*, 1952, *17*, 401–419.

TUCKER, L. R.   Relationships between multidimensional scaling and three-mode factor analysis. *Psychometrika*, 1972, *37*, 3–27.

JAMES O. RAMSAY

MULTIPLE FUNCTION PRINCIPLE

The principle of multiple function relates each manifest psychic act to a complexity of diverse underlying motivations. It supersedes Freud's concept of overdetermination and subsumes that of the ego's synthetic function. Falling within its explanatory scope are such phenomena as symptom formation, sublimation, pansexualism, and characterology.

It is held that organisms possessed of central steering tendencies (a characteristic whose emergence roughly corresponds to that of the central nervous system) are given to a collective functioning of the total organism. Man also shows—in addition to his obedience to and mastery of drive pressures, and opportunities and exigencies of the external world—the capacity to reach beyond his instinctual and immediate self-interest into the realm of self-judgment, a tendency to which, in order to survive, he must not give himself up entirely. Furthermore, his inclination to perpetuate old solutions irrespective of present circumstances, likewise demands both capitulation and active revision.

Ego Functions

The human organism, then, responds in its entirety to multiple internal and external directives, and conversely, each response or each psychic act gives evidence of multiple elemental factors. Although infinite in number, these factors converging upon a given psychic act can be reduced to two major or eight minor groups. The two major determinants are: (A) the ego's obedience to forces impinging upon it, to which it reacts as a problem-solver; and (B) the ego's active disposition to incorporate or assimilate those same forces into its very organization, as carried out under its own purposeful initiative. The eight minor groups consist of these two broad ego responses toward four sets of forces emanating from (1) the id, (2) the external world, (3) the superego, and (4) the compulsion to repeat. Since the two major responses are at variance with each other, and the four sets are likewise at variance with one another, a simultaneous, unmodified expression of all elements in one psychic act would be an impossibility, hence the compromise character of each given act. The organism's tendency toward collective functioning dictates a parsimony regarding this multiplicity of diverse elemental factors, the result of which is multiple function. The principle of multiple function is, then, that an attempted solution of a problem is possible only when it is of such a type that it in some way represents an attempted solution of other problems as well, although no act can solve all problems with equal success.

The fact that the ego operates in this harmonious manner, dealing with no demand in isolation but always in concert with the whole, brings about the cohesion otherwise ascribed to the "synthetic function of the ego." Under the principle of multiple function, the achievement of such synthesis is an inherent characteristic of ego activity rather than the result of one of its discrete functions; therefore, this principle embraces phenomena hitherto ascribed to the ego's synthetic function.

A close relationship also exists between the concept of overdetermination and the principle of multiple function. In contemporary usage the former is often taken as the term descriptive of the phenomenon for which the latter provides the theoretical explanation, namely, of the production of a given psychic event by a variable number of causes. Originally, overdetermination was explained by the fact that a given psychic trend was insufficient in isolation, and that two or more trends must combine to exceed the threshold of psychic effectiveness. It was specifically this denotation of the summation of stimuli and threshold values that was superseded by the concept of unified organismic action in response to diverse simultaneous determinants and the consequent exercise of compromise formation by the ego. There is a tendency for the term *overdetermination* to acquire the latter meaning, and a further tendency for it to be abandoned in favor of the term *multidetermination,* with which it is often taken as synonymous.

Clinical Phenomena

A number of familiar clinical phenomena are readily understandable in the light of the principle of multiple function. For example, the compromise nature of neurotic symptom formation can be seen as a special case of the general principle underlying all psychic acts. If, in addition to the compromise between impulse and defense, there is a secondary gain attached to the symptom, the latter again falls within the larger influences of the id, superego, and external world. Sublimation, by contrast, obeys the same principle, but owes its greater success to being a primarily active solution to the problem of mastering the outer world, while at the same time allowing successful gratification of strong instinctual drives. The readiness-to-hand of a sexual meaning in acts for which a realistic interpretation would yield sufficient explanation, is but a reflection of the principle that every psychic act must contain elements of instinctual gratification.

Some empirical observations on character likewise take on new clarity. Although there are a large number of possible combinations between underlying dominant impulses and observable character-types, certain combinations tend to recur with greater than random frequency, as for example the passive (male) homosexual impulse disposition and the paranoid projection mechanism. In this instance, the impulse is to experience powerful forces coming from the outside and to experience the passive surrender of the self to these forces. The projection mechanism provides, then, in addition to something of defensive value against them, a simultaneous fulfillment of these very wishes. Because it thus adheres to the principle of multiple function, the mechanism of projection is preferentially selected to coexist with these specific impulses.

BIBLIOGRAPHY

WAELDER, R. The principle of multiple function: Observations on over-determination. *Psychoanalytic Quarterly,* 1936, *5,* 45–62.

JAMES S. ROBINSON

MULTIPLE PSYCHOTHERAPY: ADLERIAN METHOD

Multiple psychotherapy is the treatment of a single patient by two or more therapists. Alfred Adler and his colleagues used this method of treatment as well as group therapy in the child guidance clinics they established in the Vienna school system in the 1920s. The practice of co-therapy continues to this day in the family education centers in the United States founded on Adlerian principles. During the 1940s Rudolf Dreikurs, a student of Alfred Adler, developed the technique of multiple therapy systematically and used it in his private practice in Chicago. Since Adlerian psychology is a socially oriented psychology, it lends itself particularly to this mode of treatment.

Clinical experience has shown there are many advantages in the use of this technique both for the patient and for the therapist, and it has also shown under what conditions the method can flourish.

Procedure

In the private practice method developed by Dreikurs in Chicago, the patient is usually seen first by one of the senior therapists who decides whether psychotherapy is appropriate. If so, the patient is referred to a colleague for testing or special history taking. Collection of this material allows the second therapist to establish rapport with the patient and to initiate a therapeutic relationship since he will be the active therapist. It is also a way of initiating multiple therapy.

The patient continues with the second therapist. Every fourth or fifth session the original intake therapist joins the group to evaluate and review. This session is called the *double interview.* They may review test results and the de-velopments which have taken place, or focus on crucial issues, and work through any therapeutic impasse. Sometimes several consecutive double interviews are used. In general, Dreikurs recommended not permitting more than four sessions without a double interview or else the "smooth cooperation between the therapists might be endangered."

Since it is part of the regular office procedure, and is established at the very beginning of the therapeutic contact, patients generally accept the arrangement without objection. For those patients who initially object to the procedure, exploration and interpretation of the psychological significance of their objections wins the patient's cooperation.

Advantages to the Therapist

Dreikurs, Shulman, and Mosak (1952) described the advantages of this method to the participating therapists as follows: Multiple therapy offers the opportunity of constant consultation between two therapists who use teamwork to check interpretations and choice of procedures. The presence of a third party interferes with the artificial atmosphere of the limited one-to-one relationship and permits the patient more chance to display his characteristic social relationships; for example, patients who maintain "good" behavior in their desire to please the active therapist find the consultant situation a deterrent to this faulty attitude. If a therapeutic impasse develops, a double interview offers a fresh approach, a reconsideration of issues, and a possible change in therapists. This accelerates therapy and avoids premature termination. When the therapist has become discouraged, the double interview can bring about recognition and correction of this situation. If the active therapist becomes oversympathetic, overprotective, wants to impress, or feels hostile toward the patient, the multiple therapy technique has the effect of interfering with the emotional involvement of the therapist. Therapists using multiple therapy find many opportunities to play different roles, thus providing a variety of experiences for the patient. One therapist may be active, forceful, and directive, while the other is permissive and nondirective. One may play "devil's advocate" while the other presents an "objective" point of view. Multiple psychotherapy is an invaluable teaching method. It facilitates the learning of therapeutic procedures by the junior therapist as he is free to develop with minimal anxiety. He shares responsibility and is highly involved.

Advantages to the Patient

Dreikurs, Mosak, and Shulman (1952) pointed out that any method that helps the therapist usually is beneficial to the patient also. They listed the following advantages of multiple psychotherapy to the patient: patients often enter psychotherapy with a false concept of what a therapist *should* be. They may idealize him/her so that the therapist seems to be omnipotent and omniscient. With the introduction of a second therapist who may disagree with the active therapist, the illusion of omniscience is destroyed. The therapists become human beings, not godlike, and the dependence normally fostered in a one-to-one relationship is inhibited. Multiple psychotherapy offers the patient the opportunity to work through his disturbed familial and social relationships by using two or more people in consort. People listen more carefully when they are subjects of discussion rather than participants in the discussion. Patients often see their own faulty perceptions when they are acted out in front of them. Interpretations which may be met by defensive behavior in individual therapy are reinforced by the concurrent interpretation of another "authority." The interpretation feels less "personal" and more objective to the patient. Multiple therapy facilitates termination because it prevents excessive dependency in the relationship. The patient's attachment is to the *situation* rather than to an *individual,* and the use of the therapist for self-indulgent gratification is diminished. The demand for excessive privacy on the part of the patient can be seen as a closing in of the social field. The use of multiple therapists avoids this and leads the patient to a more social orientation. The patient has the opportunity to observe a democratic relationship in action. Dreikurs pointed out that frank discussion of mistaken attitudes of the therapists and the patient establishes the foundation for a relationship based on a sense of equality and mutual respect. The patient observes the cooperation of the two therapists and learns one may be wrong without losing status. Multi-

ple psychotherapy exemplifies democracy in action and interferes with the cultural pattern which defines mistakes as degrading.

Limitations

Therapists should refrain from using multiple therapy unless they feel comfortable with the situation. A therapist who feels insecure may feel exposed when using a consultant. Manipulative patients often recognize competitive behavior between two therapists and exploit the lack of mutual respect to the detriment of their progress. Multiple therapy is not indicated when it is strongly against the patient's wishes or if the therapists do not clearly understand how to use the technique.

Patterns or Co-Relationships

Certain patterns of relationship between therapists are common.

The Authoritarian or Dominant/Submissive Relationship. The most common form of dominant/submissive relationship is the trainee-supervisor one. Concern with grades and lack of initiative could incapacitate therapy if no moves are made without consultation. The junior of a therapeutic team may have problems in relation to authority not only in trying to please, but by subtly fighting the senior therapist.

The Anarchic Relationship. In this form there is no structure in the relationship: Double interviews are held haphazardly, or the two therapists do not work well together or have different theoretical orientations. The absence of structure leads to poor results.

The Competitive Relationship. Two therapists may consciously or unconsciously try to outdo each other. The competitive relationship may lead to conflict rather than cooperation and the unconscious goal of the therapist may become triumph rather than therapeutic progress.

The Cooperation Between Peers in a Democratic Atmosphere. Multiple psychotherapy offers the patient an opportunity to see a democratic relationship in action. In an egalitarian relationship it is possible for the active therapist to admit mistakes, feelings of discouragement, and transference relationships openly. When the patient realizes the relationship between the two therapists is collaborative and noncompetitive, he feels free to bring up his problems with the active therapist. Since mutual criticism in an atmosphere of mutual respect can only occur in a frank, and open atmosphere, the prime requisite for the effective use of multiple psychotherapy is the democratic atmosphere.

Dreikurs and associates also pointed out that the patient is able to observe a cooperation which transcends competitiveness and status orientation. The patient can watch the therapists disagree without destroying a relationship, and learn one may be wrong without losing self-esteem. This lesson may have more far-reaching consequences than psychological interpretations of the patient's misconception that a mistake implies inadequacy or failure.

BIBLIOGRAPHY

ADLER, A. (Ed.). *Guiding the child.* New York: Greenberg, 1930.
DREIKURS, R. Techniques and dynamics of multiple psychotherapy. *Psychiatric Quarterly,* 1950, *24,* 788–799.
DREIKURS, R.; MOSAK, H.; and SHULMAN, B. Patient-therapist relationship in multiple-psychotherapy. II. Its advantages for the patient. *The Psychiatric Quarterly,* 1952, *26,* 590–596.
DREIKURS, R.; SHULMAN, B.; and MOSAK, H. Patient-therapist relationship in multiple psychotherapy. I. Its advantages to the therapist. *The Psychiatric Quarterly,* 1952, *26,* 219–227.

See also DREIKURS, RUDOLF

DOROTHY E. PEVEN

MULTIPLY HANDICAPPED CHILD

The great advances in medical science in recent years have resulted in an increase in the number of children who survive with multiple physical handicaps. Such children and their families are very much at risk for the development of behavior disorders, yet time and again professionals treat the physical problems while ignoring entirely the emotional sequelae of their handicaps. There are no clear maps of behavioral norms for different kinds of handicapped children. Furthermore, a definitive physical and behavioral diagnosis is often extremely difficult to make in early childhood,

as additional handicaps may only appear at a more advanced developmental age. Alternately, the handicapping influence of a particular defect may increase or decrease as the child grows older. Again the same handicap will affect the child differently depending on the etiology of the defect and the age of the child at the time of its occurrence. For example, the consequences of hereditary profound hearing loss are quite different from meningitic hearing loss in a ten-year-old child. The meningitic child already has speech and language competence, but is much more likely to have suffered brain damage than the congenitally deaf child. In the case of the multiply handicapped child, one must also consider the interactive effect of two or more physical defects. Finally, the child's temperament, whether "easy," "slow-to-warm-up," or "difficult," will also affect the behavioral outcome. Thus, when diagnosing such children, the therapist must avoid the hazard of identifying the physical defect as "additional findings," rather than as a part of the child's total personality and environment.

Diagnosis

The etiology of a particular defect can often alert the diagnostician to the possible presence of other handicaps with behavioral consequences. Vernon (1969) in a nine-year study of 1,468 deaf children, found that meningitic, Rh factor, premature, and rubella children all exhibited behavioral symptoms of brain damage to a much greater degree than did the genetically deaf. In addition, Vernon's study points to a much higher rate of mental retardation in these four deaf populations, a high incidence of aphasia among the premature and meningitic, and a high rate of cerebral palsy (over half) in children affected by the Rh factor. A high incidence of organic psychosis in children with congenital rubella coincides with the results of other studies (Chess, Korn, and Fernandez, 1971). The genetically deaf in Vernon's study had few multiple handicaps, and a much higher mean IQ than the rest of the study population. Vernon surmises that "Many of the learning and behavior problems that have in the past been thought of as due only to deafness probably have their basis in cerebral nervous system dysfunctions that are additional to the auditory impairment" (Vernon, 1969).

The incidence of the infantile autism syndrome was extraordinarily high (25%) in one study of congenitally blind children (Freedman, 1971). Freedman speculates that this might be a result, not of the handicap, but of the totally different mother-infant interaction created by the handicap. However, before making a diagnosis of autism in sensorially impaired children, the therapist must exercise great care in differentiating between true autistic behavior and the behavioral consequences of a sensory handicap.

For example, the visually impaired child commonly exhibits certain blindisms, such as waving his fingers in front of his face, rolling his head or body, poking at his eyes or staring fixedly at a source of light. Deaf-blind children rely heavily on their sense of smell as a means of orienting themselves in their environment, and this can sometimes result in peculiar and socially unacceptable behavior, such as smelling feet (Chess, Korn, and Fernandez, 1971). The deaf child frequently has a blank facies, with constantly scanning eyes (Lesser and Easser, 1972). Furthermore, the deaf often have a certain rigidity of action and thought which may result from, or be exaggerated by, their education. This may place heavy emphasis on rote learning, repetition and inhibition of normal gesture (Mindel and Vernon, 1971). These mannerisms, particularly in conjunction with aphasia, can lead to a misdiagnosis of autism (Lesser and Easser, 1972). Conversely an autistic child may be misdiagnosed as profoundly deaf or visually impaired when, in fact, his sensory handicap is quite mild (Elonen and Zwarensteyn, 1963).

Evaluating the intelligence and potential of a multiply handicapped child is another difficult and complex task facing the diagnostician. A number of attempts have been made to devise a standardized intelligence test for deaf children, but as yet none is entirely satisfactory (Berlinsky, 1952; Vernon and Brown, 1964). What appears to be a cognitive lack may in fact be a functional deficiency arising from the difficulty of accurately communicating the task to the child or understanding his response. The examiner must bear in mind that the congenitally handicapped child, particularly one who

is sensorially deprived, has experienced a totally different developmental environment from that of a normal child. This is particularly true of the deaf or deaf-blind child, who may have a severe experiential lack if he has been deprived of any consistent form of communication until school age. In fact, study after study points to the superior intelligence, language abilities and emotional adjustment of deaf children who have been exposed to sign or a combination of sign and oral language from birth, as against those who have experienced only oral training (Vernon, 1969; Freedman, 1971; Mindel and Vernon, 1971). As with so many development skills, it appears that there is an optimum period for the acquisition of language which cannot be compensated at a later age. Furthermore, as a result of the relative isolation imposed upon him by his handicap, the child may lack the commonplace knowledge of the world which we assume to be present in a normal child.

In order to evaluate the multiply handicapped child, one must learn a new set of norms regarding motor milestones, speech acquisition and affective responsiveness for each type of handicap in children whose other faculties are intact. Without such reference points, it is easy to assume intellectual retardation or behavioral deviance where none exists. Similarly, aberrant development may be overlooked because of a lack of knowledge of the child's developmental potential. When a child has multiple handicaps, an evaluation is manifestly more complicated.

Certain physical handicaps may have severe adverse influences on other areas of development. Rutter (1972) argues that, where perceptual and linguistic stimulation is inadequate or disorganized, cognitive development is likely to be retarded. Sensorially handicapped children are frequently deprived of such stimulation, unless their caretakers compensate for the child's failure to initiate parent-child interaction. Deafness, for example, may indirectly result in devastating cognitive and psychological effects for the child, should his parents fail to engage him in active communication. A similar lack of stimulation may result in speech retardation for the motorically impaired. Fraiberg (1971), and Williams (1968) have found that blindness leads to impairment in the areas of human object relations, adaptive hand behavior and gross motor development. Fraiberg found that when verbal and tactile stimulations were increased, and when the hands were educated to understand "graspability" and to reach for sound on cue, defects in these other areas were minimized. In other words, early developmental retardation may be a function of understimulation, resulting *indirectly* from the sensory defect.

The child's age, both at the time of impairment and at the time of diagnosis, is an important consideration in any assessment. The child who is adventitiously handicapped, particularly after age two, experiences a traumatic loss, as opposed to the lack experienced by the congenitally impaired child. On the other hand, the adventitiously deaf or blind child has a notable intellectual advantage over the child who has no memory of normal hearing or vision. Similarly, the *influence* of a given handicap may increase or decrease with time. As the child grows older and operates on a more complex cognitive level, he may be able to make progressively better use of other intact senses, with consequently greater feedback from his environment. One sense may compensate for another, as with the child whose visual acuity appears to be a positive influence over her ability to lip-read and communicate orally. The ability to read may also make up in part for experiential deprivations resulting from hearing and visual loss. Lesser and Easser (1972) point out, however, that other senses cannot compensate adequately for a sensory loss at an early age, as "Other modalities during infancy and early childhood are less developed in these handicapped children than in children who possess full range of perceptual faculties."

Reevaluations

The need for repeated evaluations as the child grows older must be emphasized. Only in this way can new defects be uncovered and taken into consideration. Such defects as sequencing problems, central language disorders, or an organic inability to control the muscles of articulation, have important consequences for the hearing impaired child and are frequently evident only by the time the child reaches school age. New audiology and vision tests may result in very different assessments of the child's degree of impairment. Reevaluation will often indicate that an earlier diagnosis was either incorrect or incomplete, due to the bias or inexperience of the examiner, the difficulty of testing a very young child, or the confusing behavioral manifestations associated with sensory defects. Mindel and Vernon (1971) point out that "Many school programs classify up to 40% of their deaf students as multiply handicapped (brain damaged, retarded), when the real problem is the inflexibility born of an orally based program."

Temperament—the way in which an individual characteristically reacts to a situation—also has an influence on the child's adaptation to his handicap. Research on temperament in normal, mentally retarded and rubella children has shown that those with signs of the "difficult child"—irregularity, withdrawal response, negative mood, intensity and slow adaptability to change—are most at risk for the development of behavior disorders. In our study of 243 rubella children, three-quarters of the children with 4 or 5 signs of the "difficult child" syndrome had behavior disorders, as opposed to only one-quarter of the "easy" or "slow-to-warm-up" children. Furthermore, half of the children with defects were classified as "difficult," as opposed to only one-sixth of the children with no defect (Chess, Korn, and Fernandez, 1971).

There can be no doubt that the multiply handicapped child is greatly at risk for behavioral disorders, through a failure of the environment, "Whether in the form of errors committed or of essential needs omitted in the child's early life" (Williams, 1968). A very real hazard in evaluating such children is a tendency to attribute all behavioral problems either to parental rejection or the handicap itself. However, the majority of parents of maladjusted, handicapped children are ordinary devoted parents with other normal children (Williams, 1968; Chess et al., 1971), and the presence of handicaps does not necessarily preclude the possibility of normal personality development. The evaluator, therefore, must assess any behavior disorder as a direct consequence either of the handicap, of concurrent brain damage, of actual emotional disturbance, of disturbance in the family, or of the interaction of any or all of these factors (Mindel and Vernon, 1971).

Impact on Family Life

We do not know precisely how chronic sensory deprivation or chronic overstimulation (e.g., the barrage of meaningless noise experienced by some deaf) affects the total development of the child. We do know, however, that their early deviant behavior often has an adverse effect on the emerging mother-infant relationship. For example, at a time when an adult approaches a normal infant of three or four months, the child will turn his head toward the person's voice, exhibit a smile response and increased body movement. Blind children, on the other hand, are delayed both in their smile response (5–6 months) and in turning their head toward a sound source. They adopt a motionless, listening attitude at the sound of a voice. Somewhat later, when the normal child begins to reach for and crawl towards sighted objects, the blind child will adopt a swivel pattern in response to sounds (Williams, 1968). The deaf child fails to turn toward the sound of his caretaker's voice. At first, he babbles and coos like a normal infant, but because he has no feedback, he soon ceases to play with his voice. By one year of age the normal child is beginning to say words, and the deaf child is mute. Often without being aware of it, the mother may feel rejected or deprived by her infant's failure to respond to her overtures. Some investigators feel that the handicapped infant's failure to elicit maternal response results in a lack of maternal stimulation (Lesser and Easser, 1972; Williams, 1968; Mindel and Vernon, 1971). The consequence may be a double deprivation resulting both from the handicap itself and from the effect of the handicap upon the environment.

The birth of a handicapped child has enormous consequences for the whole family's emotional health. The parents' first reaction is one of shock, followed by grief, anger and guilt. Many parents tend to deny the full implications of their child's handicap; they live in the present and consider problems only as they arise (Chess, Korn, and Fernandez, 1971). The child's ordinal position in the family may affect his future. For example, in a rubella project, parents of first-born handicapped children were much more devastated by their own guilt than parents who already had other normal children (Chess, Korn, and Fernandez, 1971). On the other hand, the birth of a handicapped child may be the last straw for a large family already financially and emotionally overburdened. Parents worry about neglecting their normal children, the continuing dependence of their handicapped child, and the constant financial and emotional drain.

Either because of their guilt or their own lack of knowledge of the child's abilities, parents are frequently overpermissive or inconsistent. It was found that handicapped rubella children routinely performed only half the tasks they were capable of doing (Chess, Korn, and Fernandez, 1971). In another study of multiply handicapped blind children, it was found that many of these children were grossly overprotected, with little or no consistent expectations (Elonen and Zwarensteyn, 1963).

Of all the sensory defects, deafness seems to have the most potential for damaging behavioral consequences. Parents feel greatly deprived of their traditional role as teachers and socializers. It is often difficult to determine whether the deaf child's rigidity, impulsivity and low frustration tolerance are a result of brain damage, his inability to communicate, or the methods used to counteract his defect. For example, the deaf child is constantly interrupted in his normal play by being forced to look at his caretakers' lips (Mindel and Vernon, 1971). Parents must frequently resort to physical punishment and restraint, rather than verbal discipline and explanation.

The deaf child is forced into a dependent role much more than the blind or motorically impaired child, whose whole educational impetus is directed toward increased mobility and autonomy. Because of the nature of the handicap, the deaf child must be in direct face-to-face contact with those around him in order to communicate.

As the handicapped child grows older and moves out of the relative protection of the family circle, the problems created by his handicap inevitably increase. He experiences rejection by normal peers, heavier academic demands, and a growing awareness that he will never be entirely normal. His sense of isolation and stigmatization increase as he grows older. In one study of 41 handicapped children and their families, depressions were common among 8- and 9-year-olds as they came to realize the full extent of their handicap and the limited choices the future held. Only two children who were aware of future problems were free of depression. In these two cases their parents had apparently fully accepted their child's handicap and discussed it openly and frequently with them (Minde, Hackett, Killon, and Silver, 1972).

From this overview of the problems of the multiply handicapped child, we can see that an accurate diagnosis requires considerable skill. Often the therapist must also spend a great deal of time helping the family to accept their child's handicap, showing the parents how to stimulate the child and engage him in interaction. The child must be repeatedly evaluated to ensure that a previous diagnosis and treatment plan are still effective. Above all, the child must be seen in his totality. The additional time and effort required of the professional in the evaluation and treatment of the handicapped child is often richly rewarded, however, as these children achieve an ever greater measure of their true potential.

BIBLIOGRAPHY

BERLINSKY, S. Measurement of the intelligence and personality of the deaf: A review of the literature. *Journal of Speech and Hearing Disorders*, 1952, *17*, 39–54.

CHESS, S. Autism in children with congenital rubella. *Journal of Autism and Childhood Schizophrenia*, 1971, *1*, 33–47.

CHESS, S.; KORN, S.; and FERNANDEZ, P. *Psychiatric disorders of children with congenital rubella.* New York: Brunner/Mazel, 1971.

ELONEN, A. S.; and ZWARENSTEYN, S. B. Michigan's summer program for multiple-handicapped blind children. *Outlook for the Blind*, 1963, *57*(3), 77–82.

FRAIBERG, S., and FREEDMAN, D. A. Studies in the ego development of the congenitally blind child. *Psychoanalytic Study of the Child*, 1964, *19*, 113–169.

FREEDMAN, D. A. Congenital and perinatal sensory deprivation: Some studies in early development. *American Journal of Psychiatry*, 1971, *127*(11), 115–121.

LESSER, S. R., and EASSER, B. R. Personality differences in the perceptually handicapped. *Journal of the American Academy of Child Psychiatry*, 1972, *11*, 458–466.

MINDE, K.; HACKETT, J. D.; KILLON, D.; and SILVER, S. How they grow up: 41 physically handicapped children and their families. *American Journal of Psychiatry*, 1972, *128*(12), 104–109.

MINDEL, E., and VERNON, M. *They grow in silence.* Silver Spring, Md.: National Association of the Deaf, 1971.

VERNON, M. Sociological and psychological factors associated with hearing loss. *Journal of Speech and Hearing Research*, 1969, *12*, 541–563.

WILLIAMS, C. E. Behavior disorders in handicapped children. *Developmental Medicine and Child Neurology*, 1968, *10*(6), 736–740.

STELLA CHESS

MULTIVARIATE ANALYSIS OF VARIANCE

Multivariate analysis of variance is a generalized form of analysis of variance applicable simultaneously and jointly to more than one qualitatively distinct measurement. Basically, both univariate and multivariate analysis of variance are methods for detecting and estimating differences between population means of measured variables. In some applications, the populations are naturally occurring, as in an epidemiological study, but in others the populations are created artificially by the random assignment of subjects or material to treatments, as in a clinical trial. In either case, it is assumed that the distributions of these variables may differ in mean level, but not in dispersion, skewness, or other aspects of shape. This exclusive attention to differences in means may seem unduly restrictive but is justified in applications where the economic value of an outcome measure depends only upon the population mean. In beef production, for example, the expected total return to the stockman is proportional to the average yield per animal times the number of animals in the herd. From point of view of profit, the economic value of alternative feeds or pastures, for example, may be compared in terms of mean productivities. This is precisely what the *univariate analysis of variance (anova),* which R. A. Fisher developed in the context of agricultural research, is designed to do.

The generalization of anova as represented by multivariate analysis of variance *(manova)* also focuses on means, but for several, possibly many, measured attributes or responses simultaneously. Thus, it is better suited to studies of behavioral differences, especially among human subjects, where there is no univocal economic "payoff" by which the results may be compared. In the multivariate approach, a number of qualitatively distinct measures of attributes or outcomes are analyzed and the results presented simultaneously. It is left to the investigator or the reader to assess in his own terms the meaning or total import of the possibly many differences found in the study.

General Description

In technical terms, manova is a least-squares procedure for linear estimation and tests of hypothesis in data consisting of continuously distributed, multiple, qualitatively distinct and possibly correlated dependent variables. S. S. Wilks presented the basic formulation of manova in 1932, but due to the heavy computational demands of the technique its practical applications did not begin until electronic computers became available in the 1950s. Thereafter, a rapid development of the multivariate methodology and related statistical theory ensued, with contributions by M. S. Bartlett, C. S. Rao, S. N. Roy, H. Hotelling, T. W. Anderson, and others (see Bock, 1975, for references). The essentials of some of the multivariate methods elaborated by these workers is described later.

Closely allied to manova, and often incorporated in the computational procedure, are the techniques of discriminant analysis, canonical representation, analysis of covariance, multivariate multiple regression analysis, canonical correlation, and repeated measures analysis. The relationship of these techniques to manova is discussed in the next section. Computer programs for multivariate analysis of variance and allied techniques are mentioned later. Most of the material covered in this article is discussed more fully in various textbooks on multivariate analysis.

Comparison with Univariate Analysis. The main features of manova are easily understood by comparing it, in the context of a typical application, with the more familiar technique of univariate analysis of variance. A simple but representative example is an analysis of a clinical trial in the form of a randomized experiment. Suppose that N psychiatric patients in some diagnostic category have been randomly partitioned among n different courses of drug therapy. At the end of the trial, all patients are evaluated on p distinct measures of clinical status. Univariate analysis of variance might then be applied to any one of these measures in order to detect differences in the treatment effects and to estimate the direction and magnitude of these differences.

The formal exposition of the analysis begins with the assumed model for the chosen response variable (or "variate"):

$$y_{ij} = \mu + \alpha_j + \epsilon_{ij} \qquad (1)$$

The variate y_{ij} represents the score for the clinical status measure of subject i in treatment group j. It is assumed to be an additive combination of the mean score before treatment (μ), the effect of the jth treatment (α_j), and an error (ϵ_{ij}) due to individual differences in response or to measurement error. The error is assumed to be independent from one subject to another and similarly distributed in all groups. For purposes of subsequent statistical tests, it is also assumed to be normally distributed with mean zero and unknown variance σ^2, or, in a conventional notation, $\epsilon_j \sim N(0, \sigma^2)$.

The question of whether or not differences between the treatments can be detected is posed in the form of the null hypothesis of equality of treatment effects, $H_0: \alpha_1 = \alpha_2 = \cdots = \alpha_n$. In anova, the calculations for testing this hypothesis begin with the computation of the group means,

$$y_{\cdot j} = \frac{1}{N_j} \sum_i^{N_j} y_{ij}, \qquad j = 1, 2, \ldots, n$$

and the grand mean,

$$y_{\cdot\cdot} = \frac{1}{N} \sum_j^n \sum_i^{N_j} y_{ij}$$

where

$$N = \sum_j^n N_j$$

The so-called analysis-of-variance table, in which the sum of squares of the observed scores is partitioned into additive sources, is prepared as shown in Table 1 for the case of a simple randomized experiment (one-way anova).

A statistic for testing H_0 is provided by the variance ratio

$$F = \frac{SS_b/(n-1)}{SS_w/(N-n)} \qquad (2)$$

When H_0 is true, Equation (2) follows Fisher's central F-distribution with $n-1$ degrees of freedom for the numerator and $N-n$ degrees of freedom for the denominator. Because this ratio increases monotonically with the increasing sum of squared differences among the

Table 1. Analysis of Variance for the Simple Randomized Design

Source of Variation	Degrees of Freedom	Sum of Squares
Mean	1	$SS_m = N\bar{y}_{..}^2$
Between treatments	$n-1$	$SS_b = SS_g - SS_m$
Treatment groups	n	$SS_g = \sum_{j}^{n} N_j \bar{y}_{.j}^2$
Within groups	$N-n$	$SS_w = SS_t - SS_g$
Total	$N = \sum_{j=1}^{n} N_j$	$SS_t = \sum_{j}^{n}\sum_{i}^{N_j} y_{ij}^2$

treatment effects, an observed value more extreme than the $1-\alpha$ percentile of the central F-distribution is taken as evidence of real differences among the treatment effects at the "α-level of significance." Under the assumptions of the analysis, it can be shown that this test cannot be improved upon from point of view of power (sensitivity to departure from the null hypothesis as measured by the sum of squared effect differences.)

If we accept the reality of a treatment difference, we may wish to estimate its direction and magnitude. The best (in the sense of having minimum sampling variance) linear unbiased estimator of the difference in treatment effects is given by the corresponding difference of sample means:

$$\widehat{\alpha_j - \alpha_{j'}} = y_{.j} - y_{.j'} \tag{3}$$

The sampling variance of this estimator is $\sigma^2(1/N_j + 1/N_{j'})$. The analysis-of-variance table also provides a best unbiased quadratic estimator of the unknown variance σ^2 in the form of

$$\sigma^2 = \frac{SS_w}{N-n} \tag{4}$$

Multivariate Extension of Anova. In the multivariate generalization of this procedure, the model for each of p dependent variables has the same form as the univariate model, except that each term is indexed (in this case by a superscript in parentheses) to show the variate to which it applies; that is:

$$y_{ij}^{(k)} = \mu^{(k)} + \alpha_j^{(k)} + \epsilon_{ij}^{(k)} \tag{5}$$

For each of these terms, it is customary to refer to the ordered set of values corresponding to $k = 1, 2, \ldots, p$ as a *vector*. Thus, we speak of $\{y_{ij}^{(k)}\}$ as the *vector observation,* $\{\mu^{(k)}\}$ and $\{\alpha_j^{(k)}\}$ as *vector effects,* and $\{\epsilon_{ij}^{(k)}\}$ as the *vector error.* In order to characterize the error distribution for manova, it is necessary not only to specify the mean (0) and variance—say, σ_k^2 for the kth error variate—but also to specify the *covariance* of each pair of variates as, for example, $\sigma_{kl} = \rho_{kl}\sigma_k\sigma_l$, where ρ_{kl} is the correlation between the respective variates and σ_k, σ_l the standard deviations. The $p \times p$ square symmetric array Σ containing σ_{kl} as the element in the kth row and lth column, and lth row and kth column, and containing σ_k^2 and σ_l^2 in the kth and lth diagonal position, is called the *covariance matrix* of the distribution. The multivariate normal error specification may therefore be expressed as

$$\epsilon \sim N\left(\underset{p \times 1}{\mathbf{0}}, \quad \underset{p \times p}{\Sigma}\right)$$

The computational steps in manova may be described succinctly by arithmetic operations on indexed (superscripted) numbers. Let the means of the kth element of the vector observations be

$$y_j^{(k)} = \frac{1}{N_j}\sum_{i=1}^{N_j} y_{ij}^{(k)}, \text{ for } k = 1, 2, \ldots, p \tag{6}$$

or the grand mean

$$y_{..}^{(k)} = \frac{1}{N}\sum^{n}\sum^{N_j} y_{ij}^{(k)} \tag{7}$$

Similarly, let the $p \times p$ symmetric matrix of the sum of squares and cross-products of the observations be represented as, for example, in the total sum of squares and cross-products,

$$S_t = \left[\sum_{j}^{n}\sum_{i}^{N} y_{ij}^{(k)}y_{ij}^{(l)}\right] \quad \begin{array}{l} k = 1, 2, \ldots, p \\ l = 1, 2, \ldots, p \end{array}$$

With these notational conventions, the multivariate analogue of Table 1 may be set out as shown in Table 2. The matrices of sums and cross-products in Table 2 provide the sample quantities from which is computed the test statistic for an exact test of the multivariate null-hypothesis, $H_0: \{\alpha_1^{(k)} = \alpha_2^{(k)} = \ldots = \alpha_n^{(k)}\}$ for all k. This is a composite hypothesis with respect to both treatments and variates; to reject it implies that at least one difference between treatments is significant for at least one response variable.

In the multivariate case, the statistic of choice for testing this hypothesis is not as clear-cut as in the univariate case, and no fewer than

Table 2. Multivariate Analysis of Variance for the Simple Randomized Design

Source of p-variate Variation	Degrees of Freedom	Sums of Squares and Cross-Products ($p \times p$) $k = 1, 2, \ldots, p$ $l = 1, 2, \ldots, p$
Grand mean	1	$S_m = [N y_{..}^{(k)} y_{..}^{(l)}]$
Between groups	$n - 1$	$S_b = S_g - S_m$
Group means	n	$S_g = \left[\sum\limits_{j}^{n} N_j y_{.j}^{(k)} y_{.j}^{(l)} \right]$
Within groups	$N - n$	$S_w = S_t - S_g$
Total	$N = \sum\limits_{j=1}^{n} N_j$	$S_t = \left[\sum\limits_{j}^{n} \sum\limits_{i}^{N_j} y_{ij}^{(k)} y_{ij}^{(l)} \right]$

three plausible alternatives have been proposed. Each is a function of the so-called maximal invariant statistics obtained in the solution of the polynomial in λ which results upon expansion of the determinant in the left member of Equation (8):

$$|S_b - \lambda S_w| = 0 \qquad (8)$$

The alternative test statistics computed from the $s = \min (n - 1, p)$ nonzero roots of Equation (8) are:

Wilks's criterion: $\Lambda = \prod\limits_{k=1}^{s} (1 + \lambda_k)^{-1}$

Roy's largest-root criterion: $\theta = \dfrac{\lambda_1}{1 + \lambda_1}$

Hotelling's trace criterion: $\tau = (N - n) \sum\limits_{k=1}^{s} \lambda_k$

Percentage points of the null distributions of these statistics may be obtained by computing approximations or from published tables (Bock, 1975). Roy's criterion is also the basis of a system of confidence bounds that can be used to judge the significance of all treatment contrasts for all variables simultaneously (Morrison, 1967). These bounds tend to be rather conservative, however, and many workers prefer, after the multivariate hypothesis is rejected, to examine the corresponding univariate statistic for evidence of which variates are responsible for the multivariate significance. These "protected" F- and t-tests aid in locating the variates of group differences responsible for the significant multivariate effect.

As for estimation, the point estimates of the treatment differences and of the standard errors of these differences are the same as the univariate estimates for the respective variables. The manova table also provides a minimum variance unbiased quadratic estimator of the error covariance matrix (compare Equation 4):

$$\hat{\Sigma} = \frac{1}{N - n} S_w \qquad (9)$$

The positive square roots of diagonal elements of this matrix estimate the common within-group standard deviations of the response variables, and the off-diagonal elements divided by the row and column standard deviations estimate the correlation between the respective variables. When there is one group ($n = 1$), these estimates reduce to the conventional sample covariance and correlation matrix computed from deviations about the sample means. When there is more than one group, the deviations are taken about the group means rather than the grand mean.

Allied Techniques of Multivariate Normal Analysis

Multiple-Group Discriminant Analysis. Corresponding to each of the $\min(n - 1, p)$ nonzero roots of Equation (8) is a solution of the set of linear homogeneous equations represented by

$$\sum\limits_{l=1}^{p} [S_b^{(k,l)} - \lambda_h S_w^{(k,l)}] a_{hl} = 0, \qquad \begin{array}{l} h = 1, 2, \ldots, s \\ k = 1, 2, \ldots, p \end{array} \qquad (10)$$

where $S_b^{(k,l)}$ and $S_w^{(k,l)}$ are elements in the kth row and jth column of S_b and S_w, respectively.

The quantities a_{hl} obtained from the solution of Equation (10) are estimated coefficients of so-called canonical variates defined by

$$v_h = a_{h1} y^{(1)} + a_{h2} y^{(2)} + \ldots + a_{hp} y^{(p)} \qquad (11)$$

These synthetic variables have many interesting and useful properties. The variate v_1, corresponding to the largest root of Equation (8), is that linear combination of the response variables for which the ratio of between-group to within-group sum of squares is a maximum. In that sense, it is the best single score for classifying individuals as to their group membership. In the special case of two groups, $h = s = 1$, and Equation (11) is proportional to R. A. Fisher's *discriminant function*. With a choice of a "cutting point" that takes into account the population sizes, this function provides the *Bayes classification procedure* which minimizes expected errors of misclassification (Bock, 1975, sec. 6.2).

Discriminant functions have obvious relevance for diagnostic classification based on quantitative information about the subjects. This relevance is especially apparent when there are more than two groups and the number of variables is so large that any direct use or interpretation of the data is all but impossible. By neglecting those canonical variates with insignificant or small between-group variation (as measured by the corresponding root of Equation 8), we may achieve a considerable simplification of the data by representing both the group means and individual subject's scores in terms of the first $s_0 \le s \le p$ canonical variates. In many cases, s_0 may be set as small as 2 or 3 and the mean canonical variates plotted in two or three dimensions in order to inspect the relative positions of the group centroids in the multivariate space. Because of the important property of being uncorrelated in the sample, the generalized distance (Mahalanobis distance) between any two groups may be calculated as Euclidean distance, that is, as the sum of squares of differences of canonical variate means for the groups in question.

In a similar manner, the generalized distance between any individual's score vector and the centroids of each of the groups may be calculated. After a suitable adjustment of these distances to allow for population size, the assignment of the subject to that population for which this adjusted generalized distance is a minimum is a Bayes procedure for multiple classification. This procedure could be applied, for example, to assign subjects to the diagnostic category to which their multivariate score "profile" shows them to be most similar (Tatsuoka, 1971).

Even if classification is not the main objective of a study, the canonical analysis can be useful as an aid to interpretation of the multivariate differences between groups. The standardized coefficients of the canonical variate may be inspected in order to characterize and name the dimensions of the canonical representation. Once the axes of the representation have been characterized, the relative position of the group centroids may suggest an interpretation of the variation between groups. An example of such an interpretation, illustrating also how the information for the discriminant analysis and canonical representation is extracted from the multivariate analysis of variance, is presented later ("Example").

Multivariate Analysis of Covariance. To the extent that error variation within treatment groups is due to individual differences among subjects randomly assigned within groups, it may be possible to increase appreciably the sensitivity of an experiment by an analysis of covariance with measures of the relevant background information on the subjects as covariates. In drug trials, a measure of the subject's pretrial clinical status is an obvious choice for a covariate. When the results of the trial are analyzed, this pretrial measure is included as an additional variable in the multivariate analysis of variance of the posttrial response measures, and the common within-group correlation of all pairs of measures are then computed. If the correlation between the pretrial and posttrial measures is nonzero, the regression of the latter on the former should be eliminated from the estimate of error variation required for the univariate or multivariate test statistic. Because of randomization, the corresponding adjustment of the estimated treatment effects tends to be small, and the error reduction will generally increase the magnitude of the test statistic, thus improving the prospects of detecting a significant treatment effect. The increase in sensitivity of a randomized experiment afforded by analysis of covariance is especially relevant in clinical studies in which individual difference variation within groups is typically large and for which suitable covariate measures are usually easy to obtain.

Multivariate Multiple Regression Analysis. The multivariate generalizations of regression and correlation analysis lead to useful and versatile methods for studying linear relationships between two sets of variables. When both sets contain multiple variables and are regarded asymmetrically, as when one set represents independent and the other dependent variables (or, similarly, predictors and criteria, or covariables and response variables), the generalized procedure is *multivariate multiple regression analysis.* This procedure provides an exact test of the composite null hypothesis of no association between any dependent variable and any independent variable or, equivalently, that the multiple regression coefficients between say, the p dependent variables and the q independent variables are jointly null. It is customary to require that this null hypothesis be rejected before any attempt is made to interpret the directions or magnitude of the regression effects.

If the dependent and independent variables are both included in the vector observations, the sample quantities required in the calculations for this test are contained in the estimate of the error covariance matrix extracted from the multivariate analysis of variance table (Table 2). This estimate is identical to the conventional sample covariance matrix when there is one group ($n = 1$) and, in the case of more than one group, is a pooled best estimate of the covariance matrix of multivariate normal populations that differ in their means (the group effects) but not in their variances or covariances. In either case, the maximal invariant statistics computed from this matrix provide a test of the null hypothesis of no regression of one set of variables on the other (Bock, 1975, sec. 6.1).

This test is a useful preliminary to multivariate analysis of covariance. If there is no relationship between covariables and response variables, the analysis of covariance produces no reduction of the error variance and, by reducing the number of degrees of freedom available for the error estimate, actually diminishes the power of the test of between-group effects. If the regression analysis gives evidence of such a relationship, the covariates will be useful additions to the model for predicting the group means.

Canonical Correlation. The concept of correlation, which is a symmetric relationship between two statistical variables, is generalized to two *sets* of such variables in the *canonical* correlation of Hotelling (1936). For the case of p variables in one set and q in the other, Hotelling defines the canonical correlation as the $s = \min(p, q)$ linear combinations of variables in the respective sets that are maximally correlated between sets, subject to the restriction that they are uncorrelated within sets. In fact, the discriminant functions discussed below (in the "Example") are just such linear combinations when the response measures are one set of variates and any $n - 1$ independent contrasts

among groups comprise the other set. In an exact sense, all of the multivariate normal procedures based on maximal invariant statistics are special cases of canonical correlation.

In practical work, canonical correlation is especially useful for providing a large sample test of the dimensionality of linear relationships between the two sets of variables. This test may indicate that all significant association between the two sets of variables can be explained by a small number of linear functions. The nature of these functions may be interpreted in terms of their standardized coefficients or of the first-order correlation structure between the functions and the original variables, possibly after an orthogonal rotation such as varimax.

Analysis of Repeated Measures. Multivariate data in which the score vectors consist of the same measurement made on each subject on each of several different occasions are called "repeated measures." It is assumed that the repeated measures are qualitatively similar and therefore commensurate for purposes of addition and subtraction. In particular, the scores for the several occasions will be added to obtain a sum or mean for all occasions and subtracted in order to compute gains between occasions.

Clinical experimentation in which "each subject serves as his own control" typically produces repeated measures data. The experimental procedure in such studies is to assign subjects randomly to alternative treatments and then to measure each subject on the variable of interest both *before* and *after* the assigned treatment is administered. In some applications, the measures are made several times before, during, and after the treatment. If there are p such measures, n treatment groups, N_j subjects in group j, and $N = \Sigma_j^n N_j$ subjects in total, the experiment results in an $N \times p$ ("subjects $\times$ occasions") array of scores to be analyzed. Again concentrating on the group means, the investigator examines these data to determine whether the treatments differentially affect the mean change from pretreatment to posttreatment occasions. If so, the "profile" of change in some of the groups may be more favorable than in others and the corresponding treatments more preferred for therapeutic purposes.

On certain somewhat restrictive assumptions about the covariance pattern of the repeated measures, it is possible to test for differential mean change using a univariate "mixed-model" analysis of variance. A significant group by occasion interaction rejects the null hypothesis of no differential change. Under much less restrictive assumptions, however, the same test may be carried out in a one-way multivariate analysis of variance potentially more powerful and informative than the mixed-model analysis.

In the multivariate approach, a transformation of the data, consisting of $p = 1$ contrasts of the repeated measures, is chosen in such a way as to be maximally sensitive to the expected profile of change. These contrasts play a role in the analysis similar to the discriminant functions defined above, except that they are chosen a priori rather than computed empirically. An example of such contrasts are the so-called Fisher-Tchebycheff orthogonal polynomials used in trend analysis of repeated measures data (Bock, 1975, chap. 7).

With respect to these a priori contrasts, differences between treatments are tested by means of the maximal invariant statistics or other test statistics and, where significant, are estimated and interpreted. In most cases, the interpretation becomes readily apparent when the estimated mean change profiles of the several treatments are plotted on the same graph. The statistical tests in the multivariate analysis of variances serve to establish that the apparent differences cannot be attributed to variation due to randomization.

Example

Data for this example are measures of psychiatric clinical status based on the *Kahn Mental Status Questionnaire* (MSQ) and the *Face-Hand* (F-H) *test* administered to samples of confused, psychotic, and alcoholic geriatric patients in a study by E. Kahana. An analysis of

Table 3. Diagnosis of Group Means and Within-Group Standard Deviations and Correlations for the Mental Status Questionnaire (MSQ) and Face-Hand (F-H) Test

Diagnosis-Group Means	N	Variable	
		MSQ	F-H
Confused (Conf)	22	7.624	10.085
Psychotic (Psyc)	17	1.786	1.443
Alcoholic (Alch)	16	2.214	1.366
Standard deviations	—	2.466	2.613
Correlations	—	1.000	.490
	—	.490	1.000

an experimental treatment in this study appears as a computing example in Bock (1975, p. 289). For present purposes, the experimental effect, which proved to be small, is ignored and the data are used for a small but realistic application of one-way multivariate analysis of variance. The group means $y_j^{(k)}$, the sample sizes N_j for $j = 1, 2, 3$, and the common within-group standard deviations s_k and correlations r_{kl} for $k = 1, 2$ and $l = 1, 2$ are shown in Table 3.

From the quantitities in Table 3, the within-group sums of squares and cross-products (SSPs) can be recovered by the calculation (for $n = 3$)

$$S_w^{(k,l)} = (\Sigma N_j - n) \, s_k s_l r_{kl}$$

where $r_{kl} = 1$ when $k = l$.

The between-group SSP is computed from the formula (for S_b) in Table 2. The results of these calculations appear in the partition of squares and products shown in abbreviated form in Table 4.

According to Equation (8), we obtain the maximal invariant statistics by solving the determinantal equation

$$\begin{vmatrix} 419.981 - 316.172\lambda & 644.797 - 164.106 \\ 644.797 - 164.106 & 994.416 - 355.052\lambda \end{vmatrix} = 0 \quad (11)$$

Table 4. Partition of Sums of Squares and Cross-Products

Source of Dispersion	Degrees of Freedom	Sums of Squares and Cross-Products	
Between groups	2	419.981	644.797
		644.797	994.416
Within groups	52	316.172	164.106
		164.106	355.052

Expanding Equation (11) gives the quadratic equation

$$85,326.724\lambda^2 - 251,891.522\lambda + 1,872.313 = 0$$

from which the quadratic formula yields two real roots

$$\lambda_1 = 2.945 \quad \text{and} \quad \lambda_2 = .00745$$

To test the null hypothesis of no multivariate differences between diagnostic groups, we may compute, for example, the likelihood ratio

$$\frac{1}{1 + 2.945} \times \frac{1}{1 + .00745} = .2516$$

Using Rao's F-approximation for the distribution of the likelihood ratio (which is exact for the case $p = 2$), we obtain a p-value less than .0001.

There is evidently no doubt as to the significance of differences between the groups, but the Bartlett chi-square test of the contribution of the smaller root shows it to be nonsignificant (Table 5). Thus, of the two discriminant functions shown in Table 5, only the first is useful in characterizing the score distributions of the diagnostic group. This implies that the group centroids (vector means) are essentially colinear with the axis of the first canonical variate, as is apparent in Figure 1. Also apparent is the fact that performance on the Mental Status Questionnaire and the Face-Hand test serves only to distinguish the confused from the psychotic and alcoholic groups. Although the latter test has the larger standardized coefficient in the discriminant function, both contribute significantly to discrimination. This can be verified by computing, in an analysis of covariance, the between-group F-statistic for

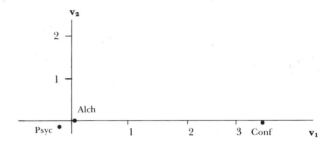

Fig. 1. Canonical representation of the diagnostic group centroids (standard score units).

the MSQ, eliminating variation due to F-H. The resulting F value of 18.0, on 2 and 51 degrees of freedom has a p-value less than .0001. This does not necessarily imply that the two tests measure different dimensions of variation, but may merely signify that they are both unreliable measures of the same dimension and that the improved discrimination due to adding either to the function is a "test-lengthening" effect.

Computer Programs

Comprehensive computer programs for multivariate analysis of variance are available in *MULTIVARIANCE* (Finn, 1974) and *MANOVA II* (Cramer, 1975). Each of these programs carries out univariate or multivariate analysis of variance for any design, balanced or unbalanced, complete or incomplete, and with or without covariates. When appropriate, the calculations include multivariate multiple regression analysis, discriminant analysis, and canonical correlation. The *MULTIVARIANCE* program also has special provisions for repeated measures analysis.

Table 5. Discriminant Functions, Canonical Variances, and Bartlett's Chi-Square

Variable	First Function (v_1) Coefficients (Standardized)	Second Function (v_2) Coefficients (Standardized)
MSQ	.1029 (.2539)	.4536 (1.1186)
F-H	.3256 (.8509)	−.2944 (−.7692)
Canonical variance	2.945	.00745
χ_B^2	71.06	.3823
df	4	1
p	$p < .0001$	$p = .5364$

BIBLIOGRAPHY

ANDERSON, T. W. *An introduction to multivariate analysis.* New York: Wiley, 1958.

BOCK, R. D. *Multivariate statistical methods in behavioral research.* New York: McGraw-Hill, 1975.

CRAMER, E. M. *MANOVA II.* Chicago: National Educational Resources, 1975.

DIXON, W. J. (Ed.). *BMDP: Biomedical computer programs.* Berkeley: University of California, 1975.

FINN, J. D. *MULTIVARIANCE: Univariate and multivariate analysis of variance, covariance, and regression.* Chicago: National Educational Resources, 1974.

HOTELLING, H. Relations between two sets of variates. *Biometrika*, 1936, *28*, 321–377.

KRAMER, C. Y. *A first course in methods of multivariate analysis.* New York: Author, 1972.

MORRISON, D. F. *Multivariate analysis.* New York: McGraw-Hill, 1967.

ROY, S. N. *Some aspects of multivariate analysis.* New York: Wiley, 1957.

TATSUOKA, M. *Multivariate analysis.* New York: Wiley, 1971.

TIMM, N. H. *Multivariate analysis with applications in education and psychology.* Monterey, Calif.: Brooks/Cole, 1975.

R. DARRELL BOCK

MÜNSTERBERG, HUGO (1863–1916)

Münsterberg was a German psychologist invited by William James to organize experimental psychology at Harvard (1897–1916). His major contribution was to applied psychology. He was also interested in psychotherapy, juristic and industrial psychology, and psychic research.

JAMES F. ADAMS

MURPHY, GARDNER (b. 1895)

Gardner Murphy, psychologist, was born at Chillicothe, Ohio, in 1895, the second son of Edgar Gardner Murphy, an Episcopal minister, and Maud King Murphy, a Vassar graduate and minor poet. An early interest in psychical research led him to study psychology, and he has maintained both interests ever since. He earned a BA degree from Yale in 1916 and an MA degree from Harvard in 1917, then joined the Yale Mobile Hospital Unit and went overseas with it. He returned in 1919, attended Columbia, earned a Ph.D. degree in 1922, and taught there until 1940, when he founded and chaired the department of psychology at the City College of New York. He built the department into a harmonious, research-oriented unit, which educated more undergraduates who earned Ph.D.s in psychology than any other department in the country; he initiated the first graduate program (an MA in clinical psychology) in the New York college system, and he gave courses that were not only very popular, but also so stimulating that the brighter students would meet with each other regularly after each lecture to discuss the ideas he had raised.

In 1952, he left to become director of research at the Menninger Foundation, where he remained until 1967. From 1967 to 1973, he was visiting professor at George Washington University. At the same time, he held many additional posts. For decades, for example, he was editor for psychology at Harper's and Richard Hodgson fellow at Harvard University; in the latter capacity he used the fellowship funds to finance parapsychological research by others. In 1950–51, he visited India for UNESCO to study the Hindu-Muslim conflict.

In 1924, he met Lois Barclay (also a Vassar graduate, then a student at Union Theological Seminary and later an eminent psychologist), and they married in 1926. Their two children are Alpen Gardner Murphy and Margaret Murphy Small. Their marriage resulted in collaboration on a number of psychological projects, including a book on developmental and social psychology and *In the Minds of Men* (1953), reporting their work in India in 1950–51.

The quality of Murphy's thinking resembles William James's in its wisdom, breadth, and depth; and his writings have helped shape psychology. His *Historical Introduction to Modern Psychology* (1929) has remained a standard text to the present. In 1929, he edited a second standard work, *An Outline of Abnormal Psychology,* and in 1931 with L. B. Murphy (Murphy, Murphy, and Newcomb, rev. 1937) he published a book that has become a classic: *Experimental Social Psychology.* He was one of the group that founded the Society for the Psychological Study of Social Issues. In 1947, he published what some consider the best book ever written on psychology, *Personality: A Biosocial Approach to Origins and Structure* (rev. 1947). This is a thousand-page compendium of psychology, enriched by relevant research from such areas as physiology, anthropology, and sociology, all integrated into a system that is both unified and also sufficiently complex to show the sources of individuals' diversity. Later major books include (with Solley) *Development of the Perceptual World* (1960), and in 1961, *Challenge of Psychical Research.*

Murphy has also been author or coauthor of several other books and of many research and theoretical papers. Especially noteworthy is a series of research articles written with students who were undergraduates at the time the research was performed, some of which helped to initiate the "new look" in perception; among them demonstrations of change in perceptual response following changes in affect, reward, or motivation.

Murphy has been president of the American Psychological Association, the Eastern Psychological Association, the Society for the Psychological Study of Social Issues, the (London) Society for Psychical Research, and the American Society for Psychical Research. Among the honors given him are the Gold Medal Award of the American Psychological Foundation; Columbia's Butler Medal; an Honorary Doctor of Science from the Graduate Faculties of the City University of New York; and the naming of the Gardner Murphy Research Building at the Menninger Foundation, and of the Gardner Murphy Research Foundation.

Whether Murphy's topic was social psychology or creativity, parapsychology or biofeedback, his approach to it has been an open, integrative one that could fuse the contributions of such diverse sources as Freud and Dewey, or Spencer, Cannon, and Klineberg with the data of hundreds of experiments to produce an orderly and creative thesis. He espouses a field theory that emphasizes both the biological and social determinants of behavior. Genetic influences are modified by environmental pressures to produce a self-structure that interprets and acts upon each new situation in its own way, and also is acted upon and influenced by the situation. His lectures and conversation have been a source of research ideas to generations of his students and colleagues. His generosity in encouraging their response to his stimulation, his initiative in finding the openings that can best further their careers, and the warmth of his interest in them

as individuals have developed their potentialities. A partial list of Murphy's publications follows:

Autobiography in E. G. Boring and G. Lindzey (Eds.), *A History of Psychology in Autobiography* (New York: Appleton-Century-Crofts, 1930); *Historical Introduction to Modern Psychology* (3rd ed., with J. Kovach; New York: Harcourt, Brace and World, 1972); (Ed.) *An Outline of Abnormal Psychology.* (Rev. ed. with A. Bachrach; New York: Modern Library, 1954); with L. B. Murphy, and T. M. Newcomb, *Experimental Social Psychology* (Rev. ed.; New York: Harper & Row, 1937); *Personality: A Biosocial Approach to Origins and Structure* (New York: Harper & Row, 1947); *In the Minds of Men: A UNESCO Study of Social Tensions in India* (New York: Basic Books, 1953); *Challenge of Psychical Research: A Primer of Parapsychology* (New York: Harper & Row, 1961); and with C. M. Solley, *Development of the Perceptual World* (New York: Basic Books, 1960).

GERTRUDE SCHMEIDLER

MUSCLE, SKELETAL: CLINICAL ASPECTS OF DISEASE

Most muscle diseases are rare and of obscure etiology, and many are inherited. While many are clinically distinct, some muscle diseases can be diagnosed only with sophisticated histochemical, biochemical, and electron microscopic evaluation of muscle tissue. Most commonly, muscle diseases produce weakness and wasting predominantly of the proximal muscles as opposed to the peripheral neuropathies where distal weakness is the rule. Exceptions are those denervating conditions involving anterior horn cells where proximal weakness is common and differentiation from myopathy can only be made with laboratory tests.

Inherited Progressive Myopathies

Inherited progressive myopathies are frequently termed "dystrophies" and are presumed to be due to some primary defect in the maintenance of skeletal muscle resulting in progressive breakdown of fibers. More specific pathogenic mechanisms have also been postulated, such as defective trophic influence of nerve or defective vascular supply.

Duchenne Dystrophy. This is a well-defined clinical entity and is the most severe of the diseases included in this category. It is fatal in early life. It is inherited in an X-linked recessive pattern and therefore occurs exclusively in males or females with Turner's syndrome. Symptoms arise in the first 3 years of life, so that patients frequently walk at a normal age yet are usually never able to run. Weakness is proximal and greatest in the pelvic region. Enlargement of the calves is a characteristic feature ("pseudohypertrophy"), as are contractures. Progression is invariable; the child becomes wheelchair-bound by the age of 12 years and rarely lives past early adulthood. The serum muscle enzymes (especially the creatinine phosphokinase or CPK) are typically markedly elevated. Associated abnormalities include cardiomyopathy and mental retardation. No treatment is known. Genetic counseling is best accomplished after female carriers have been identified in the family. These carriers may have mildly elevated serum muscle enzymes or minimal degenerative changes detectable on muscle biopsy.

Facioscapulohumeral Syndrome. This condition is characterized by progressive muscle weakness predominantly involving the muscles in the perioral, periscapular, and upper arm regions. These result in a typical appearance including "transverse smile," drooping shoulders, and inability to raise the arms over the head. It is usually inherited as an autosomal dominant but may occur sporadically. Symptoms develop late in the first decade of life and usually progress rather slowly so that a normal life span is common. Symptoms may be so mild as to be unnoticed by some patients. Rarely, there is rapid progression and severe disability. Muscle wasting is usually asymmetrical. The same pattern of muscle weakness probably results from a variety of pathological insults since the muscle biopsy may appear to be frankly denervated, myopathic, or even normal in similar-appearing patients; hence the designation facioscapulohumeral *syndrome* rather than *dystrophy*.

Limb Girdle Syndrome. This is the most vague category of primary muscle disease and includes all patients with inherited progressive proximal weakness who are not easily classified into any other category. As would be expected in a heterogenous category, the mode of inheritance, age of onset, and rate of progression are extremely variable. Most commonly, an autosomal-recessive pattern is seen although sporadic cases are frequent. An X-linked recessive form exists (Becker's muscular dystrophy) which some have thought to represent a mild form of Duchenne dystrophy. It is likely that this represents a distinct entity. Members of individual families with limb girdle weakness tend to have involvement of similar muscle groups and similar rates of progression of the disease. Serum muscle enzymes are usually moderately elevated. Cardiac involvement may occur but is unusual. Many patients previously grouped in this category are now known to have rather specific morphologically or biochemically definable conditions making muscle biopsy essential for the evaluation of any patient in this group.

Congenital Nonspecific Myopathies. These patients have infantile hypotonia and weakness, with muscle biopsies showing nonspecific myopathic changes. The condition is frequently associated with contractures (arthrogryposis multiplex).

Other Progressive Muscle Diseases. These are rare conditions in which the term *limb girdle* does not apply since other muscle groups are involved. Included in this category are patients with distal, ocular, oculopharyngeal, or oculocraniosomatic muscle weakness. Many patients in this group have rather specific muscle biopsy findings such as vacuolization or abnormal mitochondria, thus further differentiating them from the usual limb girdle variety. More recently other specific bizarre biopsy changes have been found in some patients categorized as "fingerprint" and "reducing body" myopathy. With more sophisticated evaluation techniques, better classification of these disorders will be possible.

Congenital Nonprogressive Neuromuscular Diseases

Congenital nonprogressive neuromuscular diseases are rare conditions present from birth; all clinically similar, they are commonly associated with infantile hypotonia ("floppy infant"). They are usually very slowly progressive or nonprogressive and tend to involve facial as well as limb muscles. They are diagnosed by rather distinctive changes seen on muscle biopsy, and their names are derived from the biopsy abnormalities.

Central Core Disease. Mild proximal and facial weakness are seen in this condition occasionally accompanied by infantile hypotonia. Sporadic and autosomally dominant inheritance patterns have been described.

Rod Disease (Nemaline Myopathy). This sporadically occurring disease may also be present as infantile hypotonia. Characteristically, muscle bulk is strikingly reduced and facial involvement is present. Occasionally, the weakness progresses slowly. Recently, an adult form of rod disease has been described which is also slowly progressive.

Myotubular or Centronuclear Myopathy. A rather distinct clinical picture is present in this disease. Ophthalmoparesis and facial and limb muscle weakness accompany infantile hypotonia. Slow progression is not uncommon.

Periodic Paralyses

In the category of periodic paralyses are a group of inherited conditions characterized by well-defined episodic attacks of incapacitating weakness associated with abnormal serum potassium levels. Between attacks, the patients are usually normal. In all forms the attacks are most common in the morning and are precipitated by rest following exertion or exposure to cold. All of the periodic paralyses may be associated with myotonia.

Hypokalemic Form. These patients have low serum potassium during attacks of weakness. The disease is inherited as an autosomal-dominant with incomplete penetrance in females so that many more males are affected. The attacks are variable in frequency and can be precipitated by ingestion of carbohydrates. When repeated attacks occur in close succession, a more permanent muscle weakness may become superimposed. One subvariety of this form is associated with thyrotoxicosis and occurs almost exclusively in Oriental patients. The diagnosis of the hypokalemic form is established by low serum potassium levels during an attack, provocation of an attack with glucose and insulin administration, and cessation of an attack with intravenous potassium. Therapy designed to prevent attacks includes the use of spironolactone and acetazolamide to modify serum potassium levels.

Hyperkalemic Form (Adynamia Episodica Hereditaria). This is a milder form of periodic paralysis. It is also an autosomal-dominant and is present with equal frequency in males and females. Patients have high serum potassium levels during an attack, and weakness can be precipitated by administration of potassium. The condition "paramyotonia congenita," once thought to be a specific disease entity, is now believed to be identical with hyperkalemic periodic paralysis. Treatment is accomplished with thiazide diuretics which act by lowering serum potassium and also with acetazolamide acting by an unknown mechanism probably unrelated to its effect on potassium.

Normokalemic Form. This is probably a variant of the hyperkalemic form since these patients are also made worse with potassium loading. Characteristically, they have normal potassium levels during attacks, a situation occasionally seen in the hyperkalemic form as well.

Myotonic Conditions

Myotonia is a descriptive term referring to the phenomenon of delayed muscle relaxation following voluntary or mechanically induced contraction. The patients complain of "stiffness" in that any motion is followed by an inability to relax the muscles utilized. Most typically, a patient will shake hands and then be unable to relax his grip. Percussion-induced myotonia is accomplished by a brisk tap over a muscle with a reflex hammer. If this is done on the thenar eminence, the thumb will showly adduct and remain adducted for several seconds before returning to its rest position. In severe myotonia treatment with procainamide, diphenylhydantoin (Dilantin), or quinine is often effective. Subclinical myotonia is detectable electromyographically as a characteristic form of spontaneous insertional activity (the so-called *dive-bomber phenomenon*). A variety of clinical entities have myotonia as a characteristic feature.

Myotonic Atrophy (Dystrophy). This is an autosomal, dominantly inherited disorder characterized by progressive skeletal muscle wasting associated with myotonia. It is a multisystem disease accompanied by frontal baldness, cataracts, testicular atrophy, skeletal abnormalities, mental deficiency, low serum immunoglobulin (IgG) levels, and impaired response to endogenous insulin. Typically, facial involvement accompanies diffuse limb muscle weakness so that the patients usually have ptosis and gaunt faces. Progression is variable; voluntary myotonia may be the only complaint until late adult life, or the disease may be present in early infancy manifested as infantile hypotonia.

Myotonia Congenita (Thomsen's Disease). Myotonia is often quite severe in this condition, but there is no muscle weakness or wasting. On the contrary, these patients have muscles which are larger than normal size giving them an "athletic look." The disease is inherited in an autosomal-dominant pattern, although an autosomal-recessive form is known to exist.

Chondrodystrophic Myotonia. This is a rare autosomal-recessive condition seen in infants. The disease is characterized by severe myotonia, multiple skeletal deformities, and striking hypertrophy of skeletal musculature.

Paramyotonia Congenita. This is probably identical with hyperkalemic periodic paralysis as discussed above.

Dermatomyositis/Polymyositis and Related Disorders

The category of dermatomyositis/polymyositis and related disorders includes conditions where muscle weakness is accompanied by inflammatory infiltrates noted on muscle biopsy. The muscle weakness may occur in an exacerbating-remitting pattern or be relentlessly progressive; serum muscle enzymes are usually elevated. Detection of inflammatory changes on muscle biopsy implies the possibility of treatment with corticosteroids or immunosuppressive agents and therefore should be looked for in any suspicious case since inflammatory myopathies not infrequently mimic other neuromuscular disorders. In dermatomyositis, skeletal muscle and skin undergo inflammatory change. It occurs in any age group. The skin rash is pathognomonic when it involves the periorbital and nailbed (periungual) regions. In the childhood form, the skin lesions often calcify. The muscle weakness is usually proximal and may be accompanied by muscle tenderness. Dysphagia is occasionally present. In the adult form (over age 40) there is a 10 to 50% incidence of accom-

panying malignancy. Treatment with corticosteroid and immunosuppressive agents is occasionally effective and should not be delayed once the diagnosis is established by muscle biopsy. The prognosis is fatal in approximately a third of patients. Polymyositis, aside from the absence of the skin rash, is the same as dermatomyositis. The absence of the rash makes biopsy of the muscle even more essential differentiating this relatively treatable condition from one of the other nontreatable neuromuscular diseases. Myositis frequently accompanies the so-called collagen diseases.

Other Inflammatory Diseases of Muscle

Myositis may be a manifestation of viral or bacterial infection including tuberculous, clostridial, syphilitic, and leptospiral forms. Parasitic infections include trichinosis, cysticercosis, echinococcosis, toxoplasmosis, trypanosomiasis, and schistosomiasis. Fungal infection with actinomycosis also occurs. Sarcoidosis may produce typical granulomata in muscle.

Myositis Ossificans

Myositis ossificans is a rare condition characterized by the formation of true bone deposits in regions where previous trauma has occurred. Movements become severely restricted by the deposits.

Glycogen Storage Diseases

When specific enzymes involved in glycogen metabolism are absent, glycogen may accumulate in muscle and produce varying symptoms. In any glycogen storage disease the diagnosis can only be established by biochemical demonstration of a specific enzyme deficiency.

Acid Maltase Deficiency. In the infantile form (Pompe's disease) there is hypotonia, profound weakness, organomegaly, and cardiorespiratory disease. Death usually occurs by one year of age. Electromyographic myotonia is a common feature of the disease. Milder forms also exist in which the infant may survive. An adult form of acid maltase deficiency has been reported which is clinically similar to the limb girdle form of myopathy.

Myophosphorylase Deficiency (McArdle's Disease). The typical features of this condition are weakness, easy fatigability, and characteristic painful cramping with exercise, the latter frequently being the most disabling symptom. Commonly, the cramps are accompanied by muscle breakdown and myoglobinuria. Diagnosis is likely when a patient with muscle cramps fails to produce lactate during an ischemic exercise test.

Phosphofructokinase Deficiency. This condition is clinically indistinguishable from myophosphorylase deficiency and can only be confirmed by enzymatic assay of muscle tissue.

Debrancher Enzyme Deficiency. This form also occurs in infants and is characterized by hypotonia, failure to thrive, hypoglycemia, and hepatomegaly.

Myoglobinurias

Any condition in which there is extensive muscle necrosis can result in myoglobinuria. This is most consistently found in myophosphorylase deficiency. In normal individuals, following severe exertion, there may be a breakdown of muscle and an appearance of myoglobin in the urine. This is mostly seen in untrained athletes and military recruits (so-called march gangrene). In some families myoglobinuria occurs after normal exertion; this is presumably the result of some obscure metabolic defect.

Myasthenia Gravis

This is a disorder of neuromuscular transmission characterized by fluctuating weakness which worsens with exercise. It has been found to be associated with antibodies to the acetylcholine receptor region on the muscle. Most commonly it affects the oculomotor and facial muscles, but any skeletal muscle can be involved. It may occur at any age but is mostly seen in young females and elderly males. Although usually sporadic, it rarely occurs in a familial form. Diagnosis is confirmed by the pathognomonic electromyographic and pharmacological features of the disease. Repetitive stimuli delivered to the muscle at a rate of 3 per second produce progressively smaller evoked electrical responses in the muscle (decrement response). Intravenous anticholinesterase drugs often produce dramatic improvement in strength. Defects in the immune sys-

tem are probably responsible for the weakness produced in the disease, and some forms of treatment are directed toward modification of the immune response. ACTH and corticosteroid preparations are effective in many instances. Removal of the thymus gland also has a beneficial effect in a high percentage of patients, but the mechanism is unknown. Symptomatic treatment consists of long-acting anticholinesterase drugs which probably act by increasing the effectiveness of the acetylcholine transmitter at the neuromuscular junction.

Facilitating Myasthenic (Eaton-Lambert) Syndrome

Facilitating myasthenic (Eaton-Lambert) syndrome produces weakness similar to that in myasthenia gravis, but it is milder and less frequently involves cranial muscles. The disease is almost always associated with oatcell carcinoma of the lung. Evoked muscle potentials show a decrement when stimulated at 2 to 3 per second similar to that in myasthenia gravis, but at more rapid rates (10 to 200 per second) the potentials increase in amplitude, providing the characteristic incrementing (facilitating) response. Guanidine effectively relieves the weakness, but anticholinesterase preparations are of no benefit.

BIBLIOGRAPHY

Review of current concepts of myopathies (Symposium). In W. K. Engel (Ed.), *Clinical orthopaedics and related research* (Vol. 39). Philadelphia: Lippincott, 1967.
ROWLAND, L. P., and LAYZER, R. B. Muscular dystrophies, atrophies, and related diseases. In A. B. Baker and L. H. Baker (Eds.), *Clinical neurology*. New York: Harper & Row, 1971. Chap. 37.
WALTON, J. N. (Ed.). *Disorders of voluntary muscle* (3rd ed.). Edinburgh: Churchill Livingstone, 1974.

ADAM N. BENDER

MUSCLE, SKELETAL: PATHOLOGY

Muscle tissue is rather limited in its structural reactions to injury. A diversity of clinically distinct entities may produce similar findings in the muscle biopsy and conversely, the same disease may produce different findings in the muscle biopsy of individual patients or even in different muscles in the same patient. The recent introduction of histochemical and electron microscopic evaluation of muscle biopsies has done much to clarify the situation and has added considerable information as to the pathogenesis of various disease processes involving muscle. In this article, an attempt will be made to differentiate those changes that are specific to a given disease process and those changes that are nonspecific and are seen in a variety of clinical states.

Denervation Atrophy

The three most specific changes seen in denervation are atrophy, type grouping and target fibers. Less specific is the presence of increased fat *among* (but not *in*) muscle fibers. These changes occur when any disease process disrupts the normal innervation of muscle, that is, motor neuron disease or peripheral neuropathy.

Atrophy is used to describe the state in which fibers become smaller but retain their basic internal structure. The fibers have a sharply angulated shrunken appearance as contrasted to the large rounded appearance of normal fibers. The nucleus assumes a darker, dense appearance (pyknotic). Atrophic (small angular) fibers are scattered among normal ones in early denervation but may occur in groups in chronic denervation (grouped atrophy). The end-stage of denervation atrophy is replacement of fibers by fat.

Type grouping results when previously denervated fibers become reinnervated. Whereas there is normally a random distribution of type I and type II muscle fibers, when a motor neuron of a given type is lost, all the muscle fibers previously innervated by that neuron become innervated by an adjacent normal neuron via a process known as *sprouting*. Thus many more fibers become included in the territory of the sprouting neuron. Since all of the fibers in the territory of a single motor neuron are of a given type, the process of sprouting results in large fields of uniform fibers and the usual "checkerboard" mosaic of type I and II fibers is lost. This is the phenomenon of type grouping which is rather specific for chronic denervation.

Target fibers are also characteristic of more chronic denervation. These are so named because they have three concentric zones on cross section resembling a target. The central zone is pale with disrupted myofibrils and absence of mitochondria, membranous components and glycogen; the intermediate (border) zone is excessively dark with increased mitochondria and membranous compounds. The outer zone has a normal appearance.

Nonspecific Atrophy of Type II Fibers

In some instances, muscle wasting and atrophy can occur in the absence of frank denervation. Characteristically, this form of atrophy selectively involves the type II muscle fibers. This is the change seen following disuse of the muscle (as in prolonged bed rest or immobilization with a cast). Other causes of selective type II atrophy include cachexia associated with malignancy or starvation, myasthenia gravis, corticosteroid therapy, and various endocrinopathies. In its most severe form, the changes may be indistinguishable from denervation since denervation not uncommonly will cause the type II fibers to atrophy first, thus simulating the nonspecific form. The other changes of denervation listed above are helpful in this distinction.

Nonspecific Myopathic Changes

These changes are seen in any number of neuromuscular diseases in which the primary pathological changes appear in the muscle itself and the above listed changes of denervation are absent. It must be emphasized that the term *nonspecific myopathy* is being used to define a number of conditions of obscure etiology which may be due to any of a variety of pathological insults. The most common clinical diagnosis in this group is *limb-girdle dystrophy*. With modern analytical methods, several conditions previously grouped in this category have been found to be due to specific abnormalities, such as enzyme malfunctions, mitochondrial abnormalities, or defective innervation. These changes are seen in any of the so-called dystrophies as well as the inflammatory myopathies. They merely indicate muscle fiber damage. Occasionally an element of denervation may coexist in an otherwise myopathic biopsy or vice versa since some of the changes listed below may be seen in an acute denervating process.

Degeneration. The degenerating muscle fiber appears small, round, and is stained basophilic with hematoxylin stains. There are often internally located nuclei which are large, pale, and vesicular. Regeneration usually takes place within the same fiber and is not distinguishable from the changes of degeneration. The term *degenerating-regenerating* fiber is used to describe the latter state.

Necrosis. This common myopathic change consists of a loss of the normal internal myofibrillar structure of the muscle fiber resulting in a pale appearance. The necrotic fiber frequently contains variable numbers of phagocytes.

"Moth-Eaten" Fibers. In this process there are scattered small focal areas with decreased mitochondria and membranous components giving the fiber a "moth-eaten" appearance with oxidative enzyme mitochondrial stains. This finding is quite nonspecific and is frequently seen in denervation as well as myopathic disorders.

Fiber Size Variation. Fibers which are abnormally large or small in diameter but otherwise normal are frequently seen in myopathic processes but are nonspecific and often seen in denervation as well. The small fibers are typically round as opposed to the angulated form seen in denervation. Abnormally large fibers frequently "split" and divide into smaller fibers. Membranous septae within the fiber define the site of a split.

Internal Nuclei. The usually peripherally located nuclei may migrate toward the center of a fiber. Many internal nuclei may be seen in a single cross-section of a fiber. This is nonspecific and occurs occasionally in denervation, as well, although less prominently so. It is most prominent in myotonic atrophy (dystrophy). In the latter condition the internal nuclei are most frequent in small type I fibers.

Ring Fibers and Whorls. The parallel array of myofibrils may be disrupted so that they may form a peripheral ring around the fiber. The myofibrils in the ring run perpendicular to the plane of the central myofibrils. This change is most commonly seen in myotonic atrophy. Whorls are also the results of a disrupted myofibrillar pattern but are internal rather than peripheral in location.

Vacuoles. Vacuoles form when there are focal necrotic areas within the muscle fiber. They may be relatively empty or contain breakdown products of muscle tissue.

Increased Connective Tissue. The connective issue tissue among muscle fibers is increased in myopathic processes to a much greater extent than in denervating conditions and is important in differentiating the two. This change is most striking in the Duchenne form of dystrophy and commonly accompanies contractures.

Inflammatory Myopathy

As contrasted to nonspecific myopathic changes, inflammatory myopathy has many or all of the changes mentioned above with the addition of variable numbers of inflammatory cell infiltrates. This occurs in polymyositis, dermatomyositis, and any of the so-called collagen vascular diseases having a myositic component. The infiltrates characteristically are principally around blood vessels. Since, as is mentioned above, necrotic fibers commonly contain phagocytes, it is important to ascertain that the inflammation is out of proportion to the degree of fiber necrosis before the diagnosis of inflammatory myopathy can be established.

In the childhood form of dermatomyositis, perifascicular atrophy may occur in which small rounded muscle fibers are concentrated at the periphery of muscle fascicles. Vacuoles are also common in the childhood form.

Metabolic Myopathies with Excessive Glycogen or Lipid Storage

Metabolic myopathies frequently are characterized by the presence of vacuoles indicating either excessive stored material (such as glycogen or lipid) or abnormal dilatation of membranous structures.

The glycogen storage diseases are the result of specific enzyme dysfunctions involved in glycogen metabolism. At present, four types are known to affect skeletal muscle: Cori type II (acid maltase deficiency or Pompe's disease); Cori type III (debranching enzyme deficiency); Cori type V (myophosphorylase deficiency or McArdle's disease); and Cori type VII (phosphofructokinase deficiency). Typically the muscle of these patients contains many vacuoles filled with accumulated glycogen. The most severe degree of vacuolization is seen in the Cori type II form in which the muscle fibers appear to be almost entirely filled with glycogen. Glycogen can also accumulate as evidence of a nonspecific myopathic process or when mitochondria are malfunctioning although usually to a lesser degree. To confirm the diagnosis of any of the above glycogen storage diseases, therefore, the specific enzyme deficiency must be demonstrated biochemically.

A lipid storage myopathy due to carnitine deficiency has been reported. In this condition small vacuoles which contain fat are present, reflecting the defective metabolism of this substance. Treatment with carnitine is effective.

With more effective biochemical testing procedures, it is likely that an increasing number of specific enzyme defects will be found that manifest themselves as skeletal muscle disease.

Periodic Paralyses

In both the hypo- and hyperkalemic forms of periodic paralysis, the muscle may contain characteristic vacuoles. These are usually single, large, centrally located, and represent dilated T-tubules and sacroplasmic reticulum. No storage material is contained in these vacuoles. They may be found either during or between attacks of weakness. The hypokalemic form usually produces the most prominent vacuolar change.

Specific Congenital Neuromuscular Diseases

There is a group of neuromuscular diseases of obscure etiology in which certain specific biopsy changes are so prevalent that in themselves they are sufficient to make a diagnosis. Clinically, these patients appear similar. They are weak at birth and their disease is relatively nonprogressive.

Rod Disease (Nemaline Myopathy). In this rare congenital myopathy there are numerous dense short rod-shaped structures within most of the type I fibers. Ultrastructurally, these "rods" are derived from expansion of the Z disk. Typically they have a fine periodicity. Although this disease is characteristically seen in a congenital form, rod disease beginning in adult life is also known to exist.

Central Core Disease. This disease is characterized by the presence of pale central regions ("cores") in muscle fibers which are best seen with oxidative enzyme histochemical stains. The cores represent regions of absent mitochondria and membranous structures. The change is seen only in type I fibers. The cores can be similar to target fibers in appearance but are distinguished from them by lack of an intermediate dense zone, by the large number of involved fibers, and by the absence of other denervation changes. A possible variant of this is multicore disease where multiple vertical segments of the fiber have the above changes rather than a single central horizontal region.

Myotubular or Centronuclear Myopathy. These patients are clinically distinguishable by nonprogressive facial and ocular muscle weakness in addition to limb weakness. The biopsy shows small type I fibers among normal sized type II fibers. A large percentage of the small fibers (in cross section) have single central nuclei. In longitudinal section, the nuclei line up in chains. The fibers bear a marked resemblance to those in the myotube stage of embryogenesis—hence the name *myotubular myopathy*. It has been postulated that there is a defect in the maturation of muscle fibers so that they are arrested in the myotubular stage. Occasionally, a congenitally weak patient will have small type I fibers and no central nuclei or even small type II fibers relative to type I. The latter two conditions are termed *congenital fiber type disproportion*.

Congenital Nonspecific Myopathy. This disease also produces infantile weakness and hypotonia. The biopsy here has none of the characteristic changes mentioned above but is characterized by increased connective tissue, degenerating fibers, and other nonspecific myopathic changes.

Specific Diseases Affecting Mitochondria

A growing number of patients has been reported with a variety of nonfamilial clinical symptoms in whose muscle the primary changes are seen in mitochondria. Many have eye muscle and facial weakness in addition to proximal muscle weakness (oculo-cranio-somatic neuromuscular disease). Most commonly, large increases in the number of mitochondria occur. The modified trichrome stain produces a red color in mitochondria so that a fiber thus affected has been termed a *ragged red* fiber. There are frequently large lipid droplets and glycogen accumulation within these fibers giving the central area its "ragged" red appearance. Typically, many "ragged red" fibers are present in these conditions. An occasional ragged red fiber can be a nonspecific finding seen in a variety of neuromuscular diseases. Ultrastructurally, the mitochondria may be increased in size as well as in number within the abnormal fibers. A common finding is the presence of paracrystalline structures within abnormal mitochondria. The patients occasionally have defects in oxidative metabolism as evidence for biochemically malfunctioning mitochondria.

BIBLIOGRAPHY

DUBOWITZ, V., and BROOKE, M. H. *Muscle biopsy: A modern approach.* London: Saunders, 1973.

ENGEL, W. K. Selective and nonselective susceptibility of muscle fiber types. A new approach to human neuromuscular diseases. *Archives of Neurology,* 1970, *22,* 97–117.

WALTON, J. N. (Ed.). *Disorders of voluntary muscle* (3rd ed.). Edinburgh: Churchill Livingstone, 1974.

ADAM N. BENDER

MUSCLE, SKELETAL: STRUCTURE AND FUNCTION

Structure

Skeletal muscle is the tissue by which all voluntary movements are executed. The basic unit of skeletal muscle is the striated muscle fiber. This is a long cylindrical structure averaging 50 μm in diameter and extending from tendon to tendon. Each individual fiber is actually a syncytium, the result of fusion of many primitive myoblasts during embryogenesis, so that the mature structure is multinucleated with nuclei located at the periphery. Muscle fibers occur in groups called *fascicles* which are bounded by connective tissue containing blood vessels and nerve fibers. The muscle fiber itself is surrounded by two membranes—an outer basement membrane having a hazy appearance which is composed largely of polysaccharides and an inner plasma membrane which is composed of lipoprotein.

Myofibrils. Most of the interior of the fiber is occupied by rows of myofibrils—the basic contractile units of muscle tissue. These myofibrils occur in bundles approximately 1 μm in diameter separated by membranous components and cellular organelles. The myofibrils are characterized by a repeating banded pattern. These bands give skeletal muscle its striated appearance. Each banded unit is called a sarcomere, a structure which consists of interdigitating thick and thin filaments bound on each end by a dense structure called the Z disk. The thin filaments are 2 μm long and form the light appearing I band. They are anchored on each end by the Z disk and are composed primarily of the protein actin. Two other proteins, tropomyosin and troponin are embedded in the actin superstructure and are responsible for modulating contraction. The central portion of the sarcomere is occupied by the dense A band which is composed of thick filaments 1.5 μm in length. This consists of parallel arrays of myosin molecules which are long golf club shaped structures having a single thick globular head at one end. These "heads" called cross-bridges protrude out as bumps from the thick filaments in a regular fashion and are visible on electron microscopy. They play an important part in muscle contraction. The A band of thick filaments remains constant in length during contraction, but the I band shortens during muscle contraction as the thin filaments slide in among the thick filaments. In the region where both types of filaments interdigitate, each thick filament is surrounded by an array of six thin filaments.

T-tubules and Sarcoplasmic Reticulum. Among the myofibrils are two important membranous structures: the *T-tubules* and the *sarcoplasmic reticulum.* The T-tubules are actually invaginations of the plasma membrane into the muscle fiber which penetrate perpendicular to the myofibrils, one on either side of the Z band (two per sarcomere). Analogous to the digestive tract, they are freely open to the exterior of the cell but have no anatomic opening to the interior of the cell. T-tubules function by conducting membrane action potentials into the muscle fiber. In between the two sets of T-tubules is a complex cisternal structure called the sarcoplasmic reticulum (SR) which corresponds to the smooth endoplasmic reticulum of other cells. The SR is in close appositional contact with the T-tubules via dilated lateral sacs of each end of the sarcomere (two sacs per tubule). No anatomic communication exists between the lumina of the two structures. The combination of a T-tubule and its two lateral sacs is called a triad. Toward the center of the sarcomere, the SR is composed of many small cisternae which surround the myofibrils. The SR functions as a storage area for calcium needed for contraction activation within the muscle.

Organelles. Mitochondria are large and plentiful in muscle. They are located in the I band region and serve as the muscle fiber's source of energy derived from oxidation. Numerous glycogen particles appear in the muscle fibers as clusters of dark dots 15–30 nm in diameter. Nuclei lie at the periphery of the muscle fiber just under the plasma membrane.

Fiber Types. There are at least two different muscle fiber types (referred to as types I and II) based on histochemical and ultrastructural differences. The type I fibers have proportionally more mitochondria and, therefore, are more darkly stained with oxidative enzyme histochemical reactions (such as DPNH tetrazolium reductase); glycogen is sparse and myofibrillar ATPase activity is lower. Type II fibers are the opposite, being relatively poor in oxidative enzymes and rich in glycogen and myofibrillar ATPase. It has been demonstrated experimentally that muscle fiber type is determined by innervation so that all the fibers in a single motor unit (innervated by one lower motor neuron) are of uniform fiber type. This has important significance in evaluating pathological muscle where defective innervation may be defined by the relative distribution of fiber types.

Function

Normal muscle contraction is initiated by a nerve action potential traveling down a motor neuron axon. The terminal axon contacts the muscle at a specialized region, the neuromuscular junction. Here the muscle membrane is characterized by a regular folded appearance beneath the terminal axon. The axon tip contains many small round vesicles which are thought to contain the neurotransmitter acetylcholine. When the nerve action potential arrives at the neuromuscular junction, these vesicles release the acetylcholine transmitter into the cleft between the nerve and muscle. The transmitter reacts with a specific receptor on the muscle membrane and results in depolari-

zation which, when a critical level is reached, initiates a muscle action potential. The muscle action potential travels along the muscle membrane and is conducted into the interior of the fiber by the T-tubules. The action potential in the T-tubule stimulates the lateral sacs of the sarcoplasmic reticulum to release stored calcium among the myofibrils. The calcium reacts with the modulator proteins (troponin and tropomyosin) to initiate contraction. The small cross-bridges on the myosin (thick) filaments "pull" the actin (thin) filaments in a manner similar to the action of caterpillar feet. The thin filaments slide among the thick filaments resulting in shortening of the sarcomere (the so-called *sliding filament* hypothesis). Energy for this process is derived from adenosine triphosphate (ATP) molecules via the enzyme ATPase located on the cross-bridges of the thick filaments. Relaxation results when calcium is actively taken up again by the sarcoplasmic reticulum. Energy for contraction in muscle is produced under both anaerobic (anoxic) and aerobic (oxygen dependent) conditions. The anaerobic system uses glucose derived from glycogen breakdown as an energy source. The enzyme phosphorylase starts the breakdown of glycogen to glucose resulting in a rapid source of energy at the expense of the glycogen stores in the fiber and accumulation of lactic acid as the metabolic end product. The aerobic system utilizes oxidative enzymes present in mitochondria to metabolize pyruvate and fatty acids via the Krebs cycle. It is a slower system but can maintain function for a longer time. The type II fibers have more glycogen and utilize predominantly anaerobic metabolism. Their contractions are relatively quick and in short bursts but less sustained than those in the type I fibers where oxidative metabolism provides energy for slower but more sustained contractions.

BIBLIOGRAPHY

BOURNE, G. H. (Ed.). *The structure and function of muscle* (2nd ed.). New York: Academic Press, 1973.

BRISKEY, E. J.; CASSENS, R. G.; and MARSH, B. B. *Muscle as a food* (2nd ed.). Madison: University of Wisconsin Press, 1970.

HUXLEY, H. E. The structural basis of muscular contraction. *Proceedings of the Royal Society of London*, 1971, *178*, 131–149.

ADAM N. BENDER

MUSCLE ACTION POTENTIAL (MAP)

The electrical changes accompanying muscle contraction, as typically measured by use of an electromyogram (EMG), are said to reflect *muscle action potential* (MAP) and to be an accurate indicator of muscular activity (Duffy, 1962). Increased contraction in the presence of stimulation is measurable not only when the individual responds overtly, but also when covert responding (e.g., attending or thinking) occurs. As a consequence, changes in MAP have been taken to indicate changes in the activation or arousal level of the individual.

However, there is less than perfect correspondence among measurers of muscular tension (e.g., grip or point pressure, steadiness, EMG) and, further, the magnitude of EMG change varies with (a) the locus of measurement, (b) the general state of muscle tension in the body, and (c) the nature of the stimulus situation (and, presumably, the type of response required by that situation or habitually given by a particular individual). Finally, intraindividual correlations between MAP and other measures of arousal or activation (e.g., EEG, heart rate, GSR, blood pressure) have been modest, at best, and highly variable across stimulus situations. Nevertheless, there is sufficient indication of a relationship between level of "tension" (as indicated by MAP) and performance adequacy in certain situations to warrant continued use of the measure. In addition, findings of MAP differences between normals and psychiatric patients (neurotics and psychotics) suggest the value of further investigation of muscle tension and its significance in psychopathology and personality study.

BIBLIOGRAPHY

Duffy, E. *Activation and behavior.* New York: Wiley, 1962.

See also ACTIVATION AND AROUSAL

MORTIMER H. APPLEY

MUSCLE REGENERATION

Skeletal muscle regeneration has been under study for almost a century and its occurrence in various species, including higher vertebrates and man, is fully established.

Until the early 1960s, regeneration from viable muscle fiber stumps was considered to be the sole, or at least the principle, mode of regeneration of muscle. It is generally accepted that, with minor exceptions, skeletal muscle regenerates discontinuously from single mononucleated cells, the so-called presumptive myoblasts. Following muscle injury, these cells undergo a series of mitotic divisions, at the end of which they acquire a distinct lattice of intracytoplasmic striated myofilaments which make them recognizable as myoblasts. Morphological, cytological, tissue-culture and autoradiographic studies have shown that a variable number of these mononucleated myoblasts eventually fuse to form a new myofiber, the myotube, which is a thin fiber with strongly basophilic cytoplasm, rich in newly formed RNA, and with long chains of prominent nuclei occupying its central axis. Fusion may also occur between mononucleated myoblasts and multinucleated myotubes, as well as between newly formed multinucleated myotubes. Experiments with tissue cultures of different labeled nonmyogenic cells mixed with unlabeled myoblasts have shown that a nonmyogenic cell was never incorporated into a myotube. Myoblast fusion involves the presence of molecules mediating recognition of primed homotypic cells.

A richly festooned original basement membrane continues to surround the newly regenerated fiber until replaced, in approximately five weeks, by a new one which had been forming within it it. In the absence of the scaffolding of the old basement membrane, myotubes can form by fusion of linear aggregates of myoblasts. It is within myotubes that the main part of myofilamentogenesis then takes place. This process follows a time sequence akin to that in mammalian embryonal myogenesis and in the regenerating amphibian limb, until the unique repeating periodicity of mature striated muscle is fully reached. With the appearance of the transverse tubular system and the sarcoplasmic reticulum, and with the migration of the central nuclei to a hypolemmal position, the maturation of the young muscle fiber is complete, though fiber growth in cross diameter may still proceed for a time. Insofar as the final histological and gross remolding of the regenerated muscle is concerned, it appears that mechanical tension is the the main force responsible for the histological reorganization, whereas gross molding is dependent upon tendon connections and upon pressures of the surrounding tissues.

Denervation

The effect of denervation on muscle regeneration has been extensively investigated both by Western and Soviet scientists. Denervation performed prior to the stage of myotube formation does not hinder, and possibly enhances, regeneration. If denervation occurs after myotubes are formed, it causes retardation in the maturation of the regenerate and, in the late stages, results in degeneration of the parenchymal elements of muscle followed by considerable replacement by fibrous tissue. It appears that the effects of denervation will be overcome if the regenerating muscle fibers are in continuity with segments of innervated ones. Recently introduced advanced techniques for growing tissue culture of muscle have made it possible to study more closely nerve-muscle dependence in muscle regeneration. There is solid evidence of the deleterious effect of motor denervation on muscle regeneration.

One important aspect of muscle regeneration that has not yet been adequately investigated is the effect of changes in vascular supply to muscle.

Myoblast

A major and so far unsettled dispute among investigators of muscle regeneration concerns the origin of the presumptive myoblast. There is uncertainty about where this indistinct cell comes from and what are its qualifications for presuming it to be a muscle cell progenitor. This is understandable considering that no more sophisticated an instrument than morphology has yet been utilized in identifying one cell from another in muscle regeneration, and that interpretation of relationships depends upon reconstruction of a series of static pictures. This, in the words of one prominent worker in the field, "is the problem that plagues the morphologist in studying most regenerating systems." The presumptive myoblast though it may on a genetic or molecular basis be not so undifferentiated, is morphologically indistinguishable from any macrophage.

The controversy about the origin of the presumptive myoblast is nowadays focused upon two major concepts: one maintains that it derives from a special cell in muscle, the so-called *satellite cell* first described in 1961, and another holds that it originates in the muscle fiber proper.

Satellite Cell

The first of these concepts assigns to the satellite cell the role of a "reserve" or "stem" cell for muscle regeneration. The existence and the singular localization of the satellite cell in both vertebrate and invertebrate species, have been asserted by practically all investigators in the field. It is defined as a discrete, fusiform, mononucleated cell enclosed between the basement membrane component and the plasmalemma of the muscle fiber, and directed with its long axis along the latter. It is separate from the muscle fiber proper and by definition must not contain myofilaments. Occasionally, the overlying basement membrane may invaginate around one end of the satellite cell, in which case sections at certain levels of the latter may yield the impression that it is segregated by a basement membrane "enclave" from the underlying muscle fiber. Both red and pale muscle fibers contain satellite cells and these are also present, in their typical position, in muscle spindles. They are spread rather regularly along the fibers. The capacity of satellite cells to proliferate by mitotic division is indicated by the presence of centrioles when they are at rest. Following muscle injury these undifferentiated "reserve" cells are activated into undergoing mitotic division. At this stage, that is, before they finally have demonstrated their myogenic potential by producing myofilaments, they have the appearance of ordinary macrophages and comprise a large percentage of the numerous mononucleated cells of similar appearance seen within the degenerating muscle fiber two to three days following injury. There is nothing to prevent them from being looked upon as presumptive myoblasts.

The accomplished muscle fiber is a postmitotic cellular element, and it can be anticipated that the presence in it of a cell such as the satellite cell which apparently has neither differentiated nor left the mitotic cycle, will implicate it in muscle regeneration.

Regeneration

The second major concept of muscle regeneration has largely depended on observations in amphibians and mammals. Early among the changes in injured muscle in these species there is an appearance of tiny intracytoplasmic vesicles presumably derived from broken down endoplasmic reticulum, gradually arraying themselves in chains around myonuclei, with a narrow rim of cytoplasm dividing between them and the nuclear membrane. With time individual vesicles fuse and a narrow full-circle cistern is formed, sequestering the nucleus, with a bit of cytoplasm around it, from the rest of the myofiber. That these are not degenerating nuclei of a disintegrating muscle fiber, but rather viable ones, is strongly indicated by the presence of many ribosomes, some polysomes and tiny mitochondria and a Golgi complex in the surrounding cytoplasm. Evidence of the viability of these nucleated sarcoplasmic fragments and of their ability to multiply by mitotic division has been provided by radioautography. Tritiated thymidin supplied to the injured muscle is picked up by many of the nuclei that are surrounded by the small cleaving vesicles.

Later, when myotubes are formed in the regenerating muscle, labeled nuclei are seen within them. Regeneration therefore comes from the muscle fiber itself. Such a mode of regeneration must assume that a highly differentiated element like the adult muscle fiber need not be an irreversible postmitotic element and that under appropriate stimulation, such as trauma, cold injury, amputation, or mincing, it may dedifferentiate in what is now called "depression," regaining the biological properties of an earlier state of differentiation. Such cells may then reenter the mitotic cycle and, through division, begin to differentiate anew, or be "repressed" into doing their particular bit, which is synthesizing actin and myosin, thus becoming muscle.

It should be noted that the concept of regeneration through dedifferentiation has been severely criticized by some workers.

Finally, a limited number of investigators offer alternative suggestions for the origin of myoblasts: monocytes that have migrated to the site of muscle injury; local fibroblasts, and endomysial cells have all been suggested as engaging in myogenesis, but so far little evidence has accrued in support of this view.

BIBLIOGRAPHY

ADAMS, R. D.; DENNY-BROWN, D.; and PEARSON, C. M. *Diseases of muscle—A study in pathology* (2nd ed.). New York: Harper & Row, 1962.

BETZ, E. H.; FIRKET, H.; and REZNIK, M. Some aspects of muscle regeneration. *International Review of Cytology*, 1966, *19*, 203–227.

CARLSON, B. M. The regeneration of skeletal muscle, a review. *American Journal of Anatomy*, 1975, *137*, 119–150.

FIELD, E. J. Muscle regeneration and repair. In G. H. Bourne (Ed.), *Structure and function of muscle* (Vol. 3). New York: Academic Press, 1960. Pp. 139–170.

GODMAN, G. C. On the regeneration and redifferentiation of mammalian striated muscle. *Journal of Morphology, 1957, 100*, 27–81.

HAY, E. D. Cytological studies of dedifferentiation and differentiation in regenerating amphibian limbs. In D. Rudnick (Ed.), *Regeneration.* New York: Ronald Press, 1962. Pp. 177–210.

HOLTZER, H. Myogenesis. In O. A. Schjeide and J. de Vellis (Eds.), *Cell differentiation.* New York: Van Nostrand Reinhold, 1970. Pp. 476–503.

LE GROS CLARK, W. E. An experimental study of the regeneration of mammalian striped muscle. *Journal of Anatomy*, 1946, *80*, 24–36.

MAURO, A. Satellite cells of skeletal muscle fibers. *Journal of Biophysical and Biochemical Cytology*, 1961, *9*, 493–495.

MAURO, A.; SHAFIQ, S. A.; and MILHORAT, A. T. (Eds.). *Regeneration of striated muscle and myogenesis.* Amsterdam: Exerpta Medica, 1970.

STUDITSKY, A. N., and STRIGANOVA, A. N. *Restorative processes in skeletal muscle* [Russian]. Moscow: Izdatelstvo Akademii Nauk SSSR, 1951.

ZHENEVSKAYA, R. P. The role of nervous connections on the early stages of muscle regeneration [Russian]. *Doklady Akademii Nauk SSSR*, 1958, *121*, 182–185.

ALBERT J. BEHAR

MYELIN, BIOLOGY OF

Myelin is the complex of materials that surround many of the axons in both the central (CNS) and peripheral (PNS) nervous system, particularly the large axons characterized by a rapid propagation of the nerve impulse, with which the myelin may play an important role. The presence of large quantities of myelin in the white matter imparts the white color to this tissue in contrast to the gray color of gray matter in which myelin is present to a much lesser degree. Microscopically, myelin may be stained with mordant and hematoxylin techniques, with Luxol blue, alone or with cresyl violet or the periodic acid-Schiff technique, or with phloxine, usually combined with other dyes. Ultrastructurally, myelin consists of the cell membranes of oligodendroglia in the CNS, or of Schwann cells in the PNS, wrapped around the axon in a spiral fashion.

Chemistry

Myelin is not a specific chemical substance, but a complex of substances of lipid, carbohydrate and protein character, and possibly other elements. The lipids of normal myelin include cholesterol in a free, not ester form, cerebrosides (ceramide-galactose, where ceramide is a sphingosine-fatty acid ester), sulfatides (cerebroside-sulfate), sphingomyelin (ceramide-phosphate-choline), phosphatidyl serine (where phosphatidyl refers to a triglyceride esterfied with two fatty acids and phosphoric acid) diphosphoinositide (phosphatidyl-inositol-phosphate) and phosphatidal ethanolamine (where phosphatidal refers to a phosphatidyl, in which one fatty acid is replaced by an aliphatic chain with a vinyl ether group). The sulfatides exhibit the property of metachromasia when stained with toluidine blue or cresyl violet, a property useful in the study of metachromatic leukodystrophy. The cerebrosides, sulfatides and the diphosphoinositides contain hexoses, and may be viewed as carbohydrates as well as lipids. As best can be judged, these lipid elements are present in approximately the same concentration in the myelin of the CNS (central myelin) as in that of the PNS (peripheral myelin) except for the diphosphoinositides, of which there is twice as much in the central myelin as in peripheral myelin.

Once formed, these myelin lipids are relatively stable, and only a slow, but nonetheless finite metabolic turnover is demonstrable. The protein of central myelin is bound to lipids in such fashion that they have the solubility characteristics of lipids, and have been called proteolipids. Such proteolipids are not present in peripheral myelin, in which the proteins are not soluble in fat solvents, have sometimes been termed neurokeratin, and may appear as a plexiform reticulated network in histologic sections.

The most useful distinction between central and peripheral myelin, however, lies in the solubility characteristics of the carbohydrate containing components, most probably the cerebrosides and sulfatides, which even in formalin fixed tissues, may be readily extracted by fat solvents from central myelin, but not from peripheral myelin; in consequence, they will still be present in the peripheral myelin but not in the central myelin of paraffin embedded sections. These carbohydrate substances may be readily stained in such paraffin sections by the periodic acid-Schiff (PAS) technique. Some other myelin component, presumably a phospholipid, will be stained by Luxol blue (LB) in both central and peripheral myelin. When these two staining procedures are combined, LBPAS, i.e., both staining procedures applied to the same paraffin section, peripheral myelin appears deep blue in color, this being the optical summation of the colors imparted by each stain, while central myelin appears blue-green in color, this reflecting the LB alone, the PAS coloration being absent because the carbohydrate moiety had been extracted in preparing the section.

At birth, myelin formation in the peripheral nervous system is almost completely adult in quantity and distribution, but it is far from complete in the central nervous system, in which the adult pattern is not reached for one or two years. Once formed, myelin is very susceptible to injury by a great variety of nonspecific injurious factors, such as hypoxia, inflammation, edema, and so on, as well as by the more specific injuries which characterize the "demyelinating diseases." Myelin also degenerates whenever the axon about which it lies, degenerates. As the myelin degenerates, the free cholesterol is liberated into the tissues, where it is promptly esterfied and engulfed by phagocytic mesenchymal cells. In rare conditions, e.g., coagulative necrosis, the cholesterol esters may be hydrolyzed after a long period of time, and may form cholesterol crystals. The cerebrosides are also liberated into the tissues, in which circumstance they are no longer soluble in fat solvents, will remain in the tissues and can be stained by the PAS technique in both the CNS and PNS.

Regeneration

Regeneration of myelin in the PNS is readily apparent, and may be complete. If the myelin destruction had been associated with axon loss, a regeneration of axons in the PNS will occur first, followed by a regeneration of myelin about them, since the integrity of the axon is essential for the formation and maintenance of the surrounding myelin. The regeneration of axons and myelin in the PNS may be complete, and in some instances, as in traumatic neuromas, may be overly exuberant. In cases of segmental demyelination of peripheral nerves, in which the integrity of axons is maintained, a regeneration of myelin is a natural part of the healing process.

Regeneration of axons and central myelin is very much less evident in the CNS. Although it is difficult to determine if a small number of central myelinated fibers in a lesion are residual or regenerated, it is clear that the bulk of the myelinated fibers in any lesion are permanently lost and not replaced. This applies to both axons and myelin sheaths in lesions in which both are lost, and to the myelin sheaths in lesions, such as those of multiple sclerosis, in which most axons are preserved and only the myelin is lost, apparently permanently. Regeneration of central myelin is reported more frequently in some experimental situations, often based upon ultrastructural characteristics, though the significance of these is not universally accepted as decisive evidence of such regeneration.

In contrast, the regenerative formation of peripheral myelin within the CNS is readily apparent. Peripheral myelin may be found in much larger quantities in what is essentially neuromatous tissue following injury to such nerves, as when the surrounding tissues are infarcted. In addition, peripheral myelin may be found ensheathing preserved central axons whose original central myelin sheaths had degenerated, as in plaques of multiple sclerosis. This regenerated peripheral myelin is associated with cells resembling Schwann cells, and with collagen and reticulin fibers. These cells cannot readily be traced to preexisting Schwann cells, and it is thought that they take origin by maturation and differentiation of multipotential primitive reticular cells, a concept consistent with the assumption that Schwann cells are mesenchymal, rather than neuroectodermal in character.

BIBLIOGRAPHY

ADAMS, C. W. M. *Neurohistochemistry.* Amsterdam: Elsevier, 1965.
FEIGIN, I., and OGATA, J. Schwann cells and peripheral myelin within human nervous tissues: The mesenchymal character of Schwann cells. *Journal of Neuropathology and Experimental Neurology,* 1971, *30,* 603–612.

IRWIN FEIGIN

MYELIN, CENTRAL: FINE STRUCTURAL ALTERATIONS

Morphological changes from the normal fine structure of the myelin sheath can be found associated with three categories of pathological processes: (1) errors or deviations during development, (2) responses to a variety of insults to the mature nervous system, and (3) the remyelinating process which often follows such insults.

Developmental Deviations

Normal myelin development has already been described. In humans, a number of genetic diseases are encountered in children in which myelin development does not proceed normally in the central nervous system. Generally, these conditions, metachromatic leucodystrophy, Krabbe's disease and sex-linked adrenoleucodystrophy, among others, are often due to the absence of a particular enzyme resulting in the inability of the oligodendroglial cell to form myelin. In these abortive attempts at myelin formation, the oligodendroglia often form abnormal lipid inclusions in the cytoplasm but their ability to form true myelin in certain parts of the nervous system is severely limited. The fine structure of the abnormal lipid inclusions is often characteristic of the specific disease.

At least two good experimental models for these leucodystrophies have been discovered. These are the murine mutants, jimpy and quaking. In jimpy, the mouse produces very little myelin in the central nervous system. Instead, the oligodendroglial cells ensheath the axons usually with a single layered cell process. In some instances, short lengths of a major dense line are produced but, for the most part, no myelin is synthesized. The oligodendroglia in jimpy have been reported to contain cylindrical structures reminiscent of lamellated lipid inclusions. Quaking mice also show a paucity of myelin but the severity of the lesion is much less than in jimpy. Poor myelin formation with resultant lipid accumulations in the oligodendroglial cell have also been achieved by the administration of the cholesterol inhibitor AY 9944 to the developing animal. Viral infection in the young animal also interferes with myelin formation.

Insults to CNS

The myelin sheath of the mature central nervous system shows pathological alterations as a result of insult to either the axon or the oligodendroglial cell. Severe damage to the axon, such as amputation, results in the well known phenomenon of Wallerian degeneration. In this condition, the distal portion of the axon degenerates and the associated myelin sheath subsequently disintegrates. Eventually, the debris is phagocytosed by macrophages which come to contain sudanophilic lipid inclusions.

Other insults to the axon such as may occur in motor neuron disease, various intoxications, metabolic disturbances, among others, frequently result in an initial swelling of the axon. The individual lamellae of the myelin sheath, however, show no apparent change in their thickness but the number of lamellae tend to decrease. Apparently, as the axon enlarges the myelin lamellae slip past one another much as the mainspring of a clock unwinds resulting in larger outer and inner diameters of the myelin sheath and a constant thickness of the lamellae.

If the lesion is severe enough, the axon may finally degenerate leaving an empty myelin sheath. Under these circumstances, the sheath can collapse on itself and assume a contorted and bizarre configuration. The individual lamellae, however, retain their morphological integrity for a rather long time until the sheath is finally attacked and digested by phagocytic cells.

Demyelination is the pathological process in which the myelin is affected and eventually destroyed but the axon is left apparently intact. This is the result of an effect on the oligodendroglial cell or the myelin sheath itself and, thus, exhibits a tendency towards segmental expression.

One of the early changes associated with some forms of demyelination consists of a separation of the myelin lamellae at the intraperiod line. In experimental *allergic encephalomyelitis* (EAE), sometimes considered to be a model for multiple sclerosis, one of the earliest signs of change is the separation of the outer loop from the outermost lamella providing a means of access between the intraperiod line and the extracellular space. This is followed by fairly regular separation of the lamellae until even the periaxonal space becomes confluent with extracellular spaces and eventually by myelin degeneration. The latter process is characterized by the so-called "vesicular dissolution" of myelin in which, instead of lamellar structure, the myelin takes on a configuration resulting in vesicle-shaped profiles.

In *triethyltin* (TET) intoxication, the intraperiod line also splits but the morphology is quite distinct from that seen in EAE. Instead of a fairly regular separation of the lamella, TET produces large, focal intramyelinic splits. These sometimes enormous spaces appear empty and watery and do not show any direct confluence with any other spaces in the brain. When tracer is injected directly into the brain, it is essentially excluded from the spaces and so they seem to be somehow separated from the extracellular space. Similar changes can be produced with hexachlorophene and isonicotinic hydrazide, among others.

Other alterations seen in the myelin sheath of the mature central nervous system involve the oligodendroglia: axonal interface. These changes can be seen after either axonal or glial cell damage, or both. First, the periaxonal space may become expanded. Sometimes the periaxonal space can become so greatly swollen with extracellular fluid that the axon occupies only a small portion of the enormously enlarged interior space of the sheath. Sometimes the periaxonal space remains narrow but the two apposing membranes, glial and axonal, become infolded and assume a complicated interdigitated configuration. Changes can also be seen at the paranodes where the lateral loops can become detached from the axonal membrane.

In a number of the conditions described, especially EAE, a third cell type, in addition to the oligodendroglial cell and the axon, may be encountered. These are apparently hematogenous cells such as mononuclear cells or phagocytes. Their precise role in the demyelinating process is not always entirely clear but it is assumed that at least some of them are involved in an immunological reaction.

Remyelination

While the central nervous system is not particularly noted for its regenerative capacity, the electron microscope has been able to demonstrate that remyelination does, indeed, occur in it, although often in a limited and incomplete fashion. After various lesions leading to loss of myelin, one can often observe configurations highly reminiscent of myelination in the normal, developing animal.

One of the more unusual phenomena that accompany remyelination in the central nervous system is the appearance of organelles such as mitochondria in the cytoplasmic portions of the myelin sheaths which are normally devoid of these structures. Indeed, the cytoplasmic content of the sheath is increased during remyelination by the presence of what appear to be isolated islands of cytoplasm among the lamellae. Even structures resembling the Schmidt-Lanterman cleft of the peripheral nervous system can sometimes be seen in the remyelinating central nervous system. Under these conditions, what appear to be two complete sheaths may sometimes be found around a single axon.

BIBLIOGRAPHY

HIRANO, A.   The pathology of the central myelinated axon. In G. H. Bourne (Ed.), *The structure and function of nervous tissue* (Vol. 5). New York: Academic Press, 1972. Pp. 73–162.
LAMPERT, P. W.   Fine structural changes of myelin sheaths in the central nervous system. In G. H. Bourne (Ed.), *The structure and function of nervous tissue* (Vol. 1). New York: Academic Press, 1968. Pp. 187–204.

ASAO HIRANO
JOSEFINA F. LLENA

MYELINATED AXON

It is often convenient to divide the central nervous system into two parts: the gray and the white matter. The principal structure of the gray consists of neuronal cell bodies and their processes, especially dendrites, whereas the white matter consists almost entirely of axons, many of which are covered by a white, glistening, fatty material known as myelin. To the optical microscopist, the central myelin sheath appears as a lipoidal covering on the axon, perhaps punctuated by the nodes of Ranvier. To the physiologist, the myelin sheath represented a structure which mysteriously increased the velocity of propagation of action potentials along axons provided with these devices.

With the advent of the electron microscope, the hopes of neuroanatomists were raised. It was assumed that the superior resolving power of the modern instruments would quickly settle old arguments concerning the structure of the sheath and provide some insight into the mechanism of its physiological function as well. It was soon apparent, however, that more difficulties confronted the anatomists than could have previously been anticipated. Unlike the peripheral nervous system where myelin sheaths were relatively easily accessible, the central nervous system was solidly enclosed in bone and any attempt to penetrate this protective, rigid covering, quickly led to severe artifactual changes. It was not really until the development of perfusion fixation and improved embedding techniques that the resolving power of the electron microscope could be brought to bear on the problems of the fine structure of the central myelin sheath.

Cross Sections

Low magnifications of cross sections of myelinated axons reveal dense, laminated myelin sheaths surrounding a relatively electronlucent axon. In favorably oriented longitudinal sections, the central axon is found to be bordered by the dense, laminated, myelin sheath which is divided into distinct segments separated by the nodes of Ranvier. The latter consist of short interruptions of the sheath where the axon is exposed to the extracellular space.

Higher magnifications of cross sections re-

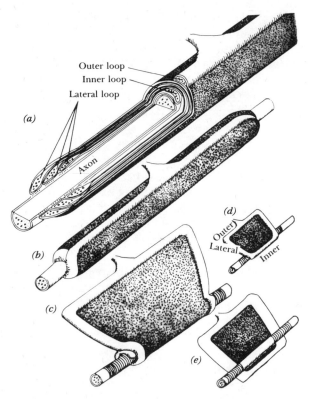

Fig. 1. *(a)* **Diagram of a myelinated axon, modified after Bunge. Part of the myelin is cut away to show the relationship between the lateral loops and the lamellae as well as between the inner loops and the axon and between the outer loop and the connection to the myelin-forming cell. Note the periodic densities, representing sections through the transverse bands between the lateral loops and the axon. *(b)* Diagram of the intact myelin sheath around an axon. *(c)* Diagram of the results of partially unrolling the intact sheath from around the axon. *(d)* Diagram of a fully unrolled myelin sheath. The resulting shovel-shaped myelin sheet is bordered on four sides by a continuous thickened rim of cytoplasm. The outer rim, when seen in section, is represented by the outer loop, and is longer than the inner rim, which is represented by the inner loop in cross section. The lateral rims are probably of equal length and are represented by the lateral loops in longitudinal sections through the nodes of Ranvier. *(e)* A diagram similar to *(d)* but showing the surface of the sheet that contacts the axon. The transverse bands are indicated by the parallel lines which trace a series of helices around the axon. (From Hirano and Dembitzer, 1967.)**

veal the well-known structure of the myelinated axon. The axon is surrounded by a plasma membrane of unit membrane construction which is itself surrounded by a narrow periaxonal space. The periaxonal space is enclosed by the myelin sheath which is a lamellated structure with a regular dense period of about 120Å. A less dense, intraperiod

line is also present midway between each pair of major dense lines. In addition to these dense components, each myelin sheath includes at least two small, tonguelike loops of cytoplasm. One of these, the inner loop, is situated in the periaxonal space while the second, the outer loop, is found at the periphery of the myelin sheath. In the rare instance when the section is cut at precisely the right angle and the preservation is very good, one can determine that the major dense line is actually a single line which originates at the inner loop and traces a spiral course around the axon until it ends at the outer loop. High resolution micrographs reveal that the major dense lines originate by the fusion of the inner leaflets of the unit membrane surrounding the inner loop and end where the fused inner leaflets once again separate and surround the outer loop of the sheath. The outer leaflet of the inner loop parallels the major dense line and since successive turns of the spiral are in contact, forming the apparently single intraperiod line. Analysis of cross sections, therefore, suggests that the myelin sheath consists of a cytoplasmic process from which most of the cytoplasm has been removed and which has been tightly wound around the axon, effectively obliterating the extracellular space between successive turns.

Longitudinal Sections

Longitudinal sections through regions near the nodes of Ranvier reveal one of the most interesting areas of the myelinated axon: the paranodal region. In this region, the individual lamellae of the sheath each end in a tongue of cytoplasm, the lateral loops, which are almost identical to the inner and outer loops seen in cross section. The innermost lamellae are not as long as the more peripheral ones and each lateral loop is in contact with the axonal membrane.

A structural analysis of the central myelin sheath, based on the longitudinal and cross-sectional observations described above, leads one to the realization that the myelin sheath consists of a single, shovel-shaped, sheet-like process surrounded on four sides by a rim of cytoplasm. When wound around the axon, jelly-roll fashion, and sectioned transversely, the outer and inner rims become apparent as the outer and inner loops respectively and the lateral loops, seen in longitudinal view, are sections through the helically wound lateral rims.

The outer, inner, and lateral loops, as might be expected from sections through a single structure, are all virtually identical to each other. They are normally devoid of organelles except for microtubules, filaments, and occasional small vesicles.

The structure of the axon within the myelin sheath is essentially the same as that of the nonmyelinated axon. It contains longitudinally oriented mitochondria, neurofilaments, microtubules, and elements of the rough endoplasmic reticulum. At the axon hillock, and initial segment as well as at the nodes of Ranvier (areas which are known to be important in the propagation of action potentials), an ill-defined dense material is found subjacent to the plasma membrane.

Axonal Membrane

Even more striking is the specialization of the axonal membrane at the paranodal region. Over most of the axonal surface, the plasma membrane appears as a typical, trilaminar unit membrane. Immediately under the lateral loops, however, the outer leaflet becomes discontinuous and forms regularly spaced densities, 150 Å wide separated by 150 Å. These densities reach to within 20 Å of the external leaflet of the lateral loops. Since they are seen in all favorably oriented sections of the paranodal regions, and since they are confined to those areas of the axonal membrane which are directly under a lateral loop and not between the loops, it has been concluded that these densities, or transverse bands, actually represent a series of helices which parallel the path of the lateral rim as it circles the axon. On three dimensional reconstruction, it becomes clear that the spaces between the bands constitute patent helical channels, over 100 Å in diameter, which can provide direct, although lengthy and winding, communication between the periaxonal space and the rest of the extracellular spaces of the central nervous system.

Myelin Formation

It has been acknowledged for many years that the myelin-forming cells of the central nervous system are *oligodendroglia*. Except during myelin formation, however, it is very unusual to find myelin sheaths in direct continuity with the perikarya of the oligodendroglial cell. It is generally assumed that this is because the connection between the sheath and the myelin-forming cell is long and tortuous and unlikely to be contained within a single section. This seems a likely explanation when one realizes that there are far more myelin sheaths in the central nervous system than oligodendroglia so that a single myelin-forming cell may be connected to as many as a few dozen sheaths, probably via their outer rims.

In developing systems, however, direct continuity between the oligodendroglial cells and the myelin sheath has, occasionally, been demonstrated. Unlike mature myelin during its formation the cytoplasmic portion of the sheath can be found to contain formed organelles, such as mitochondria. As might be expected, because of the continuity of all the cytoplasmic portions of the sheath, when such organelles are present in one cytoplasmic region, they can usually be found in all other cytoplasmic regions, as well.

Myelin formation begins with the surrounding of a naked axon by an oligodendroglial process. For the first one or two turns, the process, although thin, still contains cytoplasm but it soon begins to form short lengths devoid of cytoplasm where true myelin is formed. These regions of compacted myelin increase in extent as the wrapping continues until the mature sheath is formed and cytoplasm is normally limited to only the outer, inner, and lateral loops.

The precise means by which the wrapping progresses is not understood. Since the myelin-forming cell is connected to a number of sheaths, the outer loop cannot rotate about the axon as the Schwann cell might do in peripheral nerves. But if the inner loop proceeds around the axon producing myelin at its trailing end, one would expect that the sheath would become progressively tighter, finally impeding the movement of the inner loop. This difficulty might be overcome by assuming that, as the inner loop moves around the axon, the outer lamellae slip past each other, much as the mainspring of a watch unwinds, thus loosening the sheath and allowing the inner loop to proceed. In any event, the wrapping process goes on until maturity at which time the number of lamellae is greater or less depending on the caliber of the axon and the outer and inner loops, which are not oriented with respect to each other during development but finally come to rest, usually in the same quadrant of the circular sheath.

BIBLIOGRAPHY

BUNGE, R. P. Glial cells and the central myelin sheath. *Physiological Reviews,* 1968, *48,* 197–251.

BUNGE, R. P. Structure and function of neuroglia: Some recent observations. In F. O. Schmitt (Ed.), *The neurosciences second study program.* New York: Rockefeller University Press, 1970. Pp. 782–797.

HIRANO, A., and DEMBITZER, H. M. A structural analysis of the myelin sheath in the central nervous system. *Journal of Cell Biology,* 1967, *34,* 555–567.

HIRANO, A., and DEMBITZER, H. M. The transverse bands as a means of access to the periaxonal space of the central myelinated nerve fiber. *Journal of Ultrastructure Research,* 1969, *28,* 141–149.

PETERS, A. The morphology of axons of the central nervous system. In G. H. Bourne (Ed.), *The structure and function of nervous tissue* (Vol. 1). New York: Academic Press, 1968. Pp. 141–186.

PETERS, A., and VAUGHN, J. E. Morphology and development of the myelin sheath. In A. N. Davison and A. Peters (Eds.), *Myelination.* Springfield, Ill.: Thomas, 1970. Pp. 3–79.

ASAO HIRANO
HERBERT M. DEMBITZER

MYERS, CHARLES S. (1873–1946)

Myers was a British psychologist. A pioneer experimentalist, he expanded an early laboratory at Cambridge University; he was eminent for his work on sensation and perception, and published (with H. A. Wilson) classical research on the effect of relative phase on binaural localization of tones. Myers published the basic English text on experimental psychology, and was cofounder and first president of the British Psychological Society, and cofounder and editor of the *British Journal of Psychology.* As founder and director of the National Institute of Industrial Psychology, Myers stimulated development of applied psychology in Britain and helped reshape the policies of the British Psychological Society to recognize practitioners.

AUDREY M. SKAIFE

MYERS-BRIGGS TYPE INDICATOR

The Myers-Briggs Type Indicator (Myers, 1962) was designed to measure the personality types described by Jung (1923). Jung stated that people perceive reality differently, and they use different processes of judgment concerning their perceptions. Perception is the process by which people become aware, and judgment is the process by which they reach conclusions concerning their perceptions. The type indicator measures four different processes: (1) extraversion-introversion; (2) sensing or intuition; (3) thinking or feeling; and (4) judgment or perception. The extravert directs his perception and judgment outward upon the environment while the introvert directs his perception and judgment inward toward his own ideas. The sensing person attends more to the information that comes from his senses while the intuitive person attends more to intuition. The thinking person comes to conclusions through logical intellectual processes while the feeling person makes judgments based upon feelings. The judgment type takes a judging attitude toward the environment, while the perception type takes a perceptive attitude. Any individual is a combination of the four different processes.

There are several different forms of the scale. One of the most commonly used forms, Form F, contains 166 items of the two-choice, multiple-choice type. The reliabilities for the subscales for various kinds of subjects range from .44 to .94, with the reliabilities for senior high school and college students mostly within the .80 to .89 range.

There has been some question as to whether or not the scale actually measures the Jungian types, but it does differentiate successfully among various occupational groups. Job turnover is higher for types whose personality does not fit their job than for those whose personality and occupation are congruent. For example, thinking types in sales jobs have a higher turnover than feeling types. Extraverted-feeling types are successful in sales jobs, while architects and writers are more likely to be intuitive types. Students pursuing different curricula in school differ in type. Observation suggests that people tend to select their friends from among those of their own type.

After some experience with the scale, the authors suggest that "the Indicator, in effect, represents little more than a well-structured and standardized clinical interview" (Myers, 1962).

BIBLIOGRAPHY

Jung, C. G. *Psychological types.* London: Rutledge and Kegan Paul, 1923.
Myers, I. B. *The Myers-Briggs Type Indicator.* Princeton, N.J.: Educational Testing Service, 1962.

Clifford H. Swensen

MYOPATHIES

Definition

Myopathies are disorders of muscle function (manifesting as weakness, cramps, difficulty relaxing, myoglobinuria, or myalgia), in which there is no clinical or laboratory evidence of denervation and psychogenic causes can be excluded.

Dystrophies

These are a group of myopathies of unknown etiology, characterized by hereditary transmission and progressive course (Walton and Gardner-Medwin, 1974). On the basis of genetic and clinical analysis, several types of dystrophies have been identified.

Duchenne dystrophy is the most severe form. Genetic transmission is X-linked recessive. Onset is in early childhood, with evidence of proximal muscle weakness: waddling gait, difficulty running and difficulty rising from the ground. Pseudohypertrophy of the calves is often present. Because of increasing weakness and multiple contractures, patients are generally confined to a wheelchair in early adolescence. Involvement of respiratory muscles increases susceptibility to pulmonary infection and patients generally do not survive beyond the third decade. Heart involvement is reflected by characteristic EKG abnormalities but cardiac symptoms are rare. Serum enzymes, and particularly creatine phosphokinase (CPK), are greatly elevated in the initial stages and decline as the disease progresses. In the EMG, motor unit potentials have decreased amplitude and duration, but interference pattern is maintained. Muscle biopsy shows greater than normal variation of fiber size, signs of degeneration and (in the early stages) of regeneration and infiltration by adipose and connective tissue. There is no specific therapy. Physical therapy is aimed at preventing contractures and delaying immobilization. Prevention is based on genetic counseling and this requires detection of the female carriers. By a combination of repeated serum CPK measurements and EMG examinations, about 75% of carriers can be detected (Gardner-Medwin et al., 1971). Antenatal sex determination can identify boys with high risk if the mother is a known carrier.

Becker dystrophy is a less severe or "slow motion" variant of Duchenne dystrophy. Genetic transmission, clinical and laboratory findings are virtually identical, but onset is rarely before age five and often not until adolescence, the course is slower, and death generally does not occur before the fourth decade. No cases of Duchenne and Becker dystrophy have been reported in the same family and they are probably distinct genetic disorders.

Facioscapulohumeral (FSH) dystrophy is an autosomal dominant myopathy characterized by early involvement of facial (but not ocular) and shoulder girdle muscles. Although extent and severity of involvement vary greatly in different patients, onset is generally in adolescence and the course is more benign than in Duchenne dystrophy. Serum enzymes are normal or only slightly elevated.

Scapuloperoneal muscular dystrophy is, like FSH, a relatively benign autosomal dominant myopathy. It is characterized by involvement of the shoulder girdle and distal muscles of the legs. Facial muscles are spared.

Limb-girdle dystrophy is a wastebasket classification for genetic myopathies that do not fall into other, better-defined categories. Transmission is autosomal recessive, onset in childhood or adolescence, with slowly progressive proximal limb weakness. Serum enzymes are normal or slightly increased.

Ocular myopathy. Progressive ophthalmoplegia is a clinical syndrome of diverse etiology and uncertain classification. Differentiation between neurogenic and myopathic etiology is made particularly difficult by the peculiar morphologic and electromyographic characteristics of ocular muscles. A myopathic etiology, however, is generally accepted in those cases in which progressive external ophthalmoplegia is accompanied by proximal limb and, often, oropharyngeal muscles. Affected limb muscles show "myopathic" changes. Abnormal mitochondria are often seen in these cases in both light microscopy ("ragged red" fibers in the modified Gomori trichrome stain) and in the electron microscope. However, no specific biochemical abnormality of mitochondrial metabolism has been found and the role of mitochondrial abnormalities in the pathogenesis of these forms remains uncertain.

Pathogenetic hypothesis and biochemical studies. Muscular dystrophies have long been considered as prototypes of disorders apparently restricted to muscle, and presumably originating within the muscle. Various metabolic pathways were studied in search of a missing enzyme, but no primary metabolic defect was found, nor were there abnormalities of contractile proteins. In recent years, two hypotheses have been proposed that postulate an extramuscular etiology for the dystrophies. In 1971, on the basis of an electrophysiological technique intended to compute the number of neurones supplying a muscle, McComas et al. suggested that muscle involvement may be due to "sick motor neurones." The validity of McComas's technique, however, has been seriously challenged. W. K. Engel and collaborators have produced in animals morphological lesions resembling those of muscular dystrophy by a combination of ligation of the aorta and administration of serotonin and have suggested a vascular hypothesis for muscular dystrophy (W. K. Engel, 1973). However, no alteration of muscle microvasculature was seen in dystrophy patients in an ultrastructural investigation (Jerusalem et al., 1974). Recent research is focusing on the structure and function of membranes. Alterations of sarcoplasmic reticulum and sarcolemma have been reported. Biochemical and structural changes of the red blood cells in muscular dystrophy suggest that membrane abnormalities may not be confined to skeletal muscle (Rowland, 1976).

Myotonias

Myotonia is a defect of muscle relaxation associated with repetitive firing of motor units and persisting after curarization and peripheral nerve blocking. Myotonia is probably due to a membrane abnormality causing decreased chloride conductance (Barchi, 1975). Altera-

tions of biochemical and physicochemical properties of muscle and erythrocyte membranes were found in human myotonias (Roses and Appel, 1973, 1974; Butterfield et al., 1974). Myotonia accompanies several muscle disorders:

Myotonia congenita (Thomsen disease) is an autosomal dominant disease in which clinical symptoms are limited to myotonia. Strength is fully preserved and many patients excell in athletics.

This form should be distinguished from *autosomal recessive myotonia,* in which muscle hypertrophy is very marked, and muscle pain and sometimes weakness are seen.

Myotonic dystrophy is an autosomal dominant multisystem disorder characterized by muscle weakness and myotonia, cardiopathy, cataract, hypogonadism and baldness in men, and hyperinsulinemia without hypoglycemia.

Onset is generally in adolescence and the course is slowly progressive. Severity varies greatly from patient to patient. Involvement of facial muscles, with atrophy of temporal muscle and ptosis, causes a characteristic elongated and droopy facial appearance. The sternocleidomastoid muscles are small and limb weakness is more pronounced distally. In the infantile form, severe muscle weakness may dominate the picture, with facial diplegia and difficulty in sucking and swallowing. Mental retardation is also present in children.

Paramyotonia congenita. In some families, myotonic symptoms occur only in cold weather and, in contrast to other forms of myotonia, tend to worsen with repeated effort (myotonia paradoxica). In such families, attacks of hyperkalemic periodic paralysis may also occur and it is difficult to separate "pure paramyotonia congenita" and "familial hyperkalemic periodic paralysis with myotonia."

Treatment of myotonia. Myotonic phenomena in all these disorders are reduced by "membrane stabilizers", such as quinine, procainamide and diphenylhydantoin. Diphenylhydantoin (0.3–0.5 gram daily) is the drug of choice.

Metabolic Myopathies

Glycogen storage diseases. Five hereditary disorders of glycogen metabolism affect muscle. In all of them transmission is autosomal recessive. *Glycogenosis type II* (Pompe disease) is due to a defect of the lysosomal enzyme acid maltase (acid alpha 1,4- and 1,6-glucosidase) and was the prototype of "inborn lysosomal disease" (Hers, 1965). In the infantile, generalized form, all tissues are affected, particularly skeletal and heart muscle and also motor neurones in the spinal cord and brain. Glycogen accumulation is massive. The clinical picture, evident soon after birth, includes profound weakness ("floppy babies"), severe cardiomegaly, and sometimes, macroglossia. The course is rapidly progressive, and death occurs in most cases before age one due to cardiac failure. Glycogen is normal in structure and accumulates both free in the cytoplasm and within lysosomal sacs. There is no hypoglycemia. Unsuccessful therapeutic trials have included ketogenic diet and epinephrine, lysosomal "labilizers" (vitamin A), and enzyme replacement with bacterial or human glucosidase.

Late-onset acid maltase deficiency is a more benign form, clinically confined to skeletal muscle (A. G. Engel et al., 1973). Onset is in childhood or adult life, and the course generally slow. There is weakness of trunk and proximal limb muscles, simulating Duchenne dystrophy or polymyositis. Respiratory muscles are often involved. Serum enzymes are increased. Myotonic discharges are often seen in the EMG. No cases of infantile and late-onset acid maltase deficiency have been reported in the same family. In *glycogenosis type III* (Cori-Forbes disease, debrancher deficiency) and in *glycogenosis type IV* (Andersen disease, brancher deficiency), muscle is affected, but the clinical picture is dominated by liver disease, with hepatomegaly and hypoglycemia in debrancher deficiency, and cirrhosis in brancher deficiency.

Glycogenosis type V (McArdle disease, muscle phosphorylase deficiency) and *glycogenosis type VII* (Tarui disease, phosphofructokinase deficiency) can be described together because the clinical disorders are identical and differential diagnosis requires demonstration of the enzyme defect. Intense muscle exercise causes cramps (i.e., involuntary painful muscle shortening with electrical silence), often followed by myoglobinuria. After a brief rest, patients can resume exercise for a longer period of time ("second wind"). Aside from the exercise intolerance, patients enjoy normal lives. Muscle

glycogen is 2–4 times normal, has normal structure, and tends to form subsarcolemmal accumulations ("blebs"). The block of glycogenolysis is reflected by the failure of venous lactate to rise after ischemic exercise. There is no effective therapy for these disorders.

Disorder of lipid metabolism. Defect of the mitochondrial enzyme *carnitine palmityltransferase* was found in two patients with recurrent myoglobinuria precipitated by prolonged exercise and fasting (DiMauro and Melis-DiMauro, 1973). Utilization of long-chain, but not medium-chain, fatty acids was impaired. Muscle structure was normal. Transmission appeared to be autosomal recessive. Deficiency of muscle *carnitine,* a different disorder, was described by A. G. Engel and Angelini (1973) and five patients have been reported so far. In four of them, serum carnitine was normal and the biochemical defect may involve carnitine transport from blood into muscle. In one case, however, carnitine content was also decreased in liver and serum, suggesting a defect in hepatic synthesis of carnitine. In all these cases there was progressive muscle weakness with increased serum enzyme activity, but no myoglobinuria. Abnormal accumulation of lipid droplets within muscle fibers is the morphological hallmark of the disease. Treatment with oral carnitine was beneficial in two cases.

Mitochondrial myopathies. The diagnosis of mitochondrial myopathy is based on the observation of histological ("ragged red" fibers with a modified Gomori trichrome stain) or ultrastructural (increased number or size, presence of inclusions) abnormalities limited to or affecting predominately the mitochondria. Clinical syndromes are diverse and nonspecific, but progressive ophthalmoplegia is frequently seen. It may occur alone, associated with weakness of other cranial or limb muscles, or as part of the distinct syndrome represented by the triad of ophthalmoplegia, heart block, and pigmentary degeneration of the retina (Kearns-Sayre syndrome).

Few specific biochemical abnormalities of mitochondrial function have been discerned. Lack of respiratory control of muscle mitochondria was found in Luft disease, characterized by severe nonthyroidal hypermetabolism and mild weakness (Luft et al., 1962). In trichropoliodystrophy (Menkes disease or "steely hair disease") there is a decreased content of cytochrome a($+a_3$) in muscle, liver and brain mitochondria (French et al., 1962), secondary to a defect of intestinal copper absorption. The defects of carnitine and carnitine palmityl-transferase have been described in "metabolic myopathies."

Periodic Paralyses

These are muscle disorders of unknown pathogenesis characterized by recurrent attacks of weakness, variable in severity, extent and duration (Pearson and Kalyanaraman, 1972).

Hypokalemic familial periodic paralysis is transmitted as an autosomal dominant trait, but males are predominantly affected. Attacks are characterized by flaccid paralysis of limb or trunk muscles sparing respiratory and facial muscles and lasting from a few hours to 24 hours. Rest after strenuous exercise and large carbohydrate meals are predisposing factors. During attacks, serum enzymes are normal and electromyography shows electrical silence.

Serum potassium concentration is characteristically decreased, but there is no strict relationship between potassium levels and severity of weakness. Hypokalemia is apparently due to a shift of potassium into the muscle. Increased excretion of 17-hydroxycorticosteroids and aldosterone were reported in some cases. In the light microscope multiple vacuoles are seen during attacks and may become a permanent morphological feature in later stages of the disease. Ultrastructural studies showed that the vacuoles derive from the sarcoplasmic reticulum. Pathogenetic hypotheses include: disorder of carbohydrate metabolism, intermittent adrenocortical hypersecretion, sarcoplasmic reticulum dysfunction and a defect of muscle membrane depolarization. Attacks can be induced by administration of glucose and insulin, and this procedure is often used as a diagnostic aid. Therapy, during attacks, consists in oral administration of potassium salts. Acetazolamide is used as a prophylactic drug.

Hyperkalemic periodic paralysis is also transmitted as an autosomal dominant character. Attacks are often precipitated by rest after vigorous excercise and exposure to cold, and they rarely last more than a few hours. Clinical or electromyographic myotonia is often observed in affected families. During attacks serum potassium is moderately increased and serum enzymes are normal or slightly increased. Morphological changes are less marked than in hypokalemic periodic paralysis and consist in dilation of the sarcoplasmic reticulum. Attacks may be induced by administration of potassium. Acetazolamide is beneficial in both treatment and prevention of attacks. Pathogenesis is unknown, but electrophysiological studies and the association with myotonia suggest an abnormality of sarcolemma.

Normokalemic periodic paralysis is essentially identical to the hyperkalemic form except for the lack of serum potassium changes.

Thyrotoxic periodic paralysis. In hyperthyroidism, attacks of hypokalemic periodic paralysis are essentially identical to those of the familial variety in all respects except for the lack of genetic transmission. This disorder is more common among orientals and males are predominantly affected. There is no strict correlation between occurence of attacks and severity of hyperthyroidism, but treatment of thyroid dysfunction abolishes the attacks.

Malignant Hyperthermia

This rare and often fatal (mortality rate about 70%) disorder, generally following anesthesia with halothane or succinylcholine, is characterized by rapidly rising temperature, muscle rigidity, metabolic acidosis, high serum enzymes and, often, myoglobinuria. Susceptibility seems to be transmitted as an autosomal dominant character, but patients are generally asymptomatic prior to an attack. A dysfunction of the sarcoplasmic reticulum has been suspected, but pathogenesis remains obscure (Britt et al., 1973).

Congenital Myopathies

This is a group of benign, relatively nonprogressive myopathies, with proximal or diffuse muscle weakness and no or slight increase of serum CPK. There is debate about the role of neurogenic and myopathic factors in causation. Specific entities are defined by distinct (but not absolutely specific) structural features:

1. *Central core disease* is characterized by the presence of central areas devoid of mitochondria and glycogen and extending along the entire length of the fibers.

2. *Multicore disease.* Multiple cores are similar to those of central core disease but do not extend along the entire length of the fibers.

3. *Nemaline or rod myopathy* seems to be transmitted as an autosomal dominant trait with incomplete penetrance. The "rods" are revealed by special stains (Gomori trichrome, or phosphotungstic acid—hematoxylin). In the electron microscope they appear as ectopic accumulations of Z-line material. The patients usually have a thin, elongated face and high-arch palate. Respiratory muscles may be involved and a few lethal cases were reported in adults.

4. In *myotubular or centronuclear myopathy* there is frequent involvement of ocular and facial muscles with ptosis, squint, facial weakness. A few cases have been reported with respiratory muscle involvement and death in infancy. In most fibers, nuclei are centrally located and are surrounded by areas devoid of myofibrils, a picture reminiscent of myotubes.

5. *Fingerprint myopathy* is characterized by the presence in the electron microscope of convoluted lamellae resembling fingerprints.

6. *Reducing body myopathy* was described in two cases with death in infancy. Most fibers contained multiple eosinophilic bodies capable of reducing menadione and nitro blue tetrazolium.

Endocrine Myopathies

Hyperthyroidism can cause four muscle disorders: thyrotoxic myopathy, thyrotoxic periodic paralysis, ophthalmoplegia, and myasthenia gravis. In *thyrotoxic myopathy,* the severity of weakness is variable and not necessarily proportional to severity or duration of thyroid disfunction. Tendon reflexes are normal or hyperactive, serum CPK is normal, and EMG shows decreased duration of motor unit potentials and increased number of polyphasic potentials. Morphological alterations are minor and nonspecific. The biochemical basis of weakness is not known.

Thyrotoxic periodic paralysis is described above in "Periodic Paralyses."

Hypothroidism: Moderate weakness, cramps and muscle hypertrophy characterize hypothroid myopathy in children (Kocher-Debre-Semelaigne syndrome) and adults (Hoffman syndrome). Myoedema (mounding phenomenon) and myotonic phenomena are often present. Serum CPK is moderately elevated in most cases. Morphological changes are not specific.

In endogenous *Cushing syndrome* there is proximal muscle weakness and atrophy. Histochemistry shows predominant atrophy of type II fibers. A similar picture ("steroid myopathy") is caused by excessive steroid administration.

Acromegaly is often accompanied by moderate proximal muscle weakness and nonspecific morphological abnormalities of muscle.

Dermatomyositis and Polymyositis

Five criteria have been proposed to define polymyositis and dermatomyositis (Bohan and Peter, 1975a; 1975b).

1. Symmetrical weakness of limb-girdle muscles, generally rapid in onset and fluctuating in severity.

2. Morphological evidence of muscle degeneration, phagocytosis and regeneration.

3. Elevation of serum CPK.

4. Presence of short, small, polyphasic potentials, fibrillations, and insertional irritability in the electromyogram.

5. Skin lesions (heliotrope, periorbital edema, erythema of hands, knees, upper torso).

The major distinction between dermatomyositis and polymyositis is the presence of the rash, but there are other differences: dermatomyositis is more common and polymyositis very rare in children; dermatomyositis is clinically more uniform and often associated with malignancy; myopathy is generally more severe in dermatomyositis. Both polymyositis and dermatomyositis are immunopathological disorders, but, unlike myasthenia gravis, there is no evidence of circulating autoantibodies to muscle, although abnormal lymphocyte reactions have been reported. The initiating agent may be viral or a muscle component modified by a virus. Particles resembling myxovirus or picornavirus have been seen in muscle and other tissues in a few cases, but there is still no definite evidence of a viral etiology.

Although no controlled study is available, corticosteroids are the major drugs used in the treatment of polymyositis and dermatomyositis. In steroid-resistant patients, immunosuppressive drugs (azathioprine, methotrexate) have been used. Trichinosis and sarcoidosis are other causes of polymyositis.

Myasthenia Gravis

Myasthenia gravis is a neuromuscular disorder characterized by variably severe weakness worsened by exercise and partially relieved by cholinergic drugs (W. K. Engel et al., 1974). It involves cranial muscles, and particularly ocular, eyelids and oropharyngeal muscles (with ptosis, ophthalmoparesis, diplopia, dysphagia, nasal speech) respiratory and proximal limb muscles. The severity of weakness characteristically fluctuates in time, even within a single day. Reflexes are normal. Onset may be at any age, but more commonly in young adults. *Transient neonatal myasthenia,* lasting from a few days to several weeks, is seen in about 12% of children of myasthenic mothers.

Congenital Myasthenia. With symptoms present from birth and generally benign course, this was reported in 16 cases, many of them familial. Mothers were unaffected. Thymoma occurs in approximately 10% of cases, particularly in older patients. Pathology of muscle is limited, consisting of lymphocytic infiltrates ("lymphorhages"), group fiber atrophy and foci of myosis. Ultrastructural studies of the neuromuscular junction showed sparse and shallow synaptic clefts.

The most characteristic electromyographic abnormality is the decrement of muscle voltage responses to repetitive nerve stimulation at low rates (2.5/sec.). Diagnostic pharmacological tests are based on the use of therapeutic or provocative drugs. Edrophonium (2.0 mg) is given intravenously and, if no positive effect is seen in 30 seconds, 8.0 mg is given in two doses within the next minute. In myasthenia patients there is a dramatic amelioration of weakness, particularly of cranial muscles. Due to their abnormal sensitivity to curare, one tenth of a curarizing dose (17 micrograms d-tubocurarine/Kg body weight), administered intrave-

nously in fractional amounts (only with appropriate precautions) causes increased weakness in myasthenia patients.

The cause and site (pre- or postsynaptic) of the neuromuscular junction dysfunction in myasthenia gravis are not known. In 1960, Strauss et al., and Simpson suggested that myasthenia may be an immunopathological disorder, and abnormalities of both humoral and cellular immune mechanisms have been identified.

An experimental disease with many of the clinical and electrophysiological characteristics of myasthenia gravis has been induced in several animal species by immunization with purified electric eel or Torpedo acetylcholine receptor (Patrick and Lindstrom, 1973). Using radiolabelled α-bungarotoxin, Fambrough et al. (1973) showed decreased number and distribution of receptors in myasthenic muscle endplates.

Presence of circulating antibodies to acetylcholine receptors in myasthenic serum has been shown recently: Almon et al. (1974) and Aharonov et al. (1975) and Toyka et al. (1975) have transmitted the disorder to mice by repeated injections of serum from myasthenic patients. Therapy is based on anticholinesterase drugs administration or immunosuppression. For maintenance therapy, pyridostigmine bromide (30–60 mg, 3–4 times a day) is the anticholinesterase drug of choice. Long-term, high-single-dosage (100 mg), alternate-day oral prednisone has been beneficial in several series, although controlled studies are lacking. Thymectomy in patients without thymoma is also followed by marked improvement or complete remission in at least two thirds of the cases.

Myasthenic Syndrome

Myasthenic (Eaton-Lambert) syndrome is a rare disorder often associated with bronchogenic carcinoma, characterized clinically by weakness and easy fatigability of proximal limb muscles. Unlike myasthenia gravis, there is a decrease of the size of muscle action potentials at low rates of nerve stimulation, while muscle response is markedly increased at higher frequencies (above 10/sec). The defect of neuromuscular transmission appears to be due to a decreased number of acetylcholine quanta released by a nerve impulse. Guanidine is effective in correcting the defect.

BIBLIOGRAPHY

BARCHI, R. Myotonia. Evaluation of the chloride hypothesis. *Archives of Neurology,* 1975, *32,* 175–180.

BOHAN, A., and PETER, J. B. Polymyositis and dermatomyositis, I. *New England Journal of Medicine,* 1975a, *292,* 344–347.

BOHAN, A., and PETER, J. B. Polymyositis and dermatomyositis, II. *New England Journal of Medicine,* 1975b, *292,* 403–407.

BRITT, B. A.; KALOW W.; GORDON, A.; HUMPHREY, J. G.; and REWCASTLE, N. Malignant hyperthermia: an investigation of five patients. *Canadian Anaesthesia Society Journal,* 1973, *20,* 431–467.

DIMAURO, S., and MELIS-DIMAURO, P. M. Muscle carnitine palmityltransferase deficiency and myoglobinuria. *Science,* 1973, *182,* 929–931.

ENGEL, A. G., and ANGELINI, C. Carnitine deficiency of human skeletal muscle with associated lipid storage myopathy: A new syndrome. *Science,* 1973, *179,* 899–902.

ENGEL, W. K.; FESTOFF, B. W.; PATTEN, B. M.; SWERDLOW, M. L.; NEWBALL, H. H.; and THOMPSON, M. D. Myasthenia Gravis. *Annals of Internal Medicine,* 1974, *81,* 225–246.

ENGEL, A. G.; GOMEZ, M. R.; SEYBOLD, M. E.; and LAMBERT, E. H. The spectrum and diagnosis of acid maltase deficiency. *Neurology,* 1973, *23,* 95–106.

HERS, H. G. Inborn lysosomal diseases. *Gastroenterology,* 1965, *48,* 625–633.

LUFT, R.; IKKOS, D.; PALMIERI, G.; ERNSTER, L.; and AFZELIUS, B. A case of severe hypermetabolism of nonthyroid origin with a defect in the maintenance of mitochondrial respiratory control: A correlated clinical, biochemical, and morphological study. *Journal of Clinical Investigation,* 1962, *41,* 1776–1804.

PEARSON, C. M., and KALYANARAMAN, K. The periodic paralyses. In J. B. Stanbury, J. B. Wyngaarden, and D. S. Fredrickson (Eds.), *The metabolic basis of inherited disease.* New York: McGraw-Hill, 1972. Pp. 1181–1203.

ROWLAND, L. P. Pathogenesis of muscular dystrophies. *Archives of Neurology,* 1976, *33*(5), 315–321.

WALTON, J. N., and GARDNER-MEDWIN, D. Progressive muscular dystrophies and the myotonic disorders. In J. N. Walton (Ed.), *Disorders of voluntary muscle.* Edinburgh and London: Churchill-Livingstone, 1974. Pp. 561–613.

SALVATORE DIMAURO

MYTHOLOGY, FOLKLORE, AND PSYCHOANALYSIS

A major field of anthropology deals with the investigation of those of man's works which involve the symbolic representation of the psychological problems of individuals that find expression in culturally condoned manners. Such cultural expressions take many forms, such as religiomedical practices, folk art, folk music, folk dance, folk costume, and oral or folk literature, including mythology.

The study of folklore has been widely employed by anthropologists, who have found in expressive culture many clues for the understanding of social structure, socialization processes and aspects of the mental functioning of groups under investigation. Bascom (1954) extended Malinowski's (1926) dictum that myth serves as a charter for belief. Bascom discussed the social context of folklore, the relation of folklore to culture and the functions of folklore. Concerning the last named, he discussed its amusement factors, its role in validating culture, its educational utility, and its part in maintaining conformity to the patterns of culture. He wisely left it to psychologists to explain in depth the means by which the psychological functions of folklore operated and challenged psychoanalysts in particular to delineate those means.

Men have studied folklore since at least as long ago as the fourth century B.C., when the Sicilian philosopher Euhemeris suggested that myths are based on historical traditions, that myth heroes are real people and that man made gods in his own image. The modern systematic study of folklore and folkloristics was introduced by the brothers Grimm in 1812 (Dorson, 1963), whose work was followed by others including Deslongchamps (1838), Kuhn (1843), Müller (1888), and Steinthal (1856). Thoms introduced the term *folklore* in 1846 to replace the previously used labels *popular antiquities* and *popular literature* (Merton, 1846).

There is no commonly accepted definition of folklore. Not only do folklorists in different countries retain varying concepts of folklore but those in individual countries have different ideas concerning its nature. The *Standard Dictionary of Folklore, Mythology and Legend* (Leach, 1949–1959) presents 21 concise definitions. Incompletely successful attempts have been made to delineate folklore from the standpoint of the means of its transmission and through defining the folk. For the purposes of this presentation, folklore will be said to *be* or to be *in* oral tradition, and will by synonymized with oral or folk literature.

While the laity customarily separates mythology from the other forms of oral literature, folklorists and anthropologists include it among the major genres, along with legends, folktales, fairy tales, proverbs, and superstitions. Each of these major divisions of folk literature requires a lengthy definition (Brunvand, 1968; Róheim, 1941; Thompson, 1946; Utley, 1961). Dundes (1965) lists numerous minor genres.

Even if there were general agreement as to what constitutes folklore, discord would remain concerning its origins. The history of folkloristics is full of elaborate theories explaining how folklore arose.

The now-discarded theory of solar mythology was introduced by the philologist Müller through his study of comparative mythology (Thompson, 1946). He postulated a "mythopoeic" age when truly noble conceptions of the Aryan gods first arose. This age began not at the beginning of civilization but at a stage so early that language could not carry abstract notions. Müller compared the names of deities in various bodies of mythology with those of heavenly bodies in Sanskrit and concluded that all of the principal gods' names had originally stood for solar phenomena. His followers extended celestial explanations of myths, applying them to texts around the world. Similar research also produced a now equally debunked "zoological" interpretation that read animal symbolism into myths (DeGubernatis, 1872).

Two of the characteristics that most of the theories pertaining to the origins of folklore have sought to elucidate are irrationality and multiple existence.

It remained for psychoanalysts to demonstrate that the most satisfactory explanation for the irrationality to be found in folklore is that its formal structure fails to obey the laws of Aristotelian logic but instead follows the rules of reasoning inherent in unconscious thinking.

Among others, the Grimms, Deslongchamps, Kuhn, Müller, and Steinthal showed that the manifest content of oral literature contains themes which are to be found in the folklore of many parts of the world. Two principal explanations have been offered to explain multiple existence: polygenesis, and monogenesis and diffusion.

Polygenesis

According to the theory of polygenesis, the same item could have originated independently many times. Polygenesis is associated with the concept of psychic unity in man. Anthropologists in general have used a now-outmoded biological concept of psychic unity associated with evolutionary concepts related to Darwinism and rejected polygenesis on this basis. Following one scheme of polygenesis which was strongly supported by the English anthropological school of comparative mythologists, the foremost spokesman of which was Lang, all men evolved in one path through three identical stages of savagery, barbarism and civilization. It was believed that the ancestors of the civilized nineteenth-century Englishmen must have been aborigines like those of Australia and American Indian cultures. This supposition was crucial for folklore theory since it was also postulated that folklore arose during the stage of savagery and that as men evolved, folklore devolved. With evolution, only fragments of oral literature, called survivals, remained in civilized times. Victorian Englishmen were thought to be too sane to express themselves in the irrational manner used in the manifest content of folklore. Since the survivals were so fragmentary, they could not be understood without speculative historical reconstruction, a favorite scholarly pastime which was allied to romanticism and the worship of the past. The task of historical reconstruction was thought to be facilitated by the study of oral literature of modern "savages." This theory purportedly explained why folklore in Europe was thought to exist especially among the peasants, who were equated with barbarians.

This concept of polygenesis led to an acrimonious and erudite debate between Müller and Lang and their disciples. Müller's arguments were lethal to Lang's ideas pertaining to the idea of survivals whereas the latter destroyed the former's solar theory.

Monogenesis and Diffusion

Anthropologists today by and large prefer to explain multiple existence on the basis of monogenesis and diffusion which, applied to folklore, holds that the themes of oral literature arose in a single or at the most a few cultures and spread to and were incorporated into the folklore body of other cultures for reasons which they explained but superficially, from the viewpoint of psychoanalysts. The folkloristic and anthropological literature is replete with studies which trace avenues of diffusion (Utley, 1974).

In contrast to the prevailing anthropological view, Rooth (1962) believes the majority of today's folklorists subscribe to the theory of polygenesis.

Psychic unity has come to be conceptualized in three other ways since the introduction of the evolutionary viewpoint of the nineteenth-century anthropologists and folklorists, those of Jung, Lévi-Strauss and Freud, all of whom agree that the unconscious is the determining force behind man's production of myth. They see the symbols and motifs of folklore as consisting of disguised projections of intrapsychic conflicts.

In Jung's hypothesis, the creative power is ascribed to the impetus afforded by racially inherited *archetypes* in the collective unconscious as distinguished from the repressed conflicts of the personal unconscious, which consists of the remnants of individual life experiences (Jung, 1916, 1935). The archetypes are seen as omnipresent, unchanging and universal and to have been present from a prehistoric period in the development of mankind. There is an apparent continuity between Jung's thinking and that of the anthropologists whose ideas reflected biological Darwinian evolution transposed invalidatably into the psychological sphere. Jung considered his archetypes to determine aspects of the dreams of normal and neurotic people, the hallucinations of psychotics and certain images in the great myths and art forms of all mankind. Some Kleinian ideas seem parallel (Rascovsky et al., 1971).

For Lévi-Strauss (1967), the unconscious is empty of content but endowed with an innate structuring faculty which brings a logical order to sensory perceptions. The unconscious is reduced to a specifically human function; the structuring function of the unconscious determines the content of folklore. He does not make clear where in the mental apparatus the conflicts exist which are projected into expressive culture. He also shares with Jung, some Kleinians, and the early anthropologists the idea that the roots of oral literature are to be found in prehistory.

Freudian psychoanalysts hold that the roots of folklore are to be found in repressed conflicts pertaining to actual individual life experiences. In their thinking, humans have a species-specific genetic heritage which, because of the unfolding of innate traits depending on time-appropriate interaction with the intrafamilial environment, is essentially biosocial. Their developmental level at birth necessitates prolonged socialization before they can become acceptable adults in their societies. They have like basic biological and psychological needs and are subject to like frustrations and intrapsychic conflicts by their puericultural experiences. The vicissitudes of their innate drive derivatives are shaped by cultural requirements, reflected in child-rearing methods. Idiosyncratic psychological defensive techniques, including private dreams, hallucinations, and fantasies, do not suffice to quell their guilts and anxieties, conscious and unconscious. Those defensive techniques are supported by others which are supplied by expressive culture, including folklore.

The latent themes of dream and folklore are understood preconsciously and/or unconsciously by audiences to whom they are related, to the degree that listeners share and cathect the unresolved conflicts that are expressed in the related dream or myth. Children have wishes which they consider to be unacceptable to their parents. When those parents express their similar desires or do not react with disapproval to the revealed wish of the child, he feels less apprehension. The adult remains to some extent a child, and requires approval and reinforcement of individual psychological defensive maneuvers. Influential societal members, secular or religious, are used as parent surrogates. Religious superiors are more useful models for reduction of anxiety regarding the arcane. The public expression of their dreams, latent parts of which are preconsciously understood by their audience, permits adults of their community the use of those dreams, further disguised by secondary revision into items of oral literature, and thus altered in manners which make them culturally acceptable. Thus, because of this community of intrapsychic conflicts and primitive meanings of symbols and the limited number of defensive techniques available to the ego, all of which are reflected in dream motifs, identical or similar folklore items can arise at any time. In this view, the dream of the influential person in the group is incorporated into its existing folklore stock by diffusion.

The item of oral literature which is to be included in an existent folklore stock must contain latent elements which make it suitable to serve the individual and group functions of folklore. It may serve substitutive or supplementary purposes. If it is to be substituted for a present item, its representation of latent items may be more suitable, that is, better disguised. Or it may result from social conditions such as those which obtain when one society is more powerful than another and imposes its folklore on the weaker group. Or the members of one group may envy those of another and emulate them through the assumption of their cultural traits. Whatever the reason may be that the folklore of one group is accepted into that of another, its latent themes and symbols must present alternate means of presenting group cohesive lessons and supporting individual defensive and adaptive techniques.

According to Freudian psychoanalytic thinking, were it not for the existence of psychic unity, the dreams of influential individuals could not be incorporated into the folklore stock of his group nor could the traditional folk literature of one society be embodied into that of another. Each transmission can be viewed as resulting from diffusion.

Almost from the inception of psychoanalysis, its practitioners have been seriously involved in the study of myths and other forms of folklore, particularly the fairy tale. They studied oral literature, usually without knowledge of the cultures within which it had arisen or which had accepted it by means of diffusion. When their thinking was dominated by the topographical viewpoint or as it is commonly known, id psychology or libido psychology (Freud, 1900, Chap. 7; 1915), many psychoanalysts used the study of folklore especially to demonstrate the validity of their recently acquired knowledge concerning unconscious mechanisms and particularly symbolism. They sought simultaneously to interpret folklore from its manifest contents and then to use the same concepts they had employed in their interpretations to support those concepts. A few examples culled from the vast relevant literature suffice (Maeder, 1909; Riklin, 1908; Silberer, 1910; Storfer, 1912; Wilke, 1914). Many representatives of other disciplines have objected to this scientific method, citing regularly the voluminous contributions of Rank (1909, 1922).

Jung and his followers have continued to use this method of reasoning in their effort to demonstrate through their interpretations of folklore the concept of the effects of archetypes in the collective unconscious on its themes and symbols (Baynes, 1924; Herzog, 1967; Iandelli, 1967; Schmitz, 1932; Waters, 1950). Their work has been criticized by social scientists of various disciplines (LaBarre, 1948; Rooth, 1957).

Oedipus

Freud's (1900) interest in and analysis of the Oedipus Rex myth is the most famous example of psychoanalytic involvement in folklore. Both its analysis and the understanding of the complex which was named from the myth have been the principal foci of thousands of books and articles written by members of various social scientific disciplines. Mullahy (1948) used the myth and complex as the focus for his comparison of the psychoanalytic orientations of Freud, Jung, Adler, Sullivan, Horney, and Fromm. Lessa (1961) collected tales from Oceania and reviewed folklore literature from around the world. He concluded that diffusion rather than polygenesis explained the distribution of the Oedipus myth. With Malinowski, Lessa (1956) judged the oedipal situation to be culturally determined and not to be universal "for there are many social systems not conducive to its development" (p. 71). Fromm (1951) reanalyzed the myth, and ignoring multiple determination, decried a sexual interpretation, a stand Torres (1960) found to be irrational. The well-known Malinowski-Jones debate about the applicability of the Oedipus complex to nonpatrilineal cultures has been reviewed by Parsons (1964). Fortes's (1959) comparison of the myths of Oedipus and Job with aspects of the religion of an ancestor-worshipping tribe of West Africa is a remarkable example of the elision of multideterminism. Seeking to understand the myths and rituals solely in terms of

British social structure, he ignored the castration symbology of Orestes's biting off his own finger after killing his mother, Zipporah's having circumcized her son to avoid his being killed by Yahweh, of Oedipus's blinding of himself, and of ritual circumcision in initiation rites (Bettelheim, 1954). Reider (1960) and Reik (1923) found many medieval legends about Judas to be understandable in terms of the Oedipus myth. The Rascovskys (1969) found the filicidal behavior of Oedipus's parents to be responsible for his "acting out and psychopathic behavior." Grunberger (1962) wrote of the oedipal elements in anti-Semitism.

Aside from his interpretation of the Oedipus myth, Freud's other uses of folklore have been rarely criticized (Freud, 1912, 1913; Freud and Oppenheim, 1909). Perhaps his conservative position is responsible in part. While he was admittedly hopeful that the study of the neuroses might be destined to solve the problems inherent in the formation of myths, he recognized and complained that he and his followers were amateurs in mythology. Nor has there been adverse comment about Abraham's (1909) brilliant analysis of the Prometheus myth which remains a model of the exposition of the reasoning behind understanding oral literature in terms of the language of the dream, and whose study of Amenhotep IV (1912) was a careful and meaningful contribution to the study of religion. Similarly, other clear articles, such as Reik's (1912) *How Children Make Up Fairy Tales,* have not been censured.

While the topographical theory continued to prevail in psychoanalytic thinking, most psychoanalytic contributions to folklore continued to have as their major goal the demonstration of the coincidence of the themes and symbols of oral literature in the dreams, fantasies, and transference reactions of their patients. Occasional books and articles are seemingly still motivated by such aims. Some of the early contributions provided invaluable and as yet unmodified understanding of the meanings of symbols (Graber, 1925).

Ego Psychology

However, with the introduction of the structural theory and ego psychology, the gradually heightened interest in child analysis and a renewed interest in the possible applications of psychoanalysis to the treatment of psychotics, psychoanalysts' uses of and their comprehensions of the psychological functions of folklore have gradually shifted. Investigations have followed two routes, clinical and cross-cultural.

Psychoanalysts had long since learned that the themes which are to be found in oral literature arise in the dreams and fantasies of patients who have no knowledge of that literature. Analysts knew, too, that when individuals heard folklore themes, the tales stimulated anxiety and guilt when they reflected cathected unresolved psychic conflicts. Now, with their new interest in and understanding of the ego and its functions, psychoanalysts learned how the themes that patients heard in childhood, especially from fairy tales and religious myths, are influential in shaping their character structure and the manifest contents of their neuroses and psychoses (Balint, 1935; Bergler, 1961; Bilz, 1943; Briehl, 1937; Buhler et al., 1958; Dieckmann, 1966; Kaplan, 1963; Kris, 1932; Lubin, 1958; Müller-Erzbach, 1953; Rubenstein, 1953).

As implied in the foregoing, the cross-cultural study of folk literature by psychoanalysts began with the investigations of collections of material which had been amassed by folklorists. Until very recently, folklorists have been interested almost exclusively in the formal and historical aspects of oral literature. Marett's (1920) plea that they attempt to understand its psychological aspects was ignored. Some nineteenth-century anthropologists, notably Brinton (1896), already understood some of the projective aspects of expressive culture and deemed as necessary the examination of folklore within the context of the social and psychological structures of the people studied. However, ethnographic studies by even the most psychologically oriented anthropologists did not include systematic observational studies of socialization processes until the middle of the twentieth century so that avenues were not readily available for the type of investigation which had been recommended by Brinton. One result of this dearth of research data was that psychoanalysts did not have available information from other social scientists which would enable them to truly test their conjectures regarding the cross-cultural applicability of psychoanalytic ideas.

It is difficult to trace the relative influence of

the growing interest of psychoanalysts in ego psychology on the emergence of such systematic studies. Yet there can be no doubt that this interest offered hope to anthropologists for the understanding of the influence of social structure and puericultural practices on personality organization and its effects on the forms and themes of expressive culture. Devereux and LaBarre (1961) later suggested that psychoanalytic culture and personality studies would become one of the most effective means for the study of man in society.

Roheim appears to be the first anthropologist who entered systematic psychoanalytic training to learn what field data would be most useful to test analytic ideas cross-culturally and how to amass that information. He had been deeply interested in oral literature from the beginning of his professional work (Róheim, 1913). Folklorists of that time still held generally that keys to understanding folk literature lay in that of "savages." Róheim (1925, 1974) chose to work especially with the aborigines of Australia. Subsequently, other anthropologists and folklorists who have been especially interested in the cross-cultural understanding of expressive culture have either entered psychoanalytic training or studied psychoanalysis seriously, including R. M. Boyer (Boyer and Boyer, 1967), Carvalho-Neto (1968), Devereux (1948, 1969), DeVos (1962), Dundes (1962), D. Freeman (1967), Henry and Henry (1944), Hippler et al. (1974), LaBarre (1970), Muensterberger (1950, 1964), Posinsky (1956), and Whiting (1959).

Psychoanalysts have subsequently become involved in the formal study of anthropology and/or collaborated in cross-disciplinary field work including Erikson (1950) and Foulks (1972). Freeman (1968), Kardiner (1939), Kardiner et al. (1945), Margolin (1961) and the Parins and Morgenthaler (Parin et al., 1966, 1971). Of them, Boyer (1962, 1974) has been the most directly interested in the cross-cultural study of expressive culture.

As psychoanalytic thinking has changed from being dominated by the topographical theory in the direction of the structural hypothesis, so has the psychoanalytic view changed regarding the psychological functions of folklore. The following remarks constitute a synthesis of current psychoanalytic understanding of those functions.

Current Ideas

The myth is a special form of shared fantasy which serves to bring the individual into relationship with members of his cultural group on the basis of common psychological needs. It can be studied from the point of view of its roles in psychic and social integrations; not only does it assist in alleviating individual guilt and anxiety, but it constitutes a form of adaptation to reality; as a form of community illusion, it adds to the cohesion of the social group. Thus it influences the development of a sense of reality and the superego (Arlow, 1961).

Freud demonstrated that the type of mental activity known as unconscious fantasy is peculiarly inchoate. Drive derivatives seek immediate discharge and their dynamic force activates the mental apparatus to reproduce sensory impressions which mime previously perceived, highly gratifying impressions. A function of the ego is to delay the discharge of instinctual drive derivatives and to facilitate their expression in an adaptive, integrated manner, thus avoiding intrapsychic conflict and clash with the world of reality. Depending on the nature of the data of perception, the level of cathectic potential and the state of ego functioning, different forms of mental products emerge; out of this matrix of activity are created dreams, symptoms, fantasies, and expressive culture. Important external events become integrated into existent structures of unconsciously fantasized wishes and reality is experienced in terms of internal need.

The hierarchy in the fantasy life of each individual reflects the vicissitudes of individual experience as well as the influences of psychic differentiation and ego development. Unconscious fantasies have a systematic relationship to each other and are grouped around instinctual wishes and drive derivatives. The groups are composed of varying editions of attempts to resolve intrapsychic conflicts concerning the wishes, and each version corresponds to a different psychic movement in the history of the individual's development. At different times and under varying circumstances, one of the organized images may be brought into focus. The defensive needs of the ego may be so strong as to endow each successive set of images with such vividness that the fantasies are experienced as realities from the past.

Myths and related phenomena are group-accepted images which serve as further screening devices in the defensive and adaptive functions of the ego. They reinforce the suppression and repression of individual fantasies and personal myths (Eggan, 1955). A shared daydream is a step toward group formation and solidarity and leads to a sense of mutual identification on the basis of common needs. Myth makers serve the community alongside poets and prophets, presenting communally acceptable versions of wishes which theretofore were expressed in guilt-laden, private fantasy. Arlow (1951) showed that the same motivations operate in the realm of the ecstatic religious revelation and the prophetic calling. Idiosyncratic personal dreams are made to be forgotten. Shared daydreams are instruments of socialization and thereby character forming. The myth must be remembered and repeated. The externalization of the impulses which give rise to fantasy makes possible the process of sharing and potentiates the containment of fright and guilt through the means of art and symbolism. Myth, art, and religion are institutionalized instruments which bolster the social adaptation ordinarily made possible by the nightly abrogation of instinctual renunciation in the dream. In the genesis of myth, for both individual and group, only a kernel of realistic experience is needed. The revision or falsification of the past and its heroes by the group serves the purpose of defense, adaptation and instinctual gratification for the group and its individual constituents; they also serve in shaping personality organization.

BIBLIOGRAPHY

ABRAHAM, K. (1909). Dreams and myths: A study in folk psychology. In *Clinical papers and essays on psychoanalysis.* New York: Basic Books, 1955. Pp. 151–209.

BOYER, L. B. Remarks on the personality of shamans, with special reference to the Apaches of the Mescalero Indian reservation. In W. Muensterberger and S. Axelrad (Eds.), *Psychoanalytic study of the society.* New York: International Universities Press, 1962. Pp. 233–254.

BOYER, L. B. The man who turned into a water monster: A psychoanalytic contribution to folklore. In W. Muensterberger and A. Esman (Eds.), *Psychoanalytic study of the society.* New York: International Universities Press, 1974. Pp. 100–133.

BOYER, L. B., and BOYER, R. M. A combined anthropological and psychoanalytic contribution to folklore. *Psychopathologie Africaine,* 1967, *3,* 333–372.

DEVEREUX, G. *Essais d'ethnopsychiatrie générale.* Paris: Gallimard, 1969.

FREUD, S. (1900). The interpretation of dreams. *Standard Edition,* 1953, *4* and *5.*

FREUD, S. (1912). The theme of the three caskets. *Standard Edition,* 1958, *12,* 289–302.

FREUD, S. (1913). The occurrence in dreams of material from fairy tales. *Standard Edition,* 1958, *12,* 279–288.

FREUD, S. (1915). The unconscious. *Standard Edition,* 1957, *14,* 159–215.

FREUD, S., and OPPENHEIM, D. E. *Dreams in folklore.* New York: International Universities Press, 1909.

HIPPLER, A. E.; BOYER, L. B.; and BOYER, R. M. The psychocultural significance of the Alaska Athbascan Potlatch ceremony. In W. Muensterberger and A. Esman (Eds.), *Psychoanalytic study of the society.* New York: International Universities Press, 1974. Pp. 204–234.

JACQUES, H. P. *Mythologie et psychanalyse: Le chatment des danaides.* Montreal: Les Editions Lemeac, 1969.

MUENSTERBERGER, W. Oral trauma and taboo: A psychoanalytic study of an Indonesian tribe. In G. Róheim (Ed.), *Psychoanalysis and social science.* New York: International Universities Press, 1950. Pp. 129–172.

MUENSTERBERGER, W. Remarks on the function of mythology. In W. Muensterberger and S. Axelrad (Eds.), *Psychoanalytic study of the society.* New York: International Universities Press, 1964. Pp. 94–97.

RANK, O. *Psychoanalytische Beiträge zur Mythenforschung: Gesammelte Studien aus den Jahren 1912 bis 1914* (2nd ed.). Vienna: Internationaler Psychoanalytischer Verlag, 1922.

REIK, T. *Der eigene und der fremde Gott.* Leipzig: Internationaler Psychoanalytischer Verlag, 1923.

RÓHEIM, G. Myth and folktale. *American Imago,* 1941, *2,* 266 270.

SILBERER, H. Phantasie und Mythos. *Jahrbuch der psychoanalytischer und psychopathologischer Forschung,* 1910, *2,* 541–622.

L. BRYCE BOYER

MYTHS AND FAIRY TALES: JUNG'S VIEW

The relevance of myths and fairy tales to Jungian psychology is the proof of the reality of psychic life. In modern culture in which *myth* and *fairy tale* are popular synonyms for illusion, the *psyche* similarly has been widely devalued as unreal. It has taken psychoanalysis, and most especially Jungian psychology, to begin to restore to psychic life that primary, self-generating, and fateful power which belongs to it. This restoration represents a whole revision and reordering of human understanding; for if the psyche is a self-actualizing reality, each human is locked in a relationship with forces working within and through him, which he must heed, respect, and attempt to comprehend. The powers which he had thought resided in heaven, or in society, or in the family, or in a loved one, are more and more discovered to be moving within each person. And it is in order to grasp the nature of these inner powers that Jung called upon the myth and the fairy tale for elucidation.

There are other immediate avenues to the understanding of the inner or unconscious life: dreams, fantasies, hunches, and visions attest to that life and give working clues about it. What is unique about both the myth and the fairy tale is their collective validity. In their traditional sense, they spring from and are carried on by whole cultures; indeed, it is characteristic of fairy tales to pass beyond one culture and to become, with some variations, almost universal. Furthermore, sacred stories—which the myth and the fairy tale are—have always revealed their special power and efficacy in being ritually repeated. They have served ever and again to ground people in the deepest truth of their existence as human beings, eternally reestablishing the origins and nature of life and its link with its divine source.

Collective Unconscious

It occurred to Jung that beyond all the personal material which shapes our unconscious motivations and attitudes, there is a universal or *collective unconscious,* out of which arise intimations and images reflecting the timeless nature of human life itself. Thus each person is linked by his own inborn nature with all of humanity, as also all of humanity works within each person. The great and universally human possibilities of experience, which Jung called the *archetypes,* wait to be activated and realized in all. This fact became really clear to him when he observed that fantasies and dreams of individual patients sometimes bore an incredible resemblance to old mythological lore, of which these individual patients were quite unaware. Jung's conclusion was that the psyche retains, and can manifest, all conceivable images and reflections of what it means, and has always meant, to be human.

Concern with myths and fairy tales is therefore neither primarily historical nor primarily sociological. It is a concern with that which can illuminate the deepest psychological and spiritual problems inherent in human life. These stories have proved themselves: They have worked again and again. Their counterparts, the visions, dreams, and intuitions of modern people, also work: as the Jungian analyst observes, they bring unexpected order and meaning to an individual's experience. So the level of myth in each person is one of deep efficacy and potency. It can liberate a person from his illusion of isolation into that world which has always been shared by all, the world of archetypal experience; and in this process, it can aid in the cure of neurosis. For as one finds oneself being *bound back* to the true nature of life—in the sense of the word religion, which means "binding back"—one also finds oneself becoming free from the pervasive modern neurotic conflict, whose essence is isolation and fear. If it can be heeded, there is a level of understanding within each person which can work for, guide, and even transform him; and it is to this level that the classic myth and fairy tale bear eternal witness.

To say that these sacred stories are untrue is to speak from a point of view that denies psychological reality. Jung's dictum was: "What is real is what works." This is the pragmatic rule that governs his investigations, and it means that one ought to take seriously whatever has an undeniable effect. As he pointed out, no one has ever seen electricity, yet we are forced to grant it reality. The actual truth that is in the myth and the fairy tale is best conveyed in precisely those supernatural terms that may most offend the intellect. There is no better way to give expression to the forces, the dangers, the transformations that actually occur in the psyche, than in the "fantastic" images of myth. If there were a better way, presumably the "modern" mind would have invented it; and yet the ancient shapes and events of timeless tales continue to play through the unconscious material of the most modern.

Dreams and Myths

In the interpretation of dreams, Jung found that it often works most effectively if the figures and events portrayed are seen as different aspects of the dreamer's own psyche. This *subject level* of interpretation, in contrast to the *object level* of a literal, external view of the material, allows the dreamer to experience himself as he relives the dream, that is, to sense the power and the meaning of his own inner life. As he goes on assimilating his own nature in this way, the dreamer puts back together his split-off parts and becomes more and more the center and container of a rich, complex whole, the *self,* whose realization is the very goal of the life process of *individuation.*

Myths and fairy tales taken in the same way as dreams, as stories of our inmost psychic life, offer a new dimension for self-discovery. They enact the eternal problems and possibilities of human nature, and, like dreams, they aid in the ongoing process of integration. Myths are often used to "amplify" dream and fantasy material, that is, to enrich its meaning by comparison, since they have the whole deposit of timeless human experience within them.

A quite well known myth is the classic Greek tale of the Minotaur on the island of Crete. This was a terrible monster, part man and part bull, which inhabited a labyrinth within the earth. The king of Crete, Minos, was enraged at the people of Athens for the treacherous murder of his son, and the oracle of the god Apollo informed the Athenians that Minos could only be placated if every nine years they would send to Crete a tribute of seven youths and seven maidens to be sacrificed to the terrible Minotaur. This went on until the appearance of the hero and king's son Theseus, who, moved by the grief of his fellow Athenians, volunteered to be one of the young people to be sent to Crete, but vowed that he would overcome the Minotaur. The princess Ariadne fell in love with Theseus. She secretly gave him a ball of thread and told him to fasten one end of it to the entrance of the labyrinth so that he could find his way back out, and a magic sword, with which he could slay the Minotaur. Theseus killed the monster, found his way out, and escaped from the island with Ariadne and all of the youths and maidens.

This myth can be seen as a representation of the eternal, miraculous human process of emergence from unconsciousness. The endlessly repeated sacrifice of young lives is that constant, relentless waste of energy which always accompanies the unconscious state of life. But the hero Theseus represents the miraculous appearance of a faculty, innate in all, for penetrating that unconscious world—the tortuous labyrinth of one's own nature—getting back to the "monstrous" core of his distress, and thereby releasing him from it. This is not accomplished without help, personified by the princess Ariadne. And yet, since all the characters in this story are also ultimately oneself, it illustrates beautifully the relationship each person bears to his deeper nature. One is challenged by a state of distress, called to unravel his inner mystery, and dependent on a potent inner response and guidance in order to do so. But the myth says clearly: impossible as this task seems, it can be done.

A myth can thus act as a ground and an inspiration for one's life, making deep and ultimate sense out of the struggle in which he is engaged. In this respect, myth and fairy tale have equal validity. What distinguishes the fairy tale, in part, from the myth is its even greater universality, since it has generally lost all the topical and historical references of the myth and presents instead a beautiful abstraction. Precisely this quality gives it a peculiar potency. Its images are like a distillation of the whole wealth of experience into the most apt and perfect symbols. An examination of just one sequence from a fairy tale will help us to see these characteristics.

In a German tale called "The Hunter and the Swanmaiden," the hero, a hunter, has made a long, arduous journey to find his wife who has flown away from him in the swan-dress which she had been wearing when he first captured her. He finally comes to a glass mountain in which she, a bewitched princess, is imprisoned with all of her family. Having acquired the power to assume several animal forms, the hero can become an ant, creep up the mountain and into a crack in it, and secretly rejoin his wife inside. Here he learns that she cannot be released unless someone can overcome a twelve-headed dragon raging in the area, and he also learns details of how this might be done. He creeps back out of the mountain, goes to the nobleman in charge of feeding the dragon, and offers his services. It appears that each day the dragon requires twenty pigs to feed on, and also eats the swineherd who brings them. The hero, as the new swineherd, is advised by the nobleman to cluster the pigs together so that the dragon can eat comfortably, or else it will get very angry.

The hero drives the pigs out to the dragon, but then he scatters them here and there, so that the dragon is unable to feed. Then the hero turns into a lion and tears off two of the dragon's heads. The dragon complains bitterly: "If only I had a little of my pigs' blood, I would have more strength." The hero replies, "Yes, and if only I had a crust of bread," leaves the field of battle, returns with the pigs to the nobleman's house, eats well, and restores himself. The following day all this is repeated, except that the hero is able to tear off four of the dragon's heads. On the third and final day, it is all repeated again, and he manages to tear off the remaining six heads. Out of the very last of the heads springs a hare; the hero turns into a greyhound and bites it to death. Out of the hare flies a dove; the hero turns into an eagle and strangles it. And finally, from the head of the dove he takes a pebble. After a few days' rest, he flies, as an eagle, to the top of the glass mountain, drops the pebble into its crack, and hurries away. There is a fearful explosion, and all are released from bewitchment.

The state of bewitchment is characterized in the tale by two opposed, apparently contrary pictures. The most real and precious life (the princess and her family) is frozen and invisible behind a glass façade, but there is prodigious energy centered in the domineering twelve-headed dragon. The fairy tale says that so long as this great devourer continues to be fed, true life which is the goal of the hero's quest will remain inaccessible.

The hero represents the faculty for making a bridge between the split-off parts of one's own nature. He has penetrated to the life behind the façade of the glass mountain, and there he discovered the truth about the state of bewitchment. The truth is that there is a great potential for life locked away, which can actually be released if one can subdue one's "dragon." The dragon represents the unconscious. If, like the hero, one has a glimpse of the possibility of genuine release, he can pursue the way indicated by the fairy tale. He can live with his inner demands and terrors, and yet not give in to them, and will find, as the hero does, that they begin to lose their power and control over him.

The fairy tale does not preach withdrawal from reality. Quite the contrary, it shows psychological and spiritual reality. The "natural" human response to a terrible demand would seem to be either run from it or satisfy it im-

mediately. These were both happening in the story until the appearance of the hero. Running from the problem is reflected in the walled-off glass mountain; immediate satisfaction, in the endless sacrifices to the dragon. They are two sides of the same coin, and they can both be found acted-out in lives as long as people remain unconscious. The hero is therefore a true spiritual guide, indicating to us by his behavior that there is a middle way. It is possible to be wholly involved and at the same time wholly aware; this combination is the agent of release.

Spiritual Reality

Practical examples of the efficacy of this paradoxical teaching abound in Jungian analytical practice. Since, in this practice, great psychological forces are seen to be one's own responsibility, one needs the approach that will most aid in their integration. This approach will have to do justice to the paradoxical fact that the inner life is both "I" and "not-I," both oneself and wholly other than oneself. That special involved awareness characteristic of the hero of myth and fairy tale is the precise attitude with which one can fruitfully deal with this unconscious material. Then there is a check on onesidedness in either direction: that of being inundated by the material, and of being frightened away from it. The middle way, by which one can give full value to what is in him while remaining himself and intact, is ever and again the way of true integration and release.

The world of myth and fairy tale is clearly a special, unique kind of reality. It can be called a *spiritual* reality, and the term is adequate so long as one does not interpret it as the opposite of *natural*. The power of the myth and fairy tale lies in their capacity to encompass and transcend these opposites. These stories have indicated that fundamental human, "natural" drives, and, equally fundamental "spiritual" urges are both innately human and both are encountered in these tales in their purest symbolic form. The deepest and most abiding need reflected here seems to be the need for a final and genuine solution to the conflict of these two great directions. Jung emphasized in his theory of personality that no such solution can be genuine if it is onesided. In the tale the hero cannot succeed without the dragon, and the great antagonists are both equally indispensable.

An indicator of the popular misunderstanding of myth and fairy tale is the common assumption that, in supplying a "happy ending," they go off into unreality. In fact, they are eternally pointing to the greatest opportunity in human life, that of enduring its contradictions and coming to a state in which the opposites, including those of "happy" and "unhappy," are left behind.

BIBLIOGRAPHY

DER JÄGER UND DIE SCHWANENJUNGFRAU. In P. Zaunert (Ed.), *Deutsche Märchen seit Grimm.* Jena: Diederichs, 1964. Pp. 63–71.

JUNG, C. G. (1948). The phenomenology of the spirit in fairytales. *Collected works, 9*(1), 207–254.

JUNG, C. G. (1951). The psychology of the child archetype. *Collected works, 9*(1), 151–181.

JUNG, C. G. (1952). Symbols of transformation. *Collected works, 5.* New York: Bollingen, 1956. Pp. 26, 308, 390f.

DAVID L. HART

N

NARCISSISM

See PSYCHOANALYSIS

NARCISSISM

Freud's initial paper on narcissism was based primarily on economic considerations as he described the ebb and flow of libido starting with an infant's first awakening of interest in the outside world. Many of the phenomena of psychosis, perversions in which the individual seeks himself as a love object, important aspects of homosexuality, hypochondriasis, megalomania, and the normal reaction to organic disease were all understood in a new way by the notion that libido which had once been extended toward the outside world could under certain normal and certain pathologic conditions be withdrawn and reinvested in the individual himself. Freud's description of how one may love after the narcissistic fashion recognized that self-love is more or less a part of all of one's loving feelings, but in general it was felt that narcissistic love and object love are antithetical, that narcissism beyond the earliest phases of life is pathological.

It is important to note that relatively few new discoveries were made in the area of narcissism between the time of Freud's initial work and the late 1960s when the study of narcissistic character disorders became intense. It is as if Freud and early analysts understood important aspects of the narcissism of infancy and of the latter part of the preoedipal phase, but somehow had missed the narcissistic phenomena of the middle years of infancy. Margaret Mahler made significant contributions through her study of psychotic children. By differentiating autistic and symbiotic syndromes she added substance to Freud's concept of primary narcissism and enriched the psychoanalytic understanding of those processes by which an infant becomes aware of its environment, differentiates from its mother, develops the capacity to love and note the environment, and contemporaneously develops the capacity for self-love. Using data from successful analytic work with psychotic adults, Edith Jacobson provided theoretical constructs which converged on these same developmental processes. More recent impetus to the study of narcissism was aroused primarily by the work of two analysts, Heinz Kohut and Otto Kernberg.

There is considerable agreement between

these two men about some of the observed analytic data of narcissistic patients. The implications drawn from the data, the derived metapsychology, and the applied psychoanalytic technique have produced sharp scientific controversy. At this time the psychoanalytic understanding, treatment, and literature of narcissism is dominated by the work of these two men. In addition to their own clinical analytic experience, both of them had access to large amounts of data from analytic work done by other analysts. This suggests that the data gathered by a single analyst working alone was not sufficient to break into this new clinical area.

H. Kohut

During his years as president of the American Psychoanalytic Association and later as president of the International Psychoanalytic Association, Kohut collected observations on colleagues as they responded to those narcissistic triumphs and disappointments which are unavoidable in such organized groups. He combined this data with clinical analytic observations to make some of the most significant psychoanalytic contributions in many years. At the descriptive level he isolated four hitherto unrecognized transference configurations, and noted that one of these transferences will appear spontaneously in those patients suffering from a narcissistic personality disorder. The two major configurations may be described as follows:

The Idealizing Transference. These patients are similar to those whom Freud described as loving after the narcissistic fashion by idealizing other people and then loving them as the person they would like to be. In the psychoanalytic transference, they attribute to the analyst power, strength, sagacity, knowledge, empathy, understanding, and many other fine qualities which go far beyond human capacity. In its fullest development such a transference may progress to intense feelings of wonderment, awe, and perhaps worship. Omnipotence, omniscience, and perfection are more or less openly attributed to the analyst and largely determine the patient's analytic experience. These patients are very deficient of self-esteem. Their unconscious self-image is negative and devoid of self-love. They view themselves as depreciated, weak, and powerless. They are de-

pendent on closeness to someone who is felt to possess ideal qualities in order to provide those narcissistic supplies which they find lacking in themselves. Attaching themselves to such an idealized parental figure or analyst provides essential stability in their narcissistic economy.

The Mirror Transference. Individuals who have inordinate exhibitionistic needs and who rely for the maintenance of their self-esteem on admiration from other people may well develop this special form of transference. Just as during childhood the developing personality needs to experience the admiring eye of his parents, these patients use their analysts to reflect back approval and confirmation of their self-worth. For example, such a patient might well spend many hours describing his achievements, perhaps doing so in a subtle way that is unconsciously intended to evoke admiration and praise in the analyst. The mirror transference, in a narrow sense, may be defined by the fact that the search for approval becomes a central feature of the working-through process.

Less common forms of mirror transference were described and labeled the *alter-ego* or *twinship transference* and the *transference of merger through extension of the grandiose self.* These have in common a diminished capacity to distinguish between the self and others.

Kohut discovered the fact that in narcissistic personalities one of these four transferences will develop and that once formed it is a relatively stable configuration which may be systematically worked through as are other more neurotic transferences.

O. Kernberg

Kernberg came to the problem of narcissism through systematic study of the limits of psychoanalytic therapy and hence the study of psychoanalytic failures. In both descriptive and theoretical fashions he differentiated a more primitive level of personality functioning, one which is stable, with its own cluster of defenses, typical conflicts, and special pathology of object relations. This provided new understanding of the borderline personality, severe character disorders, impulse disorders, antisocial personalities, and addicts. The narcissistic character was seen as a special type of this characterologic group and differs from it by the presence of an unconscious grandiose self derived from a fusion of primitive ideal self, ideal object, and real self-images. The typical defenses of these individuals are: denial, projection, identification, projective identification, splitting, idealization, and omnipotence. In a new way, Kernberg differentiated the psychoneuroses and neurotic character disorders (higher-level character structure) from the narcissistic and borderline patients (lower-level character structure) by the predominance of repression in the former and splitting mechanisms in the latter. The defense of splitting was redefined and used to describe specific psychopathology of the internalized conscious and unconscious self and object representations. Instead of having a single, consolidated psychic image of a mother or father, Kernberg found multiple discrete, primitive self and object images; further, he found that though the self and object representations were separate, they could be assigned to the "real self" or the object world. In the borderline personality this allowed psychic images of an all-powerful "good" mother and a destructive, feared "bad" mother to exist side by side, either one to be activated if the psychic conditions were correct. A narcissistic individual could act and feel at one time as if he were an important, feared, powerful, demanding parent and at another time as if he were a weak, depreciated, helpless child. In contrast to the borderline patient, the splitting is more limited to the idealized and depreciated aspects of the internalized images. In the narcissistic patient, idealized internalized self and object representations are defensively activated to maintain a constantly endangered modicum of self-love. When disappointed, such a patient may become distant, aloof, withdrawn, and untouched by life's events. Typically, this represents a grandiose state, as if the individual were saying, "I am special, too important and great to bother with you," the disappointment having led to a fusion of an archaic, unmodified, grandiose parent (idealized object), an infantile ideal self-representation, and the current real self.

Most psychoanalysts once felt that patients with significant narcissistic psychopathology were unsuited for psychoanalytic treatment. Following Freud's division of neurosis into the narcissistic neuroses and the transference neuroses, it was felt either that "narcissistic pa-

tients" did not develop a transference and so did not enter into a psychoanalytic process or that the deep regressions which accompanied attempts to analyze them precluded psychoanalytic treatment. The transference-countertransference problems which arose were great, as was the potential to develop either an analytic stalemate or an outright analytic failure.

Narcissistic Character Disorder

With the development of ego psychology and most especially the systematic study of the psychic representations of the self and objects, the tools were fashioned to gain a deeper understanding of narcissistic personalities. The concept of a "self-representation" clarified confusion which had evolved from using the word *ego* to represent both the way a person conceived of himself as an individual and for part of his psychic structure. New terms like *ideal self, self-images, real self, ideal object, grandiose self,* and *self-object* stimulated inquiry and fostered new theoretical formulations. This made possible genuine analytic work with previously inaccessible patients. The analysis of narcissistic character disorders was gradually moved from the province of a few intuitive, gifted analysts to systematic analytic work done by the main body of psychoanalysts.

Descriptively, a narcissistic character disorder may be seen in an individual who superficially functions very well or perhaps even brilliantly in life. On closer observation and in the course of an analytic regression, some combination of other traits becomes apparent. Libidinally, such patients suffer greatly from an inner emptiness with strong feelings of depression, greed, envy, and rage; the balance between love and hate leans heavily toward the hateful side. Their inner life is dominated by oral aggression, turned variously toward the outside world or against themselves. In their object relations, they are found to have a tenuous hold on those whom they love. They assume others to be potentially aloof, cold, and rejecting while simultaneously displaying these same attitudes. Withdrawal from important relationships comes too easily. People who are useful to them are often admired and exploited only to be later discarded without feeling. There is a strong tendency to idealize or depreciate others and themselves. Strong exhibitionistic needs are common and seen either overtly or through derivative defensive compromises. Shame may be easily evoked and intense.

Their ego functioning may seem to be superficially good but there is an ease of regression leading to partial ego fragmentation and perhaps to transient psychotic states. Kernberg stresses the central importance of the use of splitting in these patients. Multiple mutually contradictory self and object representations are ever ready to be activated for defensive purposes. For example, a patient may see no discrepancy in reacting within a short time as if he were first a powerful, grand, important person and later as a depreciated, weak, helpless one. The defensive system is driven by fears of separation and infantile helplessness rather than by the guilt or castration anxiety seen in more neurotic patients. The superego functioning of such individuals may or may not contain significant pathology. The sense of guilt may be undeveloped, leaving them reliant on their environment for impulse control. Constant needs for admiration and reassurance stem from insufficient love in the superego introjects, so self-esteem too is externally regulated. Such patients often seem overly dependent or even addicted to the approval of others as part of a frantic search for a missing inner structure which guides their behavior and dispenses self-love for their achievements and guilt for failure to meet standards. Other superego pathology can include very early mother or father introjections, introjects acquired before all good and all bad parental images had been fused and acquired at a time when the child felt too much hostility from omnipotently perceived parents. These superego fragments now tell him that he is monstrously bad and that the punishment will be enormous and according to primitive fantasies.

Narcissistic Elements

It seems clear that there are narcissistic components to all stages of human development. Beginning with the stage of primary narcissism, there is the all-important shift to secondary narcissism, the observed grandiosity of the toddler, anal omnipotence, phallic narcissism of the oedipal stage, the narcissistic object

choice of latency, and the normal narcissistic aspects of the libidinal shift of adolescence. Kohut has well described some sublimations of narcissism as seen in the mature capacity for empathy and in creativity, humor, wisdom, and the acceptance of mortality. He views narcissism as a normal developmental line, having certain expected outcomes. Kohut emphasizes the normality and usefulness of the narcissistic aspects of personality. His approach in therapy is consistent with this when he creates an optimal analytic atmosphere for the full development of a narcissistic transference. In the idealizing transference, he accepts the patient's overvaluation of the analyst in the expectation that the patient will gradually modify his idealism through confronting himself with its unrealistic intensity. This is likened to the normal processes by which children modify their overestimation of themselves and their parents. In the course of normal development, such exaggerations would gradually change as, over a period of years, the child is repeatedly confronted with small disappointments in his omnipotent expectations of his parents. Kohut feels that traumatic disruptions in the relationship with the parent or narcissistic injuries at vulnerable times can interrupt this process, perhaps cause regression, prevent further modification, and leave the child with primitive ideal self or object representations. The analytic change in these cases is seen as being brought about by a process termed *transmuting internalization* and involves a process of repeated small identifications with an analyst who does not create further narcissistic injury but who neither participates in the patient's narcissistic fantasies. An approach like this seems to involve a different attitude on the part of the analyst. As in the analytic treatment of children and selected psychotic states, it involves a greater willingness to participate in the transference and allow a greater level of transference gratification without permanently losing an analytic stance. The patient hopefully moves on to develop higher forms of narcissism—its sublimations.

Narcissistic Pathology

Kernberg takes a very different view. He sees the narcissism of the narcissistic personality disorder as rooted in pathological early object relations. The mirror and idealizing transferences are seen as defensive positions overlying primitive conflict, rage, fear, and aggression. In terms of analytic technique, his approach is much more similar to that seen in standard psychoanalytic technique. He emphasizes the analysis of the character structure, with special attention to the defenses peculiar to this type of personality and to the intense, primitive rage which he finds in all such patients. The frustrations inherent in the psychoanalytic situation plus real or fantasy deprivation lead the patient to establish a narcissistic position toward the analyst. For example, a failure of empathy is followed by a patient treating the analyst as an omnipotent figure. Underneath this lies intense rage and vulnerability, the kind of rage that an infant might have. The rage may be handled by projection, denial, identification, or an omnipotent withdrawal. These defenses must be systematically worked through, uncovering feelings of intense emptiness, loneliness, envy, depression, and destructiveness. At bottom are wishes for love and tenderness with a fear of having destroyed the good that the analyst has had to offer.

The successful analyses are long and difficult for both partners. The patient has been repeatedly confronted with his defensive fusion of the ideal self, the ideal object, and the real self. Each of these inner representations has been explored in its pathologically independent (split) state. The patient has come to realize that both he and the analyst are neither as good or as bad, as grand or as depreciated, as he had thought. A new capacity to love has emerged and the analysis is over.

The major differences between Kohut and Kernberg should not obscure the valuable contributions each has made; however, some questions do remain. How could two reliable investigators have come to such diverse views? Is their data base the same? Does Kernberg's technique lead to unnecessary suffering due to a failure of empathy? Does Kohut produce a superficial analysis through participation in the transference? Is the ultimate goal of the analysis of narcissistic patients to replace narcissism with object love, or to replace immature narcissism with its higher form, or both? Can a complex developmental line of narcissism be formulated and then its pathological deviations identified? Answers to these ques-

tions should stimulate psychoanalysis for considerable time.

Kernberg has suggested a possible partial solution. Many analysts have evaluated some patients who tend to confirm Kohut, while others tend to confirm Kernberg. The concepts of narcissism and pathological narcissism lead to the hypothesis that in some cases there has been a fixation with blocking of further maturation along a narcissistic developmental line, while in other cases this is combined with a lower level of character structure and the formation of pathological forms of narcissism.

BIBLIOGRAPHY

Jacobson, E. *The self and the object world.* New York: International Universities Press, 1964.

Kernberg, O. Borderline personality organization. *Journal of the American Psychoanalytic Association,* 1967, *15,* 641–685.

Kernberg, O. Factors in the psychoanalytic treatment of narcissistic personalities. *Journal of the American Psychoanalytic Association,* 1970, *18,* 51–85.

Kernberg, O. Contrasting viewpoints regarding the nature and psychoanalytic treatment of narcissistic personalities: A preliminary communication. *Journal of the American Psychoanalytic Association,* 1974, *22,* 255–267.

Kohut, H. *The analysis of the self.* Psychoanalytic Study of the Child Monograph no. 4. New York: International Universities Press, 1971.

Roy N. Aruffo

NARCISSISTIC ALLIANCE

The concept of the narcissistic alliance is predicated on the clinical observation of an omnipresent narcissism and the consequent elaboration of the notion of a narcissistic ontogeny. Although the developmental hypothesis initially arose in the era of the early psychoanalytic preoccupation with instincts and their sequential vicissitudes, the advent of the structural hypothesis and the subsequent clinical and theoretical interest in the ego and its nature as well as its growth and development added a new and enormous enhancement to the developmental notion. It is not surprising then that the elaboration and extension of developmental perspectives to include lifetimes as well as infancy and childhood, the theoretical disquiet with some aspects of structural theory, and the increasing interest in the concept of the self would eventually evolve into the idea of a developmental narcissism or a narcissistic developmental line. This is opposed to the more limited, but nonetheless valid, conceptualization of narcissism as an archaic instinctual issue pertinent to an early developmental phase.

In this sense, narcissism must be seen as a sequence of narcissistic developmental phases of transmigrating issues of greatest concern and consequently of greatest sensitivity. The migration from receptive narcissistic primacy of the instinctually oral phase, through cohesive narcissistic anxieties of later development and even later phallic narcissistic concerns, is an example of this kind of sequence and development.

If narcissism is conceptualized as another developmental line, as has been postulated, with its own reflection in structure, with a protected, vulnerable narcissistic frontier or locus of importance, at any given time a considerable amount of what one deals with in the immediate clinical context can be more easily understood. It is in this respect that the concept of a narcissistic alliance was elaborated.

From this point of view, it is clear that what we call initial rapport, for example, is certainly one form of the narcissistic alliance. For example, the patient may be terrified, in the beginning of the analysis, as in any other clinical situation. It falls upon the therapist or analyst to join the patient in dealing with this anxiety so that the patient's initial massive narcissistic defenses are no longer so necessary and can be replaced, at least in part, by the involvement with the analyst himself. Only when this process has taken place can any kind of therapeutic work occur. If at this juncture however, the analyst remains only aware of the patient's initial anxieties and frights he will quickly have lost the locus of the patient's narcissistic investment as the patient moves on. This means that the empathic resonance with the patient, in terms of his current narcissism, will constantly change, and once the initial fright has quieted down, other issues will surface as the patient begins to form the relationship or to investigate some material, such that new issues of greatest current fright, greatest current anxiety, and greatest current defensive cathexis will appear.

Narcissistic Defenses

In this context the narcissistic defenses will once again be mobilized, just as they had been initially in a similarly antitherapeutic fashion. The analyst, then, must be aware of the immediate locus of the danger that confronts the patient and do whatever is necessary to dispel the patient's urgent need of mobilizing militant, narcissistic defenses in this particular area. The process of location, affectively contacting the patient in the area of his narcissistic frontier, and establishing a new relationship with the patient in this area, must be repeated once again. Each time this is done, often via interpretation, a considerable enhancement of the therapeutic alliance is made. One could say that the analyst fosters a constant transformation from the narcissistic to the therapeutic alliance.

One could repeat this description with every aspect and phase of an analysis and it would become clear that there is no moment, at any phase in any clinical situation, when the patient and the analyst escape the problem of maintaining the narcissistic alliance in such a way that the therapist's presence of the moment will allow the patient to relinquish narcissistically protective defenses sufficiently to be able to consider, to cope with, and to become involved with the issues that had been heretofore not been allowed to exist in so open a fashion.

Ordinarily the narcissistic problem in this sense, or the narcissism of the moment, never appears in the clinical situation as narcissism or as an issue unless there is a problem with it. The absence of these visible issues, however, cannot be taken as a testimony to the absence of the problem, but only to the success of the empathic and technical maintenance of the narcissistic alliance in the process of the analysis.

Therapeutic Alliance

From a conceptual point of view, one should distinguish this aspect of an alliance from what has been described as a *therapeutic alliance,* in that given the resolution of the narcissistic issues of basic trust, it is perfectly clear that there will be a propensity to form a narcissistic alliance on the part of the patient at any given time. If a narcissistic alliance is formed, it is also clear that a transference neurosis will tend to be elaborated on the basis of the relative lack of necessity of militant narcissistic protection and the relative openness of the patient in the situation. The transference neurosis in this sense represents the change of the locus of immediate narcissistic investment, and in itself can be seen as another form of narcissistic self protection when it is dealt with by interpretative means. In this way, the narcissistic alliance could be seen as a fundamental prerequisite to the elaboration of a transference neurosis.

On the other hand, the *therapeutic* alliance probably has as its developmental antecedent a form of relationship that develops quite a good deal later than the basic trust upon which it is also certainly dependent, but which in itself is not sufficient to guarantee the possibility of a therapeutic alliance. Indeed, in order to have a therapeutic alliance, as opposed to the form of initial rapport in the narcissistic alliance, a developmentally *later* form of trusting must exist that could probably be called *secondary* trust, which is a *later* form of readiness to form a narcissistic alliance. This is much more consonant with the kind of trust that a latency child still retains in his parent and which is so often absent in severely obsessional children.

It can be seen from this that the commencement of the narcissistic alliance in an ordinary analysis would antedate the development of a therapeutic alliance as well as the development of the transference neurosis. It would also be clear that during and following the resolution of the transference neurosis, the narcissistic alliance would still remain partly embodied in the therapeutic alliance as its later form, and partly unchanged in its earlier form. The well-established and regularized narcissistic alliance that is maintained successfully throughout an analysis is probably never analyzed or never dissipated completely and is potentially mobilizable at any time because of this. Certainly the question of where the internalization in the identification with the analyst resides structurally is pertinent to this, if there is at the end of the analysis an internalization of the analyst in some fashion such that the process

of analysis continues and the analytic attitude is made an integral part of the patient's mental apparatus. It is also clear that the continuing object aspect of the analyst, in the form of the narcissistic alliance which remains as a benign positive presence, is also internalized and enhances the patient's sense of well-being and sense of self.

If one considers, however, the notion of secondary autonomy as being one of only *relative* autonomy, it is then clear that under exigent circumstances, the process of internalization and structuralization that we have described can be reversed to the point where the analyst is no longer present only in terms of analytic attitude, but might be thought of as a person analyzing and in many ways may be sought out again in the service of reconstituting the external analyst in the service of the same narcissistic protection. In this way, many patients appearing for reanalysis would seem to bring a new form of transference to the new analyst, whose precursor is the old narcissistic alliance relationship with the previous therapist, or even the later form of the therapeutic alliance. This represents an attempt to reconstitute exactly the same relationship in the service of protection against the present exigent circumstances. There is some question as to whether or not this possibility would ever dissipate or disappear after a successful analysis.

BIBLIOGRAPHY

FREUD, A.   The concept of developmental lines. *Normality and pathology in childhood: Assessments of development.* New York: International Universities Press, 1966. Pp. 62–92.

FREUD, S. (1912).   The dynamics of transference. *Standard Edition.* London: Hogarth, 1958, *12,* 99–108.

FREUD, S. (1914).   On narcissism: An introduction. *Standard Edition,* 1957, *14,* 73–102.

GREENSON, R. R.   The working alliance and the transference neurosis. *Psychoanalytic Quarterly,* 1965, *24,* 135–186.

KOHUT, H.   Forms and transformations of narcissism. *Journal of the American Psychoanalytical Association,* 1966, *14,* 243–272.

ZETZEL, E. A.   Therapeutic alliance in the analysis of hysteria. *Capacity for emotional growth.* New York: International Universities Press, 1970. Pp. 182–196.

ROBERT D. MEHLMAN

NARCOTHERAPY

Narcotherapy is a general term referring to treatment of psychiatric patients with a narcotic drug. Other related terms are narcoanalysis, narcohypnosis, narcolysis, and narcosynthesis. The tendency to express oneself too freely when coming out of surgical anesthesia and the uninhibited behavior that occurs under the influence of alcohol are well known. This is really the basic process involved in narcotherapy. Alcohol, as well as other drugs such as chloroform, bromides, morphine and scopalomine, paralydehyde and medinol, methohexital (Brevital), droperidal, somnoform, ether, and carbon dioxide coma have been used in narcotherapy. More recently, amytal sodium and pentothal sodium have been the drugs of choice. Stimulants, as amphetamines, including methamphetamine (Methedrine), and methylphenidate (Ritalin) have been used along with the barbiturate to stimulate verbal expression and facilitate the therapeutic interview.

H. A. Palmer (1945) reviewed the procedure involving *continuous narcosis* in the treatment of mental disorders, using somnifane.

Clinical Application of Narcotherapy

The discrete use of narcotherapy is an effective diagnostic and therapeutic procedure in the neuroses, psychoses, and personality disorders. The approach involved in managing the different clinical entities is varied to suit the particular problem and the details elicited from the individual patient. The manic may become more coherent during narcotherapy. Personality disorders and traumatic neuroses have been treated effectively. R. R. Grinker and J. P. Spiegel (1945) treated war casualties. Organic brain disease has been differentiated from psychogenic conditions with similar symptoms. In psychogenic amnesia, pentothal is as effective as hypnosis in retrieving lost memory. F. C. Redlich, L. J. Ravitz, and G. H. Dession (1951) referred to the use of narcoanalysis in cases involving litigation. They stressed that the results included a combination of fantasy and truth, so that the productions elicited required interpretation by a psychiatrist with adequate understanding of the patient's unconscious processes. A burglar who developed a mute, withdrawn reaction to incarceration revealed the whereabouts of the stolen goods when queried under amytal sodium by H. A. Teitelbaum. Similarly, unresponsive catatonic schizophrenics may become more productive under the influence of pentothal sodium or amytal sodium. Paranoid schizophrenics have shown marked aggravation of their paranoid preoccupations as well as increased aggressiveness. Depressed patients have become more expressive and able to share their thoughts and feelings more readily. Anxious patients have become less agitated and more able to verbalize their thoughts and feelings. Psychosomatic symptoms, particularly those involving hysterical motor and sensory disturbances may respond promptly to narcotherapy. While visceral somatic symptoms respond more slowly, they are subject to improvement. As in therapy under hypnosis it is important to avoid the elimination of symptoms by direct suggestion. While this may be effective there is always the hazard of the development of other symptoms, at times more disabling than those given up by the patient.

Psychodynamics

Various psychodynamics have been suggested to explain the diagnostic and therapeutic advantages of narcotherapy. Sleep itself and suggestibility have been offered as likely explanations for the beneficial effects, while guilt and the susceptibility of the patient's pretraumatic personality are significant factors in maladaptation to stress. Grinker and Spiegel (1945) devoted considerable attention to the psychodynamics involved in war casualities they treated, and made particular reference to regression and ego disintegration, which gave rise at times to very primitive forms of global reaction. Abreaction and psychotherapy were considered to be of much importance in the reintegration of the patient's ego structure, and widening of ego boundaries. This was achieved through retrieval of the memory of very stressful experiences through hypermnesia with the help of the therapist.

L. S. Kubie and S. Margolin (1945) reviewed the psychodynamics involved in narcotherapy in great detail, stressing repression of unacceptable thoughts, feelings, and impulses with dissociation of their related energies which make inappropriate attachments. There is a natural tendency for unhealthy, excessive repression to undergo resolution, thus allowing synthesis or reintegration of the dissociated facets of personality to occur. The "psychically analgesic" drug, according to Kubie and Margolin, raises the threshold for undesirable emotions such as hate, guilt, and anxiety, making them more tolerable, so that the patients can work through the effects of their previously intolerable experiences. The drugs used also lessen the defensive significance of the patient's symptoms which play a protective role, so that the underlying conflicts can come to awareness and be subject to therapy. In the process of dissociation, as referred to above, the energy of repressed experiences becomes evident in the form of disturbing symptoms that are associated with the disruption of personality integrity and loss of self-identity. The drugs help to reestablish personality boundaries through therapeutic synthesis, with the lessening of repression. Thus the constructive, more mature reintegration of the regressive disintegrative processes takes place. The transference relationship plays a significant role in this procedure. Teitelbaum (1964) has discussed the disintegrative-reintegrative process psychodynamically and neurophysiologically.

R. M. Brickner, R. T. Porter, W. S. Homer, and J. J. Hicks (1950) elaborated on the significance of patterns of behavior that mature from the "theoretically patternless" primitive global personality of infancy to the very complex patterns of adulthood. There is regression to that earlier less patterned behavior under excessive stress. Through narcotherapy, using pentothal sodium and amytal sodium, constructive reintegration of the more mature patterns can occur.

Neurologic Processes

There has been theoretical consideration, clinical observation, and physiologic study concerning the neurologic processes involved in narcotherapy. According to Brickner and his associates (1950) the less complex, immature patterns of behavior result from subcortical neurologic integrations. These immature behavior patterns predominate when the subcortical integrations fail as a result of excessive stress, to be further integrated into the more

complex processes of the cerebral cortex. This over-all integration is essential for the more mature patterns of behavior. Grinker and Spiegel (1945) provided tangible clinical observations pertinent to this problem. They reported that the severely regressive psychosomatic reactions in some patients had characteristics of extrapyramidal disease, such as rigid, shuffling, propulsive gait; tremor; coarse nystagmoid eye movements; excessive salivation; subdued, scanning, stuttering speech; compulsive laughing and crying; and a startle reflex comparable to the Moro reflex of infancy. The authors suggested that narcosynthesis

alters the physiological status of the organism by its effect on the neural pattern of the diencephalon and cortex. One component of this effect is a greater capacity of the ego to withstand emotional discharge. . . . In fact the drug alone, with little discharge, so influences the diencephalic-cortical relations that temporary improvement takes place. (pp. 134–135)

The therapist facilitates and fortifies this improvement.

H. A. Teitelbaum, J. E. O. Newton, and W. H. Gantt (1970), in a study of the effect of pentobarbital sodium anesthesia in dogs on the cardiac orienting reflex (OR) which consisted of a transitory decrease in heart rate in response to a tone, reviewed essential data on the neurologic processes involved in barbiturate anesthesia. It was found that the cardiac OR of deceleration was more marked and that habituation did not occur during the intermediate phase of anesthesia. It is likely that during narcotherapy the patients' released reactions to barbiturates are comparable to the augmented cardiac OR, as both occur in the intermediate phase of anesthesia.

M. A. B. Brazier (1954) pointed out that barbiturates act on the neural synapse. In the early phase of barbiturate anesthesia the long fiber, specific sensory, spinothalamo-cortical pathways are partially blocked. In the intermediate phase of barbiturate narcosis there is a differential blocking action of a subcortical inhibitory system, with resultant augmentation of responses in the nonspecific, multisynaptic sensory pathways that involve the *reticular activating system* (RAS). This spontaneous inhibitory activity of the RAS is also blocked by a lesion of the RAS. In the deepest phase of barbiturate narcosis there is general inhibition with loss of differential action in the inhibitory and stimulating activities of the RAS. The disruption of balance between the RAS inhibitory and stimulating functions interferes with the subcortical integration that determines whether sensory impulses undergo elaboration essential for awareness, or not.

L. C. Johnson and A. Lubin (1967) observed that in man the various autonomic ORs to a tone, habituate or extinguish at different rates in the awake state. However, all of these ORs return during sleep with little if any habituation remaining. Sleep not only impairs the selectivity of habituation but also blocks habituation itself, as does the intermediate stage of drug narcosis.

Considering drug narcosis and sleep as related phenomena, perhaps the persistence, or lack of habituation of the ORs of the various autonomic systems during sleep, is also the result of a blocking effect by the sleep process on the spontaneous inhibitory action of the RAS. C. Fisher and W. Dement (1963) reviewed M. Jouvet's studies on the essential role of the RAS in sleep in their discussion of the psychopathology of sleep and dreams. In the above sense it can be considered that there is a release of feelings, thoughts, and impulses in dreams comparable to that occurring in narcotherapy, thus further supporting the psychotherapeutic significance of dream analysis. It would be of interest to determine whether hypnosis also augments the cardiac OR and prevents habituation of autonomic or visceral ORs, as do sleep and barbiturate anesthesia.

Drug Narcosis

Whether drug narcosis, sleep, and hypnosis have comparable underlying neurophysiologic processes, is a complex issue. The relationship between rapid eye movement (REM) sleep and dreaming is well documented and the occurrence of nystagmus during barbiturate narcosis is also well established. Is it likely that the eye movements in sleep and in narcosis have the same neurophysiologic basis that is an intrinsic part of the more complex neurologic processes involved in barbiturate narcosis augmentation of the cardiac OR as well as the failure of autonomic ORs to habituate. The above would further reinforce the similarity between sleep and narcosis. Teitelbaum (1964) has ob-

served spontaneous, nystagmoid eye movements that occur during thoughtful concentration, and interpreted these eye movements as a process that facilitated exclusion during intense preoccupation of awareness of one's environment, a function of the RAS. Are these eye movements comparable to those occurring in REM sleep and during barbiturate narcosis?

Technique and Procedure

Amytal sodium and pentothal sodium are the drugs of choice in carrying out narcotherapy. Actually pentothal has the advantage of giving rise to narcosis of rather short duration, so that if the patient reaches an unresponsive state, cessation of the injection for several minutes makes the patient available again for the therapeutic process. Amytal is used in a 5% or 10% solution. Pentothal is effective in a 2.5–5% solution. The injection is given intravenously at a slow rate of approximately 1 cc per minute. The usual procedure is to have the patient count while the injection is being delivered. Speech becomes slow, scanning, and slurred, and this is used as a gauge of the degree of narcosis that is appropriate for one's purpose. Nystagmus usually occurs, although the corneal reflex is not abolished. With amytal sodium, if narcosis becomes too deep, recovery is prolonged, so therapy may have to be delayed or even discontinued. Appropriate observation of blood pressure, pulse, and respiration is required. Respiratory obstruction is an occasional hazard, particularly due to laryngeal spasm or excessive mucous secretion. It is essential that the patient be denied food or liquid prior to the procedure.

While some patients are under the influence of the drug, mere reference to their clinical problems may initiate free flowing expression of their feelings, thoughts, and reactions. The therapist can stimulate further productivity by means of appropriate questions and remarks, facilitating free associations as well as abreactions of various degrees of aggressiveness. These responses often involve specific experiences in the patient's past life related to a significant degree to their symptoms. In some instances the productivity may be rather meager. Cautious, planned probing, depending on one's understanding of the patient's personality and clinical diagnosis, may gradually elicit associations of significance in working through the underlying conflict.

To facilitate the patient's ability to express repressed feelings, impulses, and thoughts, stimulating drugs such as amphetamines, methylphenidate, and caffeine have been administered intravenously.

Clinical Results

R. R. Grinker and J. P. Spiegel (1945) reported that 72.17% of "the main body of neuroses" in war casualities treated by means of narcotherapy returned to some type of duty. R. M. Brickner and his colleagues (1950) provided a detailed analysis of their therapeutic results in neurotic, borderline, and psychotic patients respectively, including data on brief recurrences, relapses, and prognosis in the different clinical entities. In 7 of 12 patients treated there was an increase in intelligence quotient. Of 12 neurotic patients, 11 showed better than moderate improvement, while more than half showed marked improvement. Four of 11 borderline patients showed better than moderate improvement, while 3 were markedly improved. H. A. Palmer (1937) provided detailed data on the results in patients with various diagnoses treated by means of continuous narcosis. Grinker and Spiegel (1945) did not find this procedure significantly helpful in war casualities.

BIBLIOGRAPHY

BRAZIER, M. A. B. The action of anesthetics on the nervous system, with special reference to the brain stem reticular system. In J. F. Delafresnaye (Ed.), *Brain mechanisms and consciousness.* Springfield, Ill.: Thomas, 1954. Pp. 163–199.

BRICKNER, R. M.; PORTER, R. T.; HOMER, W. S.; and HICKS, J. J. Direct reorientation of behavior patterns in deep narcosis (narcoplexis). *Archives of Neurology and Psychiatry,* 1950, *64,* 165–195.

FISHER, C., and DEMENT, W. Studies on psychopathology of sleep and dreams. *American Journal of Psychiatry,* 1963, *119,* 1160–1168.

GRINKER, R. R., and SPIEGEL, J. P. *War neuroses.* Philadelphia: Blakiston, 1945.

KUBIE, L. S., and MARGOLIN, S. The therapeutic role of drugs in the process of repression, dissociation and synthesis. *Psychosomatic Medicine,* 1945, *7,* 147–151.

PALMER, H. A. The value of continuous narcosis in the treatment of mental disorders. *Journal of Mental Science,* 1937, *83,* 636–678.

REDLICH, F. C.; RAVITZ, L. J.; and DESSION, G. H. Narcoanalysis and truth. *American Journal of Psychiatry,* 1951, *107,* 586–593.

TEITELBAUM, H. A. *Psychosomatic neurology.* New York: Grune & Stratton, 1964.

TEITELBAUM, H. A.; NEWTON, J. E. O.; and GANTT, W. H. Effects of pentobarbital sodium anesthesia and neurohumoral agents on the cardiac orienting reflex. *Conditional Reflex,* 1970, *5,* 6–26.

HARRY A. TEITELBAUM

NATIONAL INSTITUTE OF MENTAL HEALTH

The National Institute of Mental Health (NIMH), an agency of the United States government, is that nation's focal point for programs relating to mental health. NIMH's objectives are threefold: to contribute to understanding the causes of mental illness, to improve treatment and rehabilitation programs for the mentally ill, and to promote mental health.

To accomplish these objectives, the NIMH supports and conducts research into the biological and sociological causes of mental illness and mental disorders, offers financial support and professional guidance for training a variety of professional and paraprofessional personnel working or planning to work in the mental health field, and provides for the provision of a variety of mental health services.

The Institute has expended more than $4.3 billion on its programs. The NIMH budget for the fiscal year 1975 was $394 million.

History

The NIMH was created in 1946. Its rapid evolution as the major governmental instrument for the prevention, treatment, and rehabilitation of the mentally ill and the promotion of mental health in the United States reflects the rising American concern since World War II with the magnitude of the problem of mental illness.

As late as 1848, President Franklin Pierce vetoed a bill that would have provided the first federal assistance to the mentally ill. President Pierce said in essence that it was inappropriate for the federal government to be concerned about the mentally ill.

With the exception of the federal government opening Saint Elizabeths Hospital in Washington, D.C. in 1855 to treat the mentally ill, governmental concern was limited to the states' providing hospital facilities for the "insane." For many years, it was left to national, state, and local voluntary associations to arouse public attention to the needs of the mentally ill.

The mental hygiene movement in the United States is generally dated from 1908 with the publication of the autobiography of a former mental patient, Clifford Beers's *The Mind That Found Itself,* and with the establishment in the following year of the voluntary National Committee for Mental Hygiene. The book provided impetus to various volunteer organizations, but it was not until the great influx of foreign immigration from 1900 to 1920 made it necessary for the Public Health Service to establish facilities at Ellis Island, New York for the medical and psychological screening of aliens that the federal government became concerned with mental illness as a national health problem. The necessity of detecting the mentally disturbed and mentally retarded from among the thousands of immigrants and the high incidence of first admissions of foreign persons into New York State mental hospitals in those years helped to stimulate government action.

In 1930, the Public Health Service decided to bring together some of the activities in the federal mental health movement and created a Division of Mental Hygiene. This program included the study of the nature of drug addiction and methods of treatment and rehabilitation of addicts; the supervision and provision of medical and psychiatric services in federal prisons; and the study and investigation of the causes, prevalence, and means for the prevention and treatment of nervous and mental disease.

World War II sharply interrupted the development of a federal mental health program. Yet the war demonstrated to the American people the tremendous toll mental illness took in the national welfare. More men received medical discharges from the armed forces for neuropsychiatric disorders than for any other reason. By August 1945, more than one million men had been rejected for military service because of neuropsychiatric disorders. The realization that 17% of American men were unfit for military service because of such disorders gave new impetus to the mental hygiene movement.

Yet, even in 1941, before the wartime shortages of manpower had become acute and before the influx of veterans into state hospitals had begun, the state hospitals treating mental illness reported an overall deficit in personnel of nearly 50%, based on minimum recommended staffing standards.

The shortage of professional personnel was severe. There were less than 3,000 trained psychiatrists in all of the United States. Estimates of shortages of psychiatric social workers were put at 71% and of psychologists at 92%. In addition, scientific research on the etiology, treatment, and prevention of mental illness lagged far behind investigations in other fields of medical science and public health.

Legislative Foundations

In 1944, the director of the Division of Mental Hygiene, Robert Felix, presented a proposal for a national mental health program to the surgeon general of the United States. This now historic "Outline of a Comprehensive Community-Based Mental Health Program," was to form the rough basis for the subsequent National Mental Health Act of 1946.

Signed into law by President Harry S Truman on July 3, 1946, the National Mental Health Act authorized a three-fold program of research, training, and service activities. Section II of the act provided for the establishment of a National Institute of Mental Health, and authorized $7,500,000 for the erection and equipment of hospital and laboratory facilities. However, Congress adjourned before appropriating any funds to carry out the new programs authorized by the act. Thus, it was necessary for the director of the Division of Mental Hygiene to obtain a grant from a private philanthropic foundation to convene the first meeting of the National Advisory Mental Health Council (NAMHC), whose appointment the 1946 act had authorized. The NAMHC is still the principle advisory body to the NIMH, and consists of six leading medical or scientific authorities and six lay members who are authorized to make recommendations for mental health activities and functions, to review and recommend support of research and training projects, and to collect and make available information on studies in the mental health field.

On April 1, 1949, the National Institute of Mental Health (NIMH) was officially established as authorized by the National Mental Health Act, and was organizationally placed within the National Institutes of Health. In

1967, NIMH became a separate bureau of the Public Health Service (PHS) and, a year later, the agency was made a component of the PHS's Health Services and Mental Health Administration. Also in 1968, administration of programs at Saint Elizabeths Hospital was transferred from the District of Columbia to the NIMH.

In 1973, three new agencies were created from components of HSMHA which was abolished as an organizational entity. The National Institute of Mental Health became a part of the newly established Alcohol, Drug Abuse, and Mental Health Administration, along with two new institutes whose programs had formerly been administered by the NIMH: the National Institute on Alcohol Abuse and Alcoholism and the National Institute on Drug Abuse. On May 14, 1974, Public Law 93–282 officially established by statute the Alcohol, Drug Abuse, and Mental Health Administration and the three separate institutes within the agency.

Research

The National Mental Health Act and subsequent legislation created within the NIMH a variety of mechanisms for supporting research —intramural studies, research fellowships, and grants to institutions and individuals. A primary responsibility of the National Advisory Mental Health Council is to select projects that might make "valuable contributions to human knowledge with respect to the causes, prevention, or methods of diagnosis and treatment of psychiatric disorders."

Research supported by the institute ranges from small pilot studies to large international, interdisciplinary projects using the skills of many scientists. Included is work that spans the entire spectrum of behavioral science, from concern with single-cell function to broad social theory; studies that address problems of the malfunctioning brain, the sick family, and the unstable society; programs designed to shed light on the origins, diagnosis, and treatment of mental illness, and on the nature of social ills and their consequences.

A key element of the institute's extramural research program is its flexible response to human needs in contemporary society to promote the effective functioning of the family. Research and training grants are awarded by

NIMH for studies of child and family mental health, studies of crime and delinquency, minority group mental health programs, and studies of problems associated with living in crowded, urban societies.

Special projects are directed to the needs of new towns; the environmental impact on individual functioning; the extent to which work related problems are contributing to a decline in physical and mental health, decreased family stability, and a lessening of community cohesiveness; and the mental health needs of the population in times of natural disasters such as floods and earthquakes.

In addition to supporting extramural research, the NIMH conducts in its own laboratories extensive investigations into the causes, treatment, and prevention of mental disorders and into the biological and psychosocial factors that determine human behavior and development. Its scientists represent many professional disciplines concerned with mental illness and its wide-ranging effects. Neurophysiologists, neuropsychologists, biochemists, and pharmacologists undertake to understand brain function and the complex interrelations of brain and behavior; psychologists, psychiatrists, and sociologists attempt to deal with problems at the human level studying children, adolescents, and adults in their environments—the family, the school, the job, and the society. Collaboration across disciplines is frequent.

The first NIMH research grant was made in 1947 to investigate the neurological aspects of learning; in 1975 the NIMH funded approximately 1,500 research projects. More than a billion dollars—one fourth of the total NIMH budget—has been invested in research.

Among the most dramatic illustrations of the results of this research is the emergence in the mid-1950s of the era of psychopharmacology. The introduction of reserpine in 1953, and later of chlorpromazine in the treatment of mental illness brought new hope for thousands. More recently, NIMH-supported trials to evaluate the efficacy of lithium carbonate has led to the widespread use of that drug in the treatment of mania and depression.

The effectiveness of these therapeutic drugs, specifically the major and minor tranquilizers and lithium carbonate, in controlling symptoms of the two major psychoses, schizophrenia and manic-depressive psychoses, have made possible the release of thousands of patients from public mental hospitals, allowing these patients to be treated in community-based facilities after short-term inpatient care. Since 1955, the peak year for resident inpatient population in state and county mental hospitals, the number of patients in these facilities has declined for 19 consecutive years from 558,922 to 215,566, a 61% decrease.

Other major achievements of the NIMH research program include:

1. Discovery of certain brain chemicals, the neurotransmitters, whose normal function is essential for mental health. An NIMH scientist, Julius Axelrod, won a Nobel prize for his basic contributions to these findings

2. Evidence of a hereditary factor in schizophrenia and depression and considerable progress toward understanding under what conditions it is expressed

3. Development of behavior therapy based on findings from basic research on the learning process in animals and human beings which has been used successfully to alter the behavior of hitherto untreatable psychotic and retarded children, of adults suffering disabling phobias, and of long-hospitalized mental patients

4. Means of controlling through biofeedback one's own heart rate, brain waves, blood pressure, and other functions previously considered to be entirely automatic, with the resultant possibility of developing more effective treatment for psychosomatic disorders

5. Greater understanding of the phenomenon of sleep and dreams.

Prior to 1974, NIMH did extensive research in alcohol abuse and drug abuse and addiction. All research, training, and service programs connected with these two fields are now the responsibility of separate institutes, which along with NIMH are the components of the Alcohol, Drug Abuse, and Mental Health Administration in the Public Health Service of the Department of Health, Education, and Welfare.

Service

The NIMH is not a direct treatment facility. It does, however, provide a variety of nontreatment services to the general public and to the national and international scientific and professional communities.

The institute's National Clearinghouse for Mental Health Information, as part of the NIMH mission to promote mental health, collects and disseminates to the lay public, scientists, and other professionals vast amounts of information gathered from more than 40 countries on mental health programs and research findings.

Another institute service function is collecting statistics on the incidence and epidemiology of mental illness in the United States, and the utilization patterns of various mental health facilities. The collecting, analyzing, and disseminating of such data by the NIMH biometry branch aids in delineating the parameters of the problems of mental illness, provides a deeper understanding of mental health needs versus availability of resources, and facilitates planning mental health programs and allocating resources to meet anticipated needs.

The NIMH, through grants, supports a variety of direct treatment programs. The highlight of this service-support program is one which assists communities across the United States to develop mental health centers where people with emotional problems may obtain comprehensive and continuing treatment in their home communities. The community mental health centers program is the culmination of a series of events which started in 1955 with the appointment of a Joint Commission on Mental Illness to make an intensive five-year study of the mental health needs and resources of the United States. The commission's landmark report, *Action for Mental Health,* included recommendations for a variety of community-based services for the treatment and prevention of mental and emotional illness. These recommendations inspired the first Presidential message to Congress on the nation's mental health objectives. President John F. Kennedy, on February 3, 1963, appealed for new federal programs on behalf of the mentally ill. This led to the passage of the Mental Retardation Facilities and Community Mental Health Centers Act of 1963 which in turn led to a new era of federal support for mental health services.

Community mental health centers are planned and run by people in the community, with initial help from the federal government in the form of construction and staffing grants. To be eligible for such support, a center must offer inpatient and outpatient care, partial hospitalization (day, night, or weekend care), around-the-clock emergency services, and the indirect service of consultation and education to community agencies and to service professionals such as physicians, clergy, and teachers.

Many community mental health centers also provide additional services such as rehabilitation, training, research and evaluation, and special services for specific patient groups such as alcoholics, drug abusers, and rape victims.

Each center serves a distinct community or catchment area ranging in size from 75,000 to 200,000 persons. Community mental health centers are located in each of the 50 states, Guam, the Virgin Islands, Puerto Rico, and the District of Columbia. Of the 591 centers funded, 443 were in operation in 1975. When fully functioning the 591 centers will service approximately 41% of the nation's population.

At Saint Elizabeths Hospital, division of clinical and community services, NIMH professional staff and scientists provide treatment and rehabilitation for psychiatric patients. The division also operates a model comprehensive community mental health center, conducts and coordinates hospital training and research programs, and provides administrative support to other components of ADAMHA operating within the hospital.

Training

A major program goal of the NIMH is to increase the quality and quantity of personnel working in mental health and related fields. The institute's tasks in the area of manpower and training fall into two categories. The first is to plan and support programs to develop the training and utilization of mental health manpower to meet mental health service delivery systems and research needs, through manpower research and demonstration projects, training in the mental health core disciplines and related fields, and technical assistance to states, local governments, service agencies and training institutions. The second is to keep abreast of the nation's requirements in the areas of manpower planning, training, development, and utilization, through the collection and analysis of data from nationwide surveys and studies.

To increase mental health manpower resources in the United States, NIMH concentrates its program efforts on effective use of all available mental health personnel and ways to provide training for additional manpower. A variety of approaches is used—professional education and inservice training; community consultation to strengthen the mental health skills of caregivers such as religious leaders, teachers, and welfare workers; and the development of new types of mental health workers, variously designated as paraprofessionals, mental health technicians, mental health associates, and new careerists.

Through these efforts and the more traditional grant-supported fellowships and institutional-based training programs, today there are almost 90,000 professionals in organized care settings, both public and private, with an additional 20,000 in private practice. In addition, there are almost 150,000 auxiliary mental health workers employed in hospitals, community mental health centers, clinics, day care facilities, residential treatment centers, and other multi-service facilities, both private and public.

NIMH in the World Community

NIMH recognizes that the development of knowledge about mental illness and mental health has been marked by "cross fertilization" between professionals in many countries.

To facilitate this exchange of information, NIMH utilizes the skills of visiting scientists in its laboratories; sends American scientists abroad on research fellowships for advanced study; supports international conferences for the exchange of research findings; and participates in the World Health Organization.

NIMH allocates a portion of its research resources to foreign grantees and participates in collaborative international studies. These have included: a 1972 mission to assess schizophrenia research in the Soviet Union; collaboration in a World Health Organization program to set up and operate an international reference center network for psychotropic drugs; an international pilot study of schizophrenia; a six-country study of the effects of modernization; a cross national project between the U.S. and the United Kingdom; psychotherapeutic drug trials among English general practitioners; a study of autistic children in England and of suicide in Scandinavia; research on super-sensitive laboratory methods in Sweden; and three projects in Canada—megavitamin treatment, culture and tranquilizers, and drugs for the aged.

The multidisciplinary national and international programs of the NIMH are all directed toward a single, ultimate goal, to provide comprehensive and coordinated mental health services to all those in need, drawing on the fruits of research and the expertise of skilled professionals in all parts of the world.

Bertram S. Brown became Director of the National Institute of Mental Health in 1970. Previous directors were Stanley F. Yolles (1964–1970) and Robert Felix (1946–1964).

BIBLIOGRAPHY

NATIONAL INSTITUTE OF MENTAL HEALTH. *A national view of mental health.* DHEW Publication No. (NIH) 74–661. Washington, D.C.: Superintendent of Documents, U.S. Government Printing Office, 1974.

NATIONAL INSTITUTE OF MENTAL HEALTH. *Explorations in mental health training.* DHEW Publication No. (ADM) 74–109. Washington, D.C.: Superintendent of Documents, U.S. Government Printing Office, 1974.

NATIONAL INSTITUTE OF MENTAL HEALTH. *International collaboration in mental health.* DHEW Publication No. (HSM) 73–9120. Washington, D.C.: Superintendent of Documents, U.S. Government Printing Office, 1973.

NATIONAL INSTITUTE OF MENTAL HEALTH. *Mental health program reports (No. 6).* DHEW Publication No. (HSM) 73–9139. Washington, D.C.: Superintendent of Documents, U.S. Government Printing Office, 1973.

NATIONAL INSTITUTE OF MENTAL HEALTH. *National Institute of Mental Health at work for you.* DHEW Publication No. (ADM) 75–213. Washington, D.C.: Superintendent of Documents, U.S. Government Printing Office, 1975.

NATIONAL INSTITUTE OF MENTAL HEALTH. *Research in the service of mental health: Report of the research task force of the National Institute of Mental Health.* DHEW Publication No. (ADM) 75–236. Washington, D.C.: Superintendent of Documents, U.S. Government Printing Office, 1975.

NATIONAL INSTITUTE OF MENTAL HEALTH. *Lithium in the treatment of mood disorders.* DHEW Publication No. (ADM) 74–73. Washington, D.C.: Superintendent of Documents, U.S. Government Printing Office, 1974.

NATIONAL INSTITUTE OF MENTAL HEALTH. *Mental health of rural America: The rural programs of the National Institute of Mental Health.* DHEW Publication No. (HSM) 73–9035. Washington, D.C.: Superintendent of Documents, U.S. Government Printing Office, 1973.

NATIONAL INSTITUTE OF MENTAL HEALTH. *Mental illness and its treatment.* DHEW Publication No. (HSM) 73–9035. Washington, D.C.: Superintendent of Documents, U.S. Government Printing Office, 1973.

NATIONAL INSTITUTE OF MENTAL HEALTH. *Schizophrenia bulletin—Summer 1974.* DHEW Publication No. (ADM) 75–145. Washington, D.C.: Superintendent of Documents, U.S. Government Printing Office, 1975.

BERTRAM S. BROWN

NATIVISM AND EMPIRICISM IN PERCEPTION

The scientific study of perception began in the nineteenth century and proceeded at a rapid pace. In his *Physiological Optics* Helmholtz summarized an enormous body of knowledge, much of which was the result of his own investigations. It was Helmholtz who first formulated clearly the theoretical positions of the *innate* or *intuitive theory* of spatial experience on the one hand and on the other, of the *empirical theory.* The innate theory, he explained, ruled out any further investigation of the origin of spatial perceptions by regarding them simply as a function of hypothetical neural mechanisms assumed to be inborn. Helmholtz, a strong empiricist, claimed that all aspects of perception are determined by experiential factors, including memory, judgment, expectation, and reasoning. Sensations, he maintained, provide only a "sign" for external objects and events, and the interpretation of these signs is learned.

On the nativistic side, Hering explained the experience of location and depth in the visual field on the basis of fixed retinal mechanisms and proposed particular neural processes as the basis for such phenomena as color contrast and constancy. However, he never denied the role of memory factors in perception.

Helmholtz's influence on perceptual theory has remained a powerful one, and his concept of "unconscious inference" has reappeared again and again. From the establishment of Wundt's laboratory in 1879 until well into the twentieth century the empiricist outlook remained dominant. Whether the psychologist was a structuralist, functionalist, behaviorist, or act theorist, he implicitly or explicitly accepted the view that the raw sensory input had to be elaborated into a percept by psychic functions based on past learning.

Gestalt. During this period a great deal of research in perception was undertaken by ophthalmologists, physicists, and physiologists who in many cases favored nativism. In psychology, however, the main exponents of nativism (in a modified form) were members of the Gestalt school. Since the fundamental concept of Gestalt psychology is that experience is inherently organized, the idea that the experienced world is initially a mosaic or patchwork of sensations was completely unacceptable. The hundreds of pages devoted to problems of perception in Kurt Koffka's *Principles of Gestalt Psychology* (1935) constitute a polemic against empiricist concepts.

Gestalt psychologist opposed the definition of perception as the interpretation of sensation; they did not consider sensations to be part of phenomenal experience but rather products of artificial analysis. They showed that the effective stimulus for a percept is relational in nature, thus making it unnecessary to refer to past experience. In place of the innate anatomical structures of the nineteenth century nativist they substituted the concept of dynamic self-distributing processes in the brain, i.e., sensory organization. These processes of organization are not learned nor are they products of inherited neural "wiring." Gestalt theorists did not deny that past experience plays a role in perception. They insisted, however, that the empiricist provide a plausible account of how a particular perception could be learned.

"New Look." Apart from the Gestalt school, perception was not a major research area in psychology for many years. In the 1940s there occurred a remarkable revival of interest in problems of perception, mainly from an empiristic standpoint. A neofunctionalist approach called for bringing perceptual investigations from the laboratory darkroom into the light. This so-called new look psychology considered perceptual experience to be influenced by personality and learning variables such as needs, motives, emotions, reward and punishment. Many experiments were generated by this approach but most frequently the effects of these variables were found to be extremely small. Moreover, most of the research did not deal with perception in the traditional sense of the term (i.e., the experience of spatial relations, movement, form, perceptual constancy, color, etc.) but with the processes of recognition and interpretation.

Transactionalism

A different theoretical current at the same time arose from the "demonstrations" of Adalbert Ames, Jr. (1955). His distorted room was perceived from a particular viewing point as a normal rectangular room, his rotating trapezoidal window was seen to oscillate, a stationary expanding and contracting luminous balloon was perceived to approach and recede in space. Discussions of these demonstrations and conferences with psychologists, educators and philosophers led to the development of what Ames believed to be a revolutionary new interpretation of the philosophical and psychological problems of perception. This approach came to be known as transactionalism and represented a radical version of empiricism. Helmholtz's concept of unconscious inference was incorporated into the view that perception is based on assumptions developed in the course of purposive action. According to the transactionalists, the distorted room is seen as normal because most frequently in our world rooms are rectilinear and the trapezoid is seen to oscillate because of our assumption that windows are rectangular. At present, little support is given to the transactionalist theory; the demonstrations, however, are valuable. The distorted room and the chair demonstration are useful for making clear that perception is determined not by the physical object in the external world but by the retinal stimulation to which it gives rise and the trapezoidal oscillation can be explained without reference to assumptions about the rectangularity of windows.

Hebb's Theory

An empiristic account of the origin and development of form perception was presented by Hebb in his book, *Organization and Behavior* (1949). Hebb was convinced of the validity of empiricism mainly through two lines of evidence. First was the work by Riesen (1950) of vision in dark-reared chimpanzees and second, the analysis by von Senden (1960) of some 60 case reports describing visual experience in congenital cataract patients after surgery.

Riesen raised chimpanzees in complete darkness with but 90 minutes of diffuse light stimulation each day. Tests in an illuminated environment revealed serious deficiencies in the visual behavior of the subjects. For example, they were significantly retarded in mastery of visual discrimination problems as compared with normal controls.

According to Hebb, form perception in these animals was deficient because there was no opportunity for perceptual learning. A different interpretation—that darkroom rearing interfered with the normal maturation of the visual system—was later confirmed in histological studies by Riesen and others (1961). There is convincing evidence that light stimulation (in fact, even patterned light) is necessary for the normal functioning of visual structures but this fact does not support an empiristic explanation of form perception nor deny the validity of a nativistic account.

Von Senden's data have been cited by both nativists and empiricists as evidence in favor of their respective positions. Wertheimer pointed out in 1951 that it is necessary to distinguish between the first-hand data in the case reports (usually written by the surgeon), von Senden's analysis of these reports, and Hebb's interpretation of von Senden. According to Hebb, the data indicated that patients first experienced a kind of amorphous mass and gradually, with great difficulty, learned to see and discriminate shaped objects in their visual field. There is no unambiguous evidence, however, that patients could not discriminate forms. When shown a sphere and a cube and asked which was the cube and which the sphere, patients usually were unable to say. What is the source of their difficulty—that the objects are not *perceived* as different shapes or that the patients are unable to *identify* the two perceived shapes? This ambiguity is perhaps the explanation for the fact that nativists and empiricists alike have cited the cataract data, but actually neither side could rely on this evidence, for none of the case reports was based on systematic observation and experimentation. There are serious problems with visual function such as muscle cramp and nystagmus; there are motivational and emotional factors which affect the ability of the patient to adjust to a newly experienced visual world; and many patients had difficulty in verbalizing their experiences.

Current Research

The middle 1950s saw a surge of research efforts utilizing new methods and new techniques; response indicators were found which made it possible to investigate perception in animal and human infants. Walk and Gibson (1961) using the "visual cliff" apparatus obtained evidence that a wide variety of animal species and human infants by the crawling stage could discriminate depth differences. The nativistic position for distance perception was supported in studies with dark-reared rats and animals in the first day after birth. Fantz (1961) utilized a visual interest test as an indicator and investigated the development of pattern discrimination in the human infant. Reaction to novelty, changes in heart and sucking rate have also served as indicators in studies of infant perception. With a modified discrimination apparatus and training begun at 11 days of age, rhesus monkeys (Zimmermann, Torrey, 1965) required only 10 days to reach criterion on a form discrimination task. Bower (1974) in a number of ingenious experiments has analyzed various aspects of object and space perception in infants.

It is still too early to claim that the nativism-empiricism has been resolved. Perhaps the most significant advance has been a growth of theoretical sophistication which is making possible a more fruitful formulation of this ancient controversy. In the past nativists and empiricists argued about perception in general or about large areas of perceptual functioning. In recent years research questions have become more specific. For example, is a particular distance cue innately based? What is the origin of size constancy? How does form perception develop? A nativistic answer for one aspect of perception does not preclude an empiristic account of another.

Secondly, greater clarification has been achieved with respect to the concepts of learning and innateness. Traditional nativism assumed the existence of fixed structures and mechanisms which made it difficult to account for the flexibility and adaptiveness of the perceptual system. Empiricism, on the other hand, could not provide an adequate description of the learning process. A position which is emerging from the research and theorizing of the past decade can be characterized briefly as follows: What is "built-in" or innate is not fixed prewired structures but rather rules or principles which guide the learning process along certain paths. For example, Wallach (1975) has shown that position constancy is quickly reestablished when new relationships between retinal image displacements and head movements are imposed by the use of lenses. This flexibility can be understood by assuming the existence of a principle or rule which directs the perceptual system to discount image movement which covaries with head movement. A modified nativism of this kind has been proposed by Bower (1974), in order to explain how the perceptual system can adapt to the changes in proximal stimulus information produced during the course of the infant's growth.

BIBLIOGRAPHY

AMES, A., JR. *An interpretative manual.* Princeton, N.J.: Princeton University Press, 1955.

BOWER, T. G. R. *Development in infancy.* San Francisco: Freeman, 1974.

FANTZ, R. L. The origin of form perception. *Scientific American,* 1961, *204,* 66–72.

HEBB, D. O. *The organization of behavior.* New York: Wiley, 1949.

RIESEN, A. Arrested vision. *Scientific American,* 1950, *183,* 16–19.

VON SENDEN, M. *Space and sight.* London: Methuen, 1960.

WALK, R. D., and GIBSON, E. J. A comparative and analytical study of visual depth perception. *Psychological Monographs,* 1961, *75.*

WALLACH, H. *On perception.* New York: Quadrangle Books, 1975.

WERTHEIMER, M.; HEBB, D. O.; and VON SENDEN, M. On the role of learning in perception. *American Journal of Psychology,* 1951, *64,* 133–137.

ZIMMERMANN, R. R., and TORREY, C. C. Ontogeny of learning. In A. M. Schrier et al. (Eds.), *Behavior of nonhuman primates* (Vol. 2). New York: Academic Press, 1965.

See also PERCEPTUAL AFTEREFFECTS; PERCEPTUAL LEARNING; SENSATION AND PERCEPTION: AN OVERVIEW

CARL B. ZUCKERMAN

NEED

In ordinary usage *need* denotes both necessity and want or desire. These obliquely related meanings continue to inform the psychological usage of the term. The early writings of Woodworth, Freud, and Lewin use the term to refer to those appetitive necessities whose deficiency or deprivation could be counted upon to produce action that is purposive and goal-seeking. However, before 1920 there was no inclination to elevate the word *need* to conceptual status. It was simply used in ordinary discourse as synonymous with instinct, desire, and want. As greater rigor was sought in defining the attributes of motivating conditions, the necessity-want distinction emerged with greater clarity, and theorists began to differ in the emphasis they wished to give motivational terms. Those concentrating on appetitive systems settled on *drive* and relegated *need* to a physiological state of the total organism, created by deprivation and sensitizing the organism to drive stimuli. Theorists concerned with goal-seeking and purposive behavior found drive limiting and instead emphasized the *wanting, desiring* dimension.

Kurt Lewin, in his effort to portray the tension-like character of choice and strategy selection introduced need *(Bedürfnisse)* as a construct denoting biologically rooted determinants having a quasi-directional (goal-oriented) character which contributed one element to his equations designed to account for purposive action. Out of need came *tension* which, in combination with *valence,* produced flexible, adaptive, dynamic behavior (1936).

Murray

In 1938, Henry Murray's *Explorations in Personality* presented a motivational interpretation of personality function that placed the need construct at the heart of the system. It was the array and amalgam of needs that best illuminated the behavior of individuals. He defined and described need as

a construct (a convenient fiction or hypothetical concept) which stands for a force (the physico-chemical nature of which is unknown) in the brain region, a force which organizes perception, apperception, intellection, conation, and action in such a way as to transform in a certain direction an existing, unsatisfying situation. A need is sometimes provoked directly by internal processes of a certain kind (viscerogenic, endocrinogenic, thalamicogenic) arising in the course of vital sequences, but, more frequently (when in a state of readiness), by the occurrence of one of a few commonly effective *press* (or by anticipatory images of such press). Thus, it manifests itself by leading the organism to search for or to avoid encountering or, when encountered, to attend and respond to certain kinds of press. It may even engender illusory perceptions and delusory apperceptions (projections of its imaged press into unsuitable objects). Each need is characteristically accompanied by a particular feeling or emotion and tends to use certain modes (subneeds and actones) to further its trend. It may be weak or intense, momentary or enduring. But usually it persists and gives rise to a certain course of overt behavior (or fantasy), which (if the organism is competent and external opposition not insurmountable) changes the initiating circumstances in such a way as to bring about an end situation which stills (appeases or satisfies) the organism. (p. 123)

Despite the all-embracing generality of definition, Murray proceeded to investigate empirically the presence of need foci and composed a list of viscerogenic and psychogenic needs derived from objective and projective measures taken repeatedly from a group of young men. This more or less exhaustive list was combined with a similar analysis of press demands to define situations in a psychosocial manner.

Later Theories

Subsequent theorists have used need in more restricted ways. Abraham Maslow's *Motivation and Personality* (1954) organized need systems into a functional hierarchy emphasizing the growth dimension of personality from securing satisfaction of basic deficiency needs to realizing fully the unique capacities of the self. The hierarchy is composed of five classes of needs: physiological, safety, affiliative, esteem, and self-actualization. Despite the liberal use of the need construct, Maslow did not provide an explicit definition. Rather, he preferred to blend both functional (directional) and dispositional (tensional) qualities while insisting that all levels of the hierarchy were basic and constitutional in origin.

Nuttin (1968) in *Reward and Punishment in Human Learning* formally defines needs as

those organism-environment interactions that demonstrate the characteristic of requiredness, which manifests itself (a) by the existence of a coordinated hierarchy of activities within the organism's behavioral repertoire serving to maintain the required interaction, and (b) by the fact that the organism deteriorates physically or mentally if the relationships cannot be established or maintained. Needs are . . . not merely . . . states of deficiency in the organism [but include] . . . the required interactions with the environment. Since a wide variety of the organism's activities function to ensure that the state of deficiency is never, or, at best, rarely experienced, it seems appropriate to regard the deficiency state as only a phase in the total structure that constitutes the need. (p. 129)

This use captures the environmental role in a lock-and-key fashion (requiredness) having a distinct Darwinian flavor and directs attention to those cognitive and affective processes which develop in the service of needs.

The term *need* has also been adopted by theorists who prefer *motive* as their central construct. Following Murray, McClelland et al. (1953) used projective measurement to assess the preoccupation of the subject with particular themes of loss or attainment. Systems labeled need Achievement (n Ach), Affiliation (n Aff) and Power (n Power) are used to assess motive strength. These scores are then combined with indices of expectancy and value to generate estimate of motivation or action tendency. This use of need as a score label is also found in the Edwards Personal Preference Scale which uses Murray's list as the basis for a self-report personality measure.

Perhaps due to the use of need among personality theorists, the term has appeared in a formal way among learning theorists as well. Hull (1943) uses the term in his *Principles of Behavior* to refer to states of disequilibrium or deficiency which give rise to drive states, the prime motivational term. Woodworth (1958) in his *Dynamics of Behavior* refers to physiological needs as producing a set in the organism to respond. As research progresses in physiological psychology, use of the term in this way has declined and it has been returned to ordinary usage.

BIBLIOGRAPHY

Lewin, K. *Principles of topological psychology.* New York: McGraw-Hill, 1936.

McCLELLAND, D. C.; ATKINSON, J. W.; CLARK, R. A.; and LOWELL, E. L. *The achievement motive.* New York: Appleton-Century-Crofts, 1953.

WOODWORTH, R. S. *Dynamics of behavior.* New York: Holt, 1958.

ROBERT C. BIRNEY

NEEDS

See MOTIVATION

NEGATIVE THERAPEUTIC REACTION

The first reference to the negative therapeutic reaction was by Freud (1918) who, in reporting his experience with the Wolf Man, referred to the patient's "habit of producing transitory 'negative reactions'; every time something had been conclusively cleared up, he attempted to contradict the effect for a short while by an aggravation of the symptom which had been cleared up" (p. 69). He compared it to the tendency of children to respond negativistically to prohibitions when they are first invoked.

However, in *The Ego and the Id,* Freud (1923) raised such negative reactions, if they are sustained and refractory, to the level of a recognizable syndrome, the "negative therapeutic reaction," of which he wrote:

Every partial solution that ought to result, and in other people does result, in an improvement or a temporary suspension of symptoms produces in them for the time being an exacerbation of their illness; they get worse during the treatment instead of getting better. They exhibit what is known as a "negative therapeutic reaction." There is no doubt that there is something in these people that sets itself against their recovery, and its approach is dreaded as though it were a danger. We are accustomed to say that the need for illness has got the upper hand in them over the desire for recovery. (p. 49)

As Freud conceived of the syndrome of the negative therapeutic reaction, it exemplified the potential intransigence of the superego and the aggression embodied in an unconscious sense of guilt and the "masochism immanent in so many people" (Freud, 1937, p. 243). Subsequently others broadened the concept to include additional etiological determinants. Karen Horney (1936) took up ego and technical aspects in emphasizing that negative therapeutic reactions develop out of a masochistic character structure, are pervasively narcissistic, and are characterized by negative transference reactions with essential competitiveness to the analyst and to his interpretive efforts. Such patients are exceedingly vulnerable in their self-esteem and are afraid of success, which to them connotes the destruction of others. As she put it, "The negative therapeutic reaction is a special form of the fear of success. . . . Where Freud stresses feelings of guilt I have emphasized anxiety" (p. 38ff).

Joan Riviere (1936) applied the Kleinian point of view of internalized objects and the manic defense against a depressive position to a consideration of the problem of the negative therapeutic reaction. Her major emphasis was on the extent to which ambivalence exists unconsciously in the extremes of love and hate for the internalized object. Stanley Olinick (1964) suggested that

those people who display the negative therapeutic reaction were endowed from birth with greater than average funds of aggressive orality and anality. This in turn made the mothering relationship stressful (as it may later the analytic), by investing it with realistic anxieties about filling an assigned role with these masterful infants and children. (p. 544)

Both in this paper and in an updated recapitulation (1970), Olinick emphasized that

the negative therapeutic reaction is an acute, recurrent, negativistic emotional crisis in a sadomasochistic person who is prone to depression; it represents a category of superego resistance . . . denotable also as a phase of transference resistance. (p. 666)

The negativism, which he sees as highly characteristic, is oppositionally defensive against "the regressive pull towards fusion with an early, depressive, maternal object" (p. 657).

In consonance with this point of view, Anna Freud (1952) in an earlier contribution to states of negativism and emotional surrender, wrote:

Such persons see the relation to a love object exclusively in passive terms. . . . The passive surrender may signify a return from object love proper to its forerunner in the emotional development of the infant, i.e., primary identification with the love object. This is a regressive step which implies a threat to the intactness of the ego, i.e., a loss of personal characteristics which are merged with the characteristics of the love object. The individual fears this regression in terms of dissolution of the personality, loss of sanity, and defends himself against it by a complete rejection of all objects (negativism). (p. 258f)

Current Ideas

More recent formulations have underscored the significance of very early experience. Trauma during this phase is pivotal, in that it apparently influences instinctual and affective patterns, establishing a predilection for psychic pain within the self as well as in response to objects which may find later expression in the form of a negative therapeutic reaction. Loewald (1972) suggested:

In its more intractable forms the negative therapeutic reaction is rooted in preoedipal, primitive distortions of instinctual and ego development and is thus hardly amenable to interpretations in terms of guilt, conscience, and need for punishment. (p. 244)

Valenstein (1973), writing "On Attachment to Painful Feelings and the Negative Therapeutic Reaction," observed:

The attachment to pain—I might even say, in terms of masochism as well as the instinctual drives, the fixation to pain—generally suggests a major problem in object tie from the first year of life and thereafter. (p. 373)

He saw the nuclear determinant of the "negative therapeutic reaction" as being located much earlier than definitive superego formation. It originates in the very young child's failure to establish constancy in relation to a positively valued object, without which increments of pleasurable affect are neither consolidated out of object experience, nor reliably anticipated thereafter. In fact, the opposite prevails, namely, the development of an affinity for painful affect, the painful affect states connoting the inconsistently pleasure-unpleasure yielding object (p. 390).

So far as the technical difficulties encountered in the treatment of such conditions is concerned, Valenstein saw psychoanalysis as such and insight as being distinctly limited in its effect, since articulate and succinct interpretation can hardly be expected to reach the preverbal—earliest—level of development. However, if the therapist persists in working toward the possibility that the patient can and will progressively and adaptively use both what is recapitulated and articulately remembered, and what is behaviorally recapitulated and reconstructed from the time when it cannot be literally remembered, then the outcome might be the achievement of a significant measure of corrective experiential reeducation supplemented by cognitive understanding (p. 390).

BIBLIOGRAPHY

FREUD, A. (1952). Notes on a connection between the states of negativism and of emotional surrender *(Horigkeit). The writings of Anna Freud* (Vol. 4). New York: International Universities Press, 1968. Pp. 256–259.

FREUD, S. (1918). From the history of an infantile neurosis. *Standard Edition, 17.* London: Hogarth Press, 1955. Pp. 3–123.

FREUD, S. (1923). The ego and the id. *Standard Edition,* 1961, *19,* 3–66.

FREUD, S. (1937). Analysis terminable and interminable. *Standard Edition,* 1964, *23,* 209–253.

HORNEY, K. The problem of the negative therapeutic reaction. *Psychoanalytic Quarterly,* 1936, *5,* 29–44.

LOEWALD, H. W. Freud's conception of the negative therapeutic reaction, with comments on instinct theory. *Journal of the American Psychoanalytic Association,* 1972, *20,* 235–245.

OLINICK, S. L. The negative therapeutic reaction. *International Journal of Psycho-Analysis,* 1964, *45,* 540–548.

OLINICK, S. L. Panel report: Negative therapeutic reaction. *Journal of the American Psychoanalytic Association,* 1970, *18,* 665–672.

RIVIERE, J. A contribution to the analysis of the negative therapeutic reaction. *International Journal of Psycho-Analysis,* 1936, *17,* 304–320.

VALENSTEIN, A. On attachment to painful feelings and the negative therapeutic reaction. *The Psychoanalytic Study of the Child,* 1973, *28,* 365–392.

ARTHUR F. VALENSTEIN

NEOBEHAVIORISM: C. L. HULL'S SYSTEM

The term *neobehaviorism* has no clear-cut referent. It has been applied to all behavioristically oriented theorists who became prominent after about 1930: E. R. Guthrie, C. L. Hull, B. F. Skinner, and E. C. Tolman as well as their students and followers. The term has also been used in a more restricted sense, however, to refer to the *hypothetico-deductive* approach of C. L. Hull and was as such suggested by Hull himself (1952, p. 154). It is so interpreted here.

After his dissertation, which dealt with the formation of concepts (1920), he concerned himself with the effects of tobacco smoking on the efficiency of behavior (1924), the area of tests and measurement, especially aptitude testing (1928) and hypnosis and suggestibility (1933). After his appointment as research professor at Yale University in 1929, Hull turned to the development of a hypothetico-deductive behavior theory (1940; 1942; 1943; 1951; 1952). A fondness for the geometrical tradition of Euclid began during Hull's high school years:

The study of geometry proved to be the most important event of my intellectual life; it opened to me an entirely new world—the fact that thought itself could generate and really prove new relationships from previously possessed elements. Later, in the writing of a prep school paper in English composition, I tried to use the geometrical method to deduce some negative propositions regarding theology. This ultimately led to the study of Spinoza's *Ethics;* while I admired his brilliance I could not accept some of his postulates and therefore I rejected nearly all his theorems. (1952a, 144)

Newton's *Principia Mathematica* which deduced "by a rigorous process of reasoning the complex structure of (his) system" starting from "eight explicitly stated definitions and three postulates" became the chosen model at a later time (1935, p. 494).

Hull's neobehavioristic position was strongly influenced by the views of J. B. Watson "whose ideas about behavior were in the air" at the time of Hull's undergraduate work. Although "inclined to be sympathetic with Watson's views concerning the futility of introspection and the general virtues of objectivity . . . [Hull] . . . felt very uncertain about many of his dogmatic claims" (1952a, p. 153). The objectivism of early behaviorism had partly been a methodological prescription and partly a metaphysical thesis. Methodologically objectivity in science meant to insist on the intersubjective verification of definitions, procedures and observations. This stance, however, was sometimes presented along with a denial of the "existence of consciousness." For Hull the existence of consciousness was not to be denied but appeared to be "a problem needing solution" (1937, p. 30).

In his autobiography Hull acknowledges the influence of Kurt Koffka and Gestalt psychology. Koffka's criticisms of J. B. Watson's views led Hull to the conclusion

not that the Gestalt view was sound but rather that Watson had not made out as clear a case for behaviorism as the facts warranted . . . the result was a belated conversion to a kind of neo-behaviorism—a behaviorism mainly concerned with the determination of the quantitative laws of behavior and their deductive systematization. (1952a, p. 154)

Such an approach was also suggested "as a way out" of the many conflicting points of view, schools and systems of psychology around 1930. Hull (1952a) himself had come to

the definite conclusion around 1930 that psychology is a true natural science; that its primary laws are expressible quantitatively by means of a moderate number of ordinary equations; that all the complex behavior of single individuals will ultimately be derivable as secondary laws from (1) these primary laws together with (2) the conditions under which behavior occurs; and that all the behavior of groups as a whole, i.e., strictly social behavior as such, may similarly be derived as quantitative laws from the same primary equations. With these and similar views as a background, the task of psychologists obviously is that of laying bare these laws as quickly and accurately as possible, particularly the primary laws. (p. 155)

Hull's conceptual analysis of "learning," "trial and error" and rate-memorization were also much influenced by the publication of a translation of I. P. Pavlov's work on *Conditioned Reflexes* in 1927 and of which Hull at once began an intensive study (1952a, p. 154). It led to an extensive review of the then existent literature (1934), a persistent attempt to interpret all types of learning phenomena in terms of conditioning, and a long series of influential papers in the *Psychological Review,* the major theoretical journal in the field.

An early ambitious elaboration of Hull's general methodological approach was based on "the hypothesis that the remote excitatory tendencies of Ebbinghaus were essentially identical with the delayed or trace conditioned reflexes of Pavlov." Elaborating on Pavlov's concept of "inhibition of delay" Hull's theoretical analysis of "rote learning" resulted in "a formal statement of definitions and postulates together with the formal deduction of eleven theorems by a method resembling that of geometry" (1935). The latter method was possibly influenced by the axiomatics of the mathematician M. Pieri (1860–1904). Further work on the problem of rote learning convinced Hull (1938) "that the geometrical method was very clumsy" and he "abandoned it for that of ordinary mathematics." This of course required the formulation of the postulates in such a way that they could be converted into equations (1952a, p. 157). The eventual result became the "Mathematic-Deductive Theory of Rote Learning" (1940).

A few years before Hull abandoned geometry for "ordinary equations," E. C. Tolman had developed R. S. Woodworth's S-O-R formula into a program of theory construction featuring "intervening variables" as a major component of analysis. Hull's adaptation of Tolman's conception led to the systematic theory of the *Principles of Behavior* (1943), a volume which in Hull's own words "was rather different from those commonly offered to psychologists" (1952a, p. 159).

According to Tolman (1936) "Mental processes . . . will figure only in the guise of objectively definable intervening variables . . . a set of intermediating functional processes which interconnect between the initiating causes of behavior, on the one hand and the final resulting behavior itself, on the other" (p. 88). For both Hull and Tolman behavior was a function of many "initiating causes." According to Tolman (1936)

Mental processes are concepts which arise when we attempt further to elaborate the nature of this function. It is in fact so complicated that we at present seem unable to state it in any single simple statement . . . we have to handle it by conceiving it as broken down into successive sets of component functions. (p. 89)

Amalgamating his own hypothetico-deductive postulate system with Tolman's suggestion to break up the too complicated input-output function into "successive sets of component functions" produced the system described in the *Principles of Behavior* (1943) and its elaborations and modifications during the next decade (Hull, 1951; 1952).

A critical evaluation of Hull's attempt to advance psychology in this way can be found in an article by S. Koch (1954). It includes a critical discussion of Hull's method of quantifica-

tion which adapted a scaling technique devised by L. L. Thurstone (1927).

Between 1930 and 1950 Hull was regarded as one of the leading theoretical psychologists of the time. Since his death, however, his theories have been widely criticized (Koch, 1954; Marx and Hillix, 1973, pp. 297–298).

The evaluation of Hull's significance for the history of psychology is therefore likely to change with future oscillations between periods of ambitious system building followed by more modest periods of data gathering.

BIBLIOGRAPHY

HULL, C. L.   Quantitative aspects of the evolution of concepts. *Psychological Monographs,* 1920, *28* (123).

HULL, C. L.   The influence of tobacco smoking on mental and motor efficiency. *Psychological Monographs,* 1924, *33* (3), 1–160.

HULL, C. L.   *Aptitude testing.* Yonkers, New York: World, 1928.

HULL, C. L.   *Hypnosis and suggestibility: An experimental approach.* New York: Appleton-Century-Crofts, 1933.

HULL, C. L.   Learning: II. The factor of the conditioned reflex. In C. Murchison (Ed.), *A handbook of general experimental psychology.* Worcester, Mass.: Clark University Press, 1934.

HULL, C. L.   The conflicting psychologies of learning—a way out. *Psychological Review,* 1935, *42,* 491–516.

HULL, C. L.   Mind, mechanism and adaptive behavior. *Psychological Review,* 1937, *44,* 1–32.

HULL, C. L.   Conditioning: Outline of a systematic theory of learning. In *Forty-first yearbook, part II of the National Society for the Study of Education.* Chicago: University of Chicago Press, 1942. Pp. 61–95.

HULL, C. L.   *Principles of behavior: An introduction to behavior theory.* New York: Appleton-Century-Crofts, 1943.

HULL, C. L.   *Essentials of behavior.* New Haven, Conn.: Yale University Press, 1951.

HULL, C. L.   *A behavior system.* New Haven, Conn.: Yale University Press, 1952.

HULL, C. L.   Clark L. Hull. In E. G. Boring et al. (Eds.), *A history of psychology in autobiography* (Vol. 4). Worcester, Mass: Clark University Press, 1952a. Pp. 143–162.

HULL, C. L. et al.   *Mathematico-deductive theory of rote learning.* New Haven, Conn.: Yale University Press, 1940.

KOCH, S., and C. L. HULL.   In W. K. Estes et al., *Modern learning theory.* New York: Appleton-Century-Crofts, 1954. Pp. 1–176.

MARX, M. H., and HILLIX, W. A.   *Systems and theories in psychology* (2nd ed.). New York: McGraw-Hill, 1973.

THURSTONE, L. L.   A law of comparative judgment. *Psychological Review,* 1927, *34,* 273–286.

TOLMAN, E. C.   Operational behaviorism and current trends in psychology. *Proceedings of the twenty-fifth anniversary celebrating inauguration of graduate studies.* Los Angeles: University of Southern California Press, 1936. Pp. 89–103.

See also HYPOTHETICO-DEDUCTIVE METHOD; LEARNING THEORIES

THOM VERHAVE

NERVE CELLS: NORMAL

Historical Highlights

Current concepts about the morphologic characteristics of the nerve cell, first described by Purkinje (1837) and termed "neuron" by Waldeyer (1891), have evolved not only from advances in cytology in general, with the introduction of formalin (Blum, 1893) and glutaraldehyde (Sabatini et al., 1963) as fixatives, but also from the application to neuroanatomy of tissue culture (Harrison, 1907), enzyme histochemistry (Wolf et al., 1943), autoradiography (protein metabolism: Niklas and Oehlert, 1956; histogenesis: Sauer and Walker, 1959; axonal flow: Droz and Leblond, 1963), electron microscopy (Pease and Baker, 1951), scanning microscopy (Hamberger et al., 1970), and the freeze-fracture technique combined with the electron microscope (Akert et al., 1972). Of more importance has been the use of techniques designed specifically for study of the central nervous system, such as the silver impregnation method of Golgi (1873), the methylene blue vital staining method of Ehrlich (1886), the toluidine blue method of Nissl (1891), fixation by perfusion for electron microscopy by Palay et al. (1962), and fixation with formalin vapor for fluorescence microscopy by Falck and Hillarp (Falck et al., 1962).

With the toluidine blue technique, Nissl (1894) distinguished different types of nerve cells according to their content of "tigroid" substance. This substance, later referred to as Nissl substance, has been identified as ribonucleic acid in microphotometric investigations by Hydén (1943) and found to consist of ribosomes, arranged along membranes as rough endoplasmic reticulum, in electron micrographs by Palay and Palade (1955). A further distinction can be made with other techniques,

whereby some nerve cells stand out by their richer content of transmitter substances, such as acetylcholinesterase (Koelle, 1954), dopamine, 5-hydroxytryptamine and noradrenaline (Dahlström and Fuxe, 1964), or of glycogen (Shimizu and Kumamoto, 1952).

The nerve cells, numbering 2 to 10 billion in the adult human brain (Pakkenberg, 1966) and unable to multiply after reaching a fully differentiated state (Hild, 1959), are distributed according to a specific cytoarchitectonic pattern (Brodmann, 1909). The relative distance between nerve cells ("neurone density": Tower, 1954; "gray-cell" coefficient: Haug, 1963) varies with weight of the brain and mammalian species. Interconnections between regions have been elucidated by tracing the processes from Golgi-impregnated nerve cells (Ramón y Cajal, 1909) and by mapping the site of reactive changes after the experimental destruction of a group of nerve cells or fibers by methods described under "Nerve Cells in Disease." The distribution of fibers between circumscribed gray matter regions follows a distinct pattern, as demonstrated for the brain stem and cerebellum by Brodal (1939) and others. These observations have laid the foundation for an understanding of the pathways or anatomical circuitry available for electrophysiologic activity, an activity which, with sophisticated instrumentation, has been detected in single nerve cells in vivo (Forbes, 1936; Brock et al., 1952) and in vitro (Crain et al., 1953). With the aid of multidisciplinary techniques, a considerable insight has been gained with respect to the normal structure of the neuron and its metabolic properties (diagrammatically illustrated by Droz et al., 1974), and by some techniques, an association between functional state and morphology has been discerned (incorporation of isotope-tagged protein: Schultze and Oehlert, 1958; cholinesterase activity: review in Koelle, 1963).

Research Methods

Various histologic techniques are employed for morphologic studies of the nerve cell, its cell body (perikaryon), processes (axon and dendrites), and terminal endings (boutons terminaux or synaptic complex), and the procedure of fixation is determined by the method selected to visualize a specific element. For histochemical techniques, frozen sections can be prepared from either unfixed or formalin-fixed tissues. In such material, cellular elements are reproduced in their largest size, but because of the friability of the tissue, only small pieces can be cut and, furthermore, continuity of processes with individual cell bodies is broken and the topography of a region is distorted. Better definition of cellular structures is obtained if the tissue is fixed by immersion or perfusion, dehydrated and embedded in paraffin or celloidin for light microscopy or in plastic material for electron microscopy. During dehydration, the tissues undergo shrinkage, that is reduction in volume, which for the brain can amount to 40% to 50% after immersion in 10% formalin and to 10% after perfusion with rapidly acting fixatives such as Bouin's picric acid solution. The severity of shrinkage varies in different regions and between gray and white matter as well as between cytoplasm and nuclei. During cutting with the microtome, paraffin sections are compressed and nucleoli and granular material may be dislodged in the direction of cutting, whereas celloidin sections retain the form and shape of the embedded tissue; plastic material can be cut in ultrathin sections for the electron microscope without signs of dislodgment.

Morphologic Characteristics

The nerve cells are of variable size, the largest occurring in the motor region of the cerebral cortex, the ventral horns of the spinal cord, and the motor nuclei (Fig. 7) and the reticular formation of the brain stem (Fig. 5), and the smallest, represented by the granule cells, like those of the cerebellar cortex (to right of Purkinje cells, *x,* in Fig. 10). In the gray matter, which is composed mainly of nerve cells, the surfaces of the nerve cells are in contact with terminal endings (Fig. 3); these endings are surrounded by astrocytes, which by their content of glycogen can be visualized as a network on the surface of some nerve cells (arrows in Figs. 7 and 9). Oligodendrocytes, microglial cells (*m* in Fig. 10 in "Nerve Cells in Disease"), or blood vessels are often situated near the nerve cells.

The appearance of the nerve cells will vary with the staining technique used, because of differences in distribution and extent of the intracellular organelles which are electively stained, as illustrated by the following examples. With the Golgi method, a few nerve cells—1% to 10%—stand out in their entirety by a massive black metal impregnation (Fig. 1); the dendrites assume a tortuous appearance, contrasting with the tapered form demonstrable with other techniques (Fig. 2). For clarification of structural details, more delicate silver techniques are required, as, for example, Bielschowsky's or Bodian's method for neurofibrils (Fig. 2), Rasmussen's method for terminal endings (Fig. 3), and McDonald's modified technique for the Golgi apparatus (Fig. 6). With Einarson's gallocyanin technique, the Nissl substance is found to be richly developed in some nerve cells (Fig. 5) and only poorly or negligibly in others (Figs. 10 and 11); a looseness in texture of the Nissl substance and an interspersal of minute basophil granules (ribosome complex) is apparent with high-power optics (Fig. 9). When the latter technique is combined with periodic acid-Schiff, the cytoplasm becomes intensely or faintly pink in some nerve cells ("pink" nerve cells, *p* in Fig. 5) and is clear or unstained in others ("blue" nerve cells, *b* in Fig. 5). The stainability of the cytoplasm is ascribed to the diffuse occurrence of glycogen, as evidenced in sections stained for this substance (*x, y, z* in Fig. 7). The two cell types also display subtle differences in the morphology of the Nissl substance, which is coarser, less prominent and purple rather than blue in the "pink" nerve cells. Fat soluble dyes, such as sudan red, oil red O or sudan black are in frozen sections taken up by lipids aggregated in clusters of lipofuscin granules; in paraffin sections, the lipofuscin is stained pink with periodic acid-Schiff (Fig. 10) and exhibits autofluorescence when exposed to ultraviolet light. These granules, increasing with age, accumulate in some groups of nerve cells earlier than in others and irregularly in different species; simultaneously, the content of minute basophil granules is reduced (Cammermeyer, 1963), and changes in distribution of neurofibrils take place (Dayan, 1970). In electron micrographs from ultrathin sections, the various elements of the cytoplasm are distinguished by differences in arrangement of membranes and distribution of ribosomes, as in the Nissl substance and the Golgi apparatus (Fig. 13). The freeze-fracture

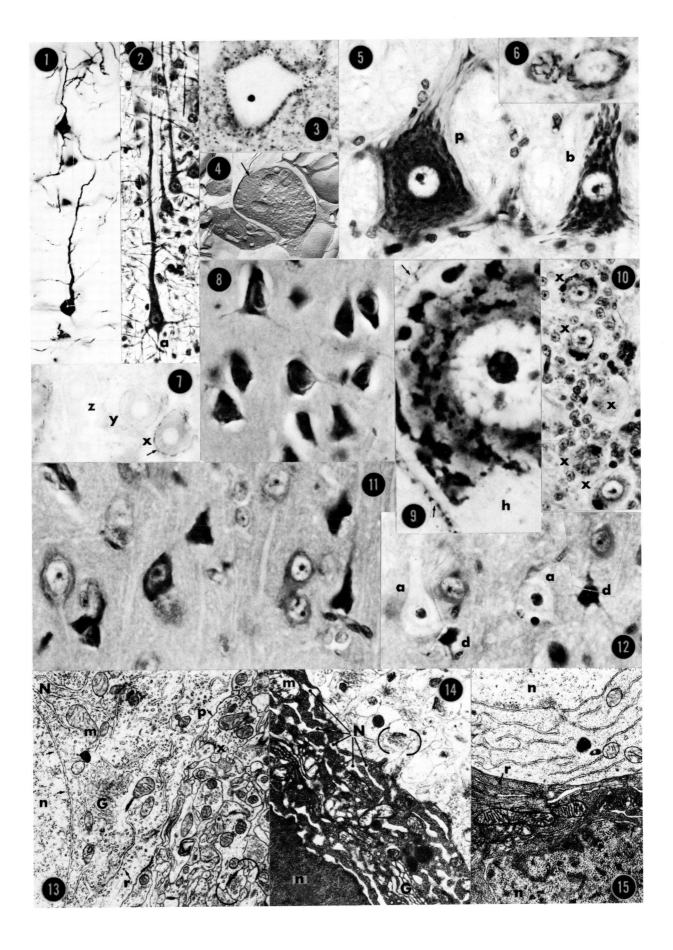

Fig. 1   Golgi silver impregnated neuron. X250.

Fig. 2.   Bodian silver impregnated neurofibrils. X250.

Fig. 3.   Rasmussen silver impregnated terminal endings. X600.

Fig. 4.   Freeze-fracture scanning electron micrograph of terminal ending (arrow). (Courtesy of Drs. L. Prescott and M. W. Brightman, Bethesda, Maryland.) X17,500.

Fig. 5.   Nissl substance in "pink" *(p)* and "blue" *(b)* neurons. X400.

Fig. 6.   McDonald silver impregnated Golgi apparatus. X800.

Fig. 7.   Glycogen in neurons *(x, y, z)* and surrounding astrocytes (arrow). X300.

Fig. 8.   Neuronal shrinkage due to hypertonic saline perfusion. X600.

Fig. 9.   Nissl substance in neuron. Pale axon hillock *(h)*. X1,500.

Fig. 10.   Lipofuscin in Purkinje cells *(x)*. X400.

Fig. 11.   Clear and "dark" neurons with fixation by immersion. X600.

Fig. 12.   Autolyzed neurons *(a)* and adjacent "dark" neurons *(d)*. Fixation delayed six hours. X600.

Fig. 13.   Electron micrograph of successfully perfused fixed neuron with rough *(N)* and smooth endoplasmic reticulum *(G)*, mitochondria *(m)*, clear nucleus *(n)*, nuclear membranes with pores (arrow), spine with axosomatic synapse *(x)*, axodendritic synapse (encircled), ribosome clusters *(r)*, and perikaryal membrane *(p)*. (Courtesy of Dr. L. J. Stensaas, Salt Lake City, Utah.) X9,600.

Fig. 14.   "Dark" nucleus *(n)* and cytoplasm with enlargement of mitochondria *(m)* and distention of nuclear membranes and rough *(N)* and smooth *(G)* endoplasmic reticulum in neuron of cerebral cortex touched prior to perfusion. (Electron micrograph by courtesy of Dr. L. J. Stensaas.) X9,600.

Fig. 15.   Pale neuron (at top) adjacent to "dark" neuron (at bottom) with compacted ribosomes (arrow) and dark nucleus *(n)*. (Electron micrograph by courtesy of Dr. L. J. Stensaas.) X9,600.

technique gives a three-dimensional view of attachments between membranes and of certain cytoplasmic elements, such as vesicles, mitochondria, etc. (Fig. 4). Since the distribution of the individual elements in the neuronal perikarya is affected by the method of preservation, the normal appearance of the neuronal population depends on the adequacy of fixation and the conditions under which the organs have been fixed.

When the organ is *fixed by perfusion,* the general appearance of nerve cells is not only uniform through the brain and spinal cord but also reproducible in animals of the same age and species. The perikaryon is round or faceted with convex sides (Figs. 5; 7; Figs. 1 and 9 in "Nerve Cells in Disease"), and its surface is separated from surrounding tissue by an extracellular space, which is visible in electron micrographs (Fig. 13) but not with the light microscope (Fig. 9). The cytoplasm extends into several processes; the axon is thin (*a* in Fig. 2) and emanates from the axon hillock, which is free of Nissl substance (*h* in Fig. 9), and the dendrites are broad-based (Fig. 5) and tapered along an even course (Fig. 2). The nucleus is large and round (Fig. 5) with well-stained membranes (Fig. 9), pale nucleoplasm and faintly stained chromatin particles, some of which cluster around a relatively large nucleolus. The appearance of normal cells is influenced by the *tonicity of the saline* used for flushing the blood; if it is hypertonic, the perikarya become shrunken, the cytoplasm assumes a dark hue and the nuclei are irregular (Fig. 8). The effect is aggravated by prolonged perfusion with larger amounts of such solutions. Hypotonicity of the solution, on the other hand, causes swelling of the tissue, with compression of the blood vessels, inadequate flow of the perfusates and incomplete fixation of the nerve cells.

When *fixed by immersion,* the population of nerve cells is heterogeneous. While most of the nerve cells are similar to those occurring in the material fixed by perfusion, a number are conspicuous by their dark appearance. In these "dark" nerve cells, the perikarya, shrunken with concave sides, are retracted from the surrounding tissue, leaving empty spaces, so-called shrinkage spaces (Fig. 11), and the dendrites are thin, tortuous and visible over a long distance by their dark color (Fig. 11). With the light microscope, the prominent traits are compaction of the Nissl substance and the neurofibrils as well as microvacuolation, and with the electron microscope, the corresponding submicroscopic features are compaction of the ribosomes (left part in Fig. 14) and dilation of the cisterns, the endoplasmic reticulum (Fig. 14) and the mitochondria. The nuclei are often shrunken, with irregular surfaces, and are darkly stained due to compaction of chromatin (Fig. 14). Typical of these neurons are aberrations in staining qualities, such as metachromasia (Heidenhain's or Mallory's azocarmine), eosinophilia (eosin alone or hematoxylin and eosin), cyanophilia (Klüver and Barrera's Luxol-fast-blue), and dark blue or yellow coloration (Baker's phospholipid method; Weil-Weigert's myelin technique). The "dark" cells develop irregularly throughout the central nervous system, but they tend to accumulate along the surfaces of gyri, around larger blood vessels entering the brain, and in the vicinity of superficial cortical damage or compression elicited during removal and cutting of the unfixed organ. Only one of two adjacent nerve cells (Fig. 15) or a larger number of nerve cells within a small area may assume the dark hue. The degree of shrinkage, the intensity of staining of nuclei and perikarya and the width of shrinkage spaces are variable; common to all, however, is shrinkage of the dendrites.

If the organ is *fixed by immersion after longer post-mortem intervals,* the heterogeneity of the neuronal population is greater. In addition to the dark nerve cells (*d* in Fig. 12), there are many nerve cells with a moderate disintegration of the Nissl substance and a few nerve cells with more severe cytoplasmic alterations attributable to post-mortem autolysis. Within 2 to 6 hours after death, scattered nerve cells display pale, foamy, vacuolated cytoplasm and moderately shrunken, darkly stained nuclei (*a* in Fig. 12), changes which are intensified with prolonged delay of fixation. These lysed nerve cells do not exhibit the tinctorial aberrations characteristic of the "dark" nerve cells. The "dark" nerve cells situated subjacent to superficial cortical damage are recognizable in material fixed 1 to 3 days after death, suggesting that these nerve cells resist the effect of post-mortem autolysis for several days.

In conclusion, the criteria for judging normality of nerve cells vary according to the conditions under which the tissues are prepared. In animals, in which the fixative can be distributed through the capillaries by a perfusion procedure, an almost instantaneous fixation after interruption of the systemic blood circulation as well as uniformity in appearance of the neuronal population are obtainable. In man, since the brain is usually removed at different intervals after death and immersed in the fixative, post-mortem autolysis and damage to the unfixed brain during its removal contribute to heterogeneity in the morphologic characteristics of the neuronal population, whereby the distribution of cytoplasmic elements is altered and cytological investigations may become equivocal. In order to obtain consistent anatomical observations and assure "equivalent cell pictures," Nissl (1895) advocated that animals of comparable age, sex, and weight be kept, sacrificed, and prepared under identical conditions. Scharrer (1933) demonstrated the necessity of using material fixed by perfusion in order to avoid the formation of "dark" neurons caused by post-mortem traumatization of the unfixed organ. Only then can reproducible histologic results be obtained.

BIBLIOGRAPHY

BRODAL, A. Experimentelle Untersuchungen über retrograde Zellveränderungen in der unteren Olive nach Läsionen des Kleinhirns. *Zeitschrift für die Gesamte Neurologie und Psychiatrie,* 1939, *166,* 646–704.

CRAIN, S. M.; GRUNDFEST H.; METTLER, F. A.; and FLINT, T. Electrical activity from tissue cultures of chick embryo spinal ganglia. *Transactions of the American Neurological Association,* 1953, 236–239.

DROZ, B.; DI GIAMBERARDINO, L.; and KOENIG, H. L. Transports axonaux de macromolécules présynaptiques. *Actualités Neurophysiologiques,* 1974, 10th Series, 236–260.

FALCK, B.; HILLARP, N. A.; THIEME, C; and THORP, A. Fluorescence of catecholamines and related compounds condensed with formaldehyde. *Journal of Histochemistry and Cytochemistry,* 1962, *10,* 348–354.

KOELLE, G. B. (Ed.) *Cholinesterases and anticholinesterase agents.* Berlin-Göttingen-Heidelberg: Springer Verlag, 1963.

PALAY, S. L.; McGEE-RUSSELL, S. M.; GORDON, S.; and GRILLO, M. A. Fixation of neural tissues for electron microscopy by perfusion with solutions of osmium tetroxide. *Journal of Cell Biology,* 1962, *12,* 385–410.

JAN CAMMERMEYER

NERVE CELLS IN DISEASE

Historical Highlights

Following the introduction in 1890 of his toluidine blue staining procedure, Nissl (1891) traced the changes in the perikaryon of the nerve cell after the axon had been severed. Such retrograde changes, referred to by Nissl (1894) as *primäre Reizung,* are encountered in both human and animal material when the axon has been damaged as the consequence of a disease process or an iatrogenic insult, and it can be induced experimentally by transection of the axon in order to determine the site of origin of nerve fibers. In addition to an acute disintegration and redistribution of Nissl substance, due to dispersal of ribosomes (electron micrographic observations: Andres, 1961), other neuronal elements are affected, in the form of displacement or "redispersion" of the Golgi apparatus (Penfield, 1920), alterations in content of enzymes (Bodian and Mellors, 1945; Kreutzberg, 1963), and separation of terminal endings from the surface of nerve cells (electron microscope: Blinzinger and Kreutzberg, 1968; scanning electron microscope: Hamberger et al., 1970). A more severe reaction with degeneration of occasional nerve cells is ascribed to a lytic action of invading microglial cells (Torvik and Skjörten, 1971). Although the retrograde reaction becomes manifest whenever the axon is damaged by any disease process, it can not be regarded as entirely specific since the morphologic reaction of *primäre Reizung* is also demonstrable in poliomyelitis (Gersh and Bodian, 1943) and in transneuronal degeneration (Torvik, 1956). Distal to a lesion, the damaged axon takes on a beaded appearance in sections impregnated by the silver method of Nauta and Gygax (1954), and the terminal endings, which become enlarged, are impregnated by the methods of Glees (1946), and Fink and Heimer (1967) for light microscopic studies and assume an increased electron density in electron micrographs, as observed by Gray and Hamlyn (1962). The development of these experimental methods has been essential for current advances in neuroanatomy, and their application to clinical material has proved to be of diagnostic value.

The systematic investigations of Spielmeyer (1922) have been indispensable for the development of neuropathology as a special discipline because they led to the definition of neuronal changes and to the establishment of uniformity in nomenclature and diagnosis. Elaborating on the pathologic forms already pointed out by Nissl (1895), Spielmeyer (1922) distinguished several types of reactions in the nerve cells, such as *swelling* (acute swelling); *shrinkage* (simple shrinkage, sclerosis); *liquefaction* (severe cell change, granular disintegration); *coagulation* (ischemic cell change, incrustation of Golgi net, homogenizing disease); *fibrillary anomalies* (Alzheimer fibrillary disease); *storage phenomena* (pigment atrophy, fatty degeneration, familial amaurotic idiocy); *vacuolation, neuronophagia,* and *incrustation* (calcium incrustation). Because of the varied conditions under which human material is handled, interpretation of the cellular changes is often equivocal. According to Scharrer (1933; 1938), shrinkage, sclerosis, and pyknosis result from trauma during extraction of the unfixed organ, and in the opinion of Camerer (1943), swelling, shrinkage, dissolution, and coagulation are consequent to post-mortem autolysis. The molecular basis of central nervous system diseases is being elucidated in an increasing number of publications based on studies with the electron microscope (Hirano, 1971), as in Tay-Sachs disease by Terry and Weiss (1963), presenile dementia by Terry (1963), adenoviral encephalitis by Gonatas et al. (1965), and so on. Again, however, some ambiguity in interpretation has arisen from difficulties in histologic preparation of clinical material for such studies. Observations in animal material fixed by perfusion have demonstrated that tissue organization is easily altered not only by a slight delay in fixation, resulting in widening of the extracellular spaces and distention of the superficial dendrites (Schultz and Karlsson, 1965; Karlsson and Shultz, 1966; Van Harreveld and Steiner, 1970), but also by postmortem trauma of the organ, resulting in the formation of "dark" neurons (Stensaas et al., 1972).

The involvement of nerve cells in different maladies expresses itself in many ways:

1. cytoarchitectural developmental anomalies of severe degree (microgyri, tuberous sclerosis, etc.) or modest degree ("wart" formation in cerebral cortex, ectopic Purkinje cells in cerebellar cortex)

2. neoplasms of benign or malignant form

3. abiotrophies (Huntington's chorea, Pick's atrophy, etc.)

4. aging processes (presenile or senile dementia)

5. genetic metabolic disorders (familial amaurotic idiocy, gargoylism, etc.)

6. viral infections (rabies, inclusion body encephalitis, poliomyelitis, "slow" virus encephalitis with Kuru disease or Creutzfeldt-Jakob disease, etc.)

7. circulatory disturbances due to organic vascular changes (arterio- and atherosclerosis, thrombosis, embolism, aneurysm, trauma, etc.) or functional anomalies in blood flow (lowered blood pressure, cardiovascular collapse, loss of blood, morphine intoxication, anesthesia, hypoglycemia, pancreasadenoma, metabolic disorders

8. central and peripheral axonal damage with retrograde and anterograde neuronal reactions (mechanical severance due to trauma, hemorrhage, infarction; hereditary metabolic disturbances in Refsum's disease, porphyria, etc.; vitamin deficiency in beriberi, etc.).

Many of these pathologic manifestations recur in veterinary medicine and can be reproduced experimentally, such as transmission of a slow virus to cause a Kuru-like condition, as demonstrated by Gajdusek et al. (1966), or topical application of alum phosphate paste with formation of neurofibrillary changes, as performed by Klatzo et al. (1965).

Research Methods. Although the material used for microscopic study of pathologic nerve cell changes is usually treated like that for study of normal nerve cells, under certain circumstances other approaches are required. Smears or frozen sections of biopsy material may be used for rapid diagnosis in the course of an operation. Human clinical material is fixed by immersion after varying post-mortem intervals, and animal material either by immersion or by perfusion for light or electron microscopic studies. The method to be selected is dictated by the object of an investigation.

Morphologic Characteristics

The purpose of the morphologic examination is.

1. to determine the site and extent of the lesions with the naked eye and low power optics
2. to assess the type of histologic aberrations with high power optics
3. to estimate the time of onset of cytologic alterations on the basis of experience as to the time required for nerve cells, neuroglial cells and vascular elements to react in a certain manner to a noxious agent
4. to correlate the anatomical changes with clinical observations
5. to interpret the mechanism underlying the pathologic manifestations.

In this review, however, only some types of histologic observations will be referred to.

For an orientation about pathomorphologic manifestations, three experimental procedures have been selected, namely severance of the axon, resulting in retrograde neuronal reaction, and embolization and compression of the blood flow supply, inducing necrosis of nerve cells. All material was fixed by perfusion with a rapidly acting fixative.

Retrograde Reaction
Following Axonal Severance

Since the operation is remote from the brain and intracerebral flow of perfusates will not be compromised by an effect of postsurgical edema or vascular damage, successful fixation of the tissue can be obtained.

The retrograde reaction in motor nerve cells is manifested within a few hours after severance of the axon by moderate changes in Nissl substance and within one to two days by disintegration or dispersal of Nissl substance along the periphery of the cell body (x in Fig. 3). Subsequently, the nerve cells undergo changes of such varied intensity that it is difficult to establish the exact sequence of the morphologic alterations, which also vary with age and region. The intensity of reaction in periodic acid-Schiff–gallocyanin-stained sections is more severe and rapid in the "pink" than in the "blue" nerve cells. On the third to fifth days,

reconstituted Nissl substance aggregates in a narrow peripheral zone (z in Fig. 3). Stainable material accumulates around the nuclei as a nuclear cap (x, z in Fig. 3). From the fifth day, the nuclei tend to be displaced toward the cell membrane, which may bulge to such a degree that an erroneous impression of nuclear expulsion arises. In some species, such as the rat, the eccentric nuclei are kidney-shaped, and in others, such as the rabbit, they are round. In this acute phase, the cytoplasm, which in normal "blue" neurons is clear (b in Fig. 1), assumes a moderate "basophilia" because of dispersal of the Nissl substance, or constituent ribosomes ("blue" neuron in center, Fig. 3). In the next days, up to the third week, formation of new Nissl substance is intense around the nucleus, leaving a widened peripheral zone free. From the second day to the third week or more, the glycogen is depleted in the nerve cells which are normally rich in this substance (Fig. 2). Even after 6–12 months, the normal distribution of Nissl substance is not completely recovered. Although most of the involved nerve cells do regenerate, a small number of them, depending on species and age of the animal and on site and type of the lesion, are permanently damaged. Such disintegration, beginning within the first week, is manifested by complete loss of Nissl substance, foamy appearance of cytoplasm (Fig. 4), destruction of nuclear membranes, with compaction of chromatin material to mimic karyorrhexis (see insert in Fig. 4), and invasion of microglial cells (m in Fig. 4); finally, the nerve cell disappears completely, leaving an empty cavity enclosing microglial cells. Thus, a reduction in the population of nerve cells takes place; in the facial nucleus it amounts to approximately 40% on the operated side, as compared with the nonoperated side, 6 months after transection of the facial nerve at its point of exit from the skull in a 15-months-old rabbit.

Nerve Cell Changes After Tissue Ischemia

In human material because of the conditions under which it is prepared, the population of nerve cells will be a mixture of cells affected not only by ischemia or anoxia, but also by postmortem autolysis and post-mortem trauma. However, even in animal material prepared by

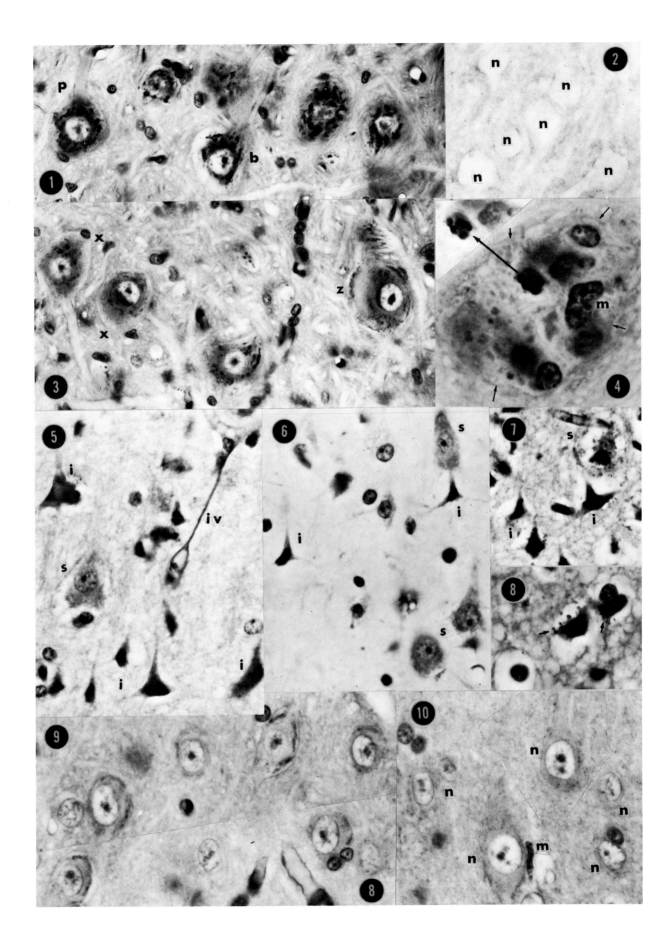

Fig. 1.   Facial nucleus with "pink" *(p)* and "blue" *(b)* neurons on unoperated side. PAS-gallocyanin. X400.

Fig. 2.   Glycogen depletion in facial nucleus 2 days after axotomy. Same microscopic section as in Fig. 7 of "Nerve Cells: Normal." X300.

Fig. 3.   Acute retrograde neuronal reaction *(x, x, z)* in facial nucleus 3 days after axotomy. Same microscopic section as in Fig. 1. X400.

Fig. 4.   Microglial cells *(m)* invading degenerated neuron (small arrow) with karyorrhexis, reproduced in insert (large arrow), 6 days after transection of facial nerve in rat. X1,500.

Fig. 5.   Embolic lesion with ischemic *(i)* and severe *(s)* neuronal changes. Intervascular strand of connective tissue *(iv)*. Duration 1 hour. PAS-gallocyanin. X600.

Fig. 6.   Same case as in Fig. 5. Gallocyanin. X600.

Fig. 7.   Embolic lesion of 3 hours' duration. PAS-gallocyanin. X600.

Fig. 8.   Incrustation of "Golgi net" (arrows). Same microscopic section as in Fig. 7. X600.

Fig. 9.   Small neurons in 3rd cortical layer. Control side. PAS-gallocyanin. X800.

Fig. 10.   Depletion of Nissl substance in small neurons *(n)* in 3rd cortical layer after 1 hour of compression of exposed hemisphere and 5 hours of survival. Microglial cell *(m)*. Same section as in Fig. 9. X800.

a perfusion procedure, fixation of the experimentally produced lesions is not always successful because of obstruction of the vascular channels by a thrombus or embolus. After temporary occlusion or compression of arteries, a no-reflow phenomenon (Ames et al., 1968) with acute endothelial changes (Hekmatpanah, 1970) will cause inadequate flow of the perfusates.

Various types of nerve cell changes are recognized in ischemic lesions, but the term ischemic neuronal change refers to a specific type described by Spielmeyer (1922). This is the most common change in clinical neuropathology, and it can be experimentally produced by embolization or clamping of the cerebral blood vessels. However, at the shortest intervals, the ischemic neuronal change may be confused with the "dark" neurons, which occur throughout the brain and aggregate in larger numbers around the lesions. After 30 to 60 minutes, the pathologic cell reaction is identifiable by disintegration or dispersal of Nissl substance (*i* in Figs. 5 and 6). Within the lesion, which has become vacuolated (periodic acid-Schiff-gallocyanin method in Fig. 5), the neuronal perikarya are shrunken and separated from the surrounding tissue by wide spaces; the cytoplasm, free of Nissl substance, is homogeneously stained and microvacuolated; the dendrites are attenuated and tortuous; the affected terminal endings exhibit abnormal stainability (Fig. 8); and the nuclei are triangular, heavily stained and eccentric (gallocyanin method in Fig. 6). At this acute stage, the perikarya exhibit the same staining aberrations as the "dark" neurons of normal tissue and likewise resist the effect of post-mortem autolysis for 24-48 hours.

In addition to the ischemic neuronal change, the severe neuronal change develops within a few hours in the same lesions. It is recognized by disintegration of the Nissl substance and coarse vacuolation of the cytoplasm; the perikaryon is fully expanded, and the dendrites retain their original width (*s* in Figs. 5 and 6). The nuclei in these cells are pale and round. The severe neuronal change progresses in severity in the next few hours (*s* in Fig. 7), terminating in formation of a cavity. At no stage do these nerve cells exhibit the staining aberrations of the ischemic nerve cells. In the textbook of Spielmeyer (1922), neuronal damage identified as the severe neuronal change in clinical material is characterized by a dark shrunken nucleus in a pale vacuolated cytoplasm; these changes resemble those which have been described in neurons undergoing post-mortem autolysis (*a* in Fig. 12 in "Nerve Cells: Normal").

After compression of the cerebral cortex, foci with ischemic and severe neuronal changes are demonstrable; in addition, the small nerve cells in the cerebral cortex exhibit subtle changes (Fig. 10) as compared with normal nerve cells (Fig. 9). These altered cells display an acute disintegration or dispersal of Nissl substance and a uniform pallor or faint blue coloration of the nonvacuolated cytoplasm (Fig. 10); the nuclei are well preserved. These neurons are regarded as properly fixed representatives of a temporary reaction to an acute impairment of oxygen supply.

In conclusion, the procedure of fixation of the tissue must be carefully considered in an analysis of the morphologic changes in nerve cells in human pathologic and animal experimental material. Since a method to obtain perfect preservation of tissue elements is usually vitiated by unforeseen or unavoidable alterations in the vasculature in this type of material, a complex of neuronal changes is inevitable, some of which may be nonspecific, such as the "dark" neurons.

BIBLIOGRAPHY

AMES, A., III; WRIGHT, R. L.; KOWADA, M.; THURSTON, J. M.; and MAJNO, G. Cerebral ischemia: II. The no-reflow phenomenon. *American Journal of Pathology,* 1968, *52,* 437–453.

BLINZINGER, K., and KREUTZBERG, G. Displacement of synaptic terminals from regenerating motoneurons by microglial cells. *Zeitschrift für Zellforschung,* 1968, *85,* 145–157.

GAJDUSEK, D. C.; GIBBS, C. J., JR.; and ALPERS, M. Experimental transmission of a kuru-like syndrome to chimpanzees. *Nature,* 1966, *209,* 794–796.

HIRANO, A. Electron microscopy in neuropathology. In H. M. Zimmerman (Ed.), *Progress in neuropathology* (Vol. 1). New York and London: Grune & Stratton, 1971. Pp. 1–61.

RUSSELL, D. S., and RUBINSTEIN, L. J. *Pathology of tumours of the nervous system* (3rd ed.). London: Edward Arnold, 1971.

SCHOLZ, W. (Ed.). Nervensystem. In O. Lubarsch, F. Henke, and R. Rössle (Eds.), *Handbuch der speziellen pathologischen Anatomie und Histologie* (Vol. 13).

Berlin-Göttingen-Heidelberg: Springer Verlag, 1955–1958.

SPIELMEYER, W. *Histopathologie des Nervensystems.* Berlin: Julius Springer, 1922.

STENSAAS, S. S.; EDWARDS, C. Q.; and STENSAAS, L. J. An experimental study of hyperchromic nerve cells in the cerebral cortex. *Experimental Neurology,* 1972, *36,* 472–487.

TORVIK, A., and SKJÖRTEN, F. Electron microscopic observations on nerve cell regeneration and degeneration after axon lesions. II. Changes in the glial cells. *Acta Neuropathologica,* 1971, *17,* 265–282.

See also NERVE CELLS: NORMAL

JAN CAMMERMEYER